Understanding Mood Disorders

Understanding Mood Disorders

Edited by Leon Chapman

hayle medical

New York

Hayle Medical,
750 Third Avenue, 9th Floor,
New York, NY 10017, USA

Visit us on the World Wide Web at:
www.haylemedical.com

ISBN: 978-1-63241-589-9

Printed in China.

Cataloging-in-Publication Data

Understanding mood disorders / edited by Leon Chapman.
p. cm.
Includes bibliographical references and index.
ISBN 978-1-63241-589-9
1. Affective disorders. 2. Depression, Mental. 3. Psychology, Pathological.
I. Chapman, Leon.

RC537 .U53 2019
616.852 7--dc23

Table of Contents

Preface

This book has been a concerted effort by a group of academicians, researchers and scientists, who have contributed their research works for the realization of the book. This book has materialized in the wake of emerging advancements and innovations in this field. Therefore, the need of the hour was to compile all the required researches and disseminate the knowledge to a broad spectrum of people comprising of students, researchers and specialists of the field.

Mood disorders are a set of psychological conditions affecting the mood of an individual. They fall under the groups of elevated mood disorders (mania or hypomania), depressive disorders and moods that cycle between mania and depression. Cyclothymic disorder, dysthymic disorder and major depression are some of the common depressive disorders. Depressive disorders can be of different types, such as atypical depression, psychotic major depression, melancholic depression, catatonic depression, seasonal affective disorder and premenstrual dysphoric disorder, besides others. A mood disorder may be induced by a substance such as alcohol, benzodiazepine, etc. Several medical conditions such as, endocrine diseases, neurological disorders, gastrointestinal diseases, cancer, pulmonary disease, etc. can also trigger mood disorders. This book is a valuable compilation of topics, ranging from the basic to the most complex advancements in the understanding of mood disorders. It presents this complex medical condition in the most comprehensible language. For someone with an interest and eye for detail, this book covers the most significant aspects of such disorders.

At the end of the preface, I would like to thank the authors for their brilliant chapters and the publisher for guiding us all-through the making of the book till its final stage. Also, I would like to thank my family for providing the support and encouragement throughout my academic career and research projects.

Editor

Occupational Noise Annoyance Linked to Depressive Symptoms and Suicidal Ideation: A Result from Nationwide Survey of Korea

Jin-Ha Yoon[1,2,3], Jong-Uk Won[1,2,3], Wanhyung Lee[1,2,3], Pil Kyun Jung[1,2,3], Jaehoon Roh[1,2,3]*

1 The Institute for Occupational Health, Yonsei University College of Medicine, Seoul, Korea, **2** Department of Preventive Medicine and Public Health, Yonsei University College of Medicine, Seoul, Korea, **3** Graduate School of Public Health, Yonsei University College of Medicine, Seoul, Korea

Abstract

Background: Noise, or undesirable sound, is one of the most common environmental stressors, and it can cause various health effects. Beyond the auditory consequences of occupational noise exposure, extra-auditory effects such as psychological problems have also been found. The aim of the current study is to elucidate the association between occupational noise annoyance and psychological symptoms, including symptoms of depression and suicidal ideation.

Methods: A total of 10,020 participants (5,410 men and 4,610 women) were included in the current analysis, using data from the fourth Korean National Health and Nutrition Examination Survey (KNHANES). Self-report questionnaires were used to assess noise annoyance levels, depressive symptoms, and suicidal ideation. Odds ratios (ORs) and 95% confidence intervals (95% CIs) for psychosocial symptoms were calculated using multiple logistic regression models.

Results: Compared to the no noise annoyance group, ORs (95% CI) of the severe annoyance groups were 1.58 (1.12–2.23) and 1.76 (1.29–2.40) in men and 1.49 (1.05–2.11) and 1.41 (1.01–1.97) in women for depressive symptoms and suicidal ideation, respectively. The ORs (95% CI) for severe noise annoyance in those with less than five hours of sleep were 2.95 (1.46–5.96) and 2.05 (1.01–4.16) in men and women, respectively, compared with those with no noise annoyance and a sleep time of more than five hours.

Conclusion: Our study shows that occupational noise annoyance is significantly related to mental health, including depressive symptoms and suicidal ideation after controlling for individual and socio-demographic characteristics even with gender stratification. However, prospective studies with quantified noise exposure assessment were needed to elucidate the causality on the association between noise annoyance and psychological symptoms.

Editor: Martin Voracek, University of Vienna, Austria

Funding: The authors have no support or funding to report.

Competing Interests: The authors have declared that no competing interests exist.

* Email: jhroh@yuhs.ac

Introduction

At its most basic, sound consists of physiological signals in the auditory system, enabling humans to communicate with both one another and the environment. However, external noise or undesirable sound is one of the most common environmental stressors, and it can result in various health consequences [1]. For example, noise-induced hearing impairment is a well-known occupational health hazard worldwide. Additionally, noise exposure is related to non-auditory effects [2], including annoyance, headache, sleep disturbance, and impaired cognitive development in children. Furthermore, acute noise exposure can cause vasoconstriction, and chronic noise exposure is related to hypertension and cardiovascular diseases [3].

The West London Survey [4] assessed 6,000 households on negative health effects related to living near a large London airport. The study revealed that high aircraft noise resulted in both acute and chronic irritability and depressive symptoms in local residents [4]. Following this discovery, additional research has suggested an association between noise exposure and mental health [5]. For example, a study from Japan identified a significant relationship between noise exposure and scores on a mental health assessment, including nervousness and depressive symptoms, with rates of mental illness increasing according to noise level [6]. This association remained significant even after adjusting for age, gender, marital status, housing type, and length of residence in the high exposure area [6]. However, another investigation that adjusted for socio-demographic variables did not find an association between aircraft noise and psychiatric hospital admission rates [7]. Additionally, the Caerphilly Study, based on prospective research, also found no association between mental disorder and traffic noise after controlling for socio-demographic factors [8]. These findings instead suggest that noisy settings reflect low socio-demographic environments, which themselves are linked to poor mental health. Thus, controversies exist as to whether noise exposure itself is related to mental illness after controlling for environmental and socio-demographic variables, such as income level and occupation. Furthermore, an epidemiology study on the topic did not include gender in a stratified analysis, despite the fact that there is a known association between gender and mental illness.

Generally, noise exposure in an occupational setting is more severe than in the general environment [9], and numerous reports exist on work-related hearing loss [10]. For example, almost one third of workers in Europe reported that, because the nose exposure was too loud, they would have to raise their voices to keep a conversation [9,11]. 30–50% of workers in Asia are exposed to noise above 90 dB [12], which is loud enough to cause occupational stress. This type of occupational noise exposure has also been linked to a high risk of death from injury [13], suggesting that high noise exposure may reduce attention in the workplace, which can lead to injury. Additionally, severe stress is known to cause psychological problems, but studies on the effects of noise on psychological symptoms are often ignored in an occupational setting.

Our study aims to examine the association between noise exposure and psychological symptoms, including depressive symptoms and suicidal ideation, in an active working population. To clarify this association, data from a national representative survey, the Korea National Health and Nutrition Examination Survey (KNHANES), were assessed, adjusting for socio-demographic characteristics and stratified for gender.

Methods

Ethics statement

Participants provided written informed consent confirming their voluntary participation. All individual identifying records were anonymized prior to analysis. This survey was approved by the Institutional Review Board (IRB) of the Korea Centers for Disease Control and Prevention (KCDC) (IRB: 2007-02-CON-04-P; 2008-04EXP-01-C; 2009-01CON-03-2C).

Fourth Korean National Health and Nutrition Examination Survey (KNHANES)

The KCDC conducted the fourth KNHANES from 2007 to 2009 [14], enrolling 13,800 households using stratified, multistage, probability sampling methods, based on 600 geographical population areas of Korea. Of the 10,067 economically active participants in the fourth KNHANES, 33 participants were excluded due to missing data on the noise exposure questionnaire, and 14 participants were excluded for missing data on depressive symptoms and suicidal ideation. Thus, data from 10,020 participants (5,410 in men, 4,610 in women) were used in the current analysis.

Annoyance from occupational noise exposure (occupational noise annoyance) and occupation

Assessment of noise exposure in an occupational setting and personal perceptions of its effects were obtained from self-report questionnaires. Question for occupational noise exposure was "Are you exposed to noise loud enough that you would raise your voices to keep a conversation during work?" [9,11], and who have answered yes to this question were asked to answer following question for personal perception of noise exposure. The answer to this question had three choices: No perception of occupational noise, perception of occupational noise without severe problems, and perception of occupational noise with severe problems. Hence, occupational noise annoyance was categorized as "none annoyance", "mild annoyance" and "severe annoyance", respectively.

Occupation type was categorized as white-, pink-, and blue-collar workers using a self-report questionnaire. White-collar workers included managers, senior officials, professionals, clerks, and skilled traders. Pink-collar workers were sales and customer service workers. Blue-collar workers included agriculture, fishery, forestry, crafts, and related trades, plant and machine operators, and elementary workers.

Depressive symptoms and suicidal ideation

A separate set of questionnaires assessed workers for the presence of depressive symptoms and suicidal ideation during the past year. For depressive symptoms, we asked, "During the past year, have you felt feelings of sadness or hopelessness that persisted for at least two weeks and that disrupted your social life?" The questionnaire for suicidal ideation asked, "During the past year, have you ever felt that you were willing to die?" There were four possible options for each questionnaire (never, rarely, yes, and always), with yes and always being categorized as symptoms of depression and suicidal ideation. Psychological symptoms workers were defined as when a worker has at least one of the two psychological symptoms of depressive symptoms or suicidal ideation.

Individual and household income and lifestyle factors

Income level was calculated using standardized methods of classifications by five-year age increments and gender compared with Korean standard income levels. Total family income was adjusted for the number of family members and was used to calculate quartile levels of household income. Hence, house hold income was categorized as low, middle-low, middle-high, and high income.

Smoking history was categorized as non-, former and current smokers. In the current study, "non-smokers" were defined as individuals who had smoked less than 100 cigarettes in their lifetime. Two or more occasions of drinking per week with seven or more glasses of alcohol in men, and two or more occasions drinking per week with five or more glasses of alcohol in women were defined as heavy alcohol drinking.

Statistical analysis

Chi-squared tests and t-tests were used to compare group differences based on the presence of psychological symptoms. The odds ratios (ORs) and 95% confidence intervals (95% CIs) for psychological symptoms were estimated using a multivariate logistic regression model. Two-tailed p-values less than 0.05 were considered statistically significant.

Results

Socio-demographic characteristics according to psychological symptoms

Results for depressive symptoms and suicidal ideation are presented in Tables 1 and 2, respectively. The average age of suicidal ideation group in men, both the depressive symptom and the suicidal ideation group in women were significantly higher than that of non-symptomatic individuals. In regards to sleep, there were significantly higher rates of psychological symptoms in those who slept for five hours or less (depressive symptoms: men = 14.4%, women = 25.1%; suicidal ideation: men = 15.3%, women = 29.6%) than in those who got six or more hours of sleep

Table 1. Basic characteristics of study population according to depressive symptom.

	Men			Women		
	Depressive symptom			Depressive symptom		
	Yes 512 (9.5%)	No 4898 (90.5%)	P	Yes 837 (18.2)	No 3773 (81.8)	P
Age	47.1±14.2	46.0±14.0	0.081	48.0±15.0	45.7±14.7	<.001
Body mass index	23.8±3.2	24.1±3.1	0.065	23.3±3.5	23.2±3.4	0.626
Sleep duration						
≤5hours	94 (14.4)	560 (85.6)	<.001	176 (25.1)	526 (74.9)	<.001
6 hours	134 (8.4)	1454 (91.6)		219 (18.7)	951 (81.3)	
7 hours	145 (9.0)	1465 (91.0)		219 (15.8)	1169 (84.2)	
≥8 hours	139 (8.9)	1419 (91.1)		223 (16.5)	1127 (83.5)	
Education						
Primary school	117 (13.2)	767 (86.8)	<.001	313 (22.3)	1094 (77.7)	<.001
Middle school	70 (10.3)	608 (89.7)		114 (19.8)	463 (80.2)	
High school	190 (9.5)	1810 (90.5)		250 (16.7)	1248 (83.3)	
Above university	135 (7.3)	1715 (92.7)		160 (14.2)	968 (85.8)	
Occupation						
White collar	142 (8.3)	1575 (91.7)	0.0713	198 (14.3)	1183 (85.7)	<.001
Pink collar	80 (9.3)	782 (90.7)		241 (18.7)	1046 (81.3)	
Blue collar	288 (10.3)	2501 (89.7)		394 (20.4)	1540 (79.6)	
House hold income						
Low	90 (13.3)	585 (86.7)	<.001	205 (24.1)	647 (75.9)	<.001
Middle low	141 (11.0)	1143 (89.0)		207 (17.3)	990 (82.7)	
Middle high	140 (8.7)	1479 (91.3)		221 (18.1)	1001 (81.9)	
High	132 (7.6)	1611 (92.4)		193 (15.2)	1075 (84.8)	
Life style						
Smoking habit						
none	108 (9.5)	1026 (90.5)	0.138	734 (17.7)	3425 (82.43)	0.023
former	144 (8.4)	1579 (91.6)		26 (21.9)	93 (78.2)	
current	260 (10.2)	2297 (89.8)		77 (23.2)	255 (76.8)	
Alcohol drinking						
Sever drinking	132 (10.2)	1159 (89.8)	0.280	783 (18.0)	3563 (82.0)	0.318
Others	380 (9.2)	3743 (90.8)		54 (20.5)	210 (79.5)	
Noise annoyance						
None	287 (8.5)	3080 (91.5)	0.001	571 (17.0)	2785 (83.0)	0.002
Mild	166 (10.3)	1452 (98.7)		215 (20.7)	826 (79.4)	
Severe	59 (13.8)	370 (86.3)		51 (23.9)	162 (76.1)	

(all p-values below 0.05). Low education was also associated with higher rates of psychological symptoms in both genders. For depression, those with education levels equal to or below primary school had rates of 13.2% and 86.8% for men and women, respectively, while those with university or above were 7.3% and 14.2%, respectively (all p-values under 0.05). Similar patterns emerged for education level and suicidal ideation. Blue-collar workers showed a higher proportion of depressive symptoms in women and higher suicidal ideation in both genders than the other types of workers (depressive symptoms: blue-collar women = 20.4%, white-collar women = 14.3%, $p<0.01$; suicidal ideation: blue-collar men = 11.5%, blue-collar women = 24.5%; white-collar men = 6.9%, white-collar women = 13.8%, all p-values under 0.05). Household income was also inversely related to both psychological conditions; the proportion of depressive symptoms in the low income group were 13.3% and 24.1% for men and women, respectively, while those in the high income group were 7.6% and 15.2%, respectively (all p values were below 0.05). Similarly, the proportion of suicidal ideation was higher in the low income group, with rates of 15.3% and 29.2% for men and women, respectively, compared with 7.2% and 13.3% in the high income group. In terms of lifestyle factors, female current smokers had higher rates of depressive symptom than non-smokers (23.2% vs. 17.7%, $p = 0.023$). The proportion of suicidal ideation in current smokers was also higher than in non-smokers in both sexes (current smoker vs. non-smoker: 10.8% vs. 9.1% in men,

Table 2. Basic characteristics of study population according to suicidal ideation.

	Men			Women		
	Suicidal ideation			Suicidal ideation		
	Yes 530 (9.8%)	No 4877 (90.2%)	P	Yes 941 (20.4%)	No 3669 (79.6%)	P
Age	48.9±15.3	45.8±13.9	<.0001	48.9±16.0	45.4±14.3	<.0001
Body mass index	23.7±3.2	24.1±3.1	0.0013	23.3±3.6	23.2±3.3	0.2269
Sleep duration				6.8±1.3	6.6±1.5	0.001
≤5hours	100 (15.3)	554 (84.7)	<.0001	208 (29.6)	494 (70.4)	<.0001
6 hours	149 (9.4)	1438 (90.6)		231 (19.7)	939 (80.3)	
7 hours	130 (8.1)	1483 (91.9)		235 (16.9)	1153 (83.1)	
≥8 hours	151 (9.7)	1402 (90.3)		267 (19.8)	1083 (80.2)	
Education						
Primary school	152 (17.2)	732 (82.8)	<.0001	383 (27.2)	1024 (72.8)	<.0001
Middle school	68 (10.0)	610 (90.0)		115 (20.0)	462 (80.1)	
High school	189 (9.5)	1811 (90.6)		280 (18.7)	1218 (81.3)	
Above university	121 (6.5)	1729 (93.5)		163 (14.4)	965 (85.6)	
Occupation						
White collar	119 (6.9)	1598 (93.1)	<.0001	190 (13.8)	1191 (86.2)	<.0001
Pink collar	87 (10.1)	775 (89.9)		273 (21.2)	1014 (78.8)	
Blue collar	321 (11.5)	2468 (88.5)		474 (24.5)	1460 (75.5)	
House hold income						
Low	103 (15.3)	572 (84.7)	0.0001	249 (29.2)	603 (70.8)	0.0001
Middle low	157 (12.2)	1127 (87.8)		280 (23.4)	917 (76.6)	
Middle high	133 (8.2)	1486 (91.8)		230 (18.8)	992 (81.2)	
High	126 (7.2)	1617 (92.8)		169 (13.3)	1099 (86.7)	
Life style						
Smoking habit						
none	103 (9.1)	1031 (90.9)	0.0477	814 (19.6)	3345 (80.4)	<.0001
former	150 (8.7)	1573 (91.3)		30 (25.2)	89 (74.8)	
current	277 (10.8)	2280 (89.2)		97 (29.2)	235 (70.8)	
Alcohol drinking						
Sever drinking	143 (11.1)	1148 (88.9)	0.0745	70 (26.5)	194 (73.5)	0.0113
Others	387 (9.4)	3736 (90.6)		871 (20.0)	3475 (80.0)	
Noise annoyance						
None	307 (9.1)	3060 (90.9)	0.0012	648 (19.3)	2708 (80.7)	0.0082
Mild	160 (9.9)	1458 (90.1)		240 (23.0)	801 (77.0)	
Severe	63 (14.7)	366 (85.3)		53 (24.9)	160 (75.1)	

p = 0.048; 29.2% vs. 19.6% in women, p<0.01). Female heavy alcohol drinkers also had significantly higher rates of suicidal ideation compared with non-heavy drinkers (26.5% vs. 20.0%, p = 0.011).

In terms of noise level perceptions, rates of depressive symptoms were 8.5% and 17.0% for those who reported no annoyance, 10.3% and 20.7 at mild annoyance, and 13.8% and 23.9% with severe annoyance for men and women, respectively (p = 0.001 in men, 0.002 in women). Similarly, the proportion of suicidal ideation increased according to the severity of noise annoyance (none, mild, and severe annoyance: 9.1%, 9.9%, and 14.7% in men, p = 0.001; 19.3%, 23.0%, and 24.9% in women, p = 0.008).

Odds ratios for depressive symptoms or suicidal ideation by noise annoyance (Table 3, 4)

Compared with the no noise annoyance group, ORs (95% CI) of the severe annoyance groups for depressive symptoms and suicidal ideation were 1.58 (1.12–2.23) and 1.76 (1.29–2.40) in men and 1.49 (1.05–2.11) and 1.41 (1.01–1.97) in women (model III), respectively, after adjusting for age, BMI, sleep time, education, occupation, household income, smoking habits, and alcohol.

In that model, all ORs (95% CI) for depressive symptoms and suicidal ideation in sleep duration less than or equal to five hours were 1.77 (1.32–2.33) and 1.76 (1.29–2.40) in men and 1.52 (1.21–1.92) and 1.41 (1.01–1.97) in women, respectively.

Table 3. Odds ratio of depressive symptoms in a multivariate logistic regression models.

		Odds ratio (95% confidence interval)					
		Men			Women		
		Model I	Model II	Model III	Model I	Model II	Model III
Noise annoyance	none	1-	1-	1-	1-	1-	1-
	mild	1.24 (1.01–1.52)	1.25 (1.01–1.54)	1.21 (0.97–1.51)	1.29 (1.08–1.55)	1.29 (1.08–1.54)	1.26 (1.04–1.52)
	severe	1.79 (1.32–2.43)	1.81 (1.32–2.48)	1.58 (1.12–2.23)	1.50 (1.07–2.10)	1.49 (1.06–2.09)	1.49 (1.05–2.11)
Seeping time	≥8 hours	1-	1-	1-	1-	1-	1-
	7 hours	1.03 (0.80–1.32)	1.08 (0.84–1.39)	1.12 (0.86–1.45)	0.93 (0.76–1.14)	0.95 (0.78–1.17)	1.00 (0.80–1.24)
	6 hours	0.97 (0.75–1.24)	1.03 (0.80–1.33)	1.09 (0.83–1.42)	1.11 (0.91–1.37)	1.15 (0.93–1.41)	1.17 (0.94–1.46)
	≤5 hours	1.77 (1.32–2.33)	1.75 (1.31–2.32)	1.73 (1.27–2.34)	1.52 (1.21–1.92)	1.53 (1.21–1.92)	1.55 (1.22–1.98)
Education	primary school		1.84 (1.27–2.67)	1.82 (1.23–2.69)		1.57 (1.10–2.24)	1.58 (1.08–2.32)
	middle school		1.39 (0.96–2.01)	1.35 (0.91–2.01)		1.30 (0.92–1.82)	1.31 (0.91–1.89)
	high school		1.27 (0.98–1.65)	1.29 (0.98–1.69)		1.13 (0.88–1.46)	1.16 (0.89–1.51)
	above university		1-	1-		1-	1-
Occupation	white collar		1-	1-		1-	1-
	pink collar		0.89 (0.65–1.21)	0.87 (0.63–1.21)		1.16 (0.90–1.49)	1.05 (0.81–1.37)
	blue collar		0.80 (0.61–1.06)	0.82 (0.61–1.08)		1.03 (0.77–1.37)	1.02 (0.76–1.37)
House hold income	low		1.59 (1.15–2.20)	1.62 (1.15–2.27)		1.43 (1.11–1.84)	1.44 (1.10–1.88)
	middle low		1.36 (1.05–1.78)	1.34 (1.01–1.77)		0.98 (0.78–1.23)	1.02 (0.80–1.29)
	middle high		1.06 (0.82–1.37)	1.11 (0.85–1.44)		1.13 (0.91–1.40)	1.17 (0.93–1.46)
	high		1-	1-		1-	1-
Smoking	never			1-			1-
	former			0.79 (0.59–1.04)			1.24 (0.76–2.01)
	current			0.99 (0.77–1.28)			1.39 (1.01–1.92)
Alcohol drinking	others			1-			1-
	severe			1.05 (0.83–1.33)			0.95 (0.66–1.36)

All models adjusted for age and body mass index.

Table 4. Odds ratio of suicidal ideation in a multivariate logistic regression models.

		Odds ratio (95% confidence interval)					
		Men			Women		
		Model I	Model II	Model III	Model I	Model II	Model III
Noise annoyance	none	1-	1-	1-	1-	1-	1-
	mild	1.10 (0.90–1.35)	1.07 (0.86–1.32)	1.06 (0.85–1.31)	1.30 (1.09–1.54)	1.29 (1.08–1.53)	1.28 (1.07–1.52)
	severe	1.81 (1.34–2.44)	1.76 (1.29–2.39)	1.76 (1.29–2.40)	1.37 (1.01–1.91)	1.40 (1.01–1.95)	1.41 (1.01–1.97)
Seeping time	≥8 hours	1-	1-	1-	1-	1-	1-
	7 hours	0.83 (0.65–1.07)	0.89 (0.69–1.15)	0.88 (0.68–1.14)	0.82 (0.68–1.01)	0.85 (0.70–1.04)	0.87 (0.70–1.06)
	6 hours	1.03 (0.80–1.31)	1.14 (0.89–1.46)	1.13 (0.88–1.44)	1.00 (0.81–1.21)	1.03 (0.84–1.26)	1.05 (0.85–1.29)
	≤5 hours	1.66 (1.25–2.18)	1.68 (1.26–2.39)	1.65 (1.24–2.18)	1.52 (1.23–1.89)	1.50 (1.21–1.87)	1.42 (1.12–1.79)
Education	primary school		2.14 (1.49–3.08)	2.07 (1.44–2.98)		1.32 (0.94–1.86)	1.25 (0.86–1.80)
	middle school		1.23 (0.85–1.79)	1.19 (0.82–1.73)		0.98 (0.70–1.37)	0.91 (0.65–1.28)
	high school		1.30 (0.99–1.70)	1.28 (0.98–1.67)		1.05 (0.82–1.35)	1.00 (0.77–1.30)
	above university		1-	1-		1-	1-
Occupation	white collar		1-	1-		1-	1-
	pink collar		1.23 (0.90–1.68)	1.21 (0.88–1.65)		1.38 (1.08–1.77)	1.32 (1.03–1.69)
	blue collar		1.01 (0.76–1.34)	1.00 (0.75–1.32)		1.28 (0.97–1.69)	1.27 (0.96–1.67)
House hold income	low		1.58 (1.15–2.17)	1.57 (1.14–2.15)		2.07 (1.61–2.65)	2.01 (1.57–2.58)
	middle low		1.45 (1.11–1.89)	1.46 (1.12–1.90)		1.65 (1.32–2.07)	1.65 (1.31–2.06)
	middle high		1.04 (1.11–1.89)	1.04 (0.80–1.35)		1.40 (1.12–1.74)	1.39 (1.11–1.74)
	high		1-	1-		1-	1-
Smoking	never			1-			1-
	former			0.84 (0.64–1.11)			1.35 (0.87–2.10)
	current			1.12 (0.87–1.44)			1.66 (1.27–2.18)
Alcohol drinking	others			1-			1-
	severe			1.28 (1.03–1.58)			1.30 (0.96–1.78)

All models adjusted for age and body mass index.

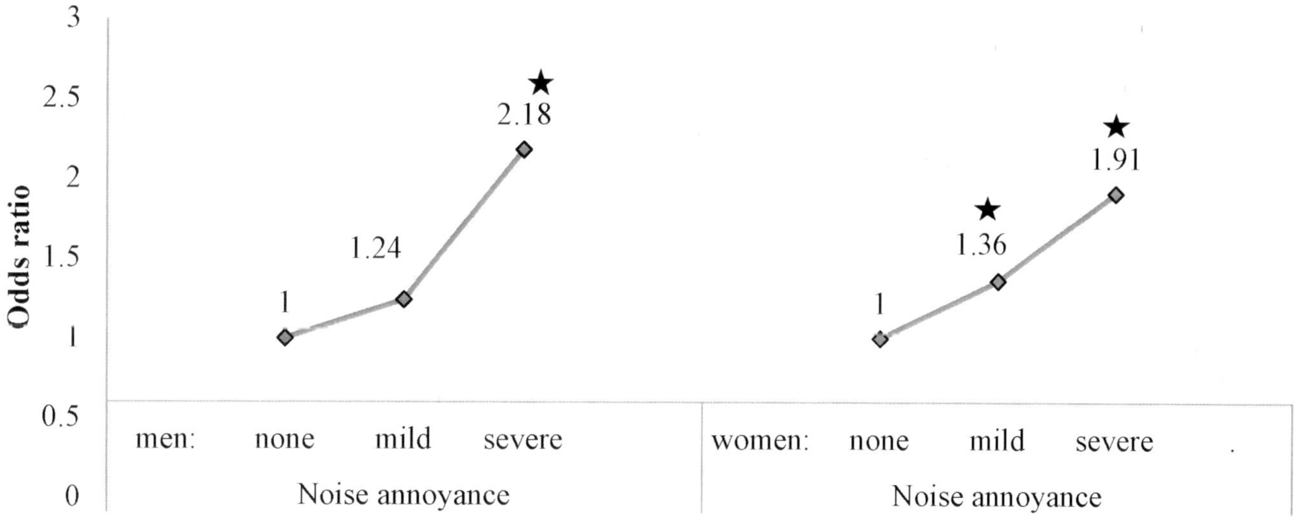

Figure 1. Odds ratio of suicidal ideation with depressed mood according to occupational noise annoyance (*p<0.05).
doi:10.1371/journal.pone.0105321.g001

Psychological symptoms (depressive symptoms or suicidal ideation) by occupational noise annoyance and sleep duration

In multivariate regression analyses controlling for age, BMI, sleep duration, education, occupation, household income, smoking habits, and alcohol use, the ORs (95% CIs) for psychological symptoms (depressive symptoms or suicidal ideation) at severe annoyance were 2.18 (1.40–3.41) in men and 1.91 (1.27–2.86) in women (Figure 1).

The interaction between sleep time and noise exposure was also calculated. In those with greater than five hours of sleep, the ORs (95% CI) of the severe noise annoyance compared with the no noise annoyance group were 1.80 (1.28–2.51) in men and 1.43 (0.98–2.07) in women. In both genders, the greatest ORs were observed in the severe noise annoyance group with less than five hours of sleep, with ORs (95% CI) of 2.95 (1.46–5.96) and 2.05 (1.01–4.16) times higher compared with the no noise annoyance with greater than five hours of sleep (Figure 2). There was no interaction effect of noise annoyance and sleep duration on psychological symptoms in the current study ($p = 0.973$ in men, 0.372 in women).

Discussion

Our large, cross-sectional, nationwide study reported an important link between occupational noise annoyance and psychological symptoms, including depression and suicidal ideation. Those associations were not attenuated by adjusting for individual characteristics such as age, BMI, smoking habits, and alcohol drinking, as well as socio-demographic characteristics including education, occupation, and household income, even with gender stratification.

The current study has several limitations. First, because of the nature of cross-sectional studies, the direction of causality of occupational noise annoyance on psychological symptoms cannot be determined. Furthermore, depressive symptoms affect the individual appraisal of the noise exposure situation, and worker who have psychological problem could experience greater annoyance from noise exposure compare to healthy workers. This current relationship could be might due to this difference in perception. Although the results of our study are supported by the potential biological explanation of the impact of noise on the arousal system, prospective studies are needed to elucidate the causal relationship. Additionally, there was no information regarding actual sound level in terms of noise frequency and decibel level. However, as discussed above, the annoyance related to occupational noise could still serve as a simple but important measure when screening for health consequences from noise exposure.

Noise can be defined as undesirable sound [1]. Both the absolute level of sound and personal perception of noise levels are important factors that can affect human health [15]. As such, noise annoyance scales (ranging from "not at all" to "extremely") are recommended by the International Commission on the Biological Effects of Noise [16]. In the current study, an assessment of noise exposure and its subjective effects (none annoyance, mild annoyance, and severe annoyance) were assigned by researchers using workers' self-report questionnaire. Although we have no information on absolute noise exposure, the subjective level of noise annoyance captured by the current questionnaire is an important means for assessing the consequence of occupational noise on mental health, particularly as this measure was significantly related to psychological symptoms including depressive symptoms and suicidal ideation.

Some studies have suggested that sustained central autonomic arousal due to chronic noise exposure might be an important risk factor for psychological disorder [17]. For instance, dopamine, an essential neurotransmitter implicated in arousal and attention [18], has been shown to be disrupted upon exposure to noise [19]. Furthermore, dopamine has been linked to the pathophysiology of depression [20]; hence, there is a biological possibility that chronic noise exposure results in psychological abnormalities by disrupting the normal processes of arousal and the dopamine pathway. Hence, our current results are potentially supported by this biological mechanism.

Depressive symptoms and suicidal ideation are important risk factors for suicide attempts. For example, depressive symptoms persisting for more than two weeks is an essential component in the diagnosis of major depressive disorder according to both the Diagnostic and Statistical Manual of Mental Disorders (DSM-5) and the International Statistical Classification of Diseases and Related Health Problems (ICD-10) [21]. Additionally, attempted

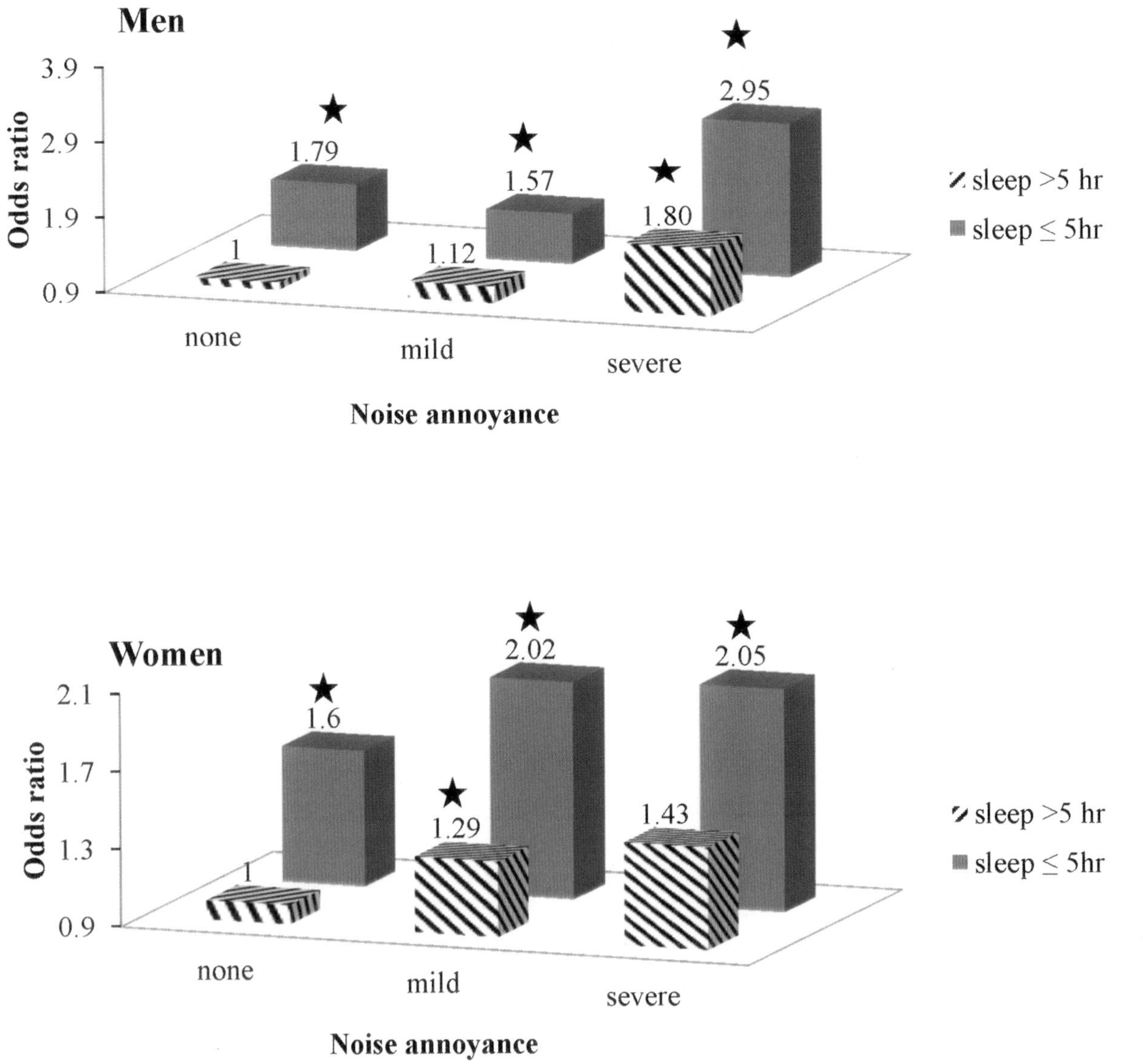

Figure 2. Risk of psychological symptoms (at least one of depressive symptoms or suicidal ideation) according to occupational noise annoyance and sleep duration (*p<0.05).

suicide is a key aspect of clinical emergency psychiatry [22]. Furthermore, the presence of suicidal ideation sharply increases the risk of a suicide attempt compared with non-suicidal ideation situations [23]. Hence, although the two questions in the current study did not cover all psychiatric diagnoses, our results suggest that these simple measures may be important psychological screening tools related to the health consequences of noise exposure.

A potential biological link has been suggested between noise exposure and poor quality of sleep [10]. In the current study, we were unable to assess sleep quality because lack of information; however, we did include sleep duration as a risk factor for psychological symptoms, with a sleep time of less than or equal to five hours related to psychological symptoms. However, there was no interaction between the effect of occupational noise annoyance and sleep duration on psychological symptoms. Hence, regardless of sleep time, our results suggest that noise exposure is an important and independent risk factor for psychological symptoms.

Previous studies have also reported that noise exposure and noise annoyance are linked to psychological symptoms [5,6]. However, other investigations have shown that the association between noise exposure and psychological symptoms are not independent of socio-demographic factors [7,8]. This might be due to the complex association between psychological abnormalities and socio-demographic characteristics [24]. Conversely, this lack of evidence might be related to the small sample size of the previous studies. However, our large cross sectional study showed that these associations were not affected after adjusting for individual and socio-demographic characteristics even with gender stratification. Moreover, these associations remained significant after stratification by sleep duration.

In general, there are gender differences associated with psychological symptoms and risk factors. For example, income level has a significant inverse relationship to suicidality in women but not in men [25,26]. However, there were no gender differences in effect of income on psychological symptoms in the current study, and overall, there were no significant gender difference between occupational noise annoyance and psychological symptoms. This may be due to our study design, which only included currently employed individuals, thus tapping into the "healthy worker effect".

In conclusion, our large, cross-sectional, nationwide study showed that occupational noise annoyance significantly related to mental health, including depressive symptoms and suicidal ideation. This link remained significant even after controlling for individual and socio-demographic characteristics even with gender stratification. However, prospective studies with quantified noise exposure assessment are needed to overcome our limitation of cross sectional design, and to elucidate the causality on the association between noise annoyance and psychological symptoms. To prevent both auditory effects and more general health consequences, such as psychological symptoms, from noise exposure, regulation strategies for occupational noise exposure are needed.

Author Contributions

Conceived and designed the experiments: JR JHY. Performed the experiments: JR JUW. Analyzed the data: JHY WL. Contributed reagents/materials/analysis tools: JHY PJ. Contributed to the writing of the manuscript: JHY WL.

References

1. Passchier-Vermeer W, Passchier WF (2000) Noise exposure and public health. Environ Health Perspect 108 Suppl 1: 123–131.
2. Stansfeld SA, Matheson MP (2003) Noise pollution: non-auditory effects on health. Br Med Bull 68: 243–257.
3. van Kempen EE, Kruize H, Boshuizen HC, Ameling CB, Staatsen BA, et al. (2002) The association between noise exposure and blood pressure and ischemic heart disease: a meta-analysis. Environ Health Perspect 110: 307–317.
4. Tarnopolsky A, Watkins G, Hand DJ (1980) Aircraft noise and mental health: I. Prevalence of individual symptoms. Psychol Med 10: 683–698.
5. Stansfeld SA, Haines MM, Burr M, Berry B, Lercher P (2000) A Review of Environmental Noise and Mental Health. Noise Health 2: 1–8.
6. Hiramatsu K, Yamamoto T, Taira K, Ito A, Nakasone T (1997) A survey on health effects due to aircraft noise on residents living around Kadena air base in the Ryukyus. Journal of Sound and Vibration 205: 451–460.
7. Kryter KD (1990) Aircraft noise and social factors in psychiatric hospital admission rates: a re-examination of some data. Psychol Med 20: 395–411.
8. Stansfeld S, Gallacher J, Babisch W, Shipley M (1996) Road traffic noise and psychiatric disorder: prospective findings from the Caerphilly Study. BMJ 313: 266–267.
9. Nelson DI, Nelson RY, Concha-Barrientos M, Fingerhut M (2005) The global burden of occupational noise-induced hearing loss. Am J Ind Med 48: 446–458.
10. Seidman MD, Standring RT (2010) Noise and quality of life. Int J Environ Res Public Health 7: 3730–3738.
11. Jeon B, Kwon S (2013) Effect of private health insurance on health care utilization in a universal public insurance system: a case of South Korea. Health Policy 113: 69–76.
12. Jiho L (2010) Occupational Diseases of Noise Exposed Workers. Hanyang Medical Reviews 30: 326–332.
13. Barreto SM, Swerdlow AJ, Smith PG, Higgins CD (1997) Risk of death from motor-vehicle injury in Brazilian steelworkers: a nested case-control study. Int J Epidemiol 26: 814–821.
14. Oh K, Lee J, Lee B, Kweon S, Lee Y, et al. (2007) Plan and operation of the 4th Korea National Health and Nutrition Examination Survey (KNHANES IV). Korean Journal of Epidemiology 29: 139–145.
15. Fields JM, De Jong RG, Gjestland T, Flindell IH, Job RFS, et al. (2001) Standardized general-purpose noise reaction questions for community noise surveys: Research and a recommendation. Journal of Sound and Vibration 242: 641–679.
16. Jakovljevic B, Paunovic K, Belojevic G (2009) Road-traffic noise and factors influencing noise annoyance in an urban population. Environ Int 35: 552–556.
17. Hardoy MC, Carta MG, Marci AR, Carbone F, Cadeddu M, et al. (2005) Exposure to aircraft noise and risk of psychiatric disorders: the Elmas survey—aircraft noise and psychiatric disorders. Soc Psychiatry Psychiatr Epidemiol 40: 24–26.
18. Robbins TW (1997) Arousal systems and attentional processes. Biol Psychol 45: 57–71.
19. Naqvi F, Haider S, Batool Z, Perveen T, Haleem DJ (2012) Sub-chronic exposure to noise affects locomotor activity and produces anxiogenic and depressive like behavior in rats. Pharmacol Rep 64: 64–69.
20. Dunlop BW, Nemeroff CB (2007) The role of dopamine in the pathophysiology of depression. Arch Gen Psychiatry 64: 327–337.
21. Stieglitz RD (2010) Assessment of depressive disorders. Ther Umsch 67: 549–553.
22. Nunes EV, Rounsaville BJ (2006) Comorbidity of substance use with depression and other mental disorders: from Diagnostic and Statistical Manual of Mental Disorders, fourth edition (DSM-IV) to DSM-V. Addiction 101 Suppl 1: 89–96.
23. Nock MK, Borges G, Bromet EJ, Alonso J, Angermeyer M, et al. (2008) Cross-national prevalence and risk factors for suicidal ideation, plans and attempts. Br J Psychiatry 192: 98–105.
24. Carter JD, Frampton CM, Mulder RT, Luty SE, Joyce PR (2010) The relationship of demographic, clinical, cognitive and personality variables to the discrepancy between self and clinician rated depression. J Affect Disord 124: 202–206.
25. Takeuchi A, Sakano N, Miyatake N (2014) Combined Effects of Working Hours, Income, and Leisure Time on Suicide in All 47 Prefectures of Japan. Ind Health.
26. Magnusson S, Makinen IH (2010) Sweden: income and suicide. Psychol Rep 107: 157–162.

2

Prevalence of Suicidal Ideation in Chinese College Students: A Meta-Analysis

Zhan-Zhan Li[1], Ya-Ming Li[2,3], Xian-Yang Lei[3], Dan Zhang[2], Li Liu[2], Si-Yuan Tang[2], Lizhang Chen[1]*

1 Department of Epidemiology and Health Statistics, School of Public Health, Central South University, Changsha, China, **2** Department of Nursing, Central South University, Changsha, Hunan Province, China, **3** The Second Affiliated Hospital, Xiangya Medical School, Central South University, Changsha, Hunan Province, China

Abstract

Background: About 1 million people worldwide commit suicide each year, and college students with suicidal ideation are at high risk of suicide. The prevalence of suicidal ideation in college students has been estimated extensively, but quantitative syntheses of overall prevalence are scarce, especially in China. Accurate estimates of prevalence are important for making public policy. In this paper, we aimed to determine the prevalence of suicidal ideation in Chinese college students.

Objective and Methods: Databases including PubMed, Web of Knowledge, Chinese Web of Knowledge, Wangfang (Chinese database) and Weipu (Chinese database) were systematically reviewed to identify articles published between 2004 to July 2013, in either English or Chinese, reporting prevalence estimates of suicidal ideation among Chinese college students. The strategy also included a secondary search of reference lists of records retrieved from databases. Then the prevalence estimates were summarized using a random effects model. The effects of moderator variables on the prevalence estimates were assessed using a meta-regression model.

Results: A total of 41 studies involving 160339 college students were identified, and the prevalence ranged from 1.24% to 26.00%. The overall pooled prevalence of suicidal ideation among Chinese college students was 10.72% (95%CI: 8.41% to 13.28%). We noted substantial heterogeneity in prevalence estimates. Subgroup analyses showed that prevalence of suicidal ideation in females is higher than in males.

Conclusions: The prevalence of suicidal ideation in Chinese college students is relatively high, although the suicide rate is lower compared with the entire society, suggesting the need for local surveys to inform the development of health services for college students.

Editor: Martin Voracek, University of Vienna, Austria

Funding: This study was supported by Hunan Province Science and Technology Project (2014FJ3093). The funder had no role in study design, data collection and analysis, decision to publish, or preparation of the manuscript.

Competing Interests: The authors have declared that no competing interests exist.

* Email: liche4005@126.com

Introduction

Suicide is usually not an isolated event, but a sequence of processes starting from death wishes, suicidal ideation, suicidal contemplation, suicide attempt, to suicide completion [1–2]. Suicidal ideation, which is defined as thoughts of self-harming or -killing [3] is a significant marker not only for mental-health problems but also for the suicide attempt and completed suicide among youths. Various suicidal cognitions (death wish, suicidal ideation, and suicide plan) and behaviors (suicide attempt, and commit suicide) are determined by common factors, such as personality characteristics, psychopathology, parenting style, family function, and substance [4–5]. Thus, it is imperative to identify the characteristics of suicidal ideation and to develop effective prevention and intervention programs.

Currently, suicide is the leading cause of death among 15- to 34-year-old in China, accounting for 19% of deaths in this age group [6]. Suicide has become an important public health issue. A tough challenge placed on top of China's higher education institutions is how to prevent college students from committing suicide and to early detect individuals at high risk of suicide. Given that about 30% of those with suicidal ideation (those who are seriously considering suicide) will attempt suicide, the first step is to determine the overall prevalence of suicidal ideation among college students [7].

Most college students in China are born after post-1980s when the "One-Child" policy switched from a promotive to a mandatory status. Consequently, the majority of them are from single-child families [8]. Hence, it has been becoming a primary argument regarding their relative impulsiveness and inability to withstand negative life events, compared with young adults with siblings. Despite many investigations into the prevalence of suicidal ideation in college students, quantitative syntheses of overall prevalence are scarce, especially in China. Primary prevention as the best and most important strategy requires a sensible plan of action for prevention and improving current policies against suicidal ideation in college students. Therefore, summarizing the prevalence of suicidal ideation in college students is the first step in developing research priorities. We performed a systematic review and meta-analysis of studies on suicidal ideation in Chinese college students with the aim to explore the prevalence of suicidal ideation in this area.

Materials and Methods

Literature Search Strategy

Databases including PubMed, Web of Knowledge, Chinese Web of Knowledge, Wangfang (Chinese database) and Weipu (Chinese database) were systematically reviewed to identify articles published between 2004 to July 2013, in either English or Chinese, reporting the estimates of suicidal ideation prevalence in Chinese college students. Articles were identified with search strategy "suicide" OR "suicidal ideation" OR "suicidal tendency" AND ("college student" OR "undergraduate"). The strategy also included a secondary search of reference lists of records retrieved from databases. Two authors screened the titles and abstracts and reviewed the full-text of the eligible articles.

Inclusion Criteria

The included studies met the following criteria: 1) an original epidemiological study aimed at Chinese college students; 2) with definition of criteria for screening methods and/or screening tools for suicidal ideation and with the provision of description of screening methods; 3) providing information about sample size and prevalence estimation for college students during the prior 12 months; 4) a cross-sectional study or a baseline survey of longitudinal study; 5) a sample size >500. 6) Language is limited to English and Chinese.

Data Extraction

Information was extracted from all selected publications by two investigators separately. Any disagreement was discussed and resolved by a third investigator. After the duplicates were removed, the following information was extracted from each article: first author, year of publication, region, area (South or North China), age range and mean age if possible, percent of males, major (medical student or not), screening method, screening tool, sample size, response rate, number of people with suicidal ideation, prevalence estimation, and sex-specific prevalence if possible.

Statistical Analysis

We first transformed proportions into a quantity (the Freeman-Tukey variant of the arcsine square root transformed proportion [9] suitable for the usual fixed and random effects summaries [10]), because the inverse variance weight in fixed-effects meta-analyses is suboptimum when dealing with binary data with low prevalence. Additionally, the transformed prevalence is weighted very slightly towards 50% and thus studies with prevalence of 0 can be included in the analysis. The pooled proportion is calculated as the back-transform of the weighted mean of the transformed proportions, using inverse arcsine variance weights for the fixed effect's model and DerSimonian-Laird weights for the random effect's model.

According to the expected heterogeneity across studies, a random-effects model was used to calculate pooled prevalence and 95% confidence interval (CIs). Between-study heterogeneity was evaluated with the Cochran chi-square (χ^2) and quantified with the I^2 statistic, which will be used to estimate total variation across studies due to heterogeneity rather than chance (<25% is considered as low heterogeneity, 25%–50% as moderate, and > 50% as high) [11,12]. In order to understand the prevalence of suicidal ideation in different sex, mean age, study year, sample, area and major and also explore the potential heterogeneity between studies, dummy-coding is used for three or more categories variables. We conducted subgroups analysis. Then the effects of these covariates on the logit prevalence of the outcome were estimated using meta-regression. Each covariate was included separately in univariate analyses, and then a multivariable meta-regression model was constructed including all covariates. Publication bias was evaluated Begg's test, the modified Egger's linear regression test and Trim-and-fill approach. Significance was set at $P<0.05$. All statistical calculations were made using Stata 11.0 (College Station, Texas) and Statsdirect 2.7.9 (http://www.statsdirect.com).

Results

Study flow and characteristics

A total of 1908 studies were identified after initial search. After removal of duplicates and an initial screening, we reviewed 177 papers in full. After exclusion of ineligible reports, 41 studies [13–53] published between January 2004 and July 20, 2013 were finally included. The flow diagram of the search process is exhibited in Figure 1. The characteristics of studies on the prevalence of suicidal ideation among college students are shown in Table 1. The sample size of the reviewed studies ranged from 610 to 21072 (median 2374), with a total of 160339 college students. Among them, 28 (68.3%) reports reported data on male ($n = 69701$), 28 (68.3%) reports on female ($n = 55140$), and 13 (31.7%) reports included mixed sex population size ($n = 35228$). In the surveys with samples, more than 54% of the individuals were men. The age ranged from 16 to 25 years old. Among them, 29 (70.7%) reports were aimed at South China ($n = 112706$), 12 reports at North China ($n = 47633$), 16 (39.0%) at medical universities ($n = 51645$), and 25 (61.0%) at non-medical students ($n = 108694$). Table 1 shows details from the 41 selected studies. Questionnaire is used to collect the information in the most of studies. 18 use the self-made scale, 9 for beck scale for suicide ideation-Chinese version, 7 for university personality inventory, and the left use other scales.

Pooled analysis in different category

Overall prevalence. The point prevalence of suicidal ideation with the 41 individual study populations ranged between 1.24% and 26.00%, with an overall meta-analysis prevalence of 10.72% (95%CI: 8.41%–13.28%, Figure 2) and evident high-level heterogeneity between studies ($I^2 = 99.6\%$, $P<0.0001$).

Sex. Pooled prevalence of all subgroups of study year, population size, male percent, area, major and sex are presented in Table 2. The summarized prevalence of females (10.32%, 95%CI: 7.17%–13.97%, Figure 3) was higher than that of males (8.84%, 95%CI: 6.45%–11.57%, Figure 4). The prevalence estimates for studies with more than 50% males were lower than estimates of groups with less than 50% males (8.84%, 95%CI: 6.45%–11.57%).

Periods. The pooled prevalence estimate decreased over time. Between 2004 and 2007, the pooled prevalence estimate was 12.10% (*95%CI:* 6.97%–18.44%), which decreased to 10.73% (95%CI: 6.16%–16.39%) between 2008 and 2009. The estimate was 10.77% (95%CI: 8.30%–13.53%) in 2010 to 2011, and 9.35% (95%CI: 5.13%–14.68%) in 2012 to 2013.

Major and area. The prevalence for the non-medical group (9.61%, 95%CI: 6.97%–12.62%) was smaller than medical group (12.58 95%CI: 10.09%–15.30%). Prevalence among college students from South and North China were 11.95% (95%CI: 9.09%–15.14%) and 8.00% (95%CI: 4.67%–12.14%) respectively.

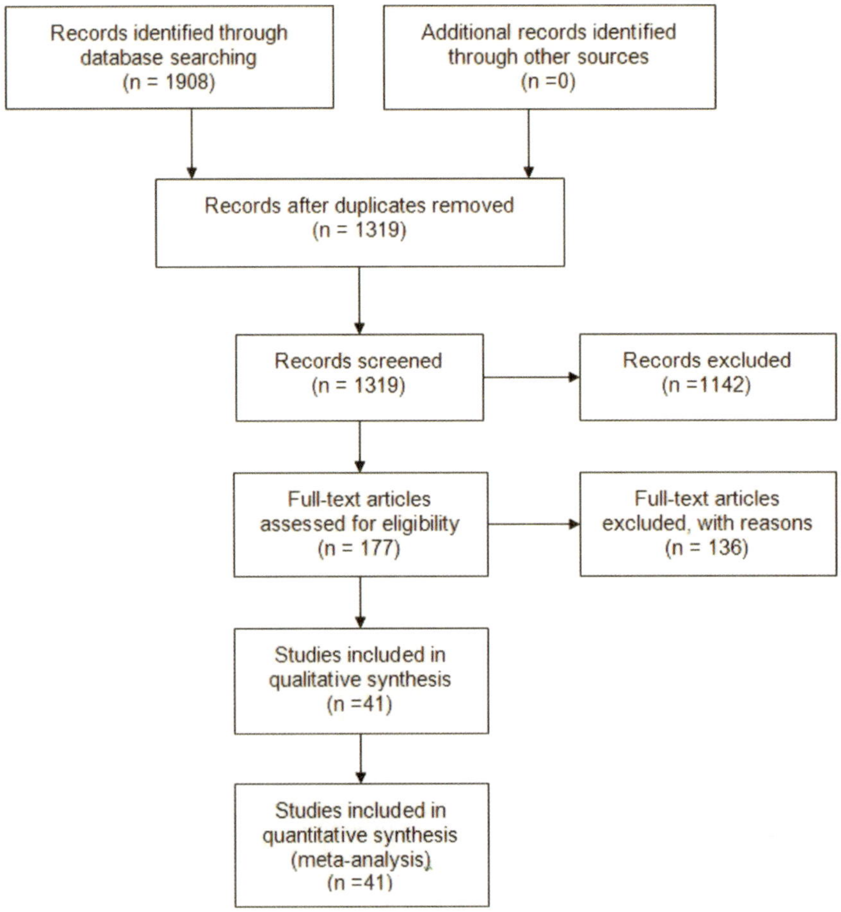

Figure 1. Flow diagram of included/excluded studies.

Population size and response rate. Regarding population size, the pooled prevalence was 11.40% (95%CI: 8.89%–14.19%) for population size <2000, 12.22% (95%CI: 9.30%–15.49%) and 7.70% (95%CI: 3.77%–12.85%) for population size >4000. Table 2 shows information about heterogeneity and publication bias. The pooled prevalence for response rate ≤90% was 12.81% (95%CI: 9.30–17.32) and 10.93 (95%CI: 9.72–12.13) for response rate >90%.

Meta-regression analysis, assessment of publication bias

We noted significant heterogeneity within studies and subgroups ($P<0.001$, $I^2 = 97.9\%–99.0\%$). In the univariate meta-regression analyses (Table 3), year of publication, male percent and major used to define suicidal ideation did not modify the estimate of prevalence. In three population size groups (<2000, 2000–4000, >4000), the prevalence estimates in population size >4000 were significantly lower compared with the other two groups. Mean age ($P = 0.017$) and response rates ($P = 0.012$) were significantly associated with the prevalence estimates. A meta-regression model was constructed including male ratio, response rate and population size (2000–4000). This model explained much of the heterogeneity between studies ($R^2 = 52.85\%$, $P = 0.016$, Table 3). We noted the prevalence of suicidal ideation decrease with response rate and male rate increase in the proportion and increase with the sample size increase. Then bias of publication was assessed using Begg's funnel plot and Egger's test. Significant publication bias was indicated by Begg's test ($P = 0.008$), but not by the modified Egger's linear regression test ($P = 0.258$). The funnel plot an apparent asymmetry that suggested the presence of a potential publication bias (Figure 5). Trim-and-Fill analyses was also used to assess publication bias. The pooled estimations for fixed and random models were −2.10 (95%CI: −2.17 to −2.02) and −2.21 (95%CI: −2.45 to −1.97). After estimated missing study was included into the meta-analysis, the pooled estimations for fixed and random models were −2.40 (95%CI: −2.47 to −2.33) and −2.43 (95%CI: −2.68 to −2.17). The estimated missing number of study is eight, which suggested the presence of publication bias.

Discussion

There is a lack of nationwide data regarding prevalence of suicidal ideation in Chinese college students at present. This is the first report attempting to synthesize the prevalence estimations of suicidal ideation among Chinese college students using meta-analysis. This comprehensive systematic review with meta-analysis of observational studies done in China in the last decade included 41 reports and more than 160 thousand college students. Therefore, it was possible to provide a reliable estimate of prevalence. This meta-analysis indicates that the prevalence of suicidal ideation in Chinese college students is 10.72% (95%CI: 8.41%–13.28%), which was close to previously reported rates [31] and fell in the range of 6%–39.2% reported in other countries [54–56].

Table 1. Characteristic of Studies on the Prevalence of Suicidal Ideation among College Students.

NO.	First author	Publication year	Region	Province	Area	Age (mean years)	Male Percent (%)	Medical student	Screening method	Screening tools	Response Rate (%)	Suicidal ideation	Sample size	Prevalence (%)
1	Wang [13]	2012	Mainland	Henan	Northern	17–22	44.2	No	Q	UPI	97.10	162	3850	4.21
2	Chen [14]	2010	Mainland	Chongqing	Southern	20.0	56.6	Yes	Q	SMQ	81.0	1279	9808	13.0
3	Xu [15]	2004	Mainland	Hunan	Southern	-	53.4	Yes	Q	SMQ	97.9	89	610	14.6
4	Chen [16]	2008	Mainland	Jilin	Northern	21.3	67.1	Yes	QI	CIDI	98.9	97	1822	5.3
5	Liu [17]	2007	Mainland	Yunnan	Southern	21.2	50.4	No	Q	SMQ	97.4	437	3313	13.2
6	Chao [18]	2008	Mainland	Jiangxi	Southern	-	51.8	No	Q	SMQ	84.2	113	1010	11.2
7	Shang [19]	2008	Mainland	Gansu	Northern	20.5	35.8	Yes	Q	SMQ	92.3	411	2678	15.4
8	Qian [20]	2008	Mainland	Beijing	Northern	-	35.4	Yes	Q	SMQ	88.2	122	2199	5.6
9	Yang [21]	2013	Mainland	Henan	Southern	20.7	33.5	Yes	Q	UPI	92.2	110	1372	8.0
10	Zhang [22]	2007	Mainland	Guangdong	Southern	-	52.8	Yes	Q	EPQ	99.3	1763	7189	24.5
11	Wang [23]	2011	Mainland	Yunnan	Southern	18.9	35.5	Yes	Q	SMQ	99.84	409	1850	22.1
12	Jiang [24]	2006	Mainland	Fujian	Southern	-	56.3	Yes	Q	SMQ	90.4	171	1254	13.6
13	Li [25]	2009	Mainland	Beijing	Northern	25.1	64.4	No	Q	UPI	97.6	380	21072	1.8
14	Li [26]	2007	Mainland	Zhejiang	Southern	18.6	40.1	No	Q	SCL-90	95.0	800	8160	9.8
15	Bao [27]	2009	Mainland	Anhui	Southern	23.1	61.0	Yes	Q	BSSI	92.7	217	1529	14.2
16	Huang [28]	2007	Mainland	Zhejiang	Southern	18.85	64.0	No	QI	SCL-90	94.2	219	3564	6.1
17	Wang [29]	2011	Mainland	Shanxi	Northern	19.2	44.9	Yes	Q	SDSS	98.3	74	1177	6.3
18	Kong [30]	2012	Mainland	Anhui	Southern	20.4	42.9	Yes	Q	SMQ	91.8	444	3030	14.7
19	Song [31]	2010	Mainland	Anhui	Southern	21.8	55.9	Yes	Q	BSSI	95.9	210	2062	10.2
20	Sun [32]	2010	Mainland	Shandong	Northern	20.4	42.4	No	Q	BSSI	94.3	228	1886	12.1
21	Yang [33]	2010	Mainland	Harbin	Northern	21.3	51.1	No	Q	SMQ	87.8	479	5240	9.1
22	Yan [34]	2009	Mainland	Guangdong	Southern	21.2	46.8	No	Q	SMQ	87.2	57	772	7.4
23	Shi [35]	2007	Mainland	Guangdong	Southern	20.6	49.8	No	Q	SMQ	98.0	297	2564	11.6
24	Shi [36]	2013	Mainland	Guangxi	Southern	20.4	52.7	No	Q	BSSI	91.0	434	2730	15.9
25	Ran [37]	2006	Mainland	Sichuan	Southern	-	70.6	No	Q	UPI	100.0	229	8850	2.6
26	Kan [38]	2013	Mainland	Zhejiang	Southern	-	46.1	No	Q	UPI	99.9	263	10138	2.6
27	Zhao [39]	2011	Mainland	Guangdong	Southern	21.7	56.6	No	Q	SMQ	96.35	98	1450	6.8
28	Yin [40]	2009	Mainland	Jiangsu	Southern	21.3	36.4	No	QI	SMQ	95.7	90	670	13.4
29	Yang [41]	2007	Mainland	Henan	Northern	16–24	74.6	No	Q	SCL-90	93.9	705	3568	19.8
30	Liu [42]	2013	Mainland	Guangdong	Southern	14–25	58.5	No	Q	SPS	100.0	585	6154	9.5
31	Tu [43]	2013	Mainland	Guangdong	Southern	21.0	60.0	No	Q	UPI	100.0	144	11603	1.24
32	Liu [44]	2008	Mainland	Beijing	Northern	-	42.5	Yes	Q	SMQ	91.4	125	1204	10.4
33	Li [45]	2008	Mainland	Beijing	Northern	20.0	55.6	No	Q	BSSI	97.6	166	2055	8.1
34	Cao [46]	2009	Mainland	Anhui	Southern	19.3	46.2	Yes	QI	BSSI	91.8	1669	10344	16.4

Table 1. Cont.

NO.	First author	Publication year	Region	Province	Area	Age (mean years)	Male Percent (%)	Medical student	Screening method	Screening tools	Response Rate (%)	Suicidal ideation	Sample size	Prevalence (%)
35	Fan [47]	2008	Mainland	Anhui	Southern	20.3	53.5	Yes	Q	BSSI	94.4	496	3517	14.1
36	Tang [48]	2011	Mainland	Hubei	Southern	10–24	54.7	No	Q	SMQ	100.0	178	2013	8.8
37	Zhang [49]	2012	Mainland	Guangdong	Southern	21.8	48.6	No	Q	SMQ	87.2	137	689	19.9
38	Zhu [50]	2011	Mainland	Jiangsu	Southern	19.6	47.1	No	Q	BSSI	98.1	430	2374	18.1
39	Zhao [51]	2012	Mainland	Guangdong	Southern	19.5	46.4	No	Q	BSSI	84.0	225	1168	19.3
40	Wang [52]	2010	Mainland	Shanxi	Northern	19.0	46.9	No	Q	UPI	93.0	46	882	5.6
41	Gau [53]	2008	Taiwan	Taiwan	Southern	19.4	48.5	No	Q	SMQ	79.2	759	2919	26.0

Screen methods: Q, questionnaire distribution; QI, questionnaire-based interview. Screening tools: UPI, University Personality Inventory, SMQ, Self-made scale; CIDI, Composite International Diagnostic Interview; BSSI, Beck Scale for Suicide Ideation-Chinese Version.

Suicidal ideation among college students is associated with various factors, which can be categorized into several domains, including physiology, suicide attitude, psychological health status, stress, and social support.

Sex may significantly affect the prevalence of suicidal ideation. A national representative population-based study from Korea found the prevalence of suicidal ideation was significantly higher among females: about 19% of females and 11% of males reported suicidal ideation [57]. In Kampala (Uganda), the prevalence of suicidal ideation was significantly higher in girls (34%) than boys (23.2%) [58]. However, other studies did not report the sex difference for suicidal ideation [59]. This meta-analysis showed that 8.84% of males and 10.32% of females had suicidal ideation, and this difference can be partially explained by the following reasons. According to the gender role socialization theory, males are expected to be independent and decisive, and display masculinity (e.g. engagement in risky behaviors). In contrast, females are expected to be dependent and indecisive, and express their stress via rumination. So females have a higher rate of suicide attempts than males, while males have a higher rate of mortality from suicide than females [60]. In China, fatal suicide rate for male was higher than females. But fatal suicide rate for females was still higher than males among population aged 15 to 34 (including college student) [61]. Suicidal ideation pattern in this meta-analysis may be similar to the pattern of fatal suicide.

Psychological health status exerts an implicit, deep and fundamental influence on suicidal ideation. About 50%–75% of children and adolescents who have suicidal ideation suffered from emotional disturbance, especially severe depression; about 1/4–2/3 of adolescents with suicidal ideation have a history of drug dependence and abuse [62]. Personality disorder in adults with suicidal ideation is more common than adolescents, indicating that adolescents with personality disorder are easily addicted to drug abuse and more likely to develop suicidal ideation [63]. Sexual orientation will greatly affect the suicidal ideation and suicidal behaviors of the youths, which is regulated by depression, hopelessness and drug abuse [64–65].

Negative life events that are a direct source of stimulation inducing suicidal ideation. College students who experience more negative life events are at increased risk for suicidal ideation. Associations between suicidal ideation and failure in love, financial problems, and divorce/separation of parents have been reported [71]. Findings also suggest that negative life events may be associated with suicidal ideation among adolescent, depressive symptoms were associated with suicidality and depressive symptoms may mediate the association of minor negative life events with suicidality [66].

Higher levels of family cohesion and family support were associated with lower levels of suicidal ideation and depression [67]. Living alone increased the risk for suicidal ideation among college students [68], suggesting that facilitating access to support resources might reduce the risk for suicidal behavior among college students. In addition, friends are also an important source of support and may be an even greater resource than the family [69]. Therefore, evaluating the support system of friends may provide further information that can help prevent suicide.

There are other factors of suicidal ideation such as cultural orientation [70], religious belief [51], history of family suicide [36], and social-economic status [46]. The factors affecting suicidal ideation in college students are not single, but multifaceted. Depression fully mediated the relationship between physical illness, interpersonal conflict and suicidal ideation, but not the relationship between financial problem and suicidal ideation [71]. Another study confirmed the hypothesis that family cohesion and

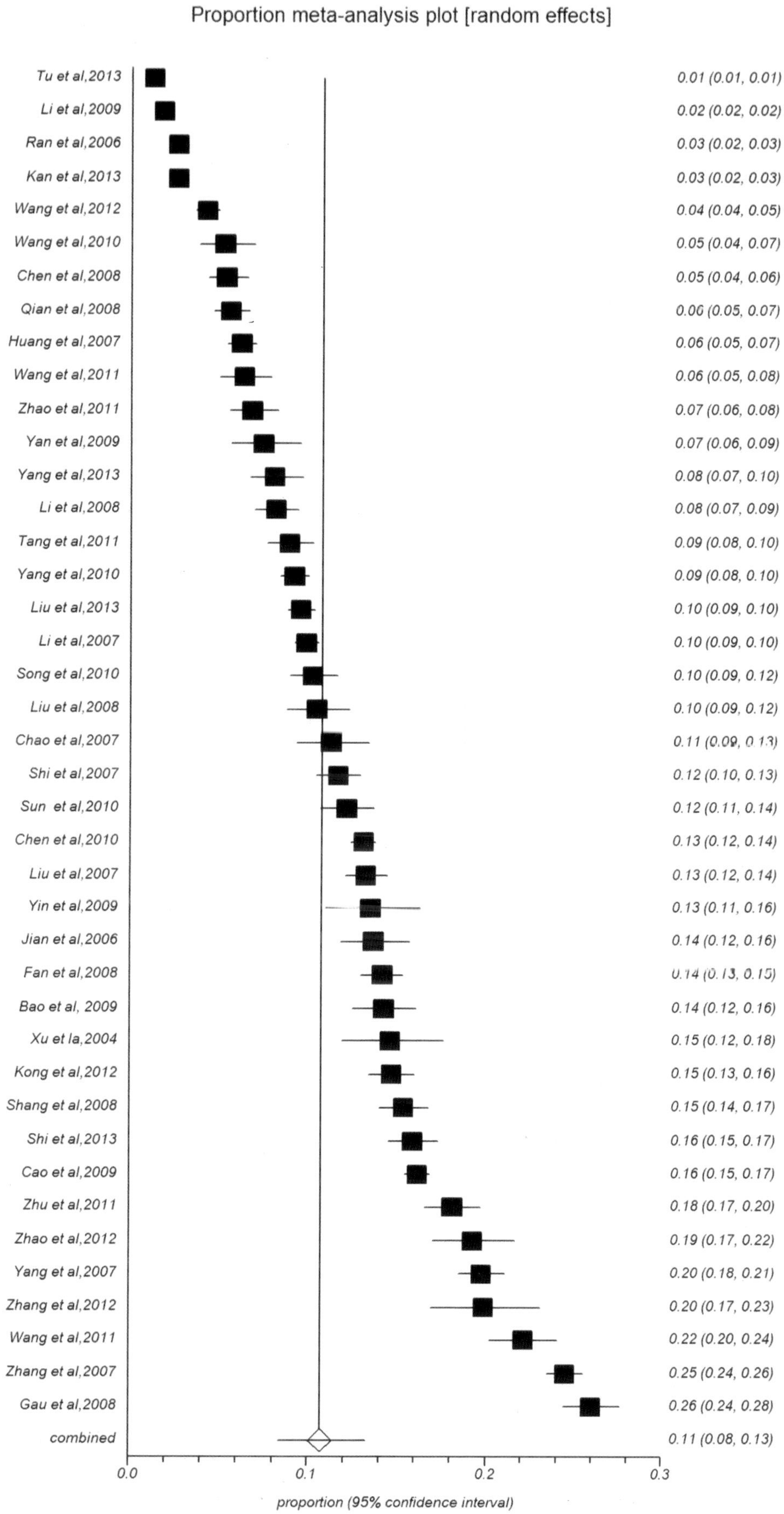

Figure 2. Forest plot of prevalence of suicidal ideation for total people.

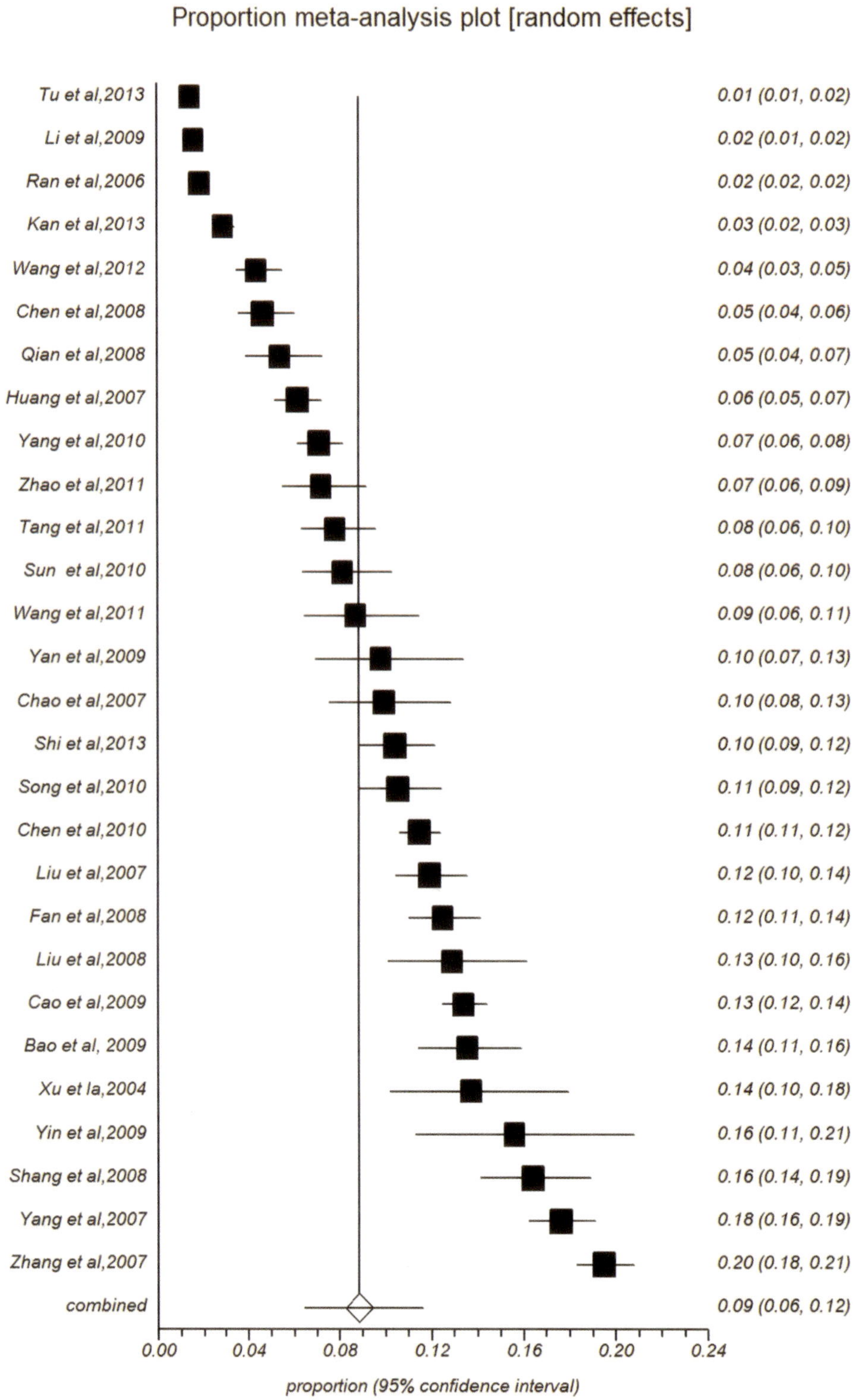

Figure 3. Forest plot of prevalence of suicidal ideation for male.

social self-concept were significant moderators for children and adolescents [70]. In sum, on an individual basis, one or all three factors could work, and even accidental factors may also contribute to suicidal ideation.

For the reasons given above, some effective measures should be taken. It is suggested that the experience of violence had a significant negative direct effect and peer support had a significant positive direct effect on their happiness. Happiness had a significant negative effect and the experience of violence had a significant positive effect on suicidal ideation. These findings demonstrate the fundamental importance of reducing exposure of violence to the youth, and that increasing peer support and their

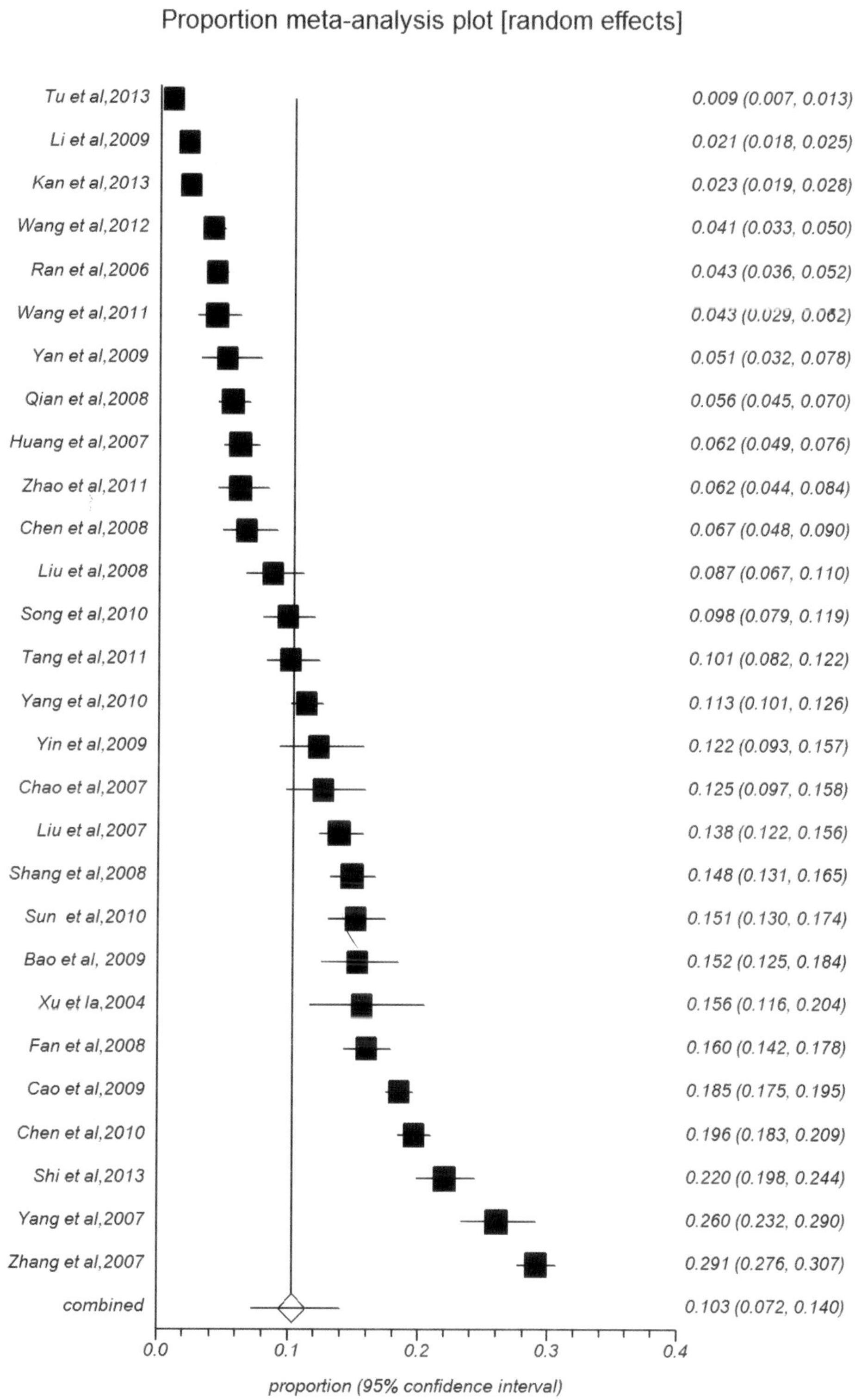

Figure 4. Forest plot of prevalence of suicidal ideation for female.

happiness may be the key to adolescent suicidal ideation prevention [72]. Sakamoto et al found that watching the video had substantial psych educational effects, which could be considered as prevention measures [73]. What is more, the lack of mental health services is an urgent problem of campus populations in China. More mental health counselors are needed [74]. College students would benefit greatly by attention to this measures.

Although this meta-analysis includes 41 studies encompassing a larger sample size than individual studies, there are still some limitations. First, the heterogeneity of both total population and subgroup was high. Most of the included studies had large sample

Table 2. Prevalence of Suicidal Ideation among College Students According to Different Category.

Category	Subgroup	NO. of Studies	Prevalence (*95%CI*)(%)	*N*	I^2 (%)	*P*	Publication Bias Test	
							P(Begg's Test)	*P*(Egger's Test)
	Total	41	10.72[8.41–13.28]	160339	99.6	<0.0001	0.258	0.008
Study year	2004–2007	9	12.10[6.97–18.44]	39072	99.7	<0.0001	0.915	0.704
	2008–2009	13	10.73[6.16–16.39]	51791	99.7	<0.0001	0.858	0.183
	2010–2011	10	10.77[8.30–13.53]	28742	97.9	<0.0001	0.600	0.942
	2012–2013	9	9.35[5.13–14.68]	47034	99.6	<0.0001	0.119	0.009
Sample size	<2000	16	11.40[8.89–14.19]	19345	97.5	<0.0001	0.003	0.001
	2000–4000	15	12.22[9.30–15.49]	42436	99.0	<0.0001	0.0001	0.0001
	>4000	10	7.70[3.77–12.85]	98558	99.9	<0.0001	0.009	0.0001
Male percent	$<50\%$	20	11.67[8.63–15.10]	59926	99.3	<0.0001	0.186	0.388
	$\geq 50\%$	21	9.85[6.68–13.57]	100413	99.7	<0.0001	0.492	0.069
Area	Northern	12	8.00[4.67–12.14]	47633	99.5	<0.0001	0.381	0.065
	Southern	29	11.95[9.09–15.14]	112706	99.6	<0.0001	0.838	0.119
Medical students	Yes	16	12.58[10.09–15.30]	51645	98.7	<0.0001	0.757	0.792
	No	25	9.61[6.97–12.62]	108694	99.6	<0.0001	0.083	0.008
Sex	Male	28	8.84 [6.45–11.57]	69701	99.3	<0.0001	0.570	0.0001
	Female	28	10.32[7.17–13.97]	55140	99.4	<0.0001	0.101	0.422
Response rate	$90\% \leq$	9	12.81[9.30–17.32]	25059	98.7	<0.0001	0.531	0.589
	$<90\%$	32	10.93[9.72–12.13]	135280	99.5	<0.0001	0.023	0.004

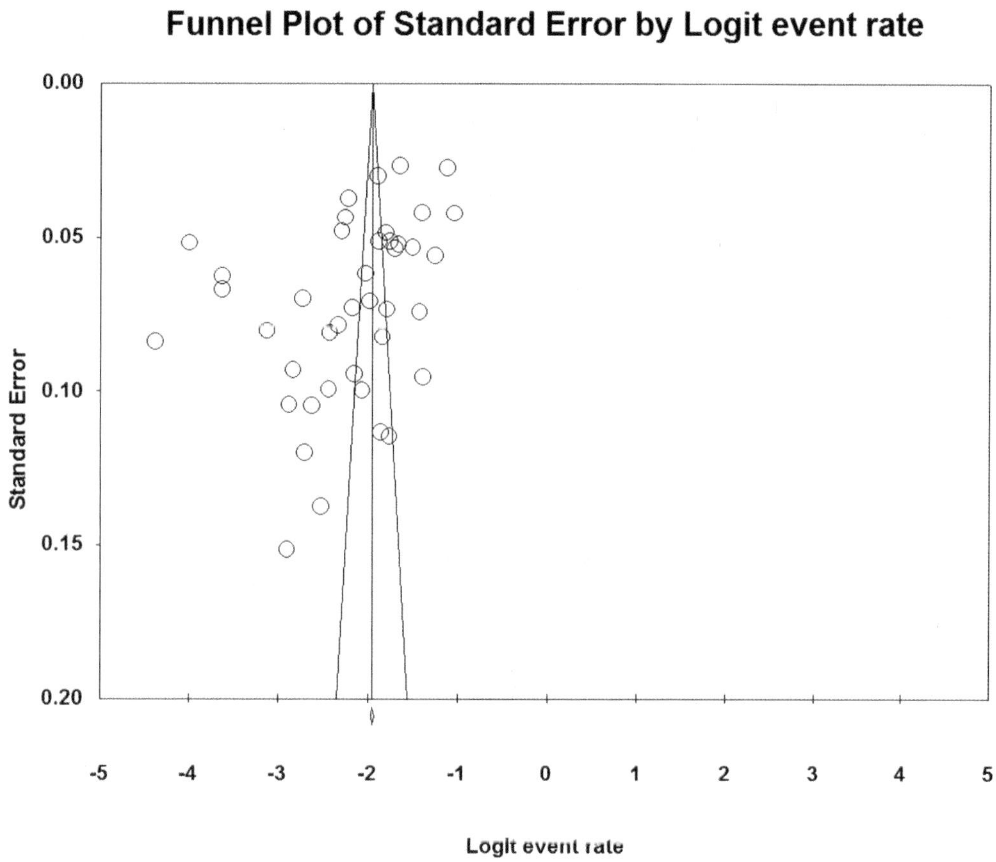

Figure 5. Funnel plot of studies included in the synthesis.

Table 3. Results of Meta-regression for Prevalence among Chinese College Students.

Covariate	Meta-regression coefficient	*95%CI*	*P* value	Variance explained (%)
Univariate analyses				
Year of publication				
2004–2007	0.176	−0.356 to 0.709	0.507	−1.40
2008–2009	0.015	−0.460 to 0.492	0.946	−2.55
2010–2011	0.078	−0.437 to 0.594	0.759	−2.31
2012–2013	−0.281	−0.809 to 0.246	0.288	0.41
Male percent	−0.235	−0.672 to 0.202	0.283	0.46
Sample size				
<2000	0.192	−0.258 to 0.642	0.394	−0.64
2000–4000	0.283	−0.168 to 0.734	0.212	1.51
>4000	−0.604	−1.082 to −0.126	0.015	12.16
Area	0.392	−0.077 to 0.863	0.099	4.43
Mean age	−0.230	−0.417 to −0.044	0.017	16.2
Screening tool	−0.435	−0.859 to −0.010	0.045	7.26
Response rate	−0.050	−0.088 to −0.011	0.012	13.01
Medical student	0.359	−0.080 to 0.799	0.106	4.16
Multivariable analyses			0.016	52.85
Response rate	−0.057	−0.10 to −0.014	0.011	
Male rate	−0.030	−0.055 to −0.004	0.024	
Sample size(2000–4000)	0.778	0.210 to 1.346	0.010	

sizes that produced very precise estimates. Meta-regression analysis showed that male ratio, sample size and response rate may be associated with the prevalence of suicidal ideation, which explained about the half of the heterogeneity between studies. But non-theory-guided selection of predictors based on an algorithm may lead to replication difficulties in future studies. We noted the prevalence of suicidal ideation decrease with response rate and male rate increase in the proportion and increase with the sample size increase. The difference of screening methods may have an influence on the heterogeneity. But this result should be carefully explained. Because some variable are associated with outcome variables in a single, and not associated with outcome variable after being combined. We call this aggregation bias, ecological bias, ecological confounding or ecological fallacy. It is acknowledged that there must be some factors affecting the heterogeneity. According to the present data, we cannot further identify the source of heterogeneity. Second, results from Begg's funnel plot and Egger's test are different but the funnel plot and Trim and Fill methods suggested the presence of a potential publication bias, a language bias, and inflated estimates by a flawed methodological design in smaller studies. The available studies had important methodological limitations, particularly related to college students with suicidal ideation selection and recruitment, which may have led to subjects included in studies differing in important ways from those excluded or ineligible for analyses, and that may have unpredictably affected prevalence estimates. Finally, the studies with a sample size less than 500 subjects were not included on the basis of the sake of representativeness of survey samples. The information bias may still affect the pooled results, although we restricted sampling methods in inclusion criteria.

In conclusion, the prevalence of suicidal ideation in Chinese college students is relatively high, although the suicide rate is lower than that of the entire society. Considering the policy of enrollment expansion of higher education in China is implemented, It is sincerely hoped that this meta-analysis synthesized within the past decade will serve as a "wake-up" call to university administration alike. The results should encourage not only more needed research in terms of the college student group as a distinct population unto itself, but also prompt colleges, society and family to develop and implement programs to address, educate and prevent those college students who are most at risk for suicidal ideation.

Supporting Information

Checklist S1 PRISMA 2009 Checklist.

Diagram S1 PRISMA 2009 Flow Diagram.

Author Contributions

Conceived and designed the experiments: ZZL YML SYT. Performed the experiments: LZC ZZL. Analyzed the data: DZ LL ZZL. Contributed reagents/materials/analysis tools: XYL ZZL LZC. Wrote the paper: ZZL YML LZC. Revised the manuscript: ZZL LZC.

References

1. Jiang M, Hu Z, Cao Y (2007) Suicide deaths concentrated in Beijing universities. Am J Psychiatry 164: 1758.
2. Perez WV (2005) The relationship between seriously considering, planning, and attempting suicide in the youth risk behavior survey. Suicide and Life-threatening Behavior 35: 35–49.
3. National Research Council (2002) Reducing Suicide: A National Imperative. Washington, DC: The National Academies Press.
4. Beautrais AL (2000) Risk factors for suicide and attempted suicide among young people. Aust N Z J Psychiatry 34: 420–436.
5. Kuo PH, Yang HJ, Soong WT, Chen WJ (2002) Substance use among adolescents in Taiwan: associated personality traits, incompetence, and behavioral/emotional problems. Drug Alcohol Depend 67:27–39.
6. Phillips MR, Li X, Zhang Y (2002) Suicide rates in China, 1995–99. Lancet 359: 835–840.
7. Kirmayer LJ, Fraser SL, Faurus V, Heather Clarke, M.A.Saucier Jean-François, et al. (2009) Cultural and Mental Health Research Unit working paper 14. Montreal, Quebec: 2009. Current approaches to Aboriginal youth suicide prevention.
8. Luo MY (2010) Social Assessment and Subdividing of After-1980s. China Youth Study 11: 32–35.
9. Stuart A, Ord JK (1994) Kendall's Advanced Theory of Statistics (6th edition). London: Edward Arnold.
10. DerSimonian R, Laird N (1986) Meta-analysis in Clinical Trials. Controlled Clinical Trials 7: 177–188.
11. Brittain EH, Fay MP, Follmann DA (2012) A valid formulation of the analysis of noninferiority trials under random effects meta-analysis. Biostatistics 13: 637–649.
12. Chootrakool H, Shi JQ, Yue R (2011) Meta-analysis and sensitivity analysis for multi-arm trials with selection bias. Stat Med 30: 1183–1198.
13. Wang BW (2012) Psychological health condition and its influence factors among freshmen with suicidal ideation. Chin J Public Health 28: 1086–1088.
14. Chen JM, Ai M, Kuang L, Wang MJ, Shen Y, et al. (2010) Suicide ideation among college students in Chongqing. Chin J Epidemiol 31: 290–293.
15. Xu HL, Xiao SY, Feng SS, Chen XX (2004) Risk factors for suicide attempt among college students at Central South University. Chin J Epidemiol 25: 288–291.
16. Chen YF, Kou CG, Zhang D, Xie B, Yu YQ, et al. (2008) Analysis on suicide tendency and its risk factors of undergraduate students[J]. Chin J Dis Control Prev 12: 450–453.
17. Liu QQ, Li H, Fang XY (2007) An investigation of suicidal ideation and suicide attempts of undergraduate in Yunnan province with their self-esteem and mental health status. China Journal of Health Psychology 15: 57–58.
18. Chao XC (2008) Different personality of undergraduate students with and without suicide ideation [J]. Health Medicine Research and Practice 5: 42–44.
19. Shang YX, Dong GQ, Liu T (2008) Analysis on prevalence of suicidal ideation and depression and its influence factors among undergraduate students in Yinchuan. Chin J Public Health 24: 934–936.
20. Qian WC, Liu BH, Huang YQ, Hao WL, Li WYTN (2008) Study on risk factors for suicidal ideation among undergraduate of medical college. Chin J Public Health 24: 1285–1286.
21. Yang CW, Shi SC, Liu JX, Jia RR, Chui WW, et al. (2013) Analysis on suicide ideation and its risk factors among medical college students. Chin J Social Medicine 30: 193–195.
22. Zhang XY, Yu SY, Zhao JB (2007) Correlation between suicidal ideation and personality, internal-external locus of control, self-esteem in medical college students. J Fourth Mil Med Univ 28: 747–749.
23. Wang T, Jiang RS, Zhou M, Huang YY, Di YX (2011) A study on influencing factors of the undergraduate suicide ideation. Journal of Kunming Medical University 12:44–47.
24. Wang XL, Xu NF, Xue HT, Jiang DW, Yang DH (2006) Analysis on suicide ideation and its factors among medical undergraduate students. Chin J Public Health 22: 653–655.
25. Li H, Huang YQ (2009) Study on the related factors of suicide ideation among graduate students in national research institutions. China Journal of Health Psychology 17: 963–966.
26. Li FH, Dai WL (2007) Analysis on suicide ideation and its factors among college students in Wenzhou. Chin J School Doctor 21: 290–291.
27. Bao DX, Fan YG, Ye DQ (2009) Correlation between suicidal ideation and Life events and social support among medical college students of Wanxi. Chin J Sch Health 30: 939–941.
28. Huang QR, Liu B, Feng TL (2007) The relationship between life event and suicide attempts among college students. China J Health Psychology 15: 210–213.
29. Wang H, Wang MX, Chu XP (2011) Study on the factors of suicidal ideation and its influences among undergraduates in Shanxi province. Foreign medical science section of med geography 32: 188–191.
30. Kong G, Sun YH, Yang LS, Zhou CX (2012) Investigation of psychosocial factors of suicide attitude among the students in a medical college. J Bengbu Med Coll 37: 1240–1243.
31. Song YM, Wan YH, Pan FM, Ye DQ (2010) Analysis on suicide ideation and its risk factors among medical college students. Chinese Journal of Health Statistics 27: 178–179.
32. Sun AY, Sun YM, Xu HL (2010) Analysis on suicide ideation and its risk factors among college students in Liao cheng. Journal of Qilu Nursing 16: 55–56.
33. Yang YJ, Qiu XH, Yang XX, Qiao ZX, Han D, et al. (2010) Study on the influencing factors of suicidal ideation among university students in Harbin. Chin J Epidemiology 31: 1103–1106.

34. Yan HH, Liu ZM, Wang SY, Yang G, Chen LF, et al. (2009) Study on the relationship between life events and suicidal ideation among undergraduates in Guangzhou. Modern Preventive Medicine 36: 476–479.
35. Shi WJ, Ma SB, Wang SY (2007) Study on prevalence of suicidal ideation and its related factors in college students in Guangzhou. Chin J Sch Health 28: 999–1000.
36. Shi XL, Liu YY, Liu SY, Zhao WS, Jiang CL (2013) Analysis of suicidal ideation and relationship with depressive disorder of Guangxi college students countermeasures research. Popular science and technology 15: 114–117.
37. Ran CF, Zhang YQ, Wang W, Tian S, Wei J, et al. (2006) Suicide-preventive and suicide-intervening mechanism for vocational college students. J Prev MedInf 22: 548–552.
38. Kan SY, Zheng XF (2013) Relationship between suicide ideation and family environment among university students. Chin J Public Health 29: 167–168.
39. Zhao GX, Jin CX, Wang SY, Chen QS, Liu GN et al. (2011) Analysis on influencing factors of suicide ideation among college students: a structural equation model study. Chin J Behv Med Brain Sci 20: 357–359.
40. Yi L (2009) Analysis on influencing factors of suicide ideation among college students. Chin J School Doctor 23: 388–390.
41. Yang XH, Zhou H, Wang SM (2007) Epidemiological investigation of suicidal ideation in college students. Chin J Sch Health 28: 527–528.
42. Liu GH, Zhang GY (2013) The relationship between personality factors and suicide ideation of undergraduates. China Journal of Health Psychology 21: 456–457.
43. Tu YM, Zhang QJ (2013) The relationship between life events, coping style and suicide ideation of undergraduates. Educational circles, 15: 60.
44. Liu BH, Huang YQ, Niu WY, Lv ZZ, Wang PY, et al. (2008) Study on the factors influencing suicidal ideation among medical students in Beijing. Chin J Epidemiol 29: 128–131.
45. Li XN, Liu HY, Liu ZR, Guo Q, Huang YQ (2008) A cross-sectional study on related factors of suicidal ideation among college students. Chinese Mental Health Journal 22: 806–815.
46. Cao HY, Sun YH, Yao YS, Zhou CX, Yang LS (2009) Suicide behavior and its factors among medical undergraduates in Anhui province. Chin J Sch Health, 30: 38–39.
47. Fan YG (2008) Study on the influencing factors of suicide ideation among underrates in Anhui Provinces. Anhui: Anhui Medical University, 2008.
48. Tang J, Yu Y, Wu Y, Du YK, Ma Y, et al. (2011) Association between non-suicidal self injuries and suicide attempts in Chinese adolescents and college students: a cross-section study. PLoS One 6: e17977.
49. Zhang X, Wang H, Xia Y (2012) Stress, coping and suicide ideation in Chinese college students. J Adolesc 35: 683–690.
50. Zhu XH, Wang CD, Zhou Q, Zhaou HF, Yang YJ, et al. (2011) Study on the factors influencing suicidal ideation among 2374 college students. Chin J Behav and Brain Sci 20: 461–462.
51. Zhao J, Yang X, Xiao R, Zhang X, Aguilera D, et al. (2012) Belief system, meaningfulness, and psychopathology associated with suicidal among Chinese college students: a cross-sectional survey. BMC Public Health 12:668.
52. Wang Y, Guo XL (2010) Survey and analysis of psychological health in 882 higher vocational freshmen. Chin J Sch Doctor 24: 202–204.
53. Gau S S, Chen YY, Tsai FJ, Li MB, Qiu YN, et al. (2008) Risk factors for suicide in Taiwanese college students. J Am Coll Health 57: 135–142.
54. Arria AM, O'Grady KE, Caldeira KM, Vincent KB, Wilcox HC, et al.(2009) Suicide ideation among college students: a multivariate analysis [J]. Arch Suicide Res 13: 230–46.
55. Garlow SJ, Rosenberg J, Moore JD, Haas AP, Koestner B, et al. (2008) Depression, desperation, and suicidal ideation in college students: results from the American Foundation for Suicide Prevention College Screening Project at Emory University. Depress Anxiety 25: 482–488.
56. Mackenzie S, Wiegel JR, Mundt M, Brown D, Saewyc E, et al. (20111) Depression and suicide ideation among students accessing campus health care. Am J Orthopsychiatry 81: 101–108.
57. Park S (2013) Gender-specific factors of suicide ideation among adolescents in the Republic of Korea: a nationally representative population-based study. Arch Psychiatr Nurs 27:253–262.
58. Swahn MS, Palmier JB, Kasirye R, Yao H (2012) Correlates of Suicide Ideation and Attempt among Youth Living in the Slums of Kampala. Int J Environ Res Public Health 9: 596–609.
59. Ellis JB, Lamis DA (2007) Adaptive characteristics and suicidal behavior: a gender comparison of young adults. Death Stud 31:845–854.
60. Canetto SS, Sakinofsky I (1998) The gender paradox in suicide. Suicide Life Threat Behav 14:1–23.
61. Cai Y, Hu N, Liu WN, Wang LJ (2012) Current situation of suicide deaths among Chinese population in 2010. Chin Pre Med 13:480–482.
62. Gunn JR, Lester D, Mcswain S (2011) Testing the warning signs of suicidal behavior among suicide ideators using the 2009 National survey on drug abuse and health. Int J Emerg Ment Health 13: 147–154.
63. Sharp C1, Green KL, Yaroslavsky I, Venta A, Zanarini MC, et al. (2012) The incremental validity of borderline personality disorder relative to major depressive disorder for suicidal ideation and deliberate self-harm in adolescents. J Pers Disord 26: 927–938.
64. Hiramura H, Shono M, Tanaka N, Nagata T, Kotamura T, et al. (2008) Prospective study on suicidal ideation among Japanese undergraduate students: correlation with stressful life events, depression, and depress genic cognitive patterns. Arch Suicide Res 12: 238–250.
65. Silenzio VM, Pena JB, Duberstein PR, Cerel J, Kerry L, et al. (2007) Sexual orientation and risk factors for suicidal ideation and suicide attempts among adolescents and young adults. Am J Public Health 97: 2017–2019.
66. Hardt J, Johnson JG (2010) Suicidality, depression, major and minor negative life events: a mediator model. Psychosoc Med 7: c5.
67. Harris TL, Molock SD (2000) Cultural orientation, family cohesion, and family support in suicide ideation and depression among African American college students. Suicide Life Threat Behav 30:341–53.
68. Lee HS, Kim S, Choi I, Lee KU (2008) Prevalence and Risk Factors Associated with Suicide Ideation and Attempts in Korean College Students. Psychiatry Investig 5: 86–93.
69. Dubow EF, Tisak J, Causey D, Hryshko A, Reid G (1991) A two-year longitudinal study of stressful life events, social support, and social problem-solving skills: contributions to children's behavioral and academic adjustment. Child Dev 62:583–599.
70. Au AC, Lau S, Lee MT (2009) Suicide ideation and depression: the moderation effects of family cohesion and social self-concept. Adolescence 44: 851–868.
71. Wu J, Wu YT, Feng SX, Meng H, Chen H (2012) Mediating effects on depression regarding the relationship between negative life events and suicide ideation among college students. Chin J Epidem 33:1111–1115.
72. Choi JH, Yu M, Kim KE (2014) Suicidal ideation in adolescents: A structural equation modeling approach. Nurs Health Sci. doi: 10.1111/nhs.12142.
73. Sakamoto S, Tanaka E, Kameyama A, Takizawa T, Takizawa S, et al. (2014) The effects of suicide prevention measures reported through a psychoeducational video: A practice in Japan. Int J Soc Psychiatry Epub ahead of print.
74. Iang M, Hu Z, Cao Y (2007) Suicide deaths concentrated in Beijing universities. Am J Psychiatry 164: 1758.

A Prospective Cohort Study to Examine the Association between Dietary Patterns and Depressive Symptoms in Older Chinese People in Hong Kong

Ruth Chan[1]*, Dicken Chan[2], Jean Woo[1]

1 Department of Medicine and Therapeutics, The Chinese University of Hong Kong, Shatin, Hong Kong, 2 The Jockey Club School of Public Health and Primary Care, The Chinese University of Hong Kong, Shatin, Hong Kong

Abstract

Introduction: Dietary patterns are culturally specific and there is limited data on the association of dietary patterns with late-life depression in Chinese. This study examined the associations between dietary patterns and baseline and subsequent depressive symptoms in community-dwelling Chinese older people in Hong Kong.

Methods: Participants aged ≥65 year participating in a cohort study examining the risk factors for osteoporosis completed a validated food frequency questionnaire at baseline between 2001 and 2003. Factor analysis was used to identify three dietary patterns: "vegetables-fruits" pattern, "snacks-drinks-milk products" pattern, and "meat-fish" pattern. Depressive symptoms were measured at baseline and 4-year using the validated Geriatric Depression Scale. Multiple logistic regression was used for cross-sectional analysis (n = 2,902) to assess the associations between dietary patterns and the presence of depressive symptoms, and for longitudinal analysis (n = 2,211) on their associations with 4-year depressive symptoms, with adjustment for socio-demographic and lifestyle factors.

Results: The highest quartile of "vegetables-fruits" pattern score was associated with reduced likelihood of depressive symptoms [Adjusted OR = 0.55 (95% CI: 0.36–0.83), p_{trend} = 0.017] compared to the lowest quartile at baseline. Similar inverse trend was observed for the highest quartile of "snacks-drinks-milk products" pattern score [Adjusted OR = 0.41 (95% CI: 0.26–0.65), p_{trend}<0.001] compared to the lowest quartile. There was no association of "meat-fish" pattern with the presence of depressive symptoms at baseline. None of the dietary patterns were associated with subsequent depressive symptoms at 4-year.

Conclusion: Higher "vegetables-fruits" and "snacks-drinks-milk products" pattern scores were associated with reduced likelihood of baseline depressive symptoms in Chinese older people in Hong Kong. The longitudinal analyses failed to show any causal relationship between dietary patterns and depressive symptoms in this population.

Editor: Robert Stewart, Institute of Psychiatry, United Kingdom

Funding: This study was supported by grants from the Research Grants Council of Hong Kong, CUHK 4101/02M; the Hong Kong Jockey Club Charities Trust; the SH Ho Centre for Gerontology and Geriatric and the Centre for Nutritional Studies, The Chinese University of Hong Kong. The funders had no role in study design, data collection and analysis, decision to publish, or preparation of the manuscript.

Competing Interests: The authors have declared that no competing interests exist.

* Email: ruthchansm@cuhk.edu.hk

Introduction

Depression is a common mental health disorder. It affects over 350 million people worldwide and it is expected that depression will become the world's leading cause of disease burden by the year 2030 [1]. Depression is less prevalent among older adults than among younger counterparts [2]. However, late-life depression is considered as an important public health problem due to its devastating consequences, including increased risk of morbidity and reduced physical, cognitive, and social functioning [3,4]. As a result, to identify modifiable risk factors for depression is inevitably important [5].

Recent evidence suggests that diet modifies key biological factors associated with the development of depression, and diet rich in fruits, vegetables, whole grains and fish is in general associated with lower risk of depression [6,7]. Studies have shown that the antioxidant compounds in fruit and vegetables could reduce neuronal damage induced by oxidative-stress whereas long-chain omega-3 polyunsaturated fatty acids could possibly affect mood by an alteration of the brain serotonergic function and its immune-neuroendocrine effects [6,7]. However, the examination of diet as a risk factor for depression has traditionally focused on the effect of single foods and nutrients, and the findings thus far are inconsistent [8]. Since diet is a combination of food and nutrients, there has been an increasing interest in using dietary pattern analysis in epidemiological studies [9]. There are two main approaches to define dietary patterns [9,10]. One approach is the *a priori* approach in which dietary indices are constructed based on prevailing dietary recommendations. Another approach is the *a posteriori* approach in which dietary patterns are derived from statistical modeling, such as factor analysis, using data from dietary records or food frequency questionnaires (FFQ).

Data on the association between dietary patterns and depression are limited. Some cross-sectional studies have been carried out in Caucasians and Japanese to evaluate the association between dietary patterns and depression or depressive symptoms in adulthood [11–16]. To our knowledge, nine prospective studies have examined the role of dietary patterns and depression or depressive symptoms in adulthood [17–25] and two prospective studies have evaluated this association in adolescents [26,27]. Few studies have investigated the association between depression and diet in Chinese older people, and these studies mainly focused on the effect of single foods and nutrients [28,29]. Only one cross-sectional study has examined the association of dietary patterns with depressive symptoms in Chinese but it was done in adolescents [27].

Since dietary patterns are culturally specific and there is limited data on the association of dietary patterns with late-life depression in Chinese, we evaluated the association between dietary patterns and baseline and subsequent depressive symptoms in older Chinese people, using data from a sample of community-dwelling men and women aged 65 and over participating in a prospective study in Hong Kong. We hypothesized that dietary patterns are associated with baseline and subsequent depressive symptoms in this population.

Methods

Study population

Subjects were participants of a cohort study examining the risk factors for osteoporosis in Hong Kong [30]. 2,000 men and 2,000 women aged 65 years and over living in the community were recruited in a health survey between August 2001 and December 2003 by recruitment notices and talks in community centers and housing estates. Participants were volunteers and were able to walk or take public transport to the study site. They were recruited using a stratified sample so that approximately 33% would be in each of these age groups: 65–69, 70–74, 75+. Compared with the official population statistics, participants had higher educational level than the overall older population in Hong Kong (12–18% vs. 3–9% with tertiary education in the age groups 80+, 75–79,70–74, and 65–69 years) [31]. The 4-year follow-up was held between August 2005 and November 2007. Follow-up was done by a mailed reminder for a follow-up body check appointment. Phone reminders were given again close to the appointment dates, and defaulters were given a second appointment to enhance attendance rates. Mean (SD) follow-up year was 3.9 (0.1) years.

We excluded participants who did not have dietary data (n = 5), those with extreme daily energy intake at the first- and last-half percentiles of the sex-specific range (n = 37), those who had missing data for the variables included for the analyses (n = 6), and those who were probable dementia defined using the cognitive part of the Community Screening Instrument for Dementia (CSI-D) with the cutoff point of ≤28.4 [32] (n = 1,050). The baseline analysis was performed on 2,902 participants. For the longitudinal analysis, we further excluded 218 participants who had depressive symptoms at baseline and 473 participants who did not attend the 4-year follow-up. 2,211 participants were therefore included for the 4-year incidence analysis (Figure 1). This study was conducted in accordance with the Declaration of Helsinki. This study was approved by the Clinical Research Ethics Committee of the Chinese University of Hong Kong. Written informed consent was obtained from all participants.

Demographic and overall health characteristics

A standardized interview was performed to collect information on age, gender, education level, marital status, smoking habit, alcohol use and medical history. Information on the duration and

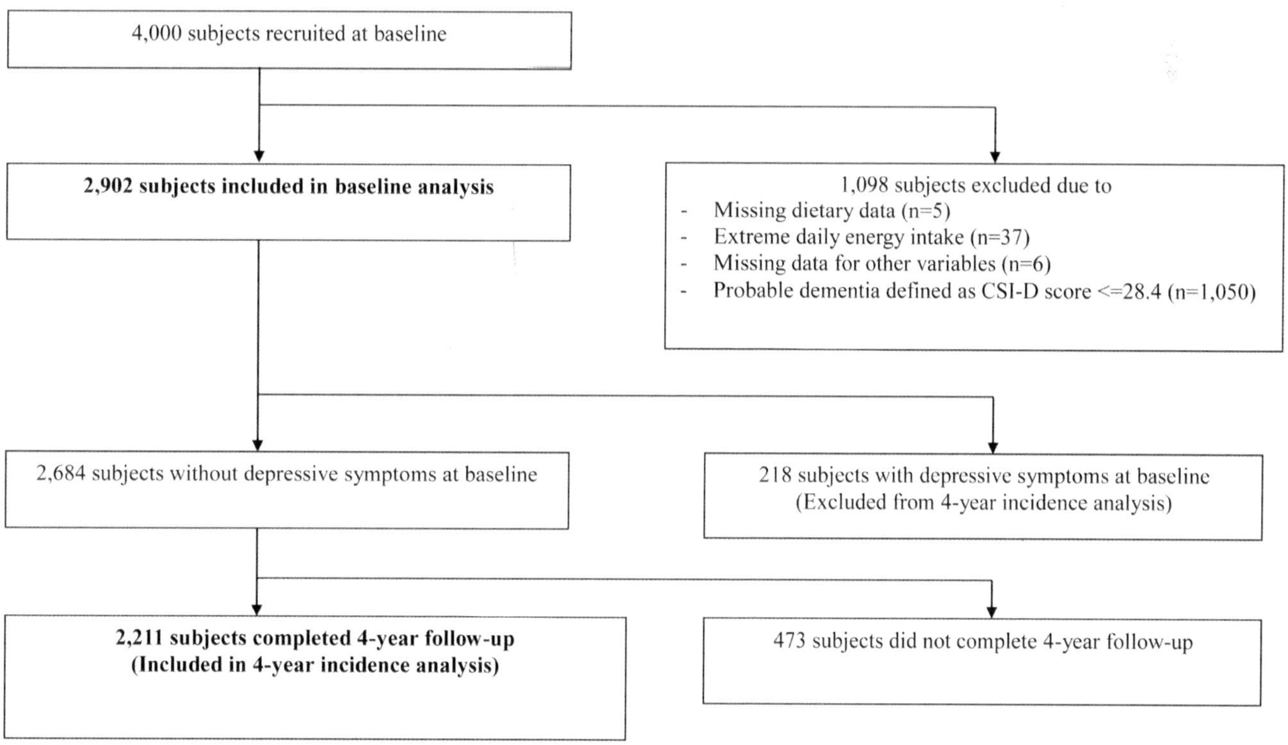

Figure 1.Number of subjects included and excluded for baseline and 4-year follow-up analyses.

level of past and current use of cigarettes, cigars and pipes was obtained. Smoking history was classified in terms of former smoking (at least 100 cigarettes smoked in a lifetime), current smoking and never smoking. Drinking status was defined as never, former (ever drank at least 5 drinks daily in a lifetime) or current drinker. Baseline disease status was obtained by self-report of their doctors' diagnoses, supplemented by the identification of drugs brought to the interviewers.

Anthropometric data

Body weight was measured to the nearest 0.1 kg with participants wearing a light gown, using the Physician Balance Beam Scale (Healthometer, Illinois, USA). Height was measured to the nearest 0.1 cm using the Holtain Harpenden stadiometer (Holtain Ltd, Crosswell, UK). Body mass index (BMI) was calculated as body weight in kg / (height in m)^2.

Physical activity assessment

Physical activity was assessed by the Physical Activity Scale for the Elderly (PASE) [33], which was adapted for use in elderly Hong Kong Chinese [34]. This is a 12-item scale measuring the average number of hours per day spent in leisure, household, and occupational physical activities over the previous 7-day period. Activity weights for each item were determined based on the amount of energy spent, and each item score was calculated by multiplying the activity weight with daily activity frequency. A composite PASE score of all the items was yielded. A higher PASE score reflects higher physical activity level.

Number of instrumental activities of daily living (IADLs) were assessed using specific questions and participants were asked to self-report of any impairment in walking two to three blocks outdoors on level ground, climbing 10 steps without resting, preparing own meals, doing heavy housework like scrubbing floors or washing windows, and shopping for groceries or clothes. A summed score from 0 to 5 was calculated from these activities as the degree of impairment in IADLs, with higher score indicating greater impairment.

Assessment of cognitive function

Since depression may be associated with cognitive impairment, in the analysis of factors associated with depression, the presence of cognitive impairment was adjusted for as a confounding factor. Cognitive function was assessed by trained research staff using the cognitive part of the Community Screening Instrument for Dementia (CSI-D) [32], validated in different cultural and educational settings [32]. The cognitive part of the CSI-D consists of 32 items in six cognitive domains: orientation to time, orientation to place, praxis, abstract thinking, language and memory. A summary score ranged from 0 to 33 was generated, with higher score meaning better cognitive function. The cutoff point for probable dementia is ≤28.4.

Assessment of depressive symptoms

Depressive symptoms was assessed by face-to-face interviews using a validated Chinese version of the Geriatric Depression Scale (GDS) [35,36]. The GDS short form was found to be a highly reliable (reliability coefficient of 0.90) and valid screening device (sensitivity of 96.3% and specificity of 87.5%) for assessing geriatric depression in Hong Kong Chinese [36]. The GDS short form consists of 15 questions relevant to depression, such as motivation, self-image, losses, agitation and mood. A yes/no format was designed for each question. A summary score ranged from 0 to 15 was generated, and a cut-off of 8 or more was used to define the presence of depressive symptoms.

Dietary assessment

Baseline dietary intake was assessed using a validated FFQ developed in a population survey [37]. Daily nutrient intake was calculated using food tables derived from McCance and Widdowson [38] and the Chinese Medical Sciences Institute [39]. The FFQ consisted of 280 food items. Each participant reported the frequency and the usual amount of consumption of each food item over the past year. For each food 9 different categories were given from never or seldom to more than once a day. Portion size was explained to participants using a catalogue of pictures of individual food portions. For seasonally consumed vegetables and fruits, participants were asked about the months of food consumption over the past year. The amount of cooking oil was estimated according to the usual cooking methods of preparing standardized portion of different foods and the usual portion of different foods consumed by the participants.

Dietary patterns derived by factor analysis

Details of dietary pattern scores derived by the factor analysis have been described elsewhere [40]. In brief, individual food items from the FFQ were aggregated into 32 food groups based on similarity of type of food and nutrient composition. The food groups were energy adjusted by dividing the energy intake from each food group by total energy intake and multiplying by 100, and were expressed as percentage contribution to total energy [41]. Factor analysis was conducted with varimax rotation using the 32 food groups [9]. Factors were retained based on an eigenvalues greater than 1.0, a scree plot, and the interpretability [42]. The factor scores for each pattern were calculated for each participant by summing intakes of food items weighted by their factor loadings. A higher score indicated greater conformity with the pattern being calculated.

Statistical analysis

Statistical analyses were performed using the statistical package SPSS version 21.0 (SPSS Inc., Illinois, US). Data were checked for normality using histograms and logarithmic transformation was applied whenever appropriate. Dietary pattern scores derived by factor analysis were stratified into quartiles based on the distribution of each sex. Pearson's correlation was used to examine the correlation between each dietary pattern score and intakes of various nutrients. Independent *t* test and chi square test were used to examine baseline differences in mean age, BMI, PASE, CSI-D score, energy intake, and also differences in the distribution of sex, education level, smoking status, alcohol use, number of IADLs, self-reported disease status, quartiles of each dietary pattern score between participants with depressive symptoms and participants without depressive symptoms at baseline. These tests were also used to examine differences in baseline characteristics between participants who included and excluded in the baseline analysis, and between participants who completed and participants who did not complete the 4-year follow-up.

Multivariate logistic regression was used to estimate the odds ratio (OR) and 95% confidence intervals (CIs) for both the baseline and the subsequent depressive symptoms according to quartiles of each dietary pattern score. Model 1 was adjusted for baseline age (years), sex, and daily energy intake (kcal). Model 2 was further adjusted for baseline BMI, PASE, number of IADLs (no difficulty/some difficulties), smoking habit (never/past/current), alcohol use (never/past/current), education level (no education/primary or below/secondary or matriculation/University or above), and marital status (married or living with a partner/ widowed, separated or divorced/single). Model 3 was further adjusted for baseline self-reported history of diabetes (yes/no), hypertension (yes/no), and CVD or stroke (yes/no), and CSI-D score. Test for trend was examined by entering quartiles of each dietary pattern score in all models. An α level of 5% was used as the level of significance. Interaction between sex and quartiles of each dietary pattern score was tested by addition of cross-product terms to the multivariate models. Interactions were not significant, thus all analyses are presented in the total population.

To check the possibility of reverse causation, a sensitivity analysis excluding participants with extreme GDS at the top two percentiles (GDS≥11) was performed for the cross-sectional data. Considering that GDS is a screening scale and may be limited as a case-defining instrument compared to other diagnostic instruments [43], multivariate logistic regression models were repeated using a group whose depressive symptom levels had clearly increased over 4-year (i.e. with an increase in GDS score at 4 and over from baseline to four years) as an outcome variable. This cut-off value was chosen because 142 participants (6.4%) could be classified as the worsening cases and this number of cases may be more sufficient and powerful for statistical analysis than using an increase in GDS score at 5 and over as a cut-off value (i.e. n = 85). All models were adjusted for the same variables mentioned above.

Results

Dietary patterns of the participants

Factor analysis identified three dietary patterns (Table 1). The first factor (vegetables-fruits pattern) was dominated by frequent intake of vegetables, fruits, soy and soy products, and legumes. The second factor (snacks-drinks-milk products pattern) was composed of a mixture of healthy and unhealthy food groups. It was characterized by frequent intake of condiments, drinks, fast food, French fries, potato chips, sweets and desserts, nuts, milk products, and whole grains. The third factor (meat-fish pattern) included frequent intake of dim sum, red and processed meats, poultry, fish and seafood, and wine.

'Vegetables-fruits' dietary pattern scores were inversely associated with total fat, saturated fat, monounsaturated fat and polyunsaturated fat intakes, and positively associated with intakes of protein, fiber, isoflavones, most vitamins and minerals. 'Snacks-drinks-milk products' dietary pattern scores were inversely associated with intakes of polyunsaturated fat and vitamin K, and positively associated with intakes of carbohydrates, protein, total fat, saturated fat, monounsaturated fat, cholesterol, fiber, most minerals and vitamins. Whilst 'snacks-drinks-milk products' dietary pattern scores were also positively associated with intakes of fiber and most minerals and vitamins, the associations were less strong than those with 'vegetables-fruits' dietary pattern scores. 'Meat-fish' dietary pattern scores were weakly positively associated with intakes of polyunsaturated fat and most micronutrients, moderately positively associated with intakes of protein, total fat and monounsaturated fat, and strongly positively associated with saturated fat and cholesterol intakes. The positive associations of protein, total fat, different kinds of fat and cholesterol with 'meat-fish' dietary pattern scores were stronger than those with 'snacks-drinks-milk products' dietary pattern scores (Table 2).

Participants' characteristics by baseline depressive status

Participants who were excluded in the cross-sectional analysis were older and less physically active, had lower education level, and were more likely to be female, widowed, separated, divorced or single, and to have self-reported history of diabetes than those who were included in the cross-sectional analysis ($p<0.05$). Those who discontinued the 4-year follow-up were older, less physically active, and were more likely to be divorced or single as compared to those who completed the 4-year follow-up ($p<0.05$) (details not shown).

Among 2,902 participants included in the cross-sectional analysis, there were 218 (7.5%) participants who were classified as having depressive symptoms at baseline. For the longitudinal analysis, 81 (3.7%) cases were newly identified as having depressive symptoms out of 2,211 participants at the 4-year follow-up. The characteristics of participants with depressive symptoms and participants without depressive symptoms at baseline are shown in Table 3. Those who had depressive symptoms had lower CSI-D score, lower education level, more impairments in IADLs, and were more likely to be widowed, separated, divorced or single, and current smokers, and were more likely to have self-reported history of heart diseases or stroke. Those who had depressive symptoms also showed lower 'vegetables-fruits' dietary pattern scores and lower 'snacks-drinks-milk products' dietary pattern scores.

Dietary patterns and the presence of depressive symptoms at baseline and 4-year

In the cross-sectional analysis, participants in the highest quartile of "vegetables-fruits" pattern score had reduced likelihood of depressive symptoms [Adjusted OR = 0.55 (95% CI: 0.36–0.83), $p_{trend} = 0.017$] compared to participants in the lowest quartile. Participants in the highest quartile of "snacks-drinks-milk products" pattern score also showed reduced likelihood of depressive symptoms [Adjusted OR = 0.41 (95% CI: 0.26–0.65), $p_{trend}< 0.001$] compared to those in the lowest quartile. There was no association of "meat-fish" pattern with depressive status at baseline (Table 4). Longitudinal analysis showed that none of the dietary patterns were associated with the presence of depressive symptoms at 4-year (Table 5).

Sensitivity analysis excluding participants with extreme GDS (i.e. GDS≥11 (n = 56)) showed similar results for the cross-sectional data (details not shown). Multivariate logistic regression models that were repeated using a group with an increase in GDS score >= 4 over four years as an outcome also showed no association between each dietary pattern and the presence of depressive symptoms at 4-year (details not shown).

Discussion

This study found an inverse association between "vegetables-fruits' and 'snacks-drinks-milk products' dietary pattern scores and baseline depressive symptoms. However, no significant associations between 'meat-fish' dietary pattern scores and baseline depressive symptoms were observed. Moreover, we did not observe significant associations between baseline dietary pattern scores and subsequent depressive symptoms at 4-year.

Previous cross-sectional studies have evaluated the association between dietary patterns and depression or depressive symptoms. However, the results are inconclusive [13–16,22]. Similar to our findings, two recent studies from Japan showed that a healthy Japanese dietary pattern characterized by high intakes of plant foods including vegetables, fruit, mushrooms and soy products was associated with fewer depressive symptoms [14,16]. Our results were also consistent with the findings from an Australian study which showed that a diet characterized by high intakes of fruits, vegetables, and plant based foods was associated with fewer depressive symptoms[13]. Compared to the "snacks-drinks-milk products" pattern and the "meat-fish" pattern, the "vegetables-fruits" pattern showed the highest correlations with fiber and other

Table 1. Food group factor loading[a] for three dietary patterns.

Food groups	Dietary patterns		
	Factor 1: Vegetables-fruits	**Factor 2: Snacks-drinks-milk products**	**Factor 3: Meat-fish**
Other vegetables	**0.60**	-0.08	0.03
Cruciferous vegetables	**0.48**	−0.08	−0.06
Tomatoes	**0.47**	0.05	−0.04
Soy	**0.43**	0.03	0.10
Dark green & leafy vegetables	**0.42**	−0.27	−0.04
Starchy vegetables	**0.42**	0.07	−0.03
Fruits	**0.39**	0.06	0.03
Legumes	**0.35**	−0.06	0.02
Mushroom & fungi	**0.25**	0.07	−0.06
Fats and oils	**−0.39**	−0.20	0.11
Condiments	−0.06	**0.48**	−0.06
Coffee	−0.15	**0.41**	−0.15
Nuts	0.12	**0.39**	−0.03
Fast food	−0.02	**0.35**	0.14
French fries and potato chips	−0.02	**0.34**	0.14
Milk and milk products	0.11	**0.33**	−0.10
Whole grains	0.16	**0.32**	−0.16
Sweets and desserts	0.01	**0.27**	0.19
Beverages	−0.02	**0.22**	0.10
Eggs	0.08	**0.22**	0.05
Dim sum	−0.17	−0.17	**0.51**
Red and processed meats	−0.07	−0.03	**0.47**
Poultry	0.06	0.03	**0.47**
Fish and seafood	0.20	−0.26	**0.33**
Cakes, cookies, pies and biscuits	0.07	0.12	**0.24**
Wine	−0.15	0.07	**0.22**
Refined grains	−0.24	−0.42	**−0.74**
Organ meats	−0.08	0.13	0.12
Others	0.01	0.07	0.05
Preserved vegetables	0	0.10	0.01
Soups	0	0	−0.01
Tea	−0.03	0.17	0.05
% variance explained	**6.5**	**5.2**	**5.2**

[a]Factor loadings with absolute value ≥0.2 are shown in bold (Field 2005). For food group loads more than one dietary pattern, only the highest absolute value of loading is bolded.

nutrients, such as vitamin C that are considered as beneficial for brain health [6]. It is possible that the "vegetables-fruits" pattern is associated with reduced oxidative stress, higher anti-inflammatory property, and higher antioxidant capacity, the potential biological mechanisms that are linked with better mood and brain health [44]. The potential protective effect of the 'vegetables-fruits" pattern could also come from folate that is rich in some cruciferous vegetables, leafy vegetables, and other green vegetables. There has been evidence to suggest that folate deficiency impairs the synthesis of homocysteine to methionine and S-adenosyl-methionine. The latter is a methyl donor and is involved in the synthesis and metabolism of neurotransmitters [45]. There is also substantial evidence from observational studies and randomized controlled trials to suggest that folate deficiency is associated with increased risk of depression [7,46].

Our study showed that 'snacks-drinks-milk products' dietary pattern was linked to a fewer depressive symptoms. Such an inverse association was less easy to interpret. In comparison to the 'vegetable-fruit' dietary pattern, the positive association of this pattern with intakes of fiber and most minerals and vitamins was less strong. However, this pattern was composed of healthy and unhealthy food groups. This pattern was dominated by the intake of condiments, drinks, sweets and desserts, fast food, French fries, potato chips, nuts, milk and milk products, and whole grains. Past studies have examined the role of these food groups in depression [47–49]. Greater intake of high-calorie sweet foods and fast foods appeared to be associated with more depressive symptoms [47,48].

Table 2. Pearson's correlations between each dietary pattern score and nutrient intakes at baseline (n = 2,902).

Nutrients	Vegetables-fruits		Snacks-drinks-milk products		Meat-fish	
	r	p	r	p	r	P
Energy (kcal)	−0.05	0.006	0.21	<0.001	0.22	<0.001
Carbohydrates (g)	−0.01	0.456	0.17	<0.001	−0.11	<0.001
Protein (g)	0.13	<0.001	0.21	<0.001	0.39	<0.001
Fat (g)	−0.12	<0.001	0.18	<0.001	0.48	<0.001
SFA (% energy)	−0.17	<0.001	0.14	<0.001	0.57	<0.001
MUFA (% energy)	−0.06	0.001	0.06	0.001	0.36	<0.001
PUFA (% energy)	−0.13	<0.001	−0.11	<0.001	0.15	<0.001
Cholesterol (mg) †	0.03	0.168	0.15	<0.001	0.55	<0.001
Fiber (g) †	0.60	<0.001	0.17	<0.001	0.04	0.019
Vitamin A (IU) †	0.57	<0.001	0.05	0.006	0.11	<0.001
Vitamin C (mg) †	0.52	<0.001	0.03	0.103	0.12	<0.001
Calcium (mg)	0.36	<0.001	0.31	<0.001	0.02	0.258
Phosphorus (mg)	0.19	<0.001	0.33	<0.001	0.07	<0.001
Iron (mg) †	0.28	<0.001	0.26	<0.001	0.18	<0.001
Potassium (mg) †	0.24	<0.001	0.08	<0.001	0.33	<0.001
Magnesium (mg) †	0.38	<0.001	0.07	<0.001	−0.01	0.645
Sodium (mg) †	0.12	<0.001	0.23	<0.001	0.31	<0.001
Zinc (mg)	0.20	<0.001	0.15	<0.001	0.28	<0.001
Isoflavones (mg) †	0.35	<0.001	0.09	<0.001	0.13	<0.001
Vitamin K (µg) †	0.52	<0.001	−0.13	<0.001	0.07	<0.001
Vitamin D (IU) †	0.10	<0.001	0.30	<0.001	0.06	0.001

SFA, Saturated fatty acids; MUFA, Monounsaturated fatty acids; PUFA, Polyunsaturated fatty acids.
† log transformed nutrient intake.

In contrast, there is evidence to suggest that increased intake of milk and dairy products, in particular the low-fat milk and dairy products is associated with better brain function and mood [49].

Our longitudinal analysis did not show significant associations between baseline dietary pattern scores and subsequent depressive symptoms at 4-year. Sensitivity analysis by repeating the multivariate logistic regression models with an outcome of a group with an increase in GDS score > = 4 over four years also confirmed these negative findings. Furthermore, in order to investigate the relationship between diet and depression persistence at 4-year, we tried to repeat the multivariate logistic regression models for participants with depressive symptoms at baseline. No association between dietary patterns and the presence of depressive symptoms was observed at 4-year among this group of baseline depressive participants and these findings further confirmed our negative longitudinal findings. Several prospective studies have examined the role of dietary patterns and incident depression or depressive symptoms in adulthood [17–25], and the findings generally support the role of dietary patterns in the development of depression. Most studies reported significant associations between dietary patterns and incident depression or depressive symptoms [17–19,21–25], but one recent study showed no clear associations between dietary patterns and depression incidence [20]. Using data of 3,486 men and women of the Whitehall II prospective cohort, Akbaraly and colleagues showed a higher odds of depressive symptoms with a "processed food pattern" which was heavily loaded by high intake of sweetened desserts, chocolates, fried food, processed meat, pies, refined grains, high-fat dairy products and condiments [18]. In the GAZEL cohort, Le Port et al. [19] reported that healthy pattern (characterized by vegetables consumption) were associated with fewer depressive symptoms in men and women, and traditional pattern (characterized by fish and fruit consumption) were associated with lower risk of incident depression in women. Furthermore, the highest quartile of low-fat, western, high snack and high fat-sweet diets in men and low-fat and high snack diets in women were associated with higher likelihood of depressive symptoms compared to the lowest quartile. However, recent findings among women in the Nurses' Health Study did not suggest clear associations between dietary Prudent and Western pattern scores and incident depression risk [20]. Differences in the study design, such as tools for assessing depression (i.e. self-reported scale vs. clinical diagnosis), inclusion and exclusion criteria for the subjects, and covariates that were included in the statistical models may account for the variations in the study findings [50]. Recent findings from a multicenter, randomized, primary prevention filed trial suggest that a Mediterranean diet supplemented with nuts could possibly reduce the risk of depression in patients with type 2 diabetes [51]. Therefore, the role of diet in depression warrants further investigation.

Strengths of our study are inclusion of both cross-sectional and longitudinal study design, and adjustment for several potential confounders. However, our study had several limitations. First, the use of the self-reported measure of depression (GDS) and cognitive impairment (CSI-D) may be one of the limitations. However, the sensitivity of these measures is high and has been validated in Chinese populations [32,36]. Second, the low number of participants with depressive symptoms at the 4-year follow-up

Table 3. Subject characteristics by baseline depressive status (n = 2,902).

	Subjects without depressive symptoms (GDS<8) (n = 2,684)		Subjects with depressive symptoms (GDS> = 8) (n = 218)		*P value*[1]
	Mean/n	**(SD/%)**	**Mean/n**	**SD/%**	
Age (years)	71.8	(4.8)	72.2	(5.0)	0.310
BMI (kg/m^2)	23.6	(3.2)	23.4	(3.3)	0.203
PASE score	94.1	(44.7)	91.5	(40.2)	0.399
CSI-D score	31.2	(0.9)	31.0	(0.8)	**0.001**
Daily energy intake (kcal)	1913.8	(571.4)	1876.3	(556.7)	0.351
Dietary pattern scores					
Vegetables-fruits	0.015	(1.002)	−0.187	(0.958)	**0.004**
Q1	651	(24.3)	76	(34.9)	**0.002**
Q2	677	(25.2)	49	(22.5)	
Q3	669	(24.9)	55	(25.2)	
Q4	687	(25.6)	38	(17.4)	
Snacks-drinks-milk products	0.022	(1.004)	−0.272	(0.915)	**<0.001**
Q1	646	(24.1)	81	(37.2)	**<0.001**
Q2	662	(24.7)	62	(28.4)	
Q3	684	(25.5)	43	(19.7)	
Q4	692	(25.8)	32	(14.7)	
Meat-fish	0.004	(0.996)	−0.045	(1.051)	0.487
Q1	669	(24.9)	56	(25.7)	0.441
Q2	665	(24.8)	61	(28.0)	
Q3	670	(25.0)	56	(25.7)	
Q4	680	(25.3)	45	(20.6)	
Female (%)	1075	(40.1)	87	(39.9)	0.967
Education level (%)					
Primary or below	1697	(63.2)	157	(72.0)	**0.014**
Secondary / Matriculation	636	(23.7)	45	(20.6)	
University or above	351	(13.1)	16	(7.3)	
Marital status (%)					
Married or living with a partner	2085	(77.7)	155	(71.1)	**0.004**
Widowed, separated or divorced	546	(20.3)	52	(23.9)	
Single	53	(2.0)	11	(5.0)	
Smoking status (%)					
Never smoke	1583	(59.0)	110	(50.5)	**0.003**
Ex-smoker	910	(33.9)	80	(36.7)	
Current smoker	191	(7.1)	28	(12.8)	
Alcohol use (%)					
Never	2203	(82.1)	181	(83.0)	0.191
Ex-drinker	55	(2.0)	8	(3.7)	
Current drinker	426	(15.9)	29	(13.3)	
Self-reported medical history (%)					
Diabetes mellitus	350	(13.0)	38	(17.4)	0.067
Hypertension	1118	(41.7)	100	(45.9)	0.225
Heart diseases or stroke	552	(20.6)	71	(32.6)	**<0.001**
IADLs					
No impairment	2141	(79.8)	138	(63.3)	**<0.001**
Some impairments	543	(20.2)	80	(36.7)	

[1]Differences between groups were assessed by independent *t* test or chi square test.

Table 4. Odds ratios (95% CI) for the cross-sectional association between dietary patterns and depressive symptoms (GDS>=8) at baseline (n=2,902).

Dietary pattern	Case / Control	Crude		P_{trend}[1]	Model 1[2]		P_{trend}	Model 2[3]		P_{trend}	Model 3[4]		P_{trend}
		OR	(95% CI)		OR	(95% CI)		OR	(95% CI)		OR	(95% CI)	
Vegetables-fruits													
Q1	76/651	1		**0.001**	1		**0.001**	1		**0.019**	1		**0.017**
Q2	49/677	0.62	0.43–0.90		0.62	0.43–0.91		0.67	0.46–0.98		0.68	0.46–0.99	
Q3	55/669	0.70	0.49–1.01		0.71	0.49–1.02		0.81	0.56–1.18		0.83	0.57–1.20	
Q4	38/687	0.47	0.32–0.71		0.48	0.32–0.72		0.56	0.37–0.84		0.55	0.36–0.83	
Snacks- drinks-milk products													
Q1	81/646	1		**<0.001**	1		**<0.001**	1		**<0.001**	1		**<0.001**
Q2	62/662	0.75	0.53–1.06		0.75	0.53–1.06		0.76	0.53–1.09		0.77	0.54–1.10	
Q3	43/684	0.50	0.34–0.74		0.51	0.34–0.74		0.51	0.34–0.76		0.52	0.35–0.78	
Q4	32/692	0.37	0.24–0.56		0.37	0.24–0.57		0.40	0.25–0.62		0.41	0.26–0.65	
Meat-fish													
Q1	56/669	1		0.221	1		0.273	1		0.269	1		0.199
Q2	61/665	1.10	0.75–1.60		1.10	0.76–1.61		1.18	0.80–1.73		1.18	0.80–1.73	
Q3	56/670	1.00	0.68–1.47		1.01	0.69–1.49		1.08	0.73–1.61		1.06	0.71–1.58	
Q4	45/680	0.79	0.53–1.19		0.81	0.54–1.22		0.80	0.53–1.22		0.77	0.51–1.18	

[1]Test for trend was examined by entering dietary pattern score quartiles as a fixed factor and testing the contrast by using the polynomial option in all models.
[2]Model 1: adjusted for age, sex and daily energy intake.
[3]Model 2: further adjusted for BMI, PASE, number of IADLs, smoking status, alcohol use, education and marital status.
[4]Model 3: further adjusted for self-reported history of diabetes mellitus, hypertension, heart disease and stroke, and CSI-D score.

Table 5. Odds ratios (95% CI) for the longitudinal association between baseline dietary patterns and 4-year incidence of depressive symptoms (GDS> = 8) (n = 2,211).

Dietary pattern	Case / Control	Crude		P_{trend}[1]	Model 1[2]		P_{trend}	Model 2[3]		P_{trend}	Model 3[4]		P_{trend}
		OR	(95% CI)		OR	(95% CI)		OR	(95% CI)		OR	(95% CI)	
Vegetables-fruits													
Q1	25/494	1		0.415	1		0.432	1		0.903	1		0.931
Q2	17/547	0.61	0.33–1.15		0.62	0.33–1.17		0.71	0.38–1.35		0.73	0.38–1.38	
Q3	18/534	0.67	0.36–1.24		0.66	0.36–1.24		0.77	0.41–1.45		0.80	0.42–1.50	
Q4	21/555	0.75	0.41–1.35		0.76	0.42–1.37		0.94	0.51–1.73		0.94	0.51–1.74	
Snacks- drinks-milk products													
Q1	24/494	1		0.430	1		0.569	1		0.845	1		0.824
Q2	13/514	0.52	0.26–1.03		0.54	0.27–1.07		0.61	0.31–1.21		0.62	0.31–1.24	
Q3	27/550	1.01	0.58–1.77		1.07	0.61–1.89		1.28	0.71–2.29		1.28	0.71–2.31	
Q4	17/572	0.61	0.33–1.15		0.65	0.34–1.24		0.84	0.43–1.65		0.85	0.43–1.68	
Meat-fish													
Q1	23/530	1		0.880	1		0.822	1		0.935	1		0.957
Q2	17/530	0.74	0.39–1.40		0.74	0.39–1.41		0.78	0.41–1.49		0.79	0.41–1.50	
Q3	16/533	0.69	0.36–1.32		0.71	0.37–1.36		0.74	0.38–1.44		0.75	0.39–1.45	
Q4	25/537	1.07	0.60–1.91		1.09	0.61–1.97		1.05	0.57–1.92		1.04	0.56–1.90	

[1]Test for trend was examined by entering dietary pattern score quartiles as a fixed factor and testing the contrast by using the polynomial option in all models.
[2]Model 1: adjusted for age, sex and daily energy intake at baseline.
[3]Model 2: further adjusted for BMI, PASE, number of IADLs, smoking status, alcohol use, education and marital status at baseline.
[4]Model 3: further adjusted for self-reported history of diabetes mellitus, hypertension, heart disease and stroke, and CSI-D score at baseline.

may have limited the power of the longitudinal analysis. Although we found significant associations between "vegetables-fruits" and "snacks-drinks-milk products" patterns and depressive symptoms in the cross-sectional analysis, the directionality of the associations was uncertain. The possibility of reverse causation may not be ruled out. People with major depression may change their eating behavior and food choices, either adopting an unhealthy diet (i.e. high-calorie foods) or reducing food intake [47,52], thus interpreting the relationship between diet and depression may be difficult in view of the bidirectional changes in diet as a consequence of mental health symptoms. We tried to conduct a sensitivity analysis excluding participants with extreme GDS (i.e. GDS≥11 (n = 56)) and the significant association between dietary patterns and depressive symptoms remained at baseline. These results possibly suggest that reverse causation seems an unlikely explanation for the significant findings in our cross-sectional analysis. Furthermore, we did not have dietary data at the 4-year follow-up whereas dietary patterns may have changed between baseline and follow-up. Moreover, although we controlled for various common factors and major chronic conditions in the analysis, residual potential confounding from some other factors related to the development of depression, such as family history of depression and recent life stress events might still be present. In addition, our sample as a whole was of a higher educational standard compared with the general Hong Kong population, and there were some differences in the baseline characteristics between those who included and those who excluded in the analysis, and between those who completed and those who discontinued the 4-year follow-up. Therefore, the results may not be generalized to the general population.

In conclusion, our cross-sectional analysis suggested significant associations between 'vegetables-fruits' dietary pattern and 'snacks-drinks-milk products' dietary pattern and the presence of depressive symptoms in the community-dwelling Chinese older people in Hong Kong. However, the longitudinal analyses did not support that dietary patterns are predictive of the occurrence of depressive symptoms.

Acknowledgments

We would like to give thanks for Ms Kay Yuen for coordination of this study.

Author Contributions

Conceived and designed the experiments: RC JW. Analyzed the data: RC DC JW. Contributed to the writing of the manuscript: RC DC JW

References

1. World Health Organization (2008) Global Burden of Disease: 2004 Update. Geneva: World Health Organization.
2. Hasin DS, Goodwin RD, Stinson FS, Grant BF (2005) Epidemiology of major depressive disorder: results from the National Epidemiologic Survey on Alcoholism and Related Conditions. Arch Gen Psychiatry 62: 1097–1106.
3. Blazer DG (2003) Depression in late life: review and commentary. J Gerontol A Biol Sci Med Sci 58: 249–265.
4. Fiske A, Wetherell JL, Gatz M (2009) Depression in older adults. Annu Rev Clin Psychol 5: 363–389.
5. Collins PY, Patel V, Joestl SS, March D, Insel TR, et al. (2011) Grand challenges in global mental health. Nature 475: 27–30.
6. Rogers PJ (2001) A healthy body, a healthy mind: long-term impact of diet on mood and cognitive function. Proc Nutr Soc 60: 135–143.
7. Stanger O, Fowler B, Piertzik K, Huemer M, Haschke-Becher E, et al. (2009) Homocysteine, folate and vitamin B12 in neuropsychiatric diseases: review and treatment recommendations. Expert Rev Neurother 9: 1393–1412.
8. Murakami K, Sasaki S (2010) Dietary intake and depressive symptoms: a systematic review of observational studies. Mol Nutr Food Res 54: 471–488.
9. Hu FB (2002) Dietary pattern analysis: a new direction in nutritional epidemiology. Curr Opin Lipidol 13: 3–9.
10. van Dam RM (2005) New approaches to the study of dietary patterns. Br J Nutr 93: 573–574.
11. Jacka FN, Pasco JA, Mykletun A, Williams LJ, Hodge AM, et al. (2010) Association of Western and traditional diets with depression and anxiety in women. Am J Psychiatry 167: 305–311.
12. Samieri C, Jutand MA, Feart C, Capuron L, Letenneur L, et al. (2008) Dietary patterns derived by hybrid clustering method in older people: association with cognition, mood, and self-rated health. J Am Diet Assoc 108: 1461–1471.
13. Crichton GE, Bryan J, Hodgson JM, Murphy KJ (2013) Mediterranean diet adherence and self-reported psychological functioning in an Australian sample. Appetite 70: 53–59.
14. Nanri A, Kimura Y, Matsushita Y, Ohta M, Sato M, et al. (2010) Dietary patterns and depressive symptoms among Japanese men and women. Eur J Clin Nutr 64: 832–839.
15. Sugawara N, Yasui-Furukori N, Tsuchimine S, Kaneda A, Tsuruga K, et al. (2012) No association between dietary patterns and depressive symptoms among a community-dwelling population in Japan. Ann Gen Psychiatry 11: 24 doi: 10.1186/1744-859X-11-24.
16. Suzuki T, Miyaki K, Tsutsum A, Hashimoto H, Kawakami N, et al. (2013) Japanese dietary pattern consistently relates to low depressive symptoms and it is modified by job strain and worksite supports. J Affect Disord 150: 490–498.
17. Sa' nchez-Villegas A, Delgado-Rodri'guez M, Alonso A, Schlatter J, Lahortiga F, et al. (2009) Association of the Mediterranean Dietary Pattern With the Incidence of Depression The Seguimiento Universidad de Navarra/University of Navarra Follow-up (SUN) Cohort. Arch Gen Psychiatry 66: 1090–1098.
18. Akbaraly TN, Brunner EJ, Ferrie JE, Marmot MG, Kivimaki M, et al. (2009) Dietary pattern and depressive symptoms in middle age. Br J Psychiatry 195: 408–413.
19. Le Port A, Gueguen A, Kesse-Guyot E, Melchior M, Lemogne C, et al. (2012) Association between dietary patterns and depressive symptoms over time: a 10-year follow-up study of the GAZEL cohort. PLOS ONE 7: e51593.
20. Chocano-Bedoya PO, O'Reilly EJ, Lucas M, Mirzaei F, Okereke OI, et al. (2013) Prospective study on long-term dietary patterns and incident depression in middle-aged and older women. Am J Clin Nutr 98: 813–820.
21. Lucas M, Chocano-Bedoya P, Shulze MB, Mirzaei F, O'Reilly EJ, et al. (2013) Inflammatory dietary pattern and risk of depression among women. Brain Behav Immun 36: 46–53.
22. Rienks R, Dobson AJ, Mishra GD (2013) Mediterranean dietary pattern and prevalence and incidence of depressive symptoms in mid-aged women: results from a large community-based prospective study. Eur J Clin Nutr 67: 75–82.
23. Hodge A, Almeida OP, English DR, Giles GG, Flicker L (2013) Patterns of dietary intake and psychological distress in older Australians: benefits not just from a Mediterranean diet. Int Psychogeriatr 25: 456–466.
24. Jacka FN, Cherbuin N, Anstey KJ, Butterworth P (2014) Dietary Patterns and Depressive Symptoms over Time: Examining the Relationships with Socioeconomic Position, Health Behaviours and Cardiovascular Risk. PLOS ONE 9: e87657.
25. Ruusunen A, Lehto SM, Mursu J, Tolmunen T, Tuomainen TP, et al. (2014) Dietary patterns are associated with the prevalence of elevated depressive symptoms and the risk of getting a hospital discharge diagnosis of depression in middle-aged or older Finnish men. J Affect Disord 159: 1–6.
26. Jacka FN, Kremer PJ, Berk M, de Silva-Sanigorski AM, Moodie M, et al. (2011) A prospective study of diet quality and mental health in adolescents. PLOS ONE 6: e24805.
27. Weng TT, Hao JH, Qian QW, Cao H, Fu JL, et al. (2011) Is there any relationship between dietary patterns and depression and anxiety in Chinese adolescents? Public Health Nutr 15: 673–682.
28. Tsai AC, Chang TL, Chi SH (2012) Frequent consumption of vegetables predicts lower risk of depression in older Taiwanese - results of a prospective population-based study. Public Health Nutr 15: 1087–1092.
29. Woo J, Lynn H, Lau WY, Leung J, Lau E, et al. (2006) Nutrient intake and psychological health in an elderly Chinese population. Int J Geriatr Psychiatry 21: 1036–1043.
30. Wong SY, Kwok T, Woo J, Lynn H, Griffith JF, et al. (2005) Bone mineral density and the risk of peripheral arterial disease in men and women: results from Mr. and Ms Os, Hong Kong. Osteoporos Int 16: 1933–1938.
31. Census and Statistics Department (2006) Hong Kong 2006 Population Bycensus Thematic Report: Older Persons. Hong Kong: Census and Statistics Department.
32. Prince M, Acosta D, Chiu H, Scazufca M, Varghese M, et al. (2003) Dementia diagnosis in developing countries: a cross-cultural validation study. Lancet 361: 909–917.
33. Washburn RA, Smith KW, Jette AM, Janney CA (1993) The Physical Activity Scale for the Elderly (PASE): development and evaluation. J Clin Epidemiol 46: 153–162.
34. Liu B, Woo J, Tang N, Ng K, Ip R, et al. (2001) Assessment of total expenditure in a Chinese population by a physical activity questionnaire: examination of validity. Int J Food Sci Nutr 52: 269–282.

35. Yesavage JA, Brink TL, Rose TL, Lum O, Huang V, et al. (1983) Development and validation of a geriatric depression screening scale. A preliminary report. J Psychiatr Res 17: 37–49.
36. Lee HB, Chiu HFK, Kwok WY, Leung CM, Kwong PK, et al. (1993) Chinese elderly and the GDS short form: a preliminary study. Clin Gerontol 14: 37–39.
37. Woo J, Leung SSF, Ho SC, Lam TH, Janus ED (1997) A food frequency questionnaire for use in the Chinese population in Hong Kong: Description and examination of validity. Nutr Res 17: 1633–1641.
38. Paul AA, Southgate DAT (1978) McCance & Widdowson's: The Composition of Foods. London: HMSO.
39. Yang Y, Wang G, Pan X (2002) China Food Composition 2002; Institute of Nutrition & Food Safety CC, editor. Peking: University Medical Press.
40. Chan R, Chan D, Woo J (2012) Associations between dietary patterns and demographics, lifestyle, anthropometry and blood pressure in Chinese community-dwelling older men and women. J Nutr Sci 1: e20 doi:10.1017/jns.2012.19
41. Reedy J, Wirfalt E, Flood A, Mitrou PN, Krebs-Smith SM, et al. (2010) Comparing 3 dietary pattern methods–cluster analysis, factor analysis, and index analysis–With colorectal cancer risk: The NIH-AARP Diet and Health Study. Am J Epidemiol 171: 479–487.
42. Field A (2005) Discovering Statistics Using SPSS; Wright DB, editor. London: Sage Publications.
43. Roman MW, Callen BL (2008) Screening instruments for older adult depressive disorders: updating the evidence-based toolbox. Issues Ment Health Nurs 29: 929–941.
44. Bodnar LM, Wisner KL (2005) Nutrition and depression: implications for improving mental health among childbearing-aged women. Biol Psychiatry 58: 679–685.
45. Bottiglieri T (2005) Homocysteine and folate metabolism in depression. Prog Neuro-Psychopharmacol Biol Psychiatry 29: 1103–1112.
46. Fava M, Mischoulon D (2009) Folate in depression: efficacy, safety, differences in formulations, and clinical issues. J Clin Psychiatry 70 Suppl 5: 12–17.
47. Jeffery RW, Linde JA, Simon GE, Ludman EJ, Rohde P, et al. (2009) Reported food choices in older women in relation to body mass index and depressive symptoms. Appetite 52: 238–240.
48. Crawford GB, Khedkar A, Flaws JA, Sorkin JD, Gallicchio L (2011) Depressive symptoms and self-reported fast-food intake in midlife women. Prev Med 52: 254–257.
49. Camfield DA, Owen L, Scholey AB, Pipingas A, Stough C (2011) Dairy constituents and neurocognitive health in ageing. Br J Nutr 106: 159–174.
50. Quirk SE, Williams;L.J.;, O'Neil A, Pasco JA, Jacka FN, et al. (2013) The association between diet quality, dietary patterns and depression in adults: a systematic review. BMC Psychiatry 175.
51. Sánchez-Villegas A, Martínez-González MA, Estruch R, Salas-Salvadó J, Corella D, et al. (2013) Mediterranean dietary pattern and depression: the PREDIMED randomized trial. BMC Medicine 11.
52. Lai JS, Hiles S, Bisquera A, Hure AJ, McEvoy M, et al. (2014) A systematic review and meta-analysis of dietary patterns and depression in community-dwelling adults. Am J Clin Nutr 99: 181–197.

4

The Efficacy of Paroxetine and Placebo in Treating Anxiety and Depression: A Meta-Analysis of Change on the Hamilton Rating Scales

Michael A. Sugarman[1]*, Amy M. Loree[1], Boris B. Baltes[1], Emily R. Grekin[1], Irving Kirsch[2]

1 Wayne State University, Department of Psychology, Detroit, Michigan, United States of America, **2** Harvard Medical School, Boston, Massachusetts, United States of America

Abstract

Background: Previous meta-analyses of published and unpublished trials indicate that antidepressants provide modest benefits compared to placebo in the treatment of depression; some have argued that these benefits are not clinically significant. However, these meta-analyses were based only on trials submitted for the initial FDA approval of the medication and were limited to those aimed at treating depression. Here, for the first time, we assess the efficacy of a selective serotonin reuptake inhibitor (SSRI) in the treatment of both anxiety and depression, using a complete data set of all published and unpublished trials sponsored by the manufacturer.

Methods and Findings: GlaxoSmithKline has been required to post the results for all sponsored clinical trials online, providing an opportunity to assess the efficacy of an SSRI (paroxetine) with a complete data set of all trials conducted. We examined the data from all placebo-controlled, double-blind trials of paroxetine that included change scores on the Hamilton Rating Scale for Anxiety (HRSA) and/or the Hamilton Rating Scale for Depression (HRSD). For the treatment of anxiety ($k=12$), the efficacy difference between paroxetine and placebo was modest ($d=0.27$), and independent of baseline severity of anxiety. Overall change in placebo-treated individuals replicated 79% of the magnitude of paroxetine response. Efficacy was superior for the treatment of panic disorder ($d=0.36$) than for generalized anxiety disorder ($d=0.20$). Published trials showed significantly larger drug-placebo differences than unpublished trials (d's$=0.32$ and 0.17, respectively). In depression trials ($k=27$), the benefit of paroxetine over placebo was consistent with previous meta-analyses of antidepressant efficacy ($d=0.32$).

Conclusions: The available empirical evidence indicates that paroxetine provides only a modest advantage over placebo in treatment of anxiety and depression. Treatment implications are discussed.

Editor: Brett Thombs, McGill University, Canada

Funding: The current study did not have any funding sources. Study design, data collection and analysis, decision to publish, and preparation of the manuscript were all done at the discretion of the study authors.

Competing Interests: The authors have declared that no competing interests exist.

* Email: Mike.Sugarman@wayne.edu

Introduction

Antidepressant medications are prescribed to 8.7% of the US population, making them the third most common class of prescription medications [1]. Antidepressants are approved for the treatment of depression and several other mental disorders, including generalized anxiety disorder [2], panic disorder, social anxiety disorder, obsessive-compulsive disorder, and post-traumatic stress disorder [3]. While several meta-analytic investigations have been conducted examining the efficacy of antidepressants in the treatment of depression, fewer analyses have focused on the efficacy of these drugs in the treatment of other conditions, including anxiety disorders. Moreover, most meta-analyses are conducted only using published studies. However, approximately 40% of the antidepressant trials conducted by pharmaceutical companies are not published [4,5]. Therefore, meta-analyses of antidepressant trials are prone to overestimations of effectiveness due to publication bias.

One strategy for avoiding publication bias is to conduct meta-analyses on data submitted to the Food and Drug Administration (FDA) in the process of obtaining drug approval, as the FDA requires that pharmaceutical companies provide information on all of the trials that they have sponsored [6]. However, analyses of data submitted to the FDA [5,7–9] only include trials conducted prior to approval of the medications. Pharmaceutical companies often conduct additional placebo-controlled double-blind trials after the medications have been approved. Thus, the data submitted to the FDA do not represent the most complete datasets of studies conducted with the medications.

The current study addresses these potential biases by evaluating the efficacy of paroxetine, a selective serotonin reuptake inhibitor (SSRI), across all placebo-controlled double-blind studies conducted by its manufacturer, GlaxoSmithKline, including those conducted following FDA approval. As part of a 2004 lawsuit settlement, GlaxoSmithKline has been required to post online the results of all clinical trials involving its drugs on its Clinical Trial Register [10,11]. Thus, unlike most other antidepressants, all studies of paroxetine can be evaluated without fear of publication bias. A recent meta-analysis reported that paroxetine did not significantly differ in overall efficacy from citalopram, escitalopram, fluoxetine, or sertraline in the treatment of depression [12]. Therefore, findings concerning the efficacy of paroxetine in the treatment of anxiety disorders could possibly generalize to other SSRIs, although further research would be necessary to support that proposition.

The current analysis is the first to evaluate the efficacy of an SSRI in the treatment of anxiety disorders using a complete dataset of sponsored placebo-controlled trials. Paroxetine and other SSRIs have been approved for the treatment of a variety of anxiety disorders, including generalized anxiety disorder, panic disorder, and social anxiety disorder [13–24]. To date, however, only two meta-analyses have investigated the degree to which SSRIs reduce symptoms of anxiety, and both of these meta-analyses focused exclusively on panic disorder [25,26]. One of these studies [25] found a moderate advantage for antidepressants compared to placebo (*Hedge's* $g = 0.41$), and the other study [26] suggested that antidepressants provide a somewhat larger benefit (Mean Effect Size = 0.55). Notably, no meta-analyses have examined anxiety disorders other than panic disorder and none have examined whether SSRIs are differentially effective in treating different types of anxiety disorders. Further, both of these meta-analyses [25,26] observed evidence for publication bias in their analyses and did not have access to a full database of published and unpublished trials, indicating that these figures may be an overestimate of the true effect sizes. The availability of the GlaxoSmithKline Clinical Trial Register provides an opportunity to evaluate the efficacy of an SSRI in the treatment of anxiety disorders without a concern for publication bias.

The availability of a complete dataset of pre-marketing and post-marketing trials also allows for the further examination of antidepressant efficacy in the treatment of depression. Previous meta-analyses of antidepressant data obtained from the FDA have consistently revealed modest differences between drug and placebo, with mean effect sizes ranging from $d = 0.31$ to 0.32 [5,7], and raw score differences in improvement on the Hamilton Rating Scale for Depression (HRSD) [27] ranging from 1.80 to 2.51 points [7,28]. The overall magnitude of the change in placebo-treated individuals duplicated greater than 80% of the antidepressant response [7]. The current study further evaluates the magnitude of benefit between an SSRI medication and placebo in the treatment of depression using the database of trials available through the GlaxoSmithKline Clinical Trial Register.

The goals of the current study are two-fold: 1) to determine the magnitude of benefit for paroxetine compared to placebo in the treatment of anxiety, and 2) to determine the magnitude of benefit for paroxetine compared to placebo in the treatment of depression, utilizing access to a complete database of clinical trials sponsored by the manufacturer. Studies examining antidepressant efficacy in the treatment of anxiety disorders have used a wide range of outcome measures. However, a commonly used measure across double-blind trials of anxiety disorders including generalized anxiety disorder and panic disorder is the Hamilton Rating Scale for Anxiety (HRSA) [29]. Therefore, the current study will focus on the HRSA as an indicator of anxiety-related outcomes. For both HRSA and HRSD analyses, we will analyze available moderator variables to determine which trial variables influence effect sizes in drug and placebo groups.

Methods

Study Retrieval

Data for all trials were obtained through the GlaxoSmithKline Clinical Trial Register [30]. According to the terms of the 2004 lawsuit, this database is required to contain every trial sponsored by GlaxoSmithKline on their medications, including paroxetine. Thus, we do not have concerns of publication bias or selective access to studies. The "result summary" files were downloaded from the website in March 2013. A total of 371 result summaries of studies on paroxetine were downloaded. Each study was evaluated for appropriateness in the current analyses. Trials were included in the current study if they met the following criteria: 1) they were a double-blind randomized intervention study containing a placebo group and at least one group receiving paroxetine; 2) they were conducted within an indicated clinical population with DSM-III or DSM-IV (depending on when the study was conducted) diagnoses of mood and/or anxiety disorders and not on healthy volunteers; 3) they included change on the HRSA and/or the HRSD from pre-treatment to post-treatment amongst their outcome measures; 4) the outcome indices were appropriately matched to the clinical diagnosis (i.e., the HRSA was evaluated in individuals with diagnoses of anxiety disorders and the HRSD was evaluated in individuals with depression); and 5) they did not include individuals who had systematically received additional treatment prior to the randomization to placebo/paroxetine. Examples meeting this last exclusion criterion include trials in which all participants were previously stabilized on another treatment and trials in which all participants simultaneously received treatment in addition to paroxetine.

Additionally, we obtained information regarding the initial approval of paroxetine from the FDA in accordance with the Freedom of Information Act [31]. This initial submission included 16 trials examining the efficacy of paroxetine in the treatment of depression and utilized the HRSD as an outcome measure. These trials have been included in previous meta-analyses of antidepressant data submitted to the FDA [7,8]. We matched these 16 trials to their respective result summary file obtained through the GSK Clinical Trial Register. However, we observed discrepancies in sample sizes for 11 of the 16 studies (ranging from $n = 1$ to $n = 12$ for each group) between the data obtained the FDA and data from the GSK Clinical Trial Register result summaries. In all of these cases, samples were larger in the FDA datasets than in those obtained from the GSK Clinical Trial Register. In the interests of using the most complete datasets and presenting results consistent with previous meta-analyses including these trials, we used the data obtained from the FDA for these 11 trials in our analyses. Further examination revealed that the differences in sample sizes in these trials did not contribute to substantial differences in trial outcome. The overall weighted meta-analytic pre-post effect sizes for both paroxetine and placebo-treated individuals across all trials were essentially identical (within $d = 0.002$) when comparing the two data sources.

Meta-Analytic Data Synthesis

For each outcome index (HRSA and HRSD), we conducted two types of data analysis: 1) an analysis of each trial's arithmetic means for both groups to determine the overall meta-analytic "effect size" [32] as a comparison between the two groups (i.e., the effect size difference between paroxetine and placebo), and 2) each group's change was calculated as the standardized mean difference, dividing the change score by the standard deviation of the change [33]. For trials that included multiple paroxetine groups compared to placebo (e.g., comparing different dosage levels or trials comparing controlled and immediate release tablets), the initial severity and change scores were combined across groups, weighted by the respective sample sizes. All analyses were conducted using the Comprehensive Meta Analysis 2.0 software package (Version 2.2.050, BIOSTAT, Englewood, NJ, USA). All analyses were conducted using both random- and fixed-effects models. Equivalent results (with regard to statistical significance) were observed for both models in almost all analyses; thus, the fixed-effects results are presented here. However, we have made the results of the random-effects models available online for interested readers (see Results S1 and Figures S1–S3). The Q [34] and I^2 [35,36] indices were used to determine the presence or absence of homogeneity and to assess the degree of inconsistency between trials.

Analysis 1 evaluated the effect size magnitude when comparing paroxetine and placebo groups in each trial, determining the benefit of paroxetine over placebo. The effect size was calculated as the difference in the change score between groups divided by the pooled standard deviation. Analysis 2 determined the absolute magnitude of change in both the placebo and paroxetine groups for each trial (i.e., the analyses were conducted separately for each group). This latter analysis allows us to evaluate and compare the magnitude of change for both treatment conditions. For both analyses, the results are presented both in raw metric (as the mean change on the respective Hamilton rating scale) and as a standardized pre-post mean difference (d). The standardized mean difference results account for variation between trials in the standard deviation of the change score [37]. Weights were determined by the sample size times the inverse of the change score variance. Note that in Analysis 1 the meta-analytic weights for each study are determined by the pooled sample size and variance across both paroxetine and placebo groups, and the weights for Analysis 2 are determined for each group separately. Thus, the overall effect sizes for Analysis 1 are slightly different than the results obtained from simply subtracting the placebo from paroxetine effect sizes in Analysis 2.

We examined several moderator variables in both analyses to determine if study characteristics influenced the standardized mean difference within each treatment and/or in the comparison between paroxetine and placebo. For the HRSA, we analyzed the following moderators: 1) Baseline severity of anxiety, as determined by the mean HRSA group score at the beginning of the trial. No previous work has examined whether antidepressant and/or placebo efficacy is superior in more severe cases of anxiety, which might be predicted based on regression to the mean effects. 2) Indication (i.e., whether the individuals in the trial were treated for panic disorder or for generalized anxiety disorder). These analyses were designed to determine if the relative efficacy of paroxetine in the treatment of symptoms of anxiety varied systematically by diagnosis. 3) Length of treatment in weeks. The double-blind trials in these analyses ranged from 8 to 12 weeks; it is possible that longer trials are associated with a larger drug-placebo difference because the drug has more time to exert its effects in longer trials. Although previous studies [7,38] have not found a significant relationship between duration of treatment and antidepressant efficacy in the treatment of depression, no previous analyses have examined this moderator variable for antidepressant efficacy in the treatment of anxiety. 4) Publication status. The current database contains all trials conducted with paroxetine, both published and unpublished; thus, publication bias is not a concern in our outcomes. Previous work [5] has demonstrated that the published literature may represent an overestimate of antidepressant efficacy in the treatment of depression, and the current analysis aimed to determine the magnitude of publication bias in the treatment of anxiety.

For the HRSD, we analyzed the following moderators: 1) Baseline severity of depression, as determined by the mean HRSD group score at the beginning of each trial. Previous analyses [7,39,40] have demonstrated that antidepressant-placebo differences increase with more severe depression. 2) Approval status (i.e., trials submitted to the FDA for the initial approval versus trials conducted post-approval). The 11 trials conducted following FDA approval have not been previously included in meta-analytic investigations. 3) Length of treatment in weeks. 4) Publication status.

Results

Study Selection

A total of 39 trials out of the original sample of 371 studies met inclusion criteria for the current analyses. The trial flow is illustrated in Figure 1. Out of the excluded studies, 121 studies did not evaluate efficacy of the drug (e.g., they evaluated the pharmacokinetics or tolerability of the drug); 153 studies were intervention studies that did not include a placebo group (e.g., they compared multiple doses of the drug, compared paroxetine against other drugs, or were open-label); 28 studies were placebo-controlled intervention studies but did not include the HRSA or HRSD in their outcome measures; 13 trials were extension studies of other trials or evaluated the efficacy of paroxetine for prevention of relapse. In nine studies, paroxetine was not the only treatment included in the intent-to-treat samples (e.g., all participants were previously stabilized on another treatment or received another simultaneous treatment in addition to paroxetine or placebo). Three studies (29060/785, 29060/251, and 29060/874) included change scores for the HRSA but the patients had a primary indication of depression rather than for anxiety disorders and thus these studies were not included. However, two of these studies (29060/251 and 29060/874) included the HRSD as an outcome measure and were included in depression analyses. Four studies included change scores on the HRSD, but the trials were for individuals with obsessive-compulsive disorder (29060/116 and 29060/118) and social phobia (29060/661 and PIR104776). The participants in these studies had low baseline severity scores (mean HRSD scores ranging from 9 to 10) and did not appear to be clinically depressed; thus, these studies were excluded. One study (29060/442) met all criteria but did not include mean change scores on the HRSD and only provided the percentage of "responders" (reduction by ≥50% on the HRSD from pre-treatment to post-treatment) in each group. Thus, we were unable to include this study in the meta-analysis.

Twelve studies were included for the HRSA, comprising 1,835 individuals randomized to paroxetine and 1,550 randomized to placebo. Twenty-seven studies were included for the HRSD, comprising 3,301 individuals randomized to paroxetine and 1,885 randomized to placebo. All studies reported their outcome measures based on "last observation carried forward" methods, meaning that the change scores for individuals who withdrew from the study were calculated based on their final data point. This method helps to control for selective attrition during the studies.

Study Characteristics

Information on all trials is presented in Table 1. The corresponding publication information is provided where applicable. All dosage levels were within the FDA-approved range for the diagnosis. For the 12 trials evaluating change on the HRSA, trial duration ranged between 8 and 12 weeks. Five trials were 8 weeks

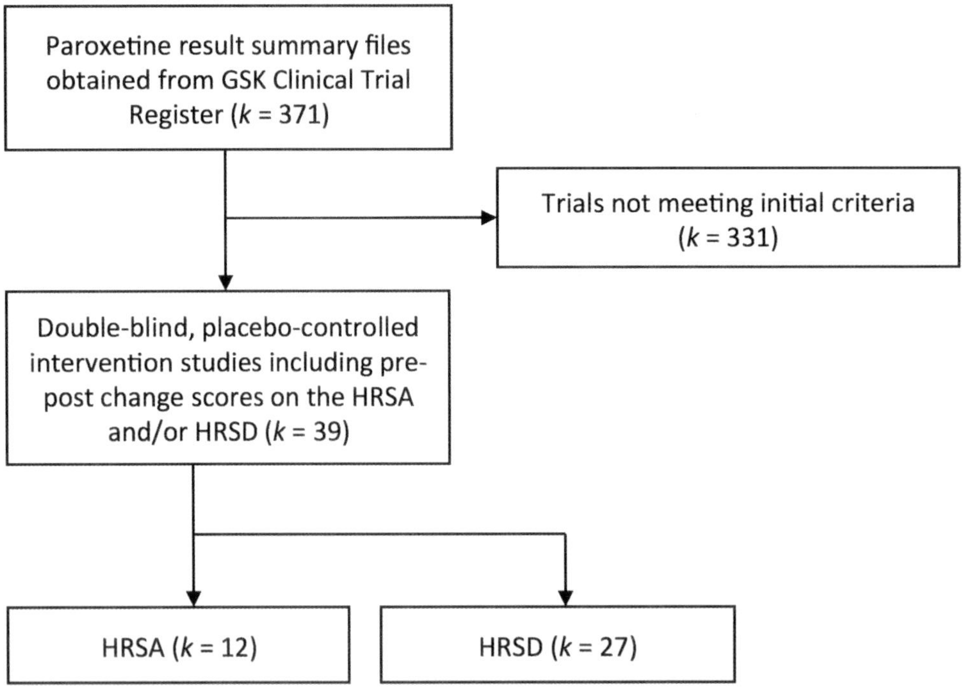

Figure 1. Trial selection Flow chart. GSK = GlaxoSmithKline, HRSA = Hamilton Rating Scale for Anxiety, HRSD = Hamilton Rating Scale for Depression. Please refer to the text for more specific information regarding specific exclusion criteria.

in duration, five were 10 weeks, and two were 12 weeks. Trials were initiated between 1991 and 2003, all following FDA approval of the medication in the treatment of depression. All trials were conducted in adults. Seven trials evaluated panic disorder and five trials evaluated generalized anxiety disorder. Flexible dose adjustment was permitted in 9 of the 12 studies (i.e., the dose of paroxetine and/or placebo could be adjusted during the trial based on therapeutic response). Eight (67%) of the studies were published in peer-reviewed journals.

For the 27 trials that included change on the HRSD as an outcome measure, trial duration ranged between 4 and 12 weeks. One trial was 4 weeks in duration, fifteen were 6 weeks, four were 8 weeks, one was 10 weeks, and six were 12 weeks. Twenty-four trials evaluated change in adults, one trial evaluated change in adolescents, and two trials evaluated change in the elderly. Twenty-six trials evaluated major depressive disorder and one trial evaluated dysthymia. Flexible dose adjustment was permitted in 21 of the 27 trials. Trials were conducted between 1982 and 2009. The trials conducted prior to 1991 ($k = 16$, 59% of trials) were included as part of the original FDA submission, and an additional 11 trials (41% of trials) were conducted following FDA approval, in 1991 or later. Sixteen (59%) of the studies were published in peer-reviewed journals.

Mean Change on the HRSA

Table 2 displays mean baseline severity, mean change, and the standardized mean difference (d) for each of the 12 trials reporting change on the HRSA. Baseline HRSA data were unavailable for two trials. Baseline severity of anxiety ranged from 18.7 to 26.0. The mean drug-placebo difference was 2.31 (95% CI: 1.72,2.91) points on the HRSA with a mean effect size difference of $d = 0.27$ (95% CI: 0.20,0.33). The weighted mean change on the HRSA was 11.11 (95% CI: 10.72,11.50) points for paroxetine and 8.77 (95% 8.35,9.20) points for placebo. The mean pre-post effect size was $d = 1.23$ (95% CI: 1.17,1.30) for paroxetine and $d = 0.96$ (95% CI: 0.90,1.02) for placebo. The differences between groups easily met statistical significance for both the raw change scores on the HRSA ($Z = 7.64$, $p < .001$) and the standardized mean difference ($Z = 7.52$, $p < .001$). The change in the placebo group duplicated 79% of the mean change score and 78% of the standardized mean difference in the paroxetine groups. These percentages are similar to those found for second-generation antidepressants in the treatment of depression [7].

A trend toward heterogeneity was observed for the mean effect size difference between paroxetine and placebo, as demonstrated by the indices of heterogeneity ($Q(11) = 17.63$, $p = .091$, $I^2 = 37.61$ [95% CI: 12.25,55.64]). A wider range of effect sizes was observed within each treatment group (Paroxetine: $Q(11) = 57.27$, $p < .001$, $I^2 = 80.79$ [95% CI: 74.98,85.25]; Placebo: $Q(11) = 65.39$, $p < .001$, $I^2 = 83.18$ [95% CI: 78.29,86.96]). These statistics indicate the necessity for moderator analyses to investigate which trial variables influenced study outcomes. Thus, we conducted moderator analyses with both analytic strategies (i.e., the paroxetine-placebo effect sizes and for paroxetine and placebo groups separately).

HRSA Moderators

The following potential moderators were analyzed: 1) baseline severity of anxiety; 2) indication (i.e., whether the individuals in the trial were treated for panic disorder or for generalized anxiety disorder); 3) length of trial in weeks; and 4) publication status.

There was no significant relationship between baseline anxiety and the paroxetine-placebo effect size difference ($Q(1) = 1.58$, $p = .208$), as shown in Figure 2. A positive relationship was observed between baseline anxiety on the HRSA and effect size for both groups (Paroxetine: $Q(1) = 21.34$, $p < .001$; Placebo: $Q(1) = 23.51$, $p < .001$). These latter effects are consistent with regression to the mean artifact. Baseline severity scores were

Table 1. List of studies.

Protocol Number	Publication	Outcome	Year	Indication	Population	Length	Dosage
29060/108	[18]	HRSA	1991	Panic	Adult	12	Flexible
29060/120	[14]	HRSA	1992	Panic	Adult	10	Fixed
29060/187	[16]	HRSA	1991	Panic	Adult	12	Flexible
29060/223		HRSA	1992	Panic	Adult	10	Flexible
29060/494	[21]	HRSA	1996	Panic	Adult	10	Flexible
29060/495	[21]	HRSA	1996	Panic	Adult	10	Flexible
29060/497	[21]	HRSA	1996	Panic	Adult	10	Flexible
29060/637		HRSA	1998	GAD	Adult	8	Flexible
29060/641	[20]	HRSA	1998	GAD	Adult	8	Fixed
29060/642	[19]	HRSA	1999	GAD	Adult	8	Flexible
29060/791		HRSA	2001	GAD	Adult	8	Flexible
29060A/856		HRSA	2003	GAD	Adult	8	Fixed
29060/01/001		HRSD	1984	Depression	Adult	6	Flexible
29060/02/001	[67,68]	HRSD	1985	Depression	Adult	6	Flexible
29060/02/002	[69,70]	HRSD	1985	Depression	Adult	6	Flexible
29060/02/003	[71]	HRSD	1985	Depression	Adult	6	Flexible
29060/02/004	[72]	HRSD	1985	Depression	Adult	6	Flexible
29060/03/001	[73,74]	HRSD	1985	Depression	Adult	6	Flexible
29060/03/002	[75,76]	HRSD	1985	Depression	Adult	6	Flexible
29060/03/003		HRSD	1985	Depression	Adult	6	Flexible
29060/03/004	[77]	HRSD	1985	Depression	Adult	6	Flexible
29060/03/005	[78]	HRSD	1985	Depression	Adult	6	Flexible
29060/03/006	[79]	HRSD	1985	Depression	Adult	6	Flexible
PAR 09	[80]	HRSD	1985	Depression	Adult	6	Fixed
UK 06	[81]	HRSD	1983	Depression	Adult	4	Fixed
UK 12		HRSD	1983	Depression	Adult	6	Fixed
UK 09		HRSD	1982	Depression	Adult	6	Fixed
PAR 07		HRSD	1986	Depression	Adult	6	Flexible
29060/115		HRSD	1991	Depression	Adult	12	Flexible
29060/128		HRSD	1991	Depression	Adult	12	Flexible
29060/251		HRSD	1992	Depression	Adult	8	Flexible
29060/327		HRSD	1994	Dysthymia	Adult	12	Flexible
29060/329	[82]	HRSD	1994	Depression	Adolescent	8	Flexible
29060/448	[83,84]	HRSD	1996	Depression	Adult	12	Flexible

Table 1. Cont.

Protocol Number	Publication	Outcome	Year	Indication	Population	Length	Dosage
29060/449	[83,84]	HRSD	1996	Depression	Adult	12	Flexible
29060/487	[85]	HRSD	1996	Depression	Elderly	12	Flexible
29060/810	[86]	HRSD	2001	Depression	Adult	8	Fixed
29060/874		HRSD	2003	Depression	Elderly	10	Fixed
112810		HRSD	2009	Depression	Adult	8	Flexible

HRSA = Hamilton Rating Scale for Anxiety. HRSD = Hamilton Rating Scale for Depression. Year: when data collection was initiated. Trials conducted prior to 1991 were submitted for the original FDA approval of the medication. Length: study duration in weeks. GAD = generalized anxiety disorder.

unavailable for two trials (29060/187 [Panic disorder] and BRL29060A/856 [Generalized anxiety disorder]) that were not included in this analysis.

The effect of indication on treatment response (Table 3) was significant. Panic disorder had a significantly larger drug-placebo difference in terms of the standardized mean difference ($Q(1) = 5.09$, $p = .024$) and the raw change score ($Q(1) = 6.77$, $p = .009$). Mean standardized difference was $d = 0.36$ (95% CI: 0.25,0.46) for panic disorder and $d = 0.20$ (95% CI: 0.11,0.29) for generalized anxiety disorder. Raw score differences were 3.24 points (95% CI: 2.32,4.15) for panic disorder and 1.64 points (95% CI: 0.86,2.42) for generalized anxiety disorder. The effect of indication was also significant within each group (Paroxetine: $Q(1) = 24.27$, $p < .001$; Placebo: $Q(1) = 32.97$, $p < .001$). However, the effects were opposite, with generalized anxiety disorder having higher effect sizes and raw change scores on the HRSA for both groups (Paroxetine: $d = 1.38$ [95% CI: 1.29,1.46] and raw change = 11.79 [95% CI: 11.29,12.30] points; Placebo: $d = 1.14$ [95% CI: 1.05,1.22] and raw change = 10.07 [95% CI: 9.49,10.64] points) compared to panic disorder (Paroxetine: $d = 1.07$ [95% CI: 0.98,1.16] and raw change = 10.06 [95% CI: 9.43,10.68] points; Placebo: $d = 0.78$ [95% CI: 0.69,0.86] and raw change = 7.17 [95% CI: 6.53,7.81] points).

Longer trial lengths were significantly associated with larger paroxetine-placebo effect sizes (Intercept = −0.40, Slope = 0.073 [95% CI: 0.023,0.124], $Q(1) = 8.02$, $p = .005$). Within each treatment group, trial length was *inversely* associated with improvement in both groups, and appeared to have a stronger relationship in the placebo group (Paroxetine: Intercept = 2.01, Slope = −0.086 [95% CI: −0.133,−0.038] $Q(1) = 12.51$, $p < .001$; Placebo: Intercept = 2.04, Slope = −0.116 [95% CI: −0.161,−0.072], $Q(1) = 26.54$, $p < .001$). However, this finding is difficult to interpret because it is confounded by differences in study indication. All five trials examining generalized anxiety disorder had a length of eight weeks, and the seven trials examining panic disorder were between 10 and 12 weeks. As described in the previous paragraph, the overall change was larger in both groups for generalized anxiety disorder, which could account for the negative slope within each group, and the drug-placebo difference was larger for panic disorder, which could account for the positive slope in the difference score. Thus, we are unable to make any firm conclusions in this analysis regarding the effect of trial length on anxiolytic response.

There was a significant effect of publication status (Table 3), with larger drug benefits in published trials ($Q(1) = 3.90$, $p = .048$). Published trials ($k = 8$) had a mean drug-placebo effect size of $d = 0.32$ (95% CI: 0.23–0.40), and unpublished trials ($k = 4$) had a mean effect size of $d = 0.17$ (95% CI: 0.06–0.29). This difference appeared to be due to a substantially smaller placebo pre-post effect sizes in published trials (Published: $d = 0.86$ [95% CI: 0.79,0.94], Unpublished: $d = 1.15$ [95% CI: 1.04,1.25], $Q(1) = 18.63$, $p = .001$). The mean pre-post effect size for the paroxetine group was actually marginally smaller for published compared to unpublished trials (Published: $d = 1.19$ [95% CI: 1.12,1.27], Unpublished: $d = 1.32$ [95% CI: 1.21,1.44], $Q(1) = 3.52$, $p = .061$).

Mean Change on the HRSD

Table 4 displays mean baseline severity, mean change, and the standardized mean difference (d) for each of the 27 trials reporting change on the HRSD. Baseline severity scores on the HRSD ranged from 19.0 to 30.5 points, all in the ranges of severe to very severe depression [41]. The weighted mean difference between paroxetine and placebo groups across all studies was 2.51 (95%

Table 2. Baseline scores, mean change, standardized mean change, and sample sizes for all studies reporting change on the Hamilton Rating Scale for Anxiety.

Protocol	Indication	Paroxetine					Placebo				Drug benefit		
		Baseline	Change	*d*	95% CI	*n*	Baseline	Change	*d*	95% CI	*n*	*d*	95% CI
29060/108	Panic	24.3	14.9	2.04	[1.57, 2.51]	58	23.5	10.0	1.62	[1.21, 2.03]	56	0.74	[0.36, 1.12]
29060/120	Panic	18.9	8.4	0.95	[0.77, 1.13]	175	19.7	6.5	0.73	[0.44, 1.02]	60	0.21	[−0.08, 0.50]
29060/187	Panic		10.1	1.10	[0.87, 1.33]	119		5.9	0.59	[0.40, 0.79]	122	0.44	[0.19, 0.70]
29060/223	Panic	20.3	10.2	1.29	[0.94, 1.64]	61	18.7	5.6	0.76	[0.48, 1.04]	55	0.61	[0.25, 0.97]
29060/494	Panic	21.9	10.0	1.08	[0.84, 1.31]	115	20.1	8.0	0.88	[0.67, 1.09]	124	0.22	[−0.04, 0.47]
29060/495	Panic	20.5	9.4	1.03	[0.79, 1.26]	112	20.4	6.6	0.74	[0.54, 0.94]	129	0.31	[0.06, 0.57]
29060/497	Panic	20.5	9.4	0.95	[0.74, 1.16]	128	20.2	6.8	0.75	[0.55, 0.95]	125	0.28	[0.03, 0.52]
29060/637	GAD	26.0	12.4	1.15	[0.96, 1.34]	181	25.9	11.3	1.04	[0.86, 1.22]	183	0.10	[−0.10, 0.31]
29060/641	GAD	23.5	12.3	1.48	[1.33, 1.63]	385	23.9	9.6	1.02	[0.84, 1.20]	180	0.32	[0.14, 0.49]
29060/642	GAD	23.9	11.8	1.32	[1.11, 1.54]	161	23.6	9.5	1.06	[0.86, 1.25]	163	0.26	[0.04, 0.48]
29060/791	GAD	24.4	11.9	1.60	[1.37, 1.84]	163	24.8	10.7	1.44	[1.22, 1.67]	162	0.17	[−0.05, 0.38]
29060A/856	GAD		10.3	1.33	[1.13, 1.53]	177		9.5	1.23	[1.04, 1.43]	181	0.10	[−0.10, 0.31]

GAD = generalized anxiety disorder. Drug benefit denotes the effect size for paroxetine compared to placebo.

CI: 2.06,2.96) points on the HRSD. The weighted mean effect size difference between the two groups was 0.32 (95% CI: 0.26,0.38). The weighted mean change on the HRSD was 11.00 (95% CI: 10.74,11.26) points for paroxetine and 8.37 (95% CI: 8.02,8.72) points for placebo. The mean pre-post effect size was 1.39 (95% CI: 1.34,1.44) for paroxetine, which was significantly greater ($Q(1) = 87.62$, $p < .001$) than the effect size for placebo ($d = 1.03$ [95% CI: 0.97,1.08]). The magnitude of change in the placebo group was equivalent to 76% of the paroxetine change scores on the HRSD and 74% of the standardized mean difference.

Indices of heterogeneity did not indicate statistically significant heterogeneity in the effect size difference between paroxetine and placebo across trials ($Q(26) = 26.54$, $p = .434$, $I^2 = 2.04$ [95% CI: −29.25,25.75]), although we did detect significant heterogeneity within each group (Paroxetine: $Q(26) = 63.21$, $p < .001$, $I^2 = 58.87$ [95% CI: 49.14–66.73]; Placebo: $Q(26) = 80.63$, $p < .001$, $I^2 = 67.75$ [95% CI: 60.63,73.59]). Nevertheless, as planned when designing the study, moderator analyses were conducted for both types of analyses.

HRSD Moderators

We analyzed the following moderators to determine whether the variables could account for variance in effect size across trials: 1) baseline severity of depression; 2) approval status; 3) length of treatment in weeks; and 4) publication status.

Figure 3 displays the relationship between baseline severity of depression on the HRSD and treatment outcome. The benefit of paroxetine over placebo was not significantly related to baseline severity ($Q(1) = 3.01$, $p = .083$), although there was a trend towards a greater benefit at higher baseline severities. The predicted paroxetine-placebo effect size at a baseline severity of HRSD = 19 was $d = 0.20$ (95% CI: 0.03,0.36) and $d = 0.48$ (95% CI: 0.29,0.68) at a baseline severity of HRSD = 30. Greater baseline severity of depression was associated with smaller pre-post effect sizes in both paroxetine ($Q(1) = 15.45$, $p < .001$) and placebo ($Q(1) = 28.23$, $p < .001$) groups. These effects are opposite from those expected based on regression to the mean artifact.

A comparison of the trials submitted for the original FDA approval (pre-approval, $k = 16$) versus trials conducted after approval (post-approval, $k = 11$), shown in Table 5, revealed that the mean paroxetine-placebo effect size did not differ significantly as a function of approval status ($Q(1) = 3.27$, $p = .077$), although there was a trend towards a greater drug-placebo benefit in pre-approval trials (Pre-Approval: $d = 0.41$ [95% CI: 0.30,0.53]; Post-Approval: $d = 0.29$ [95% CI: 0.22,0.36]). However, we observed a significant effect within both groups, with larger mean standardized differences in the post-approval trials (Table 5). For paroxetine, the mean effect size for pre-approval trials was $d = 1.24$ (95% CI: 1.15,1.33), compared to $d = 1.45$ (95% CI: 1.39,1.50) for post-approval ($Q(1) = 14.43$, $p < .001$). For placebo, the mean effect sizes were $d = 0.77$ (95% CI: 0.67,0.87) and $d = 1.14$ (95% CI: 1.07,1.21) for the pre- and post-approval trials, respectively ($Q(1) = 35.01$, $p < .001$).

An examination of the effect of trial duration on efficacy (Figure 4) revealed that the benefit of paroxetine over placebo was not significantly associated with trial duration ($Q(1) = 1.30$, $p = .254$). Likewise, the response to paroxetine did not significantly differ as a function of study length ($Q(1) = 2.62$, $p = .105$), although the mean change in the placebo group was significantly larger in longer studies ($Q(1) = 13.74$, $p < .001$).

The weighted mean difference between paroxetine and placebo was not significantly different between published and unpublished trials (Table 5; $Q(1) = 1.50$, $p = .221$). Published trials ($k = 16$) had a weighted mean effect size of $d = 0.36$ (95% CI: 0.27,0.44) and

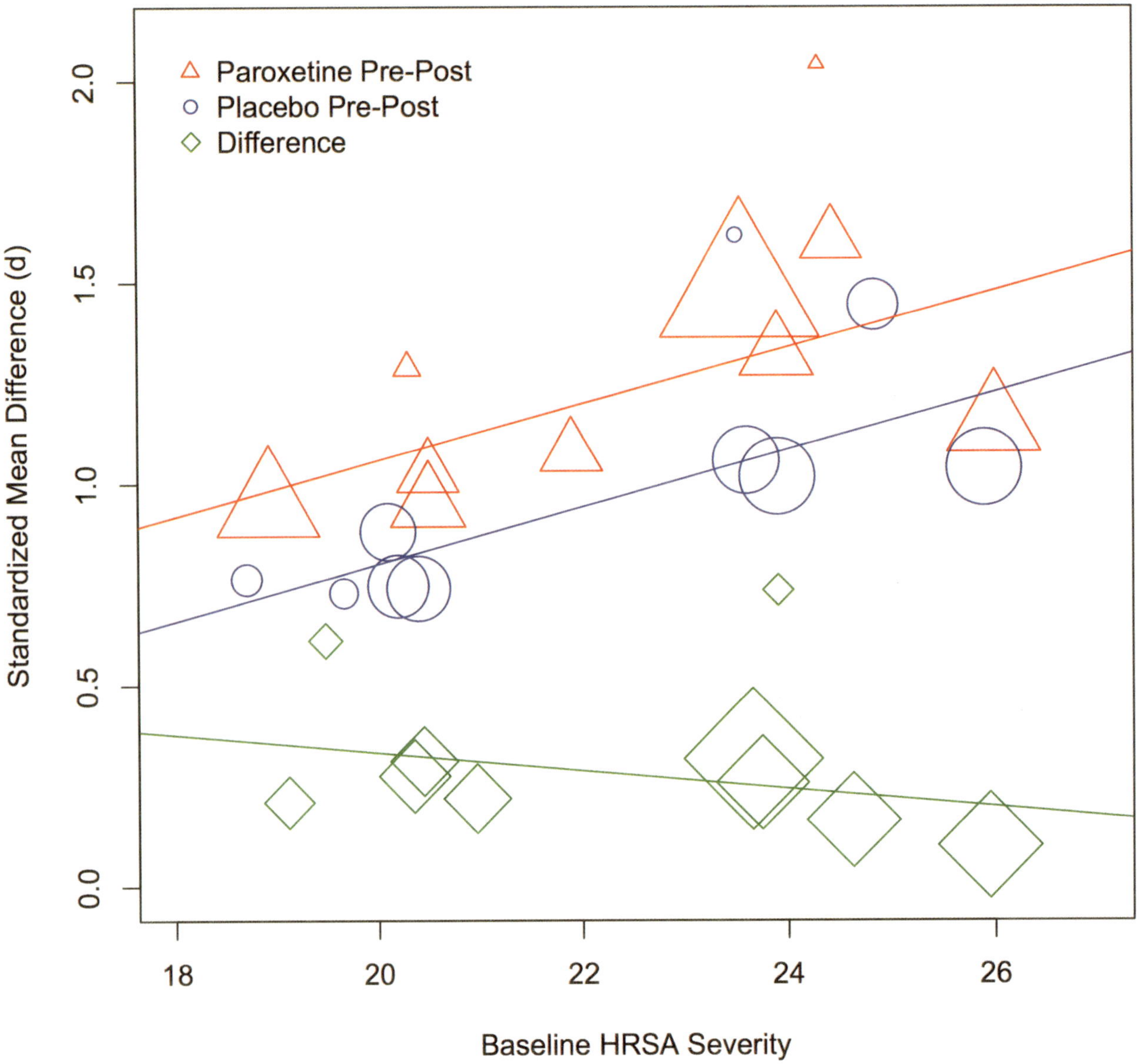

Figure 2. Baseline severity of anxiety and the mean change on the Hamilton Rating Scale for Anxiety (HRSA). The size of the marker reflects the relative weight of the study in the meta-analysis.

unpublished trials ($k = 11$) had an effect size of $d = 0.28$ (95% CI: 0.20,0.37).

Comparison of Change on the HRSA and HRSD

A comparison of the standardized mean difference between the change on the two scales indicated that the paroxetine-placebo effect size did not significantly differ between the HRSA and the HRSD (HRSA: $d = 0.27$ [95% CI: 0.20,0.33], HRSD: $d = 0.32$ [95% CI: 0.26,0.38], $Q(1) = 1.41$, $p = .235$). The mean pre-post effect size for paroxetine treatment was significantly larger ($Q(1) = 14.55$, $p < .001$) for the HRSD ($d = 1.39$ [95% CI: 1.34,1.44], $k = 27$) than for the HRSA ($d = 1.23$ [95% CI: 1.17,1.30], $k = 12$). A non-significant trend ($Q(1) = 2.38$, $p = .123$) was observed in the placebo group for larger pre-post effect sizes on the HRSD ($d = 1.03$ [95% CI: 0.97,1.08]) than on the HRSA ($d = 0.96$ [95% CI: 0.90,1.02]).

Discussion

The current analysis is the first evaluation of the efficacy of an SSRI medication in the treatment of multiple anxiety disorders, and the first to utilize a complete database of published and unpublished trials sponsored by the drug's manufacturer. Our results indicated that paroxetine presented a modest benefit over placebo in the treatment of anxiety and depression, with mean change score differences of 2.3 and 2.5 points on the HRSA and HRSD, respectively. The standardized mean difference of paroxetine over placebo was $d = 0.27$ and $d = 0.32$ for the treatment of anxiety and depression, respectively. Put another way, the average symptom reduction for an individual treated with paroxetine fell at the 61st percentile for individuals who received placebo for anxiety, and at the 63rd percentile for individuals who received placebo for depression. The difference of $d = 0.32$ in the treatment of depression is consistent with previous meta-analyses of antidepressant efficacy [5,7]. The mean treatment response did

Table 3. Moderator effects in trials examining change on the Hamilton Rating Scale for Anxiety.

Indication		Effect Size	95% CI	$Q(1)$	p
Paroxetine - Placebo	Panic	0.36	[0.25, 0.46]	5.09	*.024*
	GAD	0.20	[0.11, 0.29]		
Paroxetine	Panic	1.07	[0.98, 1.16]	24.27	*<.001*
	GAD	1.38	[1.29, 1.46]		
Placebo	Panic	0.78	[0.69, 0.86]	32.97	*<.001*
	GAD	1 14	[1.05, 1.22]		
Publication Status		**Effect Size**	**95% CI**	$Q(1)$	p
Paroxetine - Placebo	Published	0.32	[0.23, 0.40]	3.90	*.048*
	Unpublished	0.17	[0.06, 0.29]		
Paroxetine	Published	1.19	[1.12, 1.27]	3.52	.061
	Unpublished	1.32	[1.21, 1.44]		
Placebo	Published	0.86	[0.79, 0.94]	18.63	*<.001*
	Unpublished	1.15	[1.04, 1.25]		

GAD = generalized anxiety disorder.

not significantly differ between treatment of anxiety and treatment of depression. We demonstrated that individuals given placebo exhibited 79% of the magnitude of change compared to paroxetine. We also provided further support for the large magnitude of the changes in placebo groups in the treatment of depression (76% compared to paroxetine).

Several moderator variables were significantly associated with pre-post effect sizes for paroxetine and placebo on both the HRSA and the HRSD. For anxiety, we found that higher baseline severity was unrelated to drug-placebo differences, although higher severity was associated with greater changes in both paroxetine and placebo groups. Efficacy was superior in the treatment of panic disorder compared to generalized anxiety disorder; however, the overall response to both paroxetine and placebo was larger for generalized anxiety disorder. Samples with higher baseline severities were associated with lower changes in both paroxetine and placebo groups in the treatment of depression, an effect that is especially peculiar given that it is opposite to that predicted by regression toward the mean. Longer treatment was associated with larger pre-post placebo effect sizes in the treatment of depression. The increase in the symptom reduction in the placebo group in longer trials for the treatment of depression is especially interesting, given the widespread belief that placebo effects are short lived.

The magnitude of change in the placebo group was greater than 75% of the paroxetine response in the treatment of both anxiety and depression. Large effect sizes in placebo groups have been reported in the treatment of other conditions as well. However, these changes compared to the drug effect sizes do not appear to be as large as those observed in antidepressant trials in the treatment of depression and anxiety. For example, a review of the placebo effect compared to active medications (including antidepressants and anticonvulsants) in the treatment of pain associated with fibromyalgia revealed that the mean change in placebo groups accounted for 45% of the drug response [44]. This same review found that pain reduction in the placebo groups compared to the drug response in individuals with painful peripheral diabetic neuropathy was 62% [44]. Similar meta-analytic reviews have found that mean change in placebo groups replicates about 40% of drug responses in global symptom reduction during treatment of irritable bowel syndrome [45,46]. In a meta-analysis of change in placebo compared to drug groups in the treatment of symptoms of chronic fatigue syndrome, the mean placebo effect replicated only 20% of the drug response [47]. Thus, the replication of greater than 75% of the drug response indicates that the magnitude of the placebo effect is especially large in the treatment of anxiety and depression.

Given the similar efficacy between paroxetine and other second-generation antidepressants in the treatment of depression [7,12,48], it is possible that a similar magnitude of placebo effect sizes are present in the treatment of anxiety disorders with other antidepressants. However, further research will be necessary to support this proposition. The current analysis indicates that the published literature represents an overestimate of the true efficacy of paroxetine in the treatment of anxiety.

Although the differences between drug and placebo are statistically significant, whether antidepressants produce clinically significant benefits has been a topic of debate in recent years. However, to date there has been no consensus regarding what constitutes a clinically significant benefit. In their 2004 guidelines for the treatment of depression, the National Institute of Health and Clinical Excellence (NICE) proposed a mean drug-placebo standardized mean difference (SMD) ≥ 0.50 or a difference of at least three points on the HRSD as criteria for clinical significance [43]. Based on these criteria, the mean antidepressant benefit in a previous meta-analysis of trials submitted to the FDA [7] was clinically significant only in the most severe cases of depression (baseline HRSD ≥ 28). In a subsequent revision of their guidelines for the treatment of depression [42], NICE replaced the term "clinical significance" with "clinical importance." Although they did not specify their criteria for determining whether an effect was clinically important, their comparisons of SSRI-placebo differences in HRSD scores were the same as in the earlier guidelines, and the same conclusions regarding "clinical importance" were reached as had been reached with respect to "clinical significance" in 2004. Specifically, the overall difference between SSRIs and placebo (SMD = 0.34) was described as "unlikely to be of clinical importance" (pg. 317). According to these criteria, the mean

Table 4. Baseline scores, mean change, standardized mean change, and sample sizes for all studies reporting change on the Hamilton Rating Scale for Depression.

Protocol	Approval	Paroxetine					Placebo					Drug Benefit	
		Baseline	Change	*d*	95% CI	*n*	Baseline	Change	*d*	95% CI	*n*	*d*	95% CI
29060/01/001	Pre	28.0	13.5	1.66	[0.99, 2.33]	24	27.4	10.5	1.30	[0.71, 1.89]	24	0.37	[−0.20, 0.94]
29060/02/001	Pre	26.6	12.3	1.27	[0.89, 1.65]	51	25.9	6.8	0.70	[0.40, 1.01]	53	0.57	[0.18, 0.97]
29060/02/002	Pre	25.0	10.9	1.24	[0.78, 1.69]	36	24.9	5.8	0.65	[0.27, 1.04]	34	0.60	[0.12, 1.08]
29060/02/003	Pre	28.6	9.7	0.93	[0.50, 1.35]	33	28.9	7.2	0.69	[0.29, 1.08]	33	0.24	[−0.24, 0.73]
29060/02/004	Pre	28.9	12.7	1.87	[1.29, 2.44]	36	27.3	7.6	1.12	[0.70, 1.54]	38	0.76	[0.29, 1.24]
29060/03/001	Pre	24.9	10.8	1.60	[1.11, 2.09]	40	24.8	4.7	0.69	[0.33, 1.06]	38	0.92	[0.45, 1.39]
29060/03/002	Pre	24.9	8.0	1.14	[0.72, 1.55]	40	25.6	6.2	0.88	[0.51, 1.26]	40	0.26	[−0.18, 0.70]
29060/03/003	Pre	25.7	9.9	1.18	[0.76, 1.59]	41	27.0	10.0	1.19	[0.78, 1.60]	42	−0.01	[−0.44, 0.42]
29060/03/004	Pre	27.6	10.4	1.32	[0.86, 1.78]	37	27.0	6.7	0.85	[0.46, 1.24]	37	0.48	[0.02, 0.95]
29060/03/005	Pre	26.1	10.0	1.00	[0.60, 1.39]	40	26.8	4.1	0.41	[0.08, 0.73]	42	0.60	[0.16, 1.05]
29060/03/006	Pre	29.7	9.1	1.10	[0.69, 1.52]	39	28.7	3.0	0.36	[0.02, 0.71]	37	0.76	[0.29, 1.23]
PAR 09	Pre	25.2	9.1	1.28	[1.15, 1.41]	403	24.5	8.2	1.14	[0.78, 1.51]	51	0.12	[−0.17, 0.41]
UK 06	Pre	23.7	6.0	0.97	[0.38, 1.57]	19	24.2	6.2	0.83	[0.31, 1.35]	22	−0.03	[−0.64, 0.58]
UK 12	Pre	22.8	9.1	1.23	[0.57, 1.88]	19	22.3	6.7	0.86	[0.00, 1.73]	10	0.34	[−0.43, 1.11]
UK 09	Pre	26.8	8.8	0.80	[0.26, 1.35]	20	25.5	4.5	0.49	[0.01, 0.97]	21	0.45	[−0.17, 1.07]
PAR 07	Pre	30.5	13.1	1.20	[0.37, 2.03]	13	28.3	10.9	0.99	[0.19, 1.79]	12	0.22	[−0.57, 1.00]
29060/115	Post		10.6	1.23	[1.07, 1.39]	272		9.1	1.09	[0.85, 1.33]	113	0.18	[−0.04, 0.40]
29060/128	Post	25.6	11.8	1.34	[1.19, 1.48]	350	25.7	9.1	1.05	[0.84, 1.26]	136	0.31	[0.11, 0.51]
29060/251	Post	24.5	10.2	1.33	[1.08, 1.57]	120	24.4	8.3	1.07	[0.85, 1.30]	123	0.26	[0.01, 0.51]
29060/327	Post		7.3	1.14	[0.85, 1.42]	79		4.8	0.75	[0.51, 1.00]	83	0.40	[0.09, 0.71]
29060/329	Post	19.0	10.7	1.39	[1.09, 1.68]	90	19.0	9.1	1.16	[0.89, 1.44]	87	0.21	[−0.08, 0.51]
29060/448	Post	23.2	11.9	1.45	[1.25, 1.65]	206	23.4	9.9	1.22	[0.96, 1.48]	101	0.25	[0.01, 0.48]
29060/449	Post	23.8	12.7	1.54	[1.35, 1.74]	218	23.5	10.2	1.24	[0.99, 1.49]	110	0.30	[0.07, 0.53]
29060/487	Post	22.2	12.2	1.68	[1.46, 1.89]	206	22.1	9.5	1.28	[1.02, 1.54]	107	0.37	[0.14, 0.61]
29060/810	Post	23.3	12.0	1.68	[1.50, 1.86]	294	23.8	10.0	1.37	[1.14, 1.60]	142	0.28	[0.08, 0.49]
29060/874	Post	22.5	11.4	1.42	[1.27, 1.57]	334	22.4	8.9	1.10	[0.91, 1.28]	178	0.32	[0.14, 0.50]
112810	Post	22.7	12.7	1.69	[1.50, 1.89]	241	22.6	10.4	1.28	[1.07, 1.48]	171	0.30	[0.10, 0.49]

"Approval" column designates whether the study was submitted as part of the original approval submission to the FDA or whether it was conducted following FDA approval in 1991 or later. Drug benefit denotes the effect size for paroxetine compared to placebo.

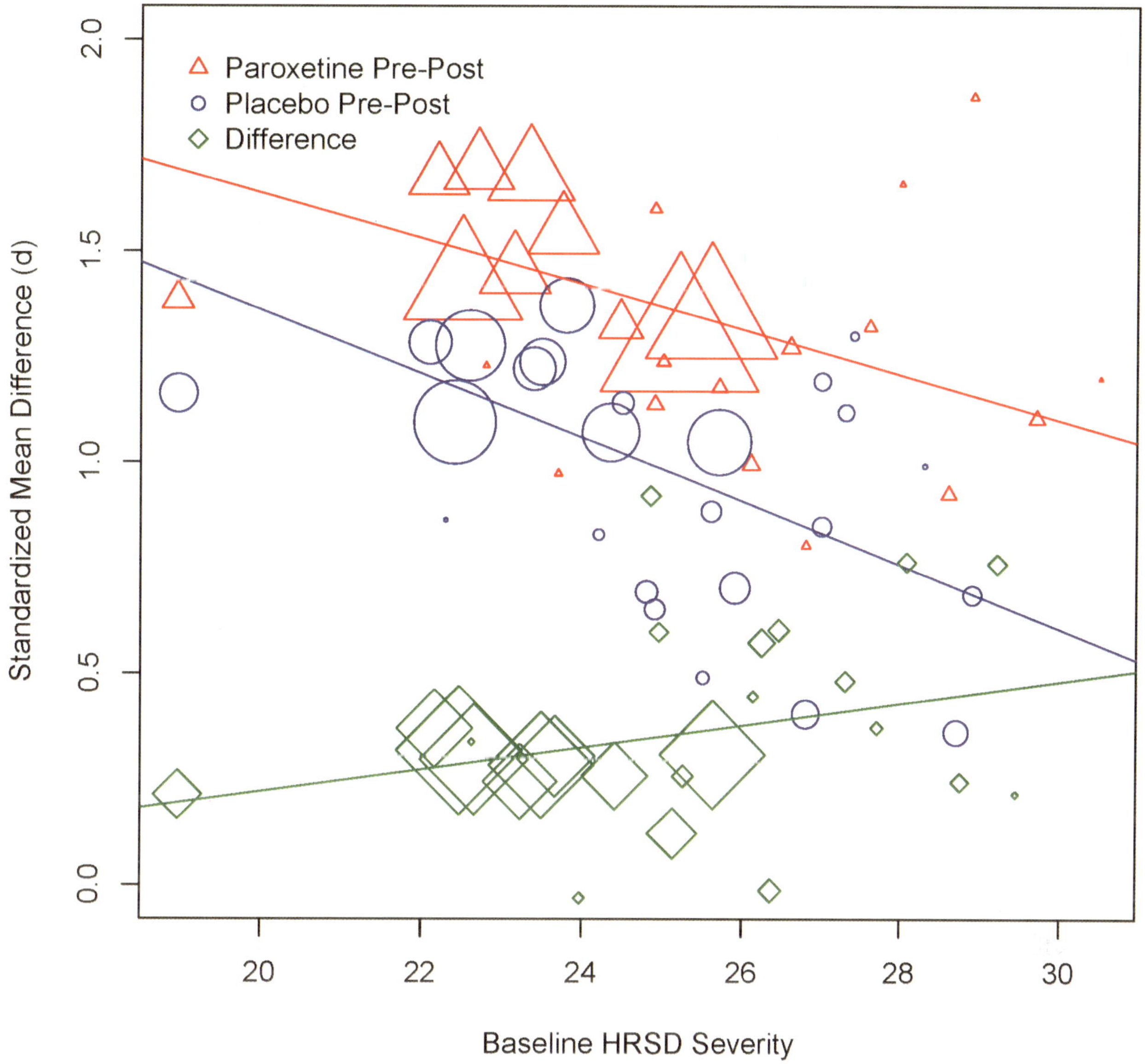

Figure 3. Baseline severity of depression and the mean change on the Hamilton Rating Scale for Depression (HRSD). The size of the marker reflects the relative weight of the study in the meta-analysis.

difference between paroxetine and placebo in the current analyses fell short of clinical significance for the treatment of both anxiety and depression.

The NICE criteria have been criticized for being arbitrary and lacking empirical justification [49]. However, a recent analysis of raw data from 43 antidepressant trials [50] compared HRSD change scores with clinician ratings of improvement on the Clinical Global Impressions Scale (CGI) [51] to establish the clinical relevance of HRSD scores. They found that change of three points or less on the HRSD corresponded to a clinician rating of "No Change" on the CGI. That is, changes of three points or less did not correspond to a clinically detectable change according to this clinician-rated measure. Thus, the drug-placebo differences that have been observed in the current and previous antidepressant meta-analyses [7,28], while statistically significant, appear to be of marginal clinical significance.

These findings have important clinical implications. The obvious alternative for the treatment of both anxiety and depression is psychotherapy intervention. However, direct comparisons of acute phase treatment for pharmacotherapy and psychotherapy in the treatment of major depression generally have yielded no significant differences between the treatment modalities [52–54]. Fewer clinical trials have directly compared antidepressants and psychotherapy in the treatment of anxiety disorders, although the available literature indicates similar comparability between antidepressants and psychotherapy. For example, one study [55] found that that acute phase cognitive-behavioral therapy yields comparable efficacy to imipramine in the treatment of panic disorder. Another study [56] found comparable 12-week efficacy between sertraline and cognitive-behavioral therapy in the treatment of childhood anxiety disorders. Overall, antidepressants, psychotherapy, and placebo all yield substantial changes in symptomatology, and are superior to no-treatment control groups [9]. Thus, in terms of treatment, the specific type of intervention may be less important than simply getting patients involved in some sort of active therapy program [53].

Table 5. Moderator effects in trials examining change on the Hamilton Rating Scale for Depression.

Pre- vs. Post-Approval		Effect Size	95% CI	$Q(1)$	p
Paroxetine - Placebo	Pre-Approval	0.41	[0.30, 0.53]	3.27	.071
	Post-Approval	0.29	[0.22, 0.36]		
Paroxetine	Pre-Approval	1.24	[1.15, 1.33]	14.43	<.001
	Post-Approval	1.45	[1.39, 1.50]		
Placebo	Pre-Approval	0.77	[0.67, 0.87]	35.01	<.001
	Post-Approval	1.14	[1.07, 1.21]		
Publication Status		**Effect Size**	**95% CI**	$Q(1)$	p
Paroxetine - Placebo	Published	0.36	[0.27, 0.44]	1.50	.221
	Unpublished	0.28	[0.20, 0.37]		
Paroxetine	Published	1.41	[1.35, 1.48]	1.45	.229
	Unpublished	1.35	[1.28, 1.43]		
Placebo	Published	0.99	[0.91, 1.07]	1.46	.227
	Unpublished	1.06	[0.98, 1.15]		

Pre-approval and Post-approval refer to whether the trial was included as part of the original approval submission to the FDA ($k = 16$) or whether it was conducted following FDA approval in 1991 or later ($k = 11$).

When given two seemingly equivalent alternatives with regard to symptom reduction, the decision may come down to patient preference and to the safety profile associated with the treatment. A meta-analysis of patient preferences when given the choice between psychological and pharmacologic treatment [57] revealed that 75% of patients prefer psychological intervention across 30 studies comprising individuals seeking treatment for depression or anxiety disorders. Paroxetine and other SSRIs have also been associated with a number of adverse events during treatment. Greater than 70% of patients report treatment-emergent symptoms of sexual dysfunction including reduced desire, arousal, and/or orgasm dysfunction, compared to less than 10% of individuals who received placebo [58]. Other adverse reported effects include drowsiness and weight gain, observed in greater than 7% of patients taking SSRIs [59]. Infrequent but severe symptoms such as serotonin syndrome [60] and increased suicidal ideation in younger adults [61,62] have also been reported. Additionally, abrupt withdrawal can result in a discontinuation syndrome in 66% of patients taking paroxetine, including symptoms of dizziness, worsened mood, agitation, headache, and nausea [63]. It is also notable that the frequency of adverse events many be underestimated in the clinical literature, as patients with depression are far more likely to self-report side effects on questionnaires than report them to physicians as is typical during clinical trials [64].

Although meta-analyses have indicated comparable efficacy between antidepressants and psychotherapy during acute stage treatment, their comparability is not as clear for long-term treatment. One study [54] found that individuals who had received "bona fide" psychotherapy from trained professionals displayed greater symptom reduction compared to those who had received SSRI treatment at post-acute phase follow-up ranging from 18 to 40 weeks ($d = 0.29$, $k = 6$). Another meta-analysis [52] of long-term naturalistic follow-up between individuals who were randomized to either acute-phase pharmacotherapy or psychotherapy in the treatment of depression across 11 studies revealed an advantage for psychotherapy at an average follow-up length of 15 months. Moreover, length of follow-up was a significant moderator such that the advantage of psychotherapy over medication was superior at longer follow-up intervals. The authors suggest that psychotherapy offers a "prophylactic effect" resulting in its long-term superiority over medications [52]. In an additional analysis of nine studies, Imel et al. [52] demonstrated that acute-phase discontinued psychotherapy was as efficacious as continued pharmacotherapy at an average follow-up interval of 14 months. That is, short-term psychotherapy (between 7 and 24 sessions) provided an equivalent long-term benefit to continuous medication usage. These findings can help to explain why antidepressants are frequently used for chronic treatment; more than 60% of individuals who take antidepressants have done so for longer than 2 years, and greater than 30% use them for 5 years or more [65]. In sum, the drawbacks to antidepressant usage and their modest benefit compared to placebo should be seriously considered before they are chosen as the primary treatment for depression or anxiety.

A limitation of the current work is that the trial database was limited to studies sponsored by GlaxoSmithKline, and does not include any additional trials that may have been conducted by independent researchers. Additionally, it is possible that GlaxoSmithKline omitted some of the outcome indices from the trial summaries posted online. A further limitation of the current analysis is that baseline severity and change were evaluated with the mean values for each group. An analysis including baseline values and response at the individual patient level would afford more power in determining a more precise estimate for the relative benefit of paroxetine over placebo at differing levels of baseline severity. The standard result summaries provided by the GlaxoSmithKline Clinical Trial Register provide baseline values and change scores only at the group level. These result summary documents also provided limited information regarding the ways in which the trials were conducted, which hindered our ability to conduct a thorough analysis for study quality. However, it appears that clinical trial sponsors are recognizing the importance of the availability of patient-level data. Several sponsors, including GlaxoSmithKline, have committed to posting patient-level study results online at Clinical Study Data Request [66]. According to

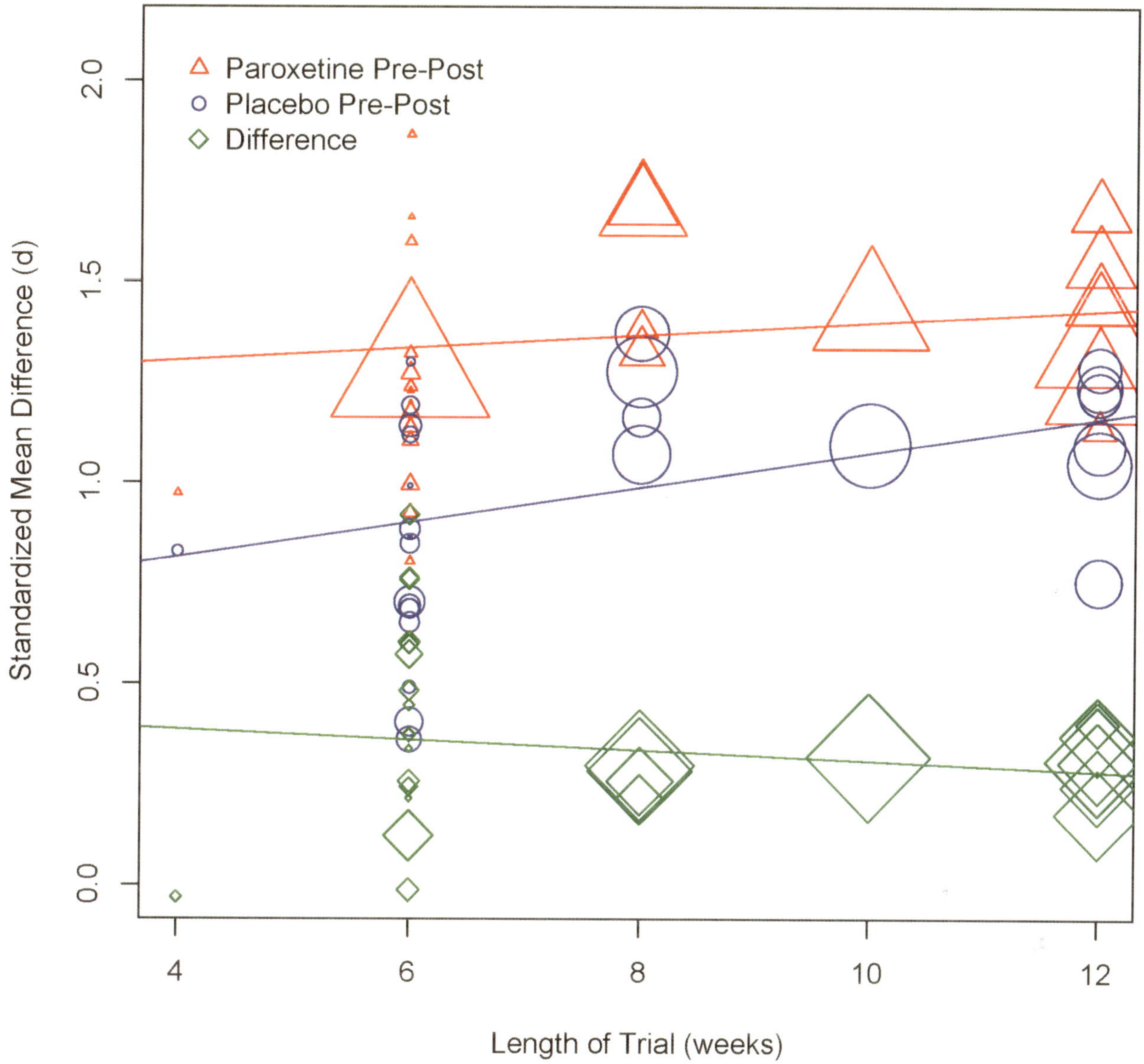

Figure 4. Trial duration (in weeks) and the mean change on the Hamilton Rating Scale for Depression (HRSD). The size of the marker reflects the relative weight of the study in the meta-analysis.

this site, GlaxoSmithKline plans to have data for all studies conducted after December 2000 freely available some time in 2015, with further studies available upon request. This site may be a valuable resource for future meta-analyses of drug efficacy.

A recent study conducted a patient-level analysis examining the relationship between baseline severity and antidepressant efficacy in the treatment of depression [39]. This study analyzed individuals from six double-blind, placebo-controlled studies of paroxetine and imipramine and found that the drug-placebo difference was greater than three points on the HRSD only at baseline severity levels of 25 and above. In fact, for individuals with mild or moderate depression (HRSD ≤ 18), the drug benefit was less than one point on the HRSD. This finding is concerning given that among Americans aged 12 years or older, approximately 19% and 28% of individuals with mild and moderate depression, respectively, take antidepressants [65].

In conclusion, paroxetine provides only a modest benefit over placebo in treating symptoms of anxiety based on the available evidence. In addition, the current study supports previous work [7] indicating that paroxetine treatment presents only a modest benefit over placebo in the treatment of depression.

Supporting Information

Checklist S1 PRISMA checklist.

Figure S1 Baseline severity of anxiety and the mean change on the Hamilton Rating Scale for Anxiety (HRSA). The size of the marker reflects the relative weight of the study in the meta-analysis. Random effects assumptions were used in the analyses. The relationship between baseline severity and effect size was marginally significant for paroxetine ($p = .069$) and statistically significant for placebo ($p = .020$), but not for the difference between paroxetine over placebo ($p = .401$).

Figure S2 Baseline severity of depression and the mean change on the Hamilton Rating Scale for Depression (HRSD). The size of the marker reflects the relative weight of the study in the meta-analysis. Random effects assumptions were used in the analyses. The relationship between baseline severity and effect size was statistically significant for paroxetine ($p = .029$) and for placebo ($p = .004$), but not for the difference between paroxetine over placebo ($p = .094$).
(TIFF)

Figure S3 Trial duration (in weeks) and the mean change on the Hamilton Rating Scale for Depression (HRSD). The size of the marker reflects the relative weight of the study in the meta-analysis. Random effects assumptions were used in the analyses. The relationship between trial length and effect size was not statistically significant for paroxetine ($p = .126$), but was statistically significant for placebo ($p = .017$). The relationship was not statistically significant for the difference between paroxetine over placebo ($p = .297$).

Results S1 Contains Table S1 and Table S2.

Author Contributions

Conceived and designed the experiments: MAS AML BBB ERG IK. Performed the experiments: MAS AML. Analyzed the data: MAS AML BBB ERG IK. Wrote the paper: MAS AML BBB ERG IK.

References

1. National Center for Health Statistics (2013) Health, United States, 2012: With special feature on emergency care. Hyattsville, MD: Centers for Disease Control and Prevention. 489 p.
2. Baldwin D, Woods R, Lawson R, Taylor D (2011) Efficacy of drug treatments for generalised anxiety disorder: Systematic review and meta-analysis. BMJ 10.1136/bmj.d1199.
3. Ravindran LN, Stein MB (2010) The pharmacologic treatment of anxiety disorders: A review of progress. J Clin Psychiatry 10.4088/JCP.10r06218blu.
4. Melander H, Ahlqvist-Rastad J, Meijer G, Beermann B (2003) Evidence b(i)ased medicine–selective reporting from studies sponsored by pharmaceutical industry: Review of studies in new drug applications. BMJ 10.1136/bmj.326.7400.1171.
5. Turner EH, Matthews AM, Linardatos E, Tell RA, Rosenthal R (2008) Selective publication of antidepressant trials and its influence on apparent efficacy. N Engl J Med 10.1056/NEJMsa065779.
6. Center for Drug Evaluation and Research (1996) Guidance for industry: Guideline for the format and content of the summary for new drug and antibiotic applications. Rockville, MD: U.S. Department of Health, Education, and Welfare. Food and Drug Administration. Available: http://www.fda.gov/downloads/Drugs/GuidanceComplianceRegulatoryInformation/Guidances/ucm072058.pdf. Accessed 31 October 2013.
7. Kirsch I, Deacon BJ, Huedo-Medina TB, Scoboria A, Moore TJ, et al. (2008) Initial severity and antidepressant benefits: A meta-analysis of data submitted to the Food and Drug Administration. PLoS Med 10.1371/journal.pmed.0050045.
8. Kirsch I, Moore TJ, Scoboria A, Nicholls SS (2002) The emperor's new drugs: An analysis of antidepressant medication data submitted to the US Food and Drug Administration. Prevention & Treatment 10.1037/1522-3736.5.1.523a.
9. Kirsch I, Sapirstein G (1998) Listening to Prozac but hearing placebo: A meta-analysis of antidepressant medication. Prevention and Treatment 10.1037/1522-3736.1.1.12a.
10. Harris G (2004) Maker of Paxil to release all trial results. New York: New York Times. Available: http://www.nytimes.com/2004/08/26/business/26CND-DRUG.html. Accessed 31 October 2013.
11. Meier B (2004) Glaxo begins posting drug trial results. New York: New York Times. Available: http://www.nytimes.com/2004/09/01/business/01registry.html?_r=0. Accessed 31 October 2013.
12. Gartlehner G, Hansen RA, Morgan LC, Thaler K, Lux L, et al. (2011) Comparative benefits and harms of second-generation antidepressants for treating major depressive disorder: An updated meta-analysis. Ann Intern Med 10.7326/0003-4819-155-11-201112060-00009.
13. Baldwin D, Bobes J, Stein DJ, Scharwachter I, Faure M (1999) Paroxetine in social phobia/social anxiety disorder. Randomised, double-blind, placebo-controlled study. Paroxetine Study Group. Br J Psychiatry 10.1192/bjp.175.2.120.
14. Ballenger JC, Wheadon DE, Steiner M, Bushnell W, Gergel IP (1998) Double-blind, fixed-dose, placebo-controlled study of paroxetine in the treatment of panic disorder. Am J Psychiatry 155: 36–42.
15. Lecrubier Y, Bakker A, Dunbar G, Judge R (1997) A comparison of paroxetine, clomipramine and placebo in the treatment of panic disorder. Collaborative Paroxetine Panic Study Investigators. Acta Psychiatr Scand 10.1111/j.1600-0447.1997.tb00388.x.
16. Lepola U, Bergtholdt B, St Lambert J, Davy KL, Ruggiero L (2004) Controlled-release paroxetine in the treatment of patients with social anxiety disorder. J Clin Psychiatry 65: 222–229.
17. Liebowitz MR, Stein MB, Tancer M, Carpenter D, Oakes R, et al. (2002) A randomized, double-blind, fixed-dose comparison of paroxetine and placebo in the treatment of generalized social anxiety disorder. J Clin Psychiatry 10.4088/JCP.v63n0113.
18. Oehrberg S, Christiansen PE, Behnke K, Borup AL, Severin B, et al. (1995) Paroxetine in the treatment of panic disorder. A randomised, double-blind, placebo-controlled study. Br J Psychiatry 10.1192/bjp.167.3.374.
19. Pollack MH, Zaninelli R, Goddard A, McCafferty JP, Bellew KM, et al. (2001) Paroxetine in the treatment of generalized anxiety disorder: Results of a placebo-controlled, flexible-dosage trial. J Clin Psychiatry 62: 350–357.
20. Rickels K, Zaninelli R, McCafferty J, Bellew K, Iyengar M, et al. (2003) Paroxetine treatment of generalized anxiety disorder: A double-blind, placebo-controlled study. Am J Psychiatry 10.1176/appi.ajp.160.4.749.
21. Sheehan DV, Burnham DB, Iyengar MK, Perera P (2005) Efficacy and tolerability of controlled-release paroxetine in the treatment of panic disorder. J Clin Psychiatry 66: 33–40.
22. Stein MB, Liebowitz MR, Lydiard RB, Pitts CD, Bushnell W, et al. (1998) Paroxetine treatment of generalized social phobia (social anxiety disorder): A randomized controlled trial. JAMA 10.1001/jama.280.8.708.
23. Wagner KD, Berard R, Stein MB, Wetherhold E, Carpenter DJ, et al. (2004) A multicenter, randomized, double-blind, placebo-controlled trial of paroxetine in children and adolescents with social anxiety disorder. Arch Gen Psychiatry 10.1001/archpsyc.61.11.1153.
24. GlaxoSmithKline (2013) Paxil Medication Guide. Research Triangle Park, NC: GlaxoSmithKline. 49 p.
25. Mitte K (2005) A meta-analysis of the efficacy of psycho- and pharmacotherapy in panic disorder with and without agoraphobia. J Affect Disord 10.1016/j.jad.2005.05.003.
26. Otto MW, Tuby KS, Gould RA, McLean RY, Pollack MH (2001) An effect-size analysis of the relative efficacy and tolerability of serotonin selective reuptake inhibitors for panic disorder. Am J Psychiatry 158: 1989–1992.
27. Hamilton M (1960) A rating scale for depression. J Neurol Neurosurg Psychiatry 10.1136/jnnp.23.1.56.
28. Khin NA, Chen YF, Yang Y, Yang P, Laughren TP (2011) Exploratory analyses of efficacy data from major depressive disorder trials submitted to the US Food and Drug Administration in support of new drug applications. J Clin Psychiatry 10.4088/JCP.10m06191.
29. Hamilton M (1959) The assessment of anxiety states by rating. Br J Med Psychol 10.1111/j.2044-8341.1959.tb00467.x.
30. GlaxoSmithKline (2014) GSK Clinical Study Register. Brentford, UK: GlaxoSmithKline. Available: http://www.gsk-clinicalstudyregister.com. Accessed 10 February 2014.
31. Freedom of Information Act (FOIA) (1994 & Supp. II 1996) Freedom of Information Act (FOIA). 5 US Congress. 552.
32. Lipsey MW, Wilson DB (2001) Practical meta-analysis (applied social research methods). Thousand Oaks, CA: Sage Publications.
33. Gibbons RD, Hedeker DR, Davis JM (1993) Estimation of effect size from a series of experiments involving paired comparisons. Journal of Educational and Behavioral Statistics 10.2307/1165136.
34. Hedges LV, Olkin I (1985) Statistical methods for meta-analysis. New York, NY: Academic Press. 369 p.
35. Higgins JPT, Thompson SG (2003) Measuring inconsistency in meta-analyses. BMJ 10.1136/bmj.327.7414.557.
36. Higgins JP, Thompson SG (2002) Quantifying heterogeneity in a meta-analysis. Stat Med 10.1002/sim.1186.
37. Bond CF Jr, Wiitala WL, Richard FD (2003) Meta-analysis of raw mean differences. Psychol Methods 10.1037/1082-989X.8.4.406.
38. Khan A, Kolts RL, Thase ME, Krishnan KR, Brown W (2004) Research design features and patient characteristics associated with the outcome of antidepressant clinical trials. Am J Psychiatry 10.1176/appi.ajp.161.11.2045.
39. Fournier JC, DeRubeis RJ, Hollon SD, Dimidjian S, Amsterdam JD, et al. (2010) Antidepressant drug effects and depression severity: A patient-level meta-analysis. JAMA 10.1001/jama.2009.1943.
40. Montgomery SA, Kasper S (2007) Severe depression and antidepressants: Focus on a pooled analysis of placebo-controlled studies on agomelatine. Int Clin Psychopharmacol 10.1097/YIC.0b013e3280c56b13.
41. American Psychiatric Association Task Force for the Handbook of Psychiatric Measures (2000) Handbook of Psychiatric Measures. Washington, DC: American Psychiatric Publishing. 864 p.

42. National Center for Health & Clinical Excellence (2010) Depression: The treatment and management of depression in adults (updated edition). London: The British Psychological Society and The Royal College of Psychiatrists. 705 p.
43. National Institute for Clinical Excellence (2004) Depression: Management of depression in primary and secondary care. London: National Institute for Clinical Excellence. 670 p.
44. Hauser W, Bartram-Wunn E, Bartram C, Reinecke H, Tolle T (2011) Systematic review: Placebo response in drug trials of fibromyalgia syndrome and painful peripheral diabetic neuropathy-magnitude and patient-related predictors. Pain 10.1016/j.pain.2011.01.050.
45. Patel SM, Stason WB, Legedza A, Ock SM, Kaptchuk TJ, et al. (2005) The placebo effect in irritable bowel syndrome trials: A meta-analysis. Neurogastroenterol Motil 10.1111/j.1365-2982.2005.00650.x.
46. Dorn SD, Kaptchuk TJ, Park JB, Nguyen LT, Canenguez K, et al. (2007) A meta-analysis of the placebo response in complementary and alternative medicine trials of irritable bowel syndrome. Neurogastroenterol Motil 10.1111/j.1365-2982.2007.00937.x.
47. Cho HJ, Hotopf M, Wessely S (2005) The placebo response in the treatment of chronic fatigue syndrome: A systematic review and meta-analysis. Psychosom Med 10.1097/01.psy.0000156969.76986.e0.
48. Kroenke K, West SL, Swindle R, Gilsenan A, Eckert GJ, et al. (2001) Similar effectiveness of paroxetine, fluoxetine, and sertraline in primary care: A randomized trial. JAMA 10.1001/jama.286.23.2947.
49. Moller HJ (2008) Isn't the efficacy of antidepressants clinically relevant? A critical comment on the results of the metaanalysis by Kirsch et al. 2008. Eur Arch Psychiatry Clin Neurosci 10.1007/s00406-008-0836-5.
50. Leucht S, Fennema H, Engel R, Kaspers-Janssen M, Lepping P, et al. (2013) What does the HAMD mean? J Affect Disord 10.1016/j.jad.2012.12.001.
51. Busner J, Targum SD (2007) The clinical global impressions scale: applying a research tool in clinical practice. Psychiatry (Edgmont) 4: 28–37.
52. Imel ZE, Malterer MB, McKay KM, Wampold BE (2008) A meta-analysis of psychotherapy and medication in unipolar depression and dysthymia. J Affect Disord 10.1016/j.jad.2008.03.018.
53. Khan A, Faucett J, Lichtenberg P, Kirsch I, Brown WA (2012) A systematic review of comparative efficacy of treatments and controls for depression. PLoS One 10.1371/journal.pone.0041778.
54. Spielmans GI, Berman MI, Usitalo AN (2011) Psychotherapy versus second-generation antidepressants in the treatment of depression: a meta-analysis. J Nerv Ment Dis 10.1097/NMD.0b013e31820caefb.
55. Barlow DH, Gorman JM, Shear MK, Woods SW (2000) Cognitive-behavioral therapy, imipramine, or their combination for panic disorder: A randomized controlled trial. JAMA 10.1001/jama.283.19.2529.
56. Walkup JT, Albano AM, Piacentini J, Birmaher B, Compton SN, et al. (2008) Cognitive behavioral therapy, sertraline, or a combination in childhood anxiety. N Engl J Med 10.1056/NEJMoa0804633.
57. McHugh RK, Whitton SW, Peckham AD, Welge JA, Otto MW (2013) Patient preference for psychological vs pharmacologic treatment of psychiatric disorders: a meta-analytic review. J Clin Psychiatry 10.4088/JCP.12r07757.
58. Serretti A, Chiesa A (2009) Treatment-emergent sexual dysfunction related to antidepressants: a meta-analysis. J Clin Psychopharmacol 10.1097/JCP.0b013e3181a5233f.
59. Cascade E, Kalali AH, Kennedy SH (2009) Real-World Data on SSRI Antidepressant Side Effects. Psychiatry (Edgmont) 6: 16–18.
60. Boyer EW, Shannon M (2005) The serotonin syndrome. N Engl J Med 10.1056/NEJMra041867.
61. Carpenter DJ, Fong R, Kraus JE, Davies JT, Moore C, et al. (2011) Meta-analysis of efficacy and treatment-emergent suicidality in adults by psychiatric indication and age subgroup following initiation of paroxetine therapy: A complete set of randomized placebo-controlled trials. J Clin Psychiatry 10.4088/JCP.08m04927blu.
62. Stone M, Laughren T, Jones ML, Levenson M, Holland PC, et al. (2009) Risk of suicidality in clinical trials of antidepressants in adults: analysis of proprietary data submitted to US Food and Drug Administration. BMJ 10.1136/bmj.b2880.
63. Rosenbaum JF, Fava M, Hoog SL, Ascroft RC, Krebs WB (1998) Selective serotonin reuptake inhibitor discontinuation syndrome: a randomized clinical trial. Biol Psychiatry 10.1016/S0006-3223(98)00126-7.
64. Zimmerman M, Galione JN, Attiullah N, Friedman M, Toba C, et al. (2010) Underrecognition of clinically significant side effects in depressed outpatients. J Clin Psychiatry 10.4088/JCP.08m04978blu.
65. Pratt LA, Brody DJ, Gu Q (2011) Antidepressant use in persons aged 12 and over: United States, 2005–2008. NCHS Data Brief 76: 1–8.
66. ideaPoint (2014) Clinical Study Data Request Site. Quincy, MA: ideaPoint, Inc. Available: https://clinicalstudydatarequest.com. Accessed 9 May 2014.
67. Rickels K, Amsterdam J, Clary C, Fox I, Schweizer E, et al. (1989) A placebo-controlled, double-blind, clinical trial of paroxetine in depressed outpatients. Acta Psychiatr Scand Suppl doi:10.1111/j.1600-0447.1989.tb07188.x.
68. Rickels K, Amsterdam J, Clary C, Fox I, Schweizer E, et al. (1992) The efficacy and safety of paroxetine compared with placebo in outpatients with major depression. J Clin Psychiatry 53(Suppl): 30–32.
69. Claghorn J (1992) A double-blind comparison of paroxetine and placebo in the treatment of depressed outpatients. Int Clin Psychopharmacol 10.1097/00004850-199206004-00006.
70. Claghorn JL (1992) The safety and efficacy of paroxetine compared with placebo in a double-blind trial of depressed outpatients. J Clin Psychiatry 53(Suppl): 33–35.
71. Smith WT, Glaudin V (1992) A placebo-controlled trial of paroxetine in the treatment of major depression. J Clin Psychiatry 53(Suppl): 36–39.
72. Kiev A (1992) A double-blind, placebo-controlled study of paroxetine in depressed outpatients. J Clin Psychiatry 53(Suppl): 27–29.
73. Feighner JP, Boyer WF (1989) Paroxetine in the treatment of depression: A comparison with imipramine and placebo. Acta Psychiatr Scand Suppl 10.1111/j.1600-0447.1989.tb07190.x.
74. Feighner JP, Boyer WF (1992) Paroxetine in the treatment of depression: A comparison with imipramine and placebo. J Clin Psychiatry 53(Suppl): 44–47.
75. Cohn JB, Crowder JE, Wilcox CS, Ryan PJ (1990) A placebo- and imipramine-controlled study of paroxetine. Psychopharmacol Bull 26: 185–189.
76. Cohn JB, Wilcox CS (1992) Paroxetine in major depression: A double-blind trial with imipramine and placebo. J Clin Psychiatry 53(Suppl): 52–56.
77. Shrivastava RK, Shrivastava SH, Overweg N, Blumhardt CL (1992) A double-blind comparison of paroxetine, imipramine, and placebo in major depression. J Clin Psychiatry 53(Suppl): 48–51.
78. Peselow ED, Filippi AM, Goodnick P, Barouche F, Fieve RR (1989) The short- and long-term efficacy of paroxetine HCl. A. Data from a 6 week double-blind parallel design trial vs. imipramine and placebo. Psychopharmacol Bull 25: 267–271.
79. Fabre LF (1992) A 6-week, double-blind trial of paroxetine, imipramine, and placebo in depressed outpatients. J Clin Psychiatry 53(Suppl): 40–43.
80. Dunner DL, Dunbar GC (1992) Optimal dose regimen for paroxetine. J Clin Psychiatry 53(Suppl): 21–26.
81. Miller SM, Naylor GJ, Murtagh M, Winslow G (1989) A double-blind comparison of paroxetine and placebo in the treatment of depressed patients in a psychiatric outpatient clinic. Acta Psychiatr Scand Suppl 10.1111/j.1600-0404.1989.tb01773.x.
82. Keller MB, Ryan ND, Strober M, Klein RG, Kutcher SP, et al. (2001) Efficacy of paroxetine in the treatment of adolescent major depression: A randomized, controlled trial. J Am Acad Child Adolesc Psychiatry 10.1097/00004583-200107000-00010.
83. Golden RN (2003) Efficacy and tolerability of controlled-release paroxetine. Psychopharmacol Bull (Suppl 1): 176–186.
84. Golden RN, Nemeroff CB, McSorley P, Pitts CD, Dube EM (2002) Efficacy and tolerability of controlled-release and immediate-release paroxetine in the treatment of depression. J Clin Psychiatry 63: 577–584.
85. Rapaport MH, Schneider LS, Dunner DL, Davies JT, Pitts CD (2003) Efficacy of controlled-release paroxetine in the treatment of late-life depression. J Clin Psychiatry 64: 1065–1074.
86. Trivedi MH, Pigotti TA, Perera P, Dillingham KE, Carfagno ML, et al. (2004) Effectiveness of low doses of paroxetine controlled release in the treatment of major depressive disorder. J Clin Psychiatry 65: 1356–1364.

5

Meloxicam Blocks Neuroinflammation, but Not Depressive-Like Behaviors, in HIV-1 Transgenic Female Rats

Christina L. Nemeth[1,2], Erica R. Glasper[5], Constance S. Harrell[1,2], Sanjana A. Malviya[2], Jeffrey S. Otis[4], Gretchen N. Neigh[1,2,3]*

1 Department of Psychiatry and Behavioral Sciences, Emory University, Atlanta, Georgia, United States of America, **2** Department of Physiology, Emory University, Atlanta, Georgia, United States of America, **3** Center for Behavioral Neuroscience, Emory University, Atlanta, Georgia, United States of America, **4** Division of Pulmonary, Allergy and Critical Care Medicine, Emory University, Atlanta, Georgia, United States of America, **5** Department of Psychology, University of Maryland, College Park, Maryland, United States of America

Abstract

Adolescents living with human immunodeficiency virus (HIV) comprise approximately 12% of the HIV-positive population worldwide. HIV-positive adolescents experience a higher rate of clinical depression, a greater risk of sexual and drug abuse behaviors, and a decreased adherence to highly active antiretroviral therapies (HAART). Using adolescent HIV-1 transgenic rats (HIV-1 tg) that display related immune response alterations and pathologies, this study tested the hypothesis that developmental expression of HIV-1-related proteins induces a depressive-like phenotype that parallels a decrease in hippocampal cell proliferation and an increase in pro-inflammatory cytokine expression in the hippocampus. Consistent with this hypothesis, adolescent HIV-1 tg rats demonstrated a depressive-like behavioral phenotype, had decreased levels of cell proliferation, and exhibited elevated expression of monocyte chemotactic protein-1 (*Mcp-1*) in the hippocampus relative to controls. Subsequently, we tested the ability of meloxicam, a selective COX-2 inhibitor, to attenuate behavioral deficits via inflammatory mechanisms. Daily meloxicam treatments did not alter the behavioral profile despite effectively reducing hippocampal inflammatory gene expression. Together, these data support a biological basis for the co-morbid manifestation of depression in HIV-positive patients as early as in adolescence and suggest that modifications in behavior manifest independent of inflammatory activity in the hippocampus.

Editor: Cheryl McCormick, Brock University, Canada

Funding: The authors would like to acknowledge the financial support of The Department of Physiology, Emory University, Atlanta, GA. Additionally, this research was supported by the Creative and Novel Ideas in HIV Research Program (CNIHR) through a supplement to the University of Alabama at Birmingham (UAB) Center For AIDS Research funding (P30 AI027767-24). This funding was made possible by collaborative efforts of the Office of AIDS Research, the National Institutes of Allergies and Infectious Diseases, and the International AIDS Society. The funders had no role in study design, data collection and analysis, decision to publish, or preparation of the manuscript.

Competing Interests: The authors have declared that no competing interests exist.

* Email: gretchen.neigh@emory.edu

Introduction

Successful highly active anti-retroviral therapy (HAART) has led to the unexpected consequence of aviremic complications of human immunodeficiency virus (HIV). In addition to the high frequency of reported HIV-Associated Dementia [1], it is estimated that 30–50% of HIV-positive patients have a mood disorder such as depression, compared to 6.5% of HIV-negative individuals [2,3]. Furthermore, adolescents living with HIV are at an even higher risk of developing a mood disorder than adults living with HIV, and adolescents in general experience a greater incidence of mental health problems, including high rates of depression [4]. Depression in HIV-positive adolescents can become life-threatening as these individuals exhibit decreased adherence to HAART and other treatment plans [4–6]. Depression has also been proposed to accelerate neurocognitive impairment in HIV-positive patients [7], which is substantially higher (67%) in perinatally infected young adults, even those on successful HAART, compared to older HIV-positive individuals (19%; [8]).

While the cause of the higher incidence of depression among HIV-positive adolescents is unknown, the stigma of being HIV-positive and the burden of lifelong medication have been proposed to account for the increased incidence of depression [9]. Despite this relationship, similar associations between external stimuli and depression have been proposed and refuted in cases of late-life depression and post-stroke depression, implicating primary changes in neuronal function [10]. We hypothesize that alterations in cerebral function may also contribute to the increased incidence of depression in HIV-positive patients. One approach that allows us to disassociate the psychosocial influences of HIV infection and the environment from the biological influences of HIV is the use of model animals.

The HIV-1 transgenic (tg) rat model is a non-replicating model of HIV infection that mimics the pathogenesis of HIV-infected patients under long-term HAART control with no detectable levels of viral replication. These rats can serve as a model of HAART-controlled HIV and are used extensively to assess the effects of HIV on various biological systems especially when the focus is on vertical transmission, as expression occurs from embryogenesis [11,12]. HIV-1 tg rats contain a gag-pol-deleted HIV-1 provirus regulated by the viral long terminal repeat. As a result, no infectious virus particles are produced, but tissues express HIV-1 proteins gp120, tat, rev, and nef in lymphoid tissues with elevated concentrations in the spleen detectable by two months of age [13]. Spleen concentrations decrease with age as HIV protein concentrations increase in other tissues, including the brain [11,13]. Viral gp120 is expressed in macrophages, B and T cells, and shed into the peripheral blood reaching concentrations of 100–200 pg/ml by the time rats develop AIDS-like pathology beyond 7 months of age [14]. The HIV-1 tg rat has proven useful for the study of neurocognitive deficits [15–18] and neuroimmune dysregulation [14,19] in adult males and females [18].

While studying the underlying neurobiology of depression in the presence of HIV is important, understanding the mechanisms related to depression in females is particularly critical. The occurrence of depression and anxiety disorders in females is two times the rate in males during adulthood and as high as two and a half times the rate observed in males during adolescence [20]. Given the potential for vertical transmission by women who are not on successful HAART and the negative impact of depression on HAART compliance [21], understanding the mechanisms that mediate depression in HIV-positive adolescent females is of serious importance and has the potential for trans-generational impact. Although psychosocial factors may account for the increased incidence of depression in adolescent females living with HIV, the potential role of biological changes has not been assessed and therefore cannot be ruled out. Here, we use the HIV-1 tg rat to directly assess the hypothesis that HIV proteins can independently precipitate depressive-like behaviors in adolescent female rats. Specifically, we assess the impact of HIV proteins on two established mediators of depressive-like behaviors: cell proliferation and neuroinflammation. Furthermore, via the use of a commonly prescribed COX-2 preferential inhibitor, we determine the extent to which inflammation mediates deficits in affective behavior in the presence of HIV-1 related proteins.

Materials and Methods

Animals

Wild-type (WT; n = 9) and HIV-1 transgenic (HIV-1 tg; n = 12) rats were bred on site (HIV-1 tg breeder males obtained from Harlan Laboratories, Indianapolis, IN) and offspring were group housed with siblings after weaning. Female rats were used for all behavioral and histological assessments. No more than two pups per genotype per litter were used in each condition. Animals were kept in an AAALAC-approved temperature- and humidity-controlled facility and maintained on a 12:12 light:dark cycle with lights on at 7 AM. Food and water were available *ad libitum* and rats were individually-housed beginning 24 hours prior to behavioral testing. Rat body mass was monitored throughout the duration of study and food consumption was recorded over a two day period. All experiments were approved and performed in accordance with the Institutional Animal Care and Use Committee of Emory University and the National Institutes of Health *Guide for the Care and Use of Laboratory Animals*.

The HIV-1 tg rat (as previously described in [13]) is hemizygous NLF-3Δgag/pol and contains functional deletions of *gag* in the 3′ region and *pol* in the 5′ region. HIV-1 tg rats manifest clinical signs and symptoms of HIV, including neurological changes, respiratory difficulty, and cataracts. Rats develop normally; however, by six months of age the rats experience poor weight gain and muscle atrophy that continues over time. The studies conducted here were completed well before 6 months of age and prior to the onset of the documented pathologies. Because these rats are hemizygous, WT littermates can be used as controls. An equal number of pups from each litter were included in all groups. Our examinations of developmental behavior and cell proliferation began at post-natal day (PND) 48 and were completed by PND 58.

Behavioral Testing

Each genotype was assessed using an extensive behavioral phenotyping schedule which included primary, secondary, and tertiary indices of behavior (adapted from Urbach *et al.* [22]). Primary behaviors were comprised of assessments of general health (appearance and weight), neurological reflexes, neuromuscular strength, and sensory function. Secondary behaviors included motor function and social behavior. Tertiary behavioral paradigms examined depressive- and anxiety-like behaviors. All behavioral observations took place during the animals' light cycle and were performed in order of increasing anxiogenesis: primary behaviors (Day 1), sucrose consumption test (Days 1–3), open field paradigm (Day 4), social interaction (Day 5), and the Porsolt forced swim test (Day 6). All rats were tested in a room separate from other animals. Behavioral tests and scoring rubric were modified from Korenova *et al.* [23].

Primary Behaviors

Surface righting: Rats were placed in a supine position and the latency to correct itself was measured (Latency <1 second = 0 points; latency ≥ 1 second = 1 point). Prehensile traction: Rats were allowed to grasp onto a wire cage lid at which point the lid is slowly inverted and the latency to fall was measured (latency $>$ 15.1 seconds = 0 points, 10.1–15 seconds = 1 point; 6.1–10 seconds = 2 points; 4.1–6.0 seconds = 3 points; 2.1–4.0 seconds = 4 points; <2 seconds = 5 points). Balance: Rats were placed in an empty cage that is rapidly moved from side to side and up and down. Normal posture is to extend all four legs and maintain an upright and balanced position (normal = 0, abnormal = 1). Audition: Two metal rods were tapped and startle response was observed (startle = 0, no startle = 1). Points for each behavior were averaged by group and compared.

Secondary Behaviors

Overall activity: Distance traveled and velocity were measured over 10 minutes in an open field arena measuring 75 cm×75 cm and scored by Cleversys automated tracking system (Reston, VA). Social interaction: The test began with the placement of the experimental rat in the center of the arena. Each rat was allowed to explore a 75 cm×75 cm arena containing a same sex and age matched stimulus rat. Latency to first interaction as well as total time interacting were measured [24].

Tertiary Behaviors

Sucrose consumption: Rats were given equal access to bottles containing a 0.9% sucrose solution or tap water. Following a 24-hour habituation, we assessed sucrose consumption by recording the volume (extrapolated from grams) of solution consumed over a 24 hour period. Presentation of bottles was reversed after the first 24 hours to prevent a side bias. A decrease in sucrose consumption relative to control rats is used as an index of anhedonic-like behaviors [25]. Open field: Rats were allowed to explore a

75 cm×75 cm arena for 10 minutes. Time spent in the center of the arena versus the periphery was used as a measure of anxiety-like behavior [26]. The test began on Day 4 with the placement of the experimental rat in the center of the arena. Behavior was videotaped and scored by Cleversys automated behavioral software. Porsolt forced swim: Rats were placed in a swim tank for 10 minutes during which time the amount of time spent struggling (defined as breaking the surface of the water with the forepaws) and time spent immobile (defined as limbs stationary for at least 2 seconds) was assessed as an index of depressive-like behaviors [27]. Latency to first bout of immobility was also recorded. As with open field, behavior was videotaped and scored automatically.

Cell Proliferation

Twenty-four hours following the last behavioral test, all rats were anesthetized and transcardially perfused with 4% paraformaldehyde. Brains were removed and stored in 4% paraformaldehyde at 4°C for at least 24 hours prior to sectioning. Brains were hemisected and one hemisphere was vibratome sectioned at 40 µm throughout the entire rostrocaudal extent of the dentate gyrus. Every 12th serial section was mounted on clear Superfrost Plus Microscope Slides (Fisher Brand Scientific, Pittsburgh, PA) and allowed to dry overnight. Slides were then incubated in a 0.1 mol/L citric acid for 40 minutes at 90°C. After a 10 minute incubation in a 3% H_2O_2 solution, slides were rinsed with phosphate buffered saline (PBS, pH 7.4) and incubated at room temperature overnight in primary (1:100; mouse monoclonal anti-Ki67 [Vector Laboratories, Burlingame, CA] in 0.3% Triton X-100 and 2% normal horse serum in PBS). Twenty-four hours later, slides were rinsed in PBS before entering secondary incubation (1:200; biotinylated horse anti-mouse, Vector Laboratories) for 1 hour. Slides were again rinsed in PBS and then reacted with a mouse Vectastain ABC Elite kit (Vector Laboratories) solution for 30 minutes according to manufacturer's instructions (Vector Laboratories) followed by a 10 minute 0.01% diaminobenzidine with 0.003% H_2O_2 (Sigma-Aldrich, St. Louis, MO) incubation. Slides were then rinsed in PBS, dried, counterstained with cresyl violet, cleared in xylene, and coverslipped with Permount (Fisher Brand Scientific).

Gene Expression

A separate cohort of rats raised under the same conditions (WT n = 10; HIV-1 tg n = 9), was used for gene expression analysis. Animals were rapidly decapitated, brain tissue was dissected frozen under RNAse-free conditions, and the hippocampus was isolated for analysis. Samples were then homogenized using the Qiagen RNeasy Mini Kit (Valencia, CA) according to manufacturer's instructions. RNA samples were reverse transcribed using Applied Biosystem's High Capacity cDNA Reverse Transcription Kit. Resulting cDNA was then quantified and normalized using the PicoGreen method (Invitrogen, Grand Island, NY). The TaqMan gene expression system was used for the detection of monocyte chemotactic protein-1 (*Mcp-1*; Rn00580555_m1), interleukin-1β (*Il-1β*; Rn00580432_m1), nuclear factor-kappa-β inhibitor, α (*Nf-κBiα*; RN01473654_g1), tumor necrosis factor (*Tnf*; Rn00562055_m1), and standardized to β-actin (Rn00667869_m1). All samples were prepared in triplicate using 1 µg of sample and carried out on an Applied Biosystems HT7900 Fast Real-Time PCR system. Data were averaged by group and analyzed via the $\Delta\Delta C_t$ method.

Meloxicam Administration

A third cohort of animals (WT n = 5; HIV-1 tg n = 9) received oral meloxicam (1 mg/kg) daily starting at weaning (PND 25) and continuing throughout the duration of the study. Behavioral testing and hippocampal gene expression of *Mcp-1* were measured as described above. Because several studies have demonstrated that daily administration of COX-2 inhibitors does not augment cell proliferation [28–30], expression of Ki-67 was not assessed in these animals.

Data Analysis

For all analyses, data were averaged by genotype and compared via one-tailed unpaired t-tests. Statistical outliers were identified by the Grubbs' outlier test and removed. Group sizes varied slightly due to the presence of statistical outliers as well as errors with video recording and/or scoring software.

For secondary and tertiary behaviors, group totals were averaged by genotype and are presented as percent of control. Rt-PCR results were averaged by genotype and analyzed via the $2^{-\Delta\Delta Ct}$ method. Specifically, fold change was calculated, standardized to a housekeeping gene (*β-actin*), and normalized to WT or vehicle treated animals.

For quantification of Ki67, slides were coded prior to data collection. The code was broken after analyses were completed. Ki67-labeled cells in the granule cell layer, subgranular zone, and hilus of the hippocampal dentate gyrus were exhaustively counted at 100× on a Zeiss Primo Star light microscope (Thornwood, NY). One hemisphere of each brain was analyzed and counts were multiplied by 24 (to account for opposite hemisphere and sampling fraction) to obtain estimates of Ki67-labeled cells in the dentate gyrus per brain.

All statistical tests were performed using GraphPad Prism 6, and differences were considered statistically significant if $p<0.05$.

Results

HIV-1 tg rats have minimal differences in general health and primary behaviors

Body mass differed between HIV-1 tg rats and WT litter-mate controls such that transgenic rats weighed less than controls ($t[15] = 7.12$, $p<0.05$); however, total food consumed over a two-day period did not differ between WT and HIV-1 tg rats ($p>0.05$; Table 1). Nominal scale results reveal few errors in HIV-1 tg rats' balance and no detected errors in surface righting or audition. Further, indices of grip strength (prehensile tension) were normal, suggesting behavioral effects were not due to signs of early muscle wasting (summarized in Table 1).

HIV-1 tg adolescent rats exhibit elevated levels of depressive-like behaviors

HIV-1 tg rats had similar latencies to first bout of floating as WT littermates ($p>0.05$); however, HIV-1 tg rats spent more time immobile than WT controls ($t[12] = 2.420$, $p<0.05$; Figure 1A). In the social interaction test, HIV-1 tg rats exhibited an increased latency to interact with a novel animal ($t[13] = 2.682$, $p<0.05$; Figure 1B). Furthermore, HIV-1 tg rats spent less time interacting with the novel stimulus rat as compared WT controls ($t[16] = 3.237$, $p<0.05$; Figure 1C).

Despite a depressive-like phenotype in the Porsolt forced swim and social interaction tests, when corrected for body mass, WT and HIV-1 tg rats consumed similar volumes of sucrose over a 24-

Table 1. Summary and mean scores of primary behaviors.

	Body Mass (g)	Food Consumption (g)	Balance (0–1)	Surface Righting (0–1)	Audition (0–1)	Prehensile Traction (0–5)
WT	120.0±4.163	10.0±1.472	0	0	0	0
HIV-1 tg	90.4±1.945*	8.25±0.250	0.2	0	0	0

Wild-type (WT) and HIV-1 transgenic (HIV-1 tg) rats were assessed using an extensive behavioral phenotyping schedule of primary, secondary, and tertiary behaviors. Mean body mass and food consumption are shown for adolescent WT and HIV-1 tg rats. Mean scores of neurologic tests, muscular strength, and sensory function are shown. Compared to WT controls, HIV-1 tg rats had decreased body mass at post-natal day 48, or the first day of behavioral testing (*$p<0.05$). Despite this, no differences were detected in any other measure.

hour test period in the sucrose consumption test (WT: 0.182±0.021 g of sucrose/g of animal; HIV-1 tg: 0.196±0.009 g of sucrose/g of animal; $p>0.05$).

HIV-1 tg rats exhibit normal activity but a trend towards increased anxiety-like behavior

Total distance traveled and central tendency were measured during the 10 minute open field test. WT and HIV-1 tg adolescent

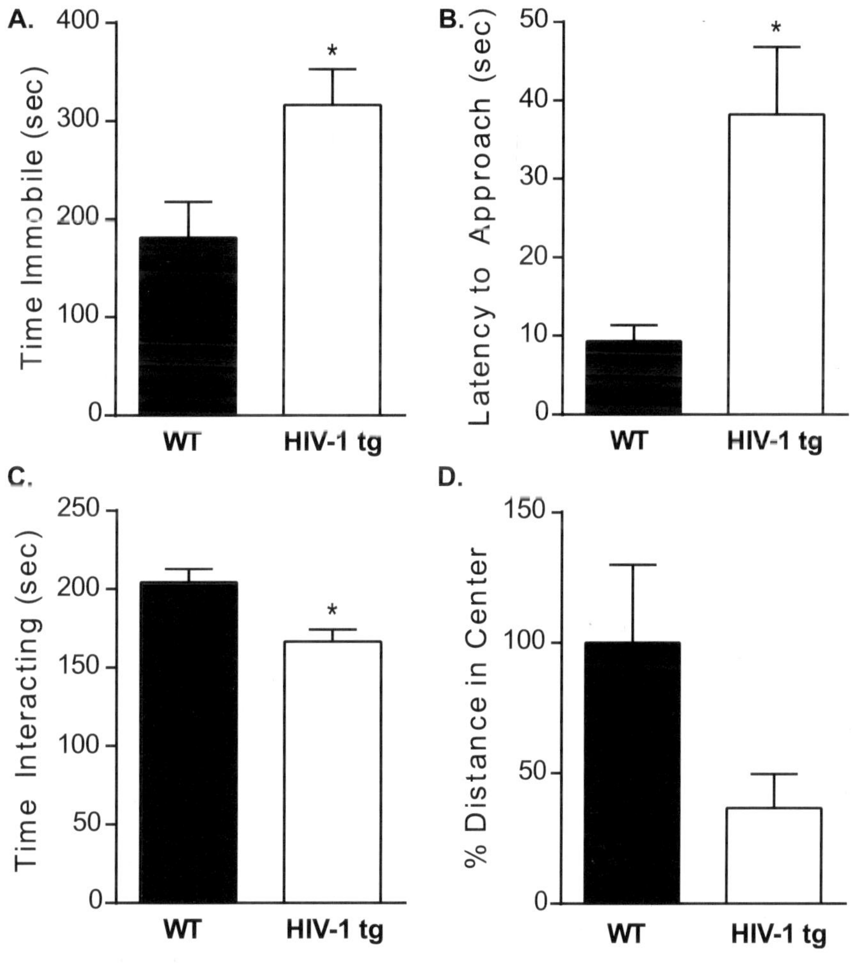

Figure 1. Rats were assessed in a battery of behavioral tests of depressive- and anxiety-like behaviors. *A,B*) In the forced swim test, latency to first immobile bout was not different between WT and HIV-1 tg rats ($p>0.05$); but HIV-1 tg rats spent significantly more time immobile in the test relative to WT controls. To measure social interaction, WT and HIV-1 tg rats were presented with an age-matched stimulus conspecific and allowed to interact for 10 minutes. *C,D*) HIV-1 tg rats had a greater latency to approach the stimulus animal (*$p<0.05$) and spent less total time interacting, relative to WT controls. The open field paradigm was used to assess anxiety-like behaviors over a 10 minute period. Total distance traveled as well as distance traveled in the center was recorded. *E*) Total activity was unchanged between WT and HIV-1 tg rats as measured in 75 cm×75 cm arena during the open field test ($p>0.05$). *F*) Compared to WT controls, HIV-1 tg rats showed decreased activity in the center of the open field suggestive of increased anxiety-like behavior. For all, *$p<0.05$ and data are presented as mean ± SEM.

rats had similar levels of activity (WT: 34.16±6.81 m; HIV-1 tg: 37.21±3.17 m); however, HIV-1 tg rats exhibit a trend towards decreased activity in the center of the open field when compared to litter-mate controls (t[14] = 2.062, $p = 0.07$; Figure 1D).

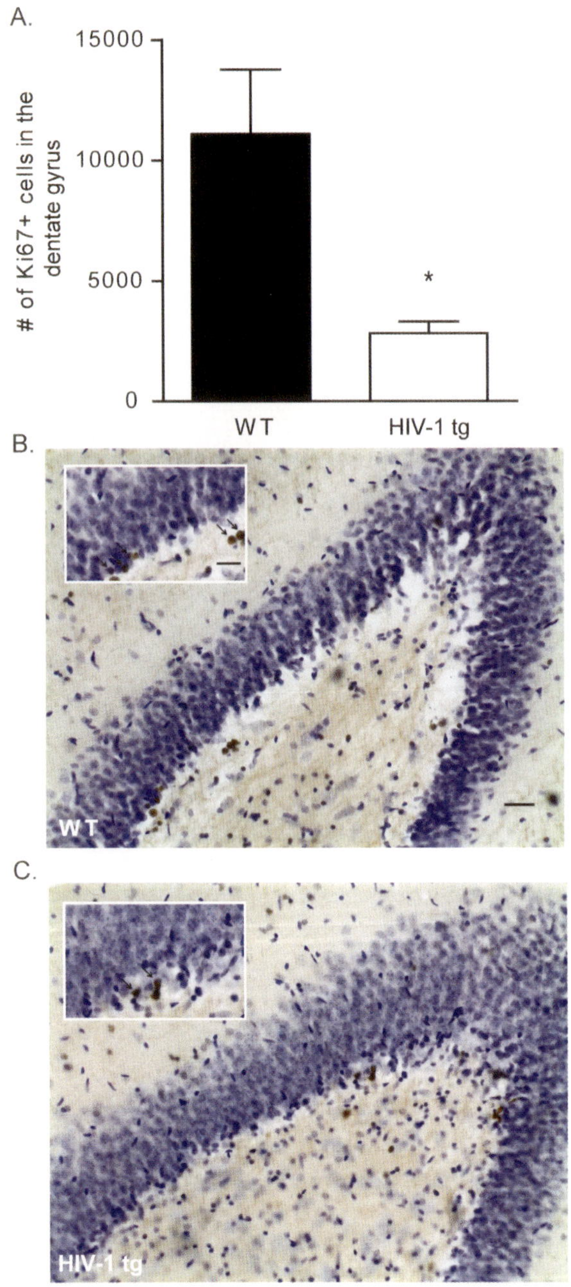

Figure 2. WT and HIV-1 tg brains were sectioned and stained for Ki-67 reactivity as a measure of cell proliferation. (A) HIV-1 tg brains had significantly decreased levels of cell proliferation in the dentate gyrus of the hippocampus as compared to WT brains (*$p < 0.05$). Data are presented as mean ± SEM. (B) Photomicrograph of hemisection containing Ki-67 stained cells in the dentate gyrus of a WT rat. Inset highlights dense region of Ki-67 positive cells, marked with arrows. (C) Photomicrograph of Ki-67 stained cells in a HIV-1 tg rat. Again, insert highlights region of Ki-67 stained cells marked with arrows. Images captured at 20x, scale bar equals 50 μM.

HIV-1 tg rats have decreased levels of hippocampal cell proliferation

Ki67 reactivity in the dentate gyrus was used as an index of cell proliferation. Data reveal that HIV-1 tg rats had significantly fewer Ki67-positively stained cells relative to WT controls (t[18] = 3.728, $p < 0.05$; Figure 2A).

HIV-1 tg rats display increased *Mcp-1* gene expression in the hippocampus

Post-mortem assessment of gene expression for inflammatory markers indicated that hippocampal expression of *Mcp-1* was significantly increased in HIV-1 tg rats as compared to WT controls (t[15] = 2.015, $p < 0.05$; Figure 3A). No group differences were detected in gene expression levels of *Il-1β* (fold change: 0.968±0.144), *NF-κBia* (fold change: 1.475±0.271), and *Tnf* (fold change: 1.007±0.353) in the hippocampus ($p > 0.05$; data not shown).

Meloxicam treatment reduces *Mcp-1*, but does not rescue behavior

Importantly, meloxicam administration attenuated expression of *Mcp-1* in the hippocampus of female adolescent HIV-1 tg rats. A t-test of *Mcp-1* gene expression revealed no difference between HIV-1 tg rats given meloxicam as compared to WT meloxicam-treated rats (t[15] = 0.718, $p > 0.05$; Figure 3B). Once daily meloxicam treatment did not alter body mass in WT (126.0±3.567 g) or HIV-1 tg (103.5±2.678 g) rats.

Conversely, daily meloxicam administration did not attenuate the behavioral deficits in the HIV-1 tg rats. Latencies to first float were comparable between WT and HIV-1 tg rats in the forced swim test (WT: 108.4±55.56 sec; HIV-1 tg: 172.1±53.03 sec); however, overall, HIV-1 tg rats spent more time immobile when compared to WT meloxicam-treated rats (t[12] = 2.207, $p < 0.05$;

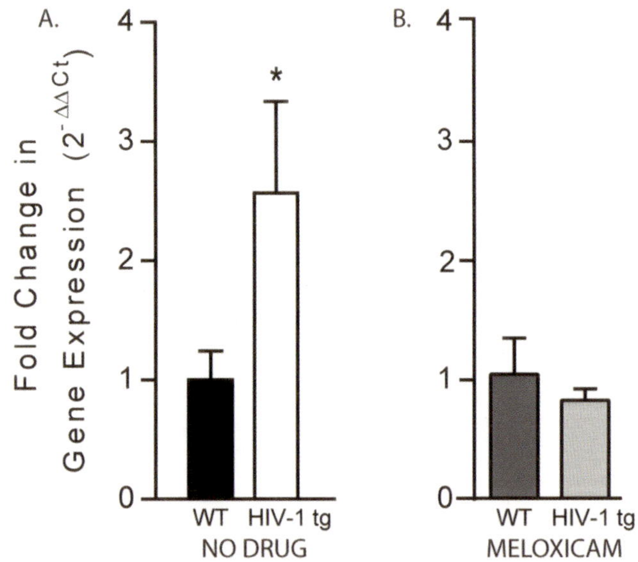

Figure 3. The effect of HIV related proteins on hippocampal inflammation was measured in adolescent WT and HIV-1 tg rats. *A)* Analysis of hippocampal gene expression of inflammatory markers showed increased expression of the potent chemokine, *Mcp-1*, in non-drug treated HIV-1 tg rats compared to WT controls (*$p < 0.05$). *B)* In contrast, once daily meloxicam administration attenuated *Mcp-1* expression in HIV-1 tg rats, normalizing inflammatory gene expression to WT levels ($p > 0.05$). Data are presented as mean ± SEM.

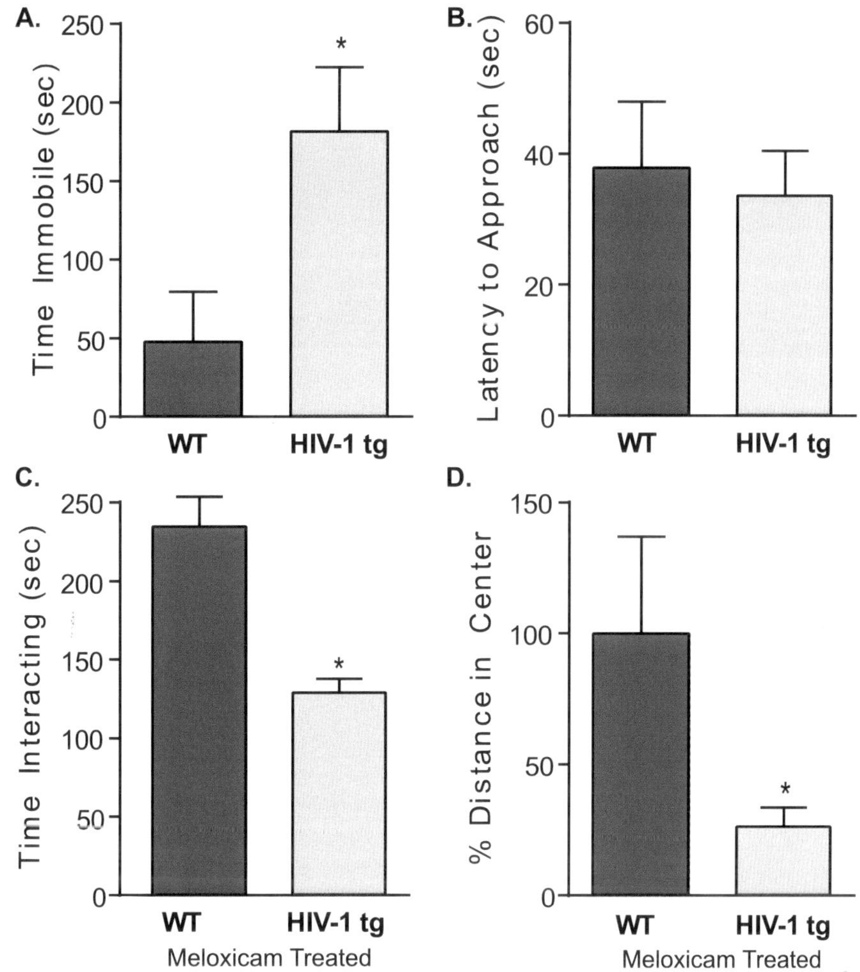

Figure 4. Depressive- and anxiety-like behaviors were measured in WT and HIV-1 tg rats receiving daily oral dosing of meloxicam. *A,B*) In the Porsolt forced swim test, meloxicam treated WT and HIV-1 tg rats showed similar latencies to first float ($p>0.05$); however, HIV-1 tg rats spent more time immobile compared to WT controls (*$p<0.05$). *C,D*) Similarly, in the social interaction test, meloxicam treated WT and HIV-1 tg rats showed no differences in their time to approach a stimulus rat ($p>0.05$); however, overall, meloxicam-treated HIV-1 tg rats spend less time interacting (*$p<0.05$). *E,F*) In the open field test, meloxicam treated HIV-1 tg rats showed no differences in overall locomotion ($p>0.05$), but did show a significant decrease in distance traveled in the center of the open field, as compared to WT rats (*$p<0.05$). Data are presented as mean ± SEM.

Figure 4A). WT and HIV-1 tg rats had similar latencies to approach a novel conspecific (Figure 4B); but, HIV-1 tg rats spent less overall time interacting compared to meloxicam-treated WT controls (t[12] = 2.564, $p<0.05$; Figure 4C).

In terms of anxiety-like behaviors, total distance traveled did not statistically differ between WT and HIV-1 tg meloxicam-treated rats (WT: 26.15±5.39 m; HIV-1 tg: 15.77±2.99 m; $p>0.05$); however, meloxicam-treated rats traveled less in the center of the open field compared to WT controls (t[11] = 2.859, $p<0.05$; Figure 4D).

Discussion

Expression of HIV-1 proteins triggered depressive-like and anxiety-like behaviors in adolescent female rats and reduced cell proliferation in the dentate gyrus of the hippocampus, concomitant with increased expression of *Mcp-1*. Given that *Mcp-1* is increased in the hippocampi of HIV-1 tg adolescent female rats, and given the potential role of neuroinflammation in altered affective-like behavior, we tested the hypothesis that affective-like behavior was driven by inflammatory mechanisms. Meloxicam, frequently prescribed for osteoarthritis, was selected to block inflammation in the current set of experiments due to its highly potent inhibition of prostaglandin synthetase and low level of gastrointestinal toxicity as demonstrated in both humans and model animal systems [31,32]. While inhibition of *Mcp-1* in the hippocampus of HIV-1 tg rats by oral meloxicam treatment does not attenuate the presence or degree of behavioral disruption, future work is necessary to determine if there is a functional link between the observed decreased basal rate of cell proliferation and the increased depressive- and anxiety-like behavior in the HIV-1 tg rat. At present, we can conclude that expression of HIV-1 proteins during development is sufficient, in the absence of stress or other psychosocial and environmental factors, to precipitate increased depressive-like and anxiety-like behaviors in adolescent females. This finding is important because it draws attention to a potential neurobiological basis for the increased incidence of depression in HIV-positive individuals. Furthermore, the HIV-1 tg rat may provide a model system in which novel antidepressant therapies can be assessed.

Although rodents are incapable of experiencing depression to the same extent as humans, core symptoms of the disease can be manipulated and assessed in a rodent model. Social withdrawal is a hallmark symptom of clinical depression and is an ethologically relevant metric of depressive-like behaviors in rodent models [33,34]. When presented with a stimulus animal in the social interaction task, HIV-1 tg rats exhibit a greater latency to approach a novel conspecific, in addition to a decrease in the total time interacting with the novel conspecific. Importantly, this behavior is not confounded by an overall deficit of motor ability or activity. Furthermore, this social withdrawal is consistent with performance in the Porsolt forced swim test, the most widely used paradigm of depressive-like behaviors [35], in which HIV-1 tg rats spent more time immobile compared to WT controls. The same pattern is apparent for rats receiving daily meloxicam administration. However, it may be important to note that meloxicam-treated rats show an insignificant decrease in overall activity, suggestive of an interaction between drug treatment and locomotor ability, despite no change in body mass compared to non-treated animals and reports that meloxicam is well tolerated by rodents [36]. Finally, depressive behaviors in the social interaction test and Porsolt forced swim paradigm were apparent in the absence of altered sucrose consumption, which may be due to differences in metabolic rates between WT and HIV-1 tg rats. When corrected for weight, HIV-1 tg rats consumed similar volumes of a sucrose solution compared to WT rats and similar amounts of chow in the home cage, despite a more than 30 g difference in body weight between WT and HIV-1 tg rats.

In adulthood, HIV-1 tg rats develop pathology consistent with human AIDS [13]; however, in the current study, increases in depressive- and anxiety-like behavior are detectable before such pervasive alterations in general health and mobility occur. Our testing began on PND 48, and at this time, neurological reflexes, neuromuscular strength, and sensory function were indistinguishable from WT litter-mate controls. Therefore, these data support the sufficiency of HIV-1 related proteins, in the absence of additional stressors or active virus replication, to precipitate deficits in affective-like behavior.

Increased peripheral circulating inflammatory biomarkers are well established in major depressive disorders as well as other disease states [37,38]. Similarly, given that HIV in humans is marked by a pronounced inflammatory response in the brain and periphery that is believed to contribute to the neuropathology of the disease [39,40] and HIV-associated dementias [41], we examined inflammatory activity in the hippocampus as a potential mechanism driving behavior. Measures of inflammatory cytokines in the hippocampi of adolescent HIV-1 tg rats reveals increased expression of *Mcp-1*, a pro-inflammatory biomarker produced by macrophages and endothelial cells that is elevated in cases of major depression [42–44]. However, no differences were observed in the expression of *Il-1β*, *Nf-κBia*, or *Tnf* in the hippocampus. Despite the involvement of proinflammatory cytokines in HIV-1 related pathology, depressive disorders, [42,43,45] and decreased cell proliferation [30,46], daily administration of meloxicam, a selective COX-2 inhibitor, had no effect on affective behavior notwithstanding the attenuation of increased expression of *Mcp-1* in the hippocampus. These findings suggest that the manifestation of altered affective-like behaviors in the presence of HIV-1 related proteins does not stem from inflammatory mechanisms and that dysregulation of other systems may play a larger role in the HIV-1 related behavioral phenotype. Previous groups have associated inflammatory activity in the presence of HIV-1 proteins, either in adult whole brain lysate immediately following *tat* administration [47] or in frontal cortex brain lysate of the adult male tg rat [48]. With this said, inflammatory activation in adolescent HIV-1 tg rats appears to be limited to the expression of *Mcp-1* and rampant HIV-related inflammation may not be apparent at this early stage. As such, *Mcp-1* may serve as an early indicator of HIV-1 associated disease progression independent of behavior. Alternatively, it has been hypothesized that inflammatory activation in HIV rodent models is due to the neurotoxic effects of gp120 and tat on neurons and astrocytes and is not a result of HIV-1 related pathology [48]. However, due to the limited inflammatory response observed in adolescent HIV-1 tg rats and sustained altered affective-like behavior in the absence of *Mcp-1* activation, it is unlikely that inflammation drives behavioral change in the HIV-1 tg rat.

Consistent with the manifestation of depressive-like behaviors observed in adolescent HIV-1 tg rats, the current study demonstrates that developmental expression of HIV-1 related proteins results in decreased levels of cell proliferation in the dentate gyrus of the hippocampus. Ki67 is present in almost all phases of the cell cycle, with the exception of G_0, making it a suitable marker for proliferating progenitor cells [49], a precursor for neurogenesis in regions of the hippocampus [50]. Decreases in cell proliferation, as indicated by Ki67, have been recorded in other instances of depressive-like states in rodents, including in dams who have experienced repeated separation from their pups [50] and in rats who have experienced chronic stress [51]. Furthermore, morphologic and volumetric differences observed in the hippocampi of patients with major depressive disorders [52–54] are paralleled by a decrease of adult hippocampal neurogenesis [55]. The neurogenesis hypothesis of major depression suggests that decreases in cell proliferation may underlie structural alterations within the adult brain, an effect that has been reversed by the administration of classic anti-depressant treatments in the dentate gyrus of the human, rodent, and non-human primate brain [56,57].

The rates of clinical depression and depressive symptomatology among the adult HIV-positive population are higher than observed in the general population [58] and adolescents living with HIV-1 are at a higher risk of psychiatric illness and risk-taking behaviors [59]. We show here that the developmental expression of HIV-1 related proteins is sufficient to induce depressive-like behaviors in adolescent rats, cause a decrease in cellular proliferation in the dentate gyrus of the hippocampus, and lead to increased expression of hippocampal *Mcp-1*. Further, blockade of *Mcp-1* in the adolescent female HIV-1 tg rat fails to attenuate the presence or degree of depressive-like behavioral disruption. These findings are important because they demonstrate that depressive-like behaviors, decreased cell proliferation, and increased neuroinflammation can be induced by the presence of HIV proteins in the absence of active virus and that behavioral despair is not driven by *Mcp-1* activation. These data suggest that HIV-associated depression may have a neurobiological basis that is separate from either the psychosocial impact of the disease or the rampant neuroinflammation characteristic of neuroAIDS.

Acknowledgments

The authors would also like to thank Sean D. Kelly and Leah Chisholm for their assistance with this work.

Author Contributions

Conceived and designed the experiments: GNN CLN. Performed the experiments: CLN CSH SAM ERG. Analyzed the data: CLN CSH SAM ERG. Contributed reagents/materials/analysis tools: JSO. Contributed to the writing of the manuscript: CLN GNN.

References

1. Simioni S, Cavassini M, Annoni J-M, Rimbault A, Bourquin I, et al. (2010) Cognitive dysfunction in HIV patients despite long-standing suppression of viremia. AIDS: 1243–1250. doi:10.1097/QAD.0b013e3283354a7b.
2. Hinkin C, Castellon S, Durvasula R, Hardy D, Lam M, et al. (2002) Medication adherence among HIV+ adults. Neurology 59: 1944–1950.
3. Lopes M (2012) Gender, HIV Status, and Psychiatric Disorders: Results From the National Epidemiologic Survey on Alcohol and Related Conditions. Psychiatry Interpers Biol Process: 384–391. doi:10.4088/JCP.10m06304.
4. Williams PL, Leister E, Chernoff M, Nachman S, Morse E, et al. (2010) Substance use and its association with psychiatric symptoms in perinatally HIV-infected and HIV-affected adolescents. AIDS Behav 14: 1072–1082. doi:10.1007/s10461-010-9782-0.
5. Mellins CA, Tassiopoulos K, Malee K, Moscicki A-B, Patton D, et al. (2014) Behavioral health risks in perinatally HIV-exposed youth: co-occurrence of sexual and drug use behavior, mental health problems, and nonadherence to antiretroviral treatment. AIDS Patient Care STDS 25: 413–422. doi:10.1089/apc.2011.0025.
6. Byakika-Tusiime J, Crane J, Oyugi JH, Ragland K, Kawuma A, et al. (2009) Longitudinal antiretroviral adherence in HIV+ Ugandan parents and their children initiating HAART in the MTCT-Plus family treatment model: role of depression in declining adherence over time. AIDS Behav 13 Suppl 1: 82–91. doi:10.1007/s10461-009-9546-x.
7. Bragança M, Palha A (2011) Depression and neurocognitive performance in Portuguese patients infected with HIV. AIDS Behav 15: 1879–1887. doi:10.1007/s10461-011-9973-3.
8. Paramesparan Y, Garvey L, Ashby J, Foster C, Fidler S, et al. (2010) High Rates of Asymptomatic Neurocogntivie Impairment in Vertically Acquired HIV-1-Infected Adolescents Surviving to Adulthood. J Acquir Immune Defic Syndr 55: 132–136.
9. Chaudoir SR, Norton WE, Earnshaw VA, Moneyham L, Mugavero MJ, et al. (2011) Coping with HIV Stigma: Do Proactive Coping and Spiritual Peace Buffer the Effect of Stigma on Depression? AIDS Behav 16: 2382–2391. doi:10.1007/s10461-011-0039-3.
10. Neigh GN, Karelina K, Zhang N, Glasper ER, Owens MJ, et al. (2009) Cardiac arrest and cardiopulmonary resuscitation dysregulates the hypothalamic-pituitary-adrenal axis. J Cereb Blood Flow Metab 29: 1673–1682. doi:10.1038/jcbfm.2009.85.
11. Peng J, Vigorito M, Liu X, Zhou D, Wu X, et al. (2010) The HIV-1 transgenic rat as a model for HIV-1 infected individuals on HAART. J Neuroimmunol 218: 94–101. doi:10.1016/j.jneuroim.2009.09.014.
12. Ray P, Liu X-H, Robinson L, Reid W, Xu L, et al. (2003) A novel HIV-1 transgenic rat model of childhood HIV-1– associated nephropathy. Kidney Int 63: 2242–2253.
13. Reid W, Sadowska M, Denaro F, Rao S, Foulke J, et al. (2001) An HIV-1 transgenic rat that develops HIV-related pathology and immunologic dysfunction. P Natl Acad Sci USA 98: 9271–9276. doi:10.1073/pnas.161290298.
14. Reid W, Abdelwahab S, Sadowska M, Huso D, Neal A, et al. (2004) HIV-1 transgenic rats develop T cell abnormalities. Virology 321: 111–119. doi:10.1016/j.virol.2003.12.010.
15. Vigorito M, LaShomb AL, Chang SL (2007) Spatial learning and memory in HIV-1 transgenic rats. J Neuroimmune Pharmacol 2: 319–328. doi:10.1007/s11481-007-9078-y.
16. Lashomb AL, Vigorito M, Chang SL (2009) Further characterization of the spatial learning deficit in the human immunodeficiency virus-1 transgenic rat. J Neurovirol 15: 14–24. doi:10.1080/13550280802232996.
17. Moran L, Aksenov M, Booze R, Webb K, Mactutus C (2013) Adolescent HIV-1 transgenic rats: Evidence for dopaminergic alterations in behavior and neurochemistry revealed by methamphetamine challenge. Curr HIV Res 10: 415–424.
18. Moran LM, Booze RM, Webb KM, Mactutus CF (2013) Neurobehavioral alterations in HIV-1 transgenic rats: evidence for dopaminergic dysfunction. Exp Neurol 239: 139–147. doi:10.1016/j.expneurol.2012.10.008.
19. Rao JS, Kim H-W, Kellom M, Greenstein D, Chen M, et al. (2011) Increased neuroinflammatory and arachidonic acid cascade markers, and reduced synaptic proteins, in brain of HIV-1 transgenic rats. J Neuroinflamm 8: 101. doi:10.1186/1742-2094-8-101.
20. National Survey on Drug Use and Health (2012) Depression triples between the ages of 12 and 15 among adolescent girls.
21. Kacanek D, Jacobson DL, Spiegelman D, Wanke C, Isaac R, et al. (2010) Incident depression symptoms are associated with poorer HAART adherence: a longitudinal analysis from the Nutrition for Healthy Living study. J Acquir Immune Defic Syndr 53: 266–272. doi:10.1097/QAI.0b013e3181b720e7.
22. Urbach YK, Bode FJ, Nguyen HP, Riess O, Hörsten S Von (2010) Rat Genomics. Methods 597. doi:10.1007/978-1-60327-389-3.
23. Korenova M, Zilka N, Stozicka Z, Bugos O, Vanicky I, et al. (2009) NeuroScale, the battery of behavioral tests with novel scoring system for phenotyping of transgenic rat model of tauopathy. J Neurosci Methods 177: 108–114. doi:10.1016/j.jneumeth.2008.09.027.
24. File SE, Hyde JR (1978) Can social interaction be used to measure anxiety? Br J Pharmacol 62: 19–24.
25. Willner P, Towell A, Sampson D, Sophokleous S, Muscat R (1987) Reduction of sucrose preference by chronic unpredictable mild stress, and its restoration by a tricyclic antidepressant. Psychopharmacology (Berl) 93: 358–364.
26. Prut L, Belzung C (2003) The open field as a paradigm to measure the effects of drugs on anxiety-like behaviors: a review. Eur J Pharmacol 463: 3–33. doi:10.1016/S0014-2999(03)01272-X.
27. Porsolt R, Anton G, Blavet N, Jalfre M (1978) Behavioral despair in rats: A new model sensitive to antidepressant treatments. Eur J Pharmacol 47: 379–391.
28. Goncalves MB, Williams E-J, Yip P, Yáñez-Muñoz RJ, Williams G, et al. (2010) The COX-2 inhibitors, meloxicam and nimesulide, suppress neurogenesis in the adult mouse brain. Br J Pharmacol 159: 1118–1125. doi:10.1111/j.1476-5381.2009.00618.x.
29. Jung K-H, Chu K, Lee S-T, Kim J, Sinn D-I, et al. (2006) Cyclooxygenase-2 inhibitor, celecoxib, inhibits the altered hippocampal neurogenesis with attenuation of spontaneous recurrent seizures following pilocarpine-induced status epilepticus. Neurobiol Dis 23: 237–246. doi:10.1016/j.nbd.2006.02.016.
30. Russo I, Amornphimoltham P, Weigert R, Barlati S, Bosetti F (2011) Cyclooxygenase-1 is involved in the inhibition of hippocampal neurogenesis after lipopolysaccharide-induced neuroinflammation. Cell Cycle 10: 2568–2573. doi:10.4161/cc.10.15.15946.
31. Ahmed M, Khanna D, Furst DE (2005) Meloxicam in rheumatoid arthritis. Expert Opin Drug Metab Toxicol 1: 739–751. doi:10.1517/17425255.1.4.739.
32. Engelhardt G (1996) Pharmacology of meloxicam, a new non-steroidal anti-inflammatory drug with an improved safety profile through preferential inhibition of COX-2. Br J Rheumatol 35 Suppl 1: 4–12.
33. Fischer CW, Liebenberg N, Elfving B, Lund S, Wegener G (2012) Isolation-induced behavioural changes in a genetic animal model of depression. Behav Brain Res 230: 85–91. doi:10.1016/j.bbr.2012.01.050.
34. Derntl B, Seidel E-M, Eickhoff SB, Kellermann T, Gur RC, et al. (2011) Neural correlates of social approach and withdrawal in patients with major depression. Soc Neurosci 6: 482–501. doi:10.1080/17470919.2011.579800.
35. Detke MJ, Rickels M, Lucki I (1995) Active behaviors in the rat forced swimming test differentially produced by serotonergic and noradrenergic antidepressants. Psychopharmacology (Berl) 121: 66–72.
36. Bourque SL, Adams MA, Nakatsu K, Winterborn A (2010) Comparison of buprenorphine and meloxicam for postsurgical analgesia in rats: effects on body weight, locomotor activity, and hemodynamic parameters. J Am Assoc Lab Anim Sci 49: 617–622.
37. Miller AH (2010) Depression and immunity: a role for T cells? Brain Behav Immun 24: 1–8. doi:10.1016/j.bbi.2009.09.009.
38. Frank-Cannon TC, Alto LT, McAlpine FE, Tansey MG (2009) Does neuroinflammation fan the flame in neurodegenerative diseases? Mol Neurodegener 4: 47. doi:10.1186/1750-1326-4-47.
39. Zanin V, Delbue S, Marcuzzi A, Tavazzi E, Del Savio R, et al. (2012) Specific protein profile in cerebrospinal fluid from HIV-1-positive cART-treated patients affected by neurological disorders. J Neurovirol 18: 416–422. doi:10.1007/s13365-012-0109-y.
40. Merrill JE, Chen ISY (1991) HIV-1, macrophages, glial cells and cytokines in AIDS nervous system disease. FASEB J 5: 2391–2397.
41. Kipnis J, Derecki NC, Yang C, Scrable H (2008) Immunity and cognition: what do age-related dementia, HIV-dementia and "chemo-brain" have in common? Trends Immunol 29: 455–463. doi:10.1016/j.it.2008.07.007.
42. Piletz JE, Halaris A, Iqbal O, Hoppensteadt D, Fareed J, et al. (2009) Pro-inflammatory biomakers in depression: treatment with venlafaxine. World J Biol Psychiatry 10: 313–323. doi:10.3109/15622970802573246.
43. Raison CL, Capuron L, Miller AH (2006) Cytokines sing the blues: inflammation and the pathogenesis of depression. Trends Immunol 27: 24–31. doi:10.1016/j.it.2005.11.006.
44. Suarez EC (2003) The Relation of Severity of Depressive Symptoms to Monocyte-Associated Proinflammatory Cytokines and Chemokines in Apparently Healthy Men. Psychosom Med 65: 362–368. doi:10.1097/01.PSY.0000035719.79068.2B.
45. Brabers NACH, Nottet HSLM (2006) Role of the pro-inflammatory cytokines TNF- α and IL-1 β in HIV-associated dementia. Eur J Clin Invest: 447–458.
46. Taupin P (2008) Adult neurogenesis, neuroinflammation and therapeutic potential of adult neural stem cells. Int J Med Sci 5: 127–132.
47. Lawson MA, Kelley KW, Dantzer R (2011) Intracerebroventricular administration of HIV-1 Tat induces brain cytokine and indoleamine 2,3-dioxygenase expression: A possible mechanism for AIDS comorbid depression. Brain Behav Immun 25: 1569–1575. doi:10.1016/j.bbi.2011.05.006.
48. Royal W, Zhang L, Guo M, Jones O, Davis H, et al. (2012) Immune activation, viral gene product expression and neurotoxicity in the HIV-1 transgenic rat. J Neuroimmunol 247: 16–24. doi:10.1016/j.jneuroim.2012.03.015.
49. Scholzen T, Gerdes J (2000) The Ki-67 protein: From the known and the unknown. J Cell Phys 182: 311–322.
50. Sung Y-H, Shin M-S, Cho S, Baik H-H, Jin B-K, et al. (2010) Depression-like state in maternal rats induced by repeated separation of pups is accompanied by a decrease of cell proliferation and an increase of apoptosis in the hippocampus. Neurosci Lett 470: 86–90. doi:10.1016/j.neulet.2009.12.063.
51. Heine VM, Maslam S, Zareno J, Joels M, Lucassen PJ (2004) Suppressed proliferation and apoptotic changes in the rat dentate gyrus after acute and

chronic stress are reversible. Eur J Neurosci 19: 131–144. doi:10.1046/j.1460-9568.2003.03100.x.
52. Campbell S, Macqueen G (2004) The role of the hippocampus in the pathophysiology of major depression. J Psych Neurosci 29: 417–426.
53. Sheline YI, Gado MH, Kraemer HC (2004) Untreated depression and hippocampal volume loss. Am J Psychiatry 161: 1309–1310.
54. Stockmeier CA, Mahajan GJ, Konick LC, Overholser JC, Jurjus GJ, et al. (2004) Cellular changes in the postmortem hippocampus in major depression. Biol Psych 56: 640–650. doi:10.1016/j.biopsych.2004.08.022.
55. Kempermann G, Kronenberg G (2003) Depressed new Neurons?–Adult hippocampal neurogenesis and a cellular plasticity hypothesis of major depression. Biol Psych 54: 499–503. doi:10.1016/S0006-3223(03)00319-6.
56. Boldrini M, Underwood MD, Hen R, Rosoklija GB, Dwork AJ, et al. (2009) Antidepressants increase neural progenitor cells in the human hippocampus. Neuropsychopharmacology 34: 2376–2389. doi:10.1038/npp.2009.75.
57. Duman RS, Nakagawa S, Malberg J (2001) Regulation of adult neurogenesis by antidepressant treatment. Neuropsychopharmacology 25: 836–844. doi:10.1016/S0893-133X(01)00358-X.
58. Walkup J, Wei W, Sambamoorthi U, Crystal S (2008) Antidepressant treatment and adherence to combination antiretroviral therapies among patients with AIDS and diagnosed depression. Psychiatr Q 79: 43–53. doi:10.1007/s11126-007-9055-x.
59. Koenig LJ, Nesheim S, Abramowitz S (2011) Adolescents with perinatally acquired HIV: emerging behavioral and health needs for long-term survivors. Curr Opin Obstet Gynecol 23: 321–327. doi:10.1097/GCO.0b013e32834a581b.

6

Gender-Specific Effects of Depression and Suicidal Ideation in Prosocial Behaviors

Ricardo Cáceda[1]*, Tori Moskovciak[2], Stefania Prendes-Alvarez[2], Justyna Wojas[2], Anzhelika Engel[2], Samantha H. Wilker[2], Jorge L. Gamboa[3], Zachary N. Stowe[1]

1 Psychiatric Research Institute, University of Arkansas for Medical Sciences, Little Rock, Arkansas, United States of America, **2** Department of Psychiatry and Behavioral Sciences, University of Miami Miller School of Medicine, Miami, Florida, United States of America, **3** Department of Medicine, Vanderbilt University, Nashville, Tennessee, United States of America

Abstract

Background: Prosocial behaviors are essential to the ability to relate to others. Women typically display greater prosocial behavior than men. The impact of depression on prosocial behaviors and how gender interacts with those effects are not fully understood. We explored the role of gender in the potential effects of depression on prosocial behavior.

Methods: We examined prosocial behaviors using a modified version of the Trust Game in a clinical population and community controls. Study participants were characterized on the severity of depression and anxiety, presence of suicidal ideation, history of childhood trauma, recent stressful life events, and impulsivity. We correlated behavioral outcomes with gender and clinical variables using analysis of variance and multiple regression analysis.

Results: The 89 participants comprised four study groups: depressed women, depressed men, healthy women and healthy men (n = 16–36). Depressed men exhibited reciprocity more frequently than healthy men. Depression induced an inversion of the gender-specific pattern of self-centered behavior. Suicidal ideation was associated with increased reciprocity behavior in both genders, and enhancement of the effect of depression on gender-specific self-centered behavior.

Conclusions: Depression, particularly suicidal ideation, is associated with reversal of gender-specific patterns of prosocial behavior, suggesting abnormalities in sexual hormones regulation. This explanation is supported by known abnormalities in the hypothalamus-pituitary-adrenal and hypothalamus-pituitary-gonadal axes found in depression.

Editor: Frank Krueger, George Mason University/Krasnow Institute for Advanced Study, United States of America

Funding: This work was funded partly by the Arsht Foundation and partly by internal funds from the Department of Psychiatry, University of Miami. The funders had no role in study design, data collection and analysis, decision to publish, or preparation of the manuscript.

Competing Interests: The authors have declared that no competing interests exist.

* Email: rcaceda@uams.edu

Introduction

Prosocial behaviors, defined as voluntary behaviors intended to benefit others, are central to the formation and maintenance of healthy interpersonal relationships, and for integration into society [1]. They are viewed as virtues in many cultures and include altruism, reciprocity and cooperation. Gender differences in prosocial behaviors have been well characterized. For example, women display greater and more frequent generosity and altruistic behavior than men [2–5]. Growing evidence supports that these gender differences in behavior are linked to sex hormones [6,7].

Depression affects 10–15% of adults in the US and 350 million worldwide [8]. Patients with major depression frequently experience impaired social functioning, defined as an individual's ability to perform and fulfill normal social roles [9]. The interaction between depression and prosocial behavior is unclear, at least partly because of the methodological challenge to establish causality and its directionality. Prosociality has been suggested to promote healthy development when appropriately regulated, but to increase the risk for psychopathology when overly low or high [10]. Whereas low prosocial behavior is associated with antisocial traits [11], high prosocial orientation may lead to over concern for others and high anxiety [12]. For instance, the differential gender rates for depression have been associated with preadolescent differences in prosociality associated with empathy and compliance [13]. Depression has also been associated with increased altruism and decreased self-centeredness, which can be explained by feelings of worthlessness, anxiety, and submissive behavior [14], leading to situations in which the depressed person is taken advantage of by others. On the other hand, depression can be seen as a state of increased anhedonia and self-centeredness [15], in which a person is unable to love him or herself and, as corollary, unable to care for somebody else. In contrast, it has been proposed that prosocial behaviors play a protective role against mood and anxiety disorders [16,17]. Likewise, suicide has been seen as the product of both altruistic impetus (i.e., to spare my family or for the greater good of the community), and egoistic motivation (associated with low social integration) [18].

The purpose of the current study is to examine the impact of depression on prosocial behavior using a well validated behavioral economic tool: the Trust Game [19,20], which involves a sequential economic exchange between two parties. We sought to extend previous investigations of depression by interrogating the impact of gender on the differences in prosocial behavior in depressed patients. Given the interaction of depression and hypothalamus function and the evidence that gonadal hormones mediate prosocial behaviors, we hypothesized that gender has an influence on the expression of prosocial behavior, which is reversed in depressed subjects.

Methods

Participants

We recruited four groups of adult (20–60 years old) volunteers: healthy women, healthy men, depressed women, and depressed men (See Table 1). Inclusion criteria for the depressed patient group were: a) meeting DSM-IV criteria for Major Depressive Disorder; and b) ability to provide written informed consent. Exclusion criteria were: a) history of schizophrenia, schizoaffective disorder or bipolar disorder; b) active substance use disorders, other than tobacco, by self-report; and c) suicide attempts in the last year. Depressed patients were recruited from the University of Miami and Jackson Memorial Hospital psychiatric outpatient clinics. Healthy participants were recruited from the Miami community.

Ethics Statement

All procedures were approved by the University of Miami and Jackson Memorial Hospital Institutional Review Boards. Participants were remunerated for their participation.

Procedures

After written informed consent, participants' demographics, psychiatric history, and medical history were obtained. Next, participants completed the Beck Depression Inventory (BDI-2) [21], Beck Anxiety Inventory (BAI) [22], Columbia Suicide Severity Rating Scale (C-SSRS) [23], Barratt Impulsiveness Scale (BIS-11) [24], Childhood Trauma Questionnaire (CTQ) [25], and the Survey for Recent Life Experiences (SRLE) [26]. We measure suicidal ideation (SI) with the severity of suicidal ideation subscale of the C-SSRS applied to "currently" in order to identify current suicidal ideation. Following completion of these scales study participants were trained and then participated in a modified version of the Trust Game.

The Trust Game is a standard two-person reciprocal exchange game widely employed to model interpersonal trust and willingness to reciprocate trust [19]. We used two computer-based trials in which each involved 30 rounds of one-time interactions between each study participant and different anonymous individuals. In the first trial or baseline condition, the participant (trustee role) and the other anonymous individual (the investor) were endowed with an initial pot of money ($X), then the investor sent a certain amount of money ($X) to the participant. Next, the participant received three times what the investor sent ($3X), and was asked to choose how much money he/she wanted to give back to the investor, either $1.5X or $0. During the second trial or "emotionally challenging condition," the participant first played the role of the investor, and by design, in 50% of the rounds received some money back from the other player (trustee). Next, the roles were reversed with the participant playing the role of the trustee. (See Figure 1) The goal of the emotionally challenging condition was to expose a participant to either a fair or unfair

Table 1. Demographic and clinical characteristics of depressed patients and healthy participants.

	Healthy women	Depressed women	Healthy men	Depressed men	F	P
N	16	36	17	20		
Age (years)	29.9±2.3	34.0±2.1	33.8±2.9	41.2±3.1	1.31	0.28
Education (years)	16.1±0.6	13.9±0.4^{c}	16.1±0.9^{d,b}	13.5±1.3^{c}	2.2	0.09
Student or working/unemployed, disabled or retired	12/0	15/14	10/1	6/8	11.06	<0.001*
Receiving antidepressant medication	0	24 (67%)	0	15 (75%)	32	<0.0001*
BDI-2	4.9±0.5^{b,d}	27.0±2.0^{a,c}	2.7±0.6^{b,d}	27.7±3.6^{a,c}	26.33	<0.001
Suicidal ideation	0	17	0	11	33.0	<0.0001*
Childhood trauma	33.2±4.2	45.5±4.3^{c}	28.8±3.5^{b}	34.9±6.6	2.02	0.118
Socio cultural stress	16.3±1.9^{b,d}	34.5±6.4^{a,c}	18.1±3.5^{b,d}	26.4±2.7^{a,c}	3.30	0.036
Social acceptability stress	8.0±0.5^{b,d}	12.7±0.7^{a,c}	7.6±0.6^{b,d}	12.3±1.3^{a,c}	8.60	<0.001
Social victimization stress	5.6±0.5^{b,d}	9.0±0.6^{a,c}	5.3±0.5^{b,d}	9.4±0.9^{a,c}	7.75	0.001
Work stress	10.0±0.6^{b}	14.9±0.9^{a}	10.6±0.8	13.4±1.2	4.57	0.016
Time pressure stress	18.0±1.4	19.7±1.0	15.2±2.0	18.8±1.8	0.85	0.513
Finances stress	10.5±1.6	14.4±1.0	8.5±1.0	14.6±1.0	3.57	0.037
Attentional impulsivity	14.6±0.8	19.1±0.9^{c}	15.3±1.7^{b}	17.3±0.9	3.41	0.032
Motor impulsivity	23.4±1.1	23.8±1.0	20.6±1.1	23.9±1.7	1.03	0.448
Nonplanning impulsivity	16.6±1.3	26.7±2.4^{c}	16.6±1.2^{b,d}	26.7±2.4^{c}	6.33	0.002

Bonferroni correction was used for multiple comparison;
[a]compared to suicide attempter group;
[b]compared to suicidal ideation group;
[c]compared to depressed control group;
[d]compared to healthy control group;
*Yates chi square.

experience, aiming to elicit an emotional response and detect its influence on the participant's subsequent choice as trustee. In our study, reciprocity was operationally measured by the number of times participants gave money back in the first trial or baseline condition (expressed as a percentage of the total 30 rounds). This behavior has also been described as trustworthiness [4]. In the emotionally-challenging condition altruism was defined as the number of times participants gave money back despite not receiving any in the first round (expressed as a percentage of the number of times not receiving money back in the first round). Degree of self-centered behavior was measured by the number of times participants did not give money back on the second round after receiving money (expressed as a percentage of the number of times receiving money back in the first round).

Data analysis

We used a two-way analysis of variance (ANOVA) to examine the main effects of either depression (depressed or healthy controls) or suicidal ideation (present or absent) status and gender and their interaction, and clinical measures and outcomes of the Trust Game as dependent variables. We also created dummy variables (healthy/non-suicidal females, healthy/non-suicidal males, depressed/suicidal females, and depressed/suicidal males) to compare differences among these four groups using ANOVA and Bonferroni correction for multiple comparisons. We also evaluated the effect of these four different groups and the offer amount on reciprocity behavior using a generalized lineal model. Model selection was based in the lower Akaike's information criterion (AIC).

To examine individual variability of prosocial behavior with gender, depression, and other clinical variables we performed linear regression using reciprocity behavior in the baseline condition and self-centered behavior in the emotionally challenging condition as dependent variables, and depression severity, antidepressant use, presence of SI, anxiety, and recent social acceptability stress as independent variables. When a multiple regression was performed with these three variables it was non-significant.

Significance level was set at $P \leq 0.05$. We reported corrected P values [27].

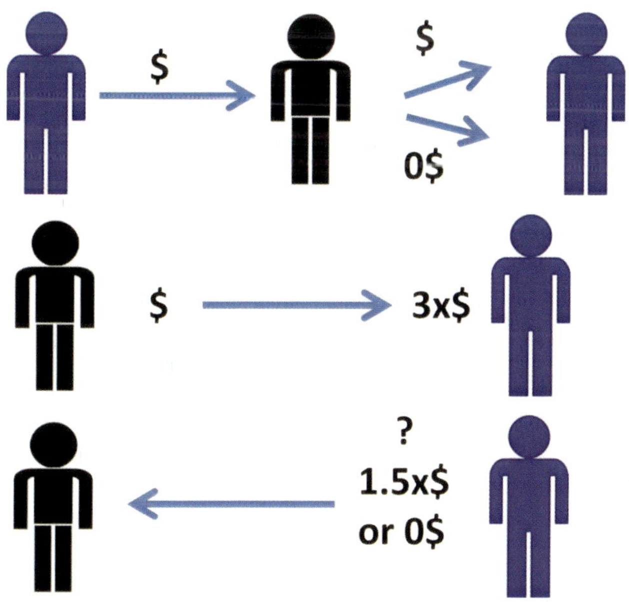

Figure 1. Depiction of the variations of the trust game. A. Baseline condition, the participant plays the role of trustee (blue) who receives a certain amount of money from the investor (3X) and needs to decide whether to give back some (1.5X) or none; B. Emotionally challenging condition, the participant plays two rounds with the same player. In the first, he/she plays the role of the investor who receives some money back only in half of the rounds; immediately afterwards roles are switched and the participant plays the role of trustee who must decide how much money to return.

Results

Composition of the four study groups (healthy women, healthy men, depressed women, and depressed men) did not differ in age, racial composition or educational years. Depression severity ($F(3,89) = 26.33$, $df = 86$, $P < 0.001$), presence of SI (Yates chi-squared test, $X^2 = 37.13$, $P < 0.0001$), recent sociocultural stress ($F(3,89) = 3.30$, $df = 85$, $P = 0.024$), social acceptability stress ($F(3,89) = 8.60$, $df = 86$, $P < 0.001$), and social victimization ($F(3,89) = 7.75$, $df = 85$, $P = 0.001$) were higher among the depressed groups than in the healthy control groups. (See Table 1).

Baseline condition

In the baseline condition, the main effect of depression ($F(3,89) = 5.81$, $df = 86$, $P < 0.001$) and the interaction of gender × depression ($P = 0.035$) were significant. *Post-hoc* analysis revealed that healthy men displayed reciprocity behavior less frequently than depressed men and both women groups (Figure 2A). There was no SI in the healthy control groups. There was a significant main effect of SI on depressed patients' reciprocity behavior ($F(3,56) = 5.6$, $df = 54$, $P = 0.002$). *Post-hoc* analysis revealed that reciprocity behavior was higher in men with SI than in those without SI (See Table 2 and Figure 2B).

Emotionally challenging condition

In the emotionally challenging condition, no difference was observed between the four groups in altruistic behavior. For self-centered behavior (not giving after receiving), the main effect of gender ($F(3,89) = 3.47$, $df = 86$, $P = 0.02$) and the interaction of gender × depression was significant ($P = 0.001$). *Post-hoc* analysis revealed that healthy women exhibited less frequent self-centered behavior compared to all the other groups (See Table 2 and Figure 2C).

Closer scrutiny of the effects of SI on prosocial behavior revealed no effect on altruistic behavior. Regarding self-centered behavior, we observed a significant interaction of gender × SI ($F(3,56) = 7.38$, $df = 54$, $P < 0.001$). *Post-hoc* analysis revealed that women with SI exhibited more frequent self-centered behavior than women without SI. However, men showed the opposite pattern: suicidal men displayed less self-centered behavior compared to non-suicidal men (Figure 2D).

Effect of amount offered

In healthy women, the amount of money offered modulated baseline reciprocity behavior, as women were more generous when smaller amounts (<$12) were involved than when larger amounts ($15–$90) were considered ($P < 0.001$, Figure 3). The amount offered had no significant influence in the other studied groups. Healthy men displayed less reciprocity behavior across all offer values compared with the other studied groups ($P < 0.001$, Figure 3).

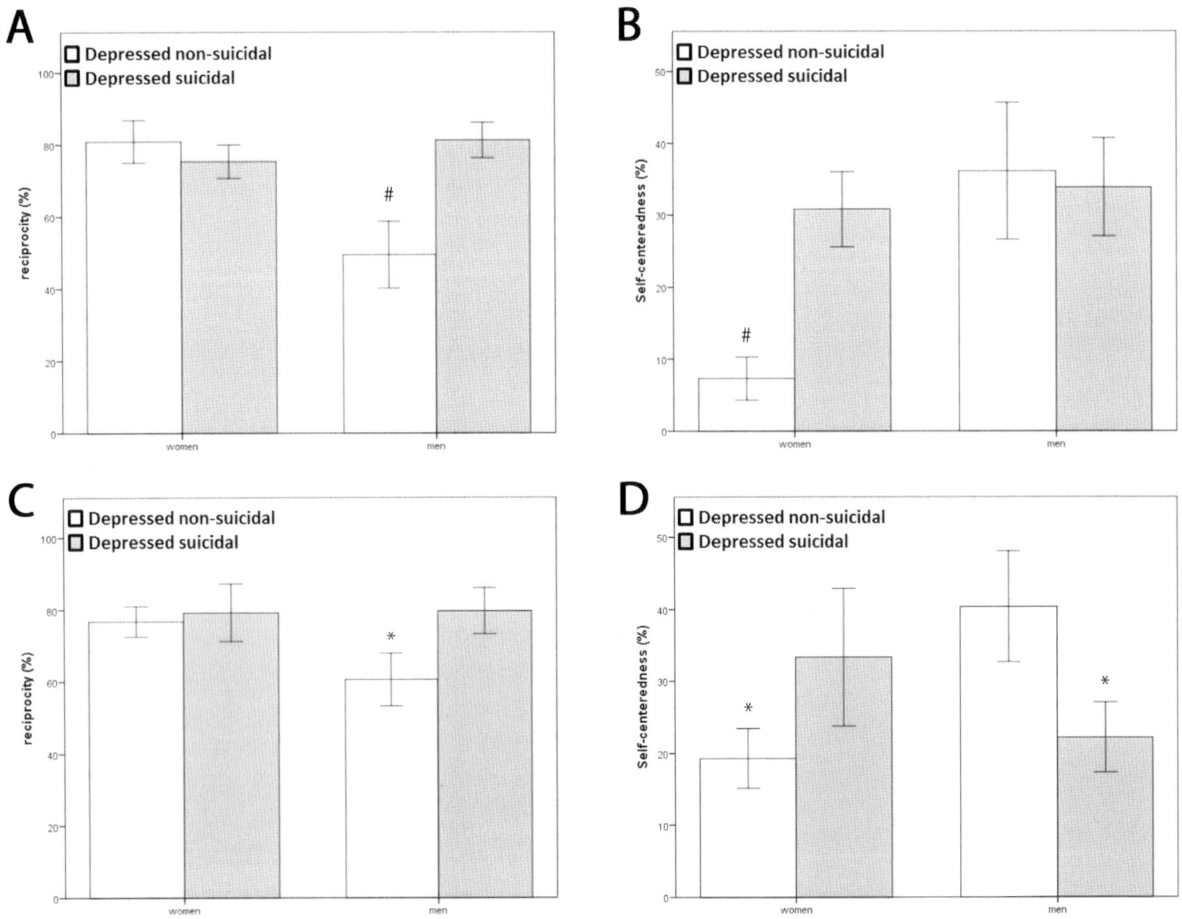

Figure 2. Effect of depression and presence of suicidal ideation in prosocial behavior in men and women. A. Reciprocity behavior during baseline condition in healthy participants and depressed patients. B. Self-centered behavior during emotionally challenging condition in healthy participants and depressed patients. C. Reciprocity behavior during baseline condition in depressed non suicidal and depressed suicidal patients. D. Self-centered behavior during emotionally challenging condition in in depressed non suicidal and depressed suicidal patients. * Different between healthy and depressed participants, # different from all other groups; $p<0.05$.

Antidepressant effect

Prosocial behavior was not associated with antidepressant therapy, presence of SI, or interaction between these variables.

Other factors associated with prosocial behavior

To further identify factors influencing behavior in the baseline and the emotionally challenging conditions, we performed linear regressions using either reciprocity or self-centered behavior as dependent variables, and gender, anxiety, emotional abuse, and recent life events as independent variables. Reciprocity behavior correlated positively with anxiety severity ($R^2=0.188$, $P=0.012$), social victimization ($R^2=0.082$, $P=0.024$), and recent social acceptability stress ($R^2=0.073$, $P=0.033$). On the other hand, history of childhood trauma was positively correlated with self-centered behavior ($R^2=0.067$, $P=0.022$).

Discussion

Our main finding was a gender-specific effect of depression on prosocial behavior: a) healthy men displayed less reciprocity behavior than healthy women; b) depressed men exhibited reciprocity behavior more frequently than healthy men, whereas reciprocity behavior in women did not change with depression; c) depressed women were more self-centered than healthy women; and d) SI induced an inversion of the gender-specific pattern of self-centered behavior: suicidal depressed women were more self-centered, whereas suicidal depressed men were less self-centered.

Gender differences in prosocial behavior in healthy individuals

Our findings are consistent with previous reports of lower reciprocity in the Trust Game in men compared with women in the general population [5,28–30]. Gender-specific differences in social behavior are mediated by the action of sex hormones and the degree of dimorphic brain structure and function associated with expression of X chromosome-linked genes [31]. For example, estrogen levels are positively correlated with aggression and resentment in women, and progesterone is negatively correlated with suspiciousness and resentment in the luteal phase of the menstrual cycle [32]. Physical violence and sexual aggression are suppressed with estradiol administration [33,34]. The Ultimatum Game, another monetary exchange task, has provided valuable insight in differential prosocial behavior across genders. In the Ultimatum Game participants are asked to respond to a wide range of offers and reject or punish unsatisfactory offers from another player [35]. Additionally, men with low testosterone are more likely to accept low offers in the Ultimatum Game [36].

Table 2. Behavior of depressed patients and healthy participants in the modified Trust Game.

	Healthy women[(a)]	Depressed women[(b)]	Healthy men[(c)]	Depressed men[(d)]	F	P		
						Gender effect	Depression effect	Gender × depression interaction
N	16	36	17	20				
Reciprocity	80.4±6.2[c]	75.6±4.5[c]	46.4±9.3[a,b,d]	81.2±4.9[c]	3.68	0.178	0.073	0.026
Altruistic behavior	62.5±9.4	56.1±5.0	46.3±9.6	52.3±7.4	0.34	0.223	0.622	0.371
Self-centered behavior	7.2±3.2[b,c,d]	30.2±5.1[a]	39.6±9.8[a]	21.4±4.0[a]	2.45	0.085	0.042	0.201

Bonferroni correction was used for multiple comparison;
[a]compared to suicide attempter group;
[b]compared to suicidal ideation group;
[c]compared to depressed control group;
[d]compared to healthy control group.

Similarly, men with high testosterone levels tend to be more aggressive and display less prosocial behavior [37]. Cooperativeness, a proxy measure of altruism, is higher in women than in men, and is correlated with increased grey matter volume in the posterior inferior frontal and left anterior medial prefrontal cortices [38]. The neural network underlying altruistic behavior has been shown to involve the anterior insular cortex [39] and the amygdala [40] in addition to striatal reward centers [41]. These brain regions have also been shown to be affected in major depression [42,43]. Hence, it is reasonable to hypothesize that gender differences in prosocial behaviors associated with depression may be related to distinct pattern of neural activation in the limbic system (i.e. insula, amygdala and striatum).

Comparison with previous studies

We found a gender role reversal in self-centered behavior with depression, but only men showed increased prosocial behavior with depression. To our knowledge gender-specific effects of depression and SI on prosocial behavior have not been previously explored. A recent administration of the Trust Game to adult depressed Chinese women who played the role of the trustee reported less frequency of both altruistic and self-centered behavior than healthy women [44]. However, meaningful comparisons between this study and ours are precluded by major differences in design including a higher number of potential response and outcomes, but mostly a considerable element of risk (the opposing player may find out about the participant's response) with potential negative consequences to the participant. In contrast, in our study the participant only had the dichotomic choice to reciprocate or not, and he/she was aware that these answers will be known to the other player, but without possibility of payback from the other player. We explicitly followed this design to avoid confounding effects of payback or reputation on the decision whether to reciprocate or not. Increases in prosocial behavior in depressed patients have been demonstrated in a different economic social interaction using the Ultimatum Game. Individuals with depression tended to show strong negative reaction to unfair offers [45,46]. However, depressed patients tended to offer significantly larger amounts of money than controls [46,47]. This result is in line with the view of increased prosocial behavior in depressed men as an exaggerated need to accommodate to others, particularly during socially stressful situations, which may reflect an overanxious anticipation of rejection due to inappropriate feelings of guilt and worthlessness [48] and fear of negative evaluation [14]. This explanation is supported by our finding of correlation of increased anxiety and recent social stress with reciprocity behavior. On the other hand, decreased prosocial behavior in depressed women may be associated with negative affect, self-centeredness and decreased ability to care for others.

The explanation for at least part of the gender-specific effect of depression in prosocial behavior could lie in gender-specific abnormalities in guilt and reward processing [49,50]. Changes in the frequency of engagement in prosocial behaviors may reflect variations in their subjective value compared to that of monetary rewards. Guilt, almost ubiquitously present in severe depression, can be a strong motivator for altruistic behavior [14,51]. However, further research is warranted to test the role of guilt and anhedonia on the effects of depression on prosocial behavior.

Gender differences in prosocial behavior in depression

Our study found that depression and SI resulted in reversal of gender differences in prosocial behaviors. The most parsimonious explanation would be that these findings are associated with decreased functional gonadotropin-releasing hormone (GnRH) in

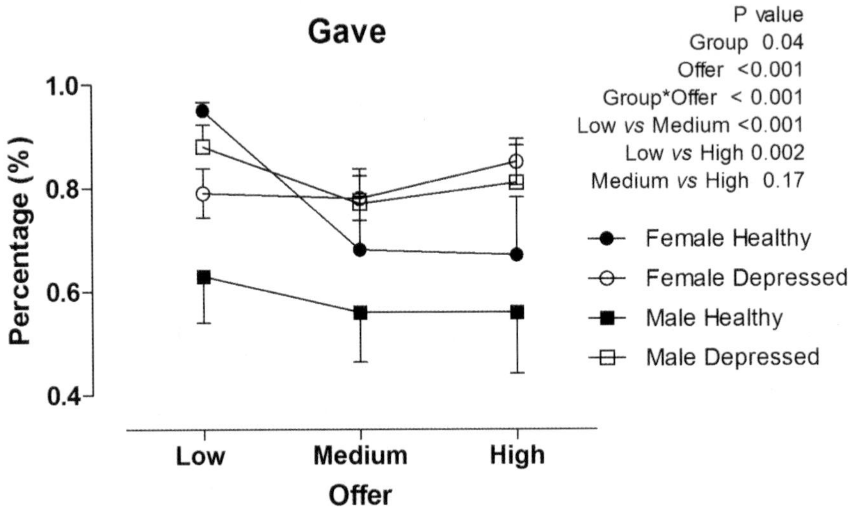

Figure 3. Relationship between offer amount during the baseline condition and reciprocity behavior in healthy women, depressed women, healthy men and depressed men.

depressed suicidal patients [52]. Supporting that connection are studies showing that bioavailable testosterone levels are lower in severely depressed men [53], and administration of GnRH agonist to healthy women is associated with increases in depressive symptoms [54].

Germane to studies of gender-specific behavior and depression, previous reports have found depressed women more often have an anxious and atypical symptom profiles, endorsing more somatic and affective symptoms compared to men [55–59]. Depressed women also display a higher tendency to ruminate about problems [60], higher stress, and lower fulfillment associated with traditional gender roles [61].

Suicidal ideation

There is debate whether suicide represents a severe manifestation of depression or an independent phenomenon. Suicide in the context of mood disorders has been associated with positive and negative moral connotations. Regardless of these differentiations, the reversal of the gender-specific pattern of prosocial behavior in depressed suicidal patients seems to be related to a disruption of HPG axis. For instance, low testosterone levels have been reported in cerebrospinal fluid and serum in suicide attempters [62,63]. Furthermore, suicide attempters that jumped off heights showed a trend toward lower testosterone levels without increases in luteinizing hormone, suggestive of dysfunction at the hypothalamus-pituitary level [64]. Lastly, suicidal ideation has been associated with cognitive abnormalities including executive function deficits [65] and increased impulsive choice [66]. The potential gender specific role of these cognitive factors in suicidal thinking and their influence on prosocial behavior will need to be further elucidated.

Possible antidepressants effect

Our results did not show an effect of antidepressant usage on prosocial behavior, although this may be explained by the lack of power since the study was not primarily designed for this purpose. Antidepressants such as selective serotonin reuptake inhibitors (SSRIs), tricyclics, and monoamine oxidase inhibitors are known to induce sexual side effects including decreased libido and anorgasmia. These side effects seem to be GnRH independent [67]; however, antidepressants are associated with increased salivary testosterone in both men and women receiving SSRIs [68]. Further exploration of the effect of antidepressant medication on prosocial behavior is warranted.

Causality

Even though we did not test for a causal relationship, we believe that the most likely explanation for the observed reversal of gender differences in prosocial behaviors is that depression drives changes in prosocial behavior by modulation of sexual hormones. This hypothesis is based on: a) the association of gender-specific social behavior with sexual hormones in healthy individuals [2–4]; b) the hypogonadal state caused by depression via HPA axis hyperactivity and suppression of GnRH secretion [52]; and c) these behavioral changes are more pronounced in the presence of SI, which supports a dose-response relationship with depression severity. However, it is possible that certain coping styles such as masochism [16,69] lead to pseudoaltruistic behaviors that predispose an individual to the development of mood disorders [17,70].

Limitations

In this study we did not use a structured clinical interview, which prevented exploring the role of gender difference in comorbidities including anxiety and personality disorders. Even though we used a widely used behavioral economic tool [71], it is still a simplified model of human social interaction. The interaction in this exchange took place via a computer screen, with no direct personal contact between the players. We did not record income of participants, which has been described as a strong predictor of charitable contributions [72]. Additionally, the majority of the depressed patients were receiving antidepressant pharmacotherapy, and we cannot account for the effect of medication on behavior. Lastly, we did not measure sexual hormones levels.

Conclusions

We confirmed and expanded gender differences in prosocial behavior in healthy individuals. Depression increased reciprocity behavior in depressed men while increasing self-centered behavior in depressed women. The presence of SI enhanced the effects of depression on self-centered behavior in both genders. Social stress and anxiety in depressed male patients are likely drivers of an exaggerated need to accommodate to others. The pattern of gender-specific changes in social behavior in depressed suicidal patients is suggestive of abnormalities in GnRH secretion and a hypogonadal state. Understanding gender differences in depression may facilitate the design of more efficacious treatments. Further prospective and longitudinal studies are warranted to better confirm our findings, and to relate clinical outcomes to HPA dysfunction.

Acknowledgments

We thank Ms. Christine Oots for her critical review of this manuscript.

Author Contributions

Conceived and designed the experiments: RC SPA. Performed the experiments: TM SPA JW AE SW. Analyzed the data: RC TM SPA JLG ZNS. Contributed reagents/materials/analysis tools: JLG. Wrote the paper: RC TM SPA AE JW SW JLG ZNS.

References

1. Fehr E, Fischbacher U (2003) The nature of human altruism. Nature 425: 785–791.
2. London P, Bower RK (1968) Altruism, extraversion, and mental illness. J Soc Psychol 76: 19–30.
3. Glynn SA, Kleinman SH, Schreiber GB, Zuck T, Combs SM, et al. (2002) Motivations to donate blood: demographic comparisons. Transfusion 42: 216–225.
4. Zak PJ, Borja K, Matzner WT, Kurzban R (2005) The neuroeconomics of distrust: Sex differences in behavior and physiology. American Economic Review 95: 360–363.
5. Innocenti A, Pazienza MG (2008) Gender Differences in Altruism. In: Innocenti A, Sbriglia P, editors. Games, Rationality and Behaviour. New York: Palgrave Macmillan. 134–158.
6. Zak PJ, Kurzban R, Ahmadi S, Swerdloff RS, Park J, et al. (2009) Testosterone administration decreases generosity in the ultimatum game. PLoS One 4: e8330.
7. Schultheiss OC, Campbell KL, McClelland DC (1999) Implicit power motivation moderates men's testosterone responses to imagined and real dominance success. Horm Behav 36: 234–241.
8. WHO (2008) The Global Burden of Disease.
9. Hirschfeld RM, Montgomery SA, Keller MB, Kasper S, Schatzberg AF, et al. (2000) Social functioning in depression: a review. J Clin Psychiatry 61: 268–275.
10. Hay DF (1994) Prosocial development. J Child Psychol Psychiatry 35: 29–71.
11. Hastings PD, Zahn-Waxler C, Robinson J, Usher B, Bridges D (2000) The development of concern for others in children with behavior problems. Dev Psychol 36: 531–546.
12. Hay DF, Pawlby S (2003) Prosocial development in relation to children's and mothers' psychological problems. Child Dev 74: 1314–1327.
13. Keenan K, Hipwell AE (2005) Preadolescent clues to understanding depression in girls. Clin Child Fam Psychol Rev 8: 89–105.
14. O'Connor LE, Berry JW, Weiss J, Gilbert P (2002) Guilt, fear, submission, and empathy in depression. J Affect Disord 71: 19–27.
15. Isen AM (2000) Some perspectives on positive affect and self-regulation. Psychol Inq 184–187.
16. Schwartz C, Meisenhelder JB, Ma Y, Reed G (2003) Altruistic social interest behaviors are associated with better mental health. Psychosom Med 65: 778–785.
17. Fujiwara T (2007) The role of altruistic behavior in generalized anxiety disorder and major depression among adults in the United States. J Affect Disord 101: 219–225.
18. Durkheim E (1992) Suicide and fertility: a study of moral statistics. Eur J Popul 8: 175–197.
19. McCabe K, Houser D, Ryan L, Smith V, Trouard T (2001) A functional imaging study of cooperation in two-person reciprocal exchange. Proc Natl Acad Sci U S A 98: 11832–11835.
20. King-Casas B, Tomlin D, Anen C, Camerer CF, Quartz SR, et al. (2005) Getting to know you: reputation and trust in a two-person economic exchange. Science 308: 78–83.
21. Beck AT, Steer RA, Ball R, Ranieri W (1996) Comparison of Beck Depression Inventories -IA and -II in psychiatric outpatients. J Pers Assess 67: 588–597.
22. Beck AT, Steer RA (1990) BAI, Beck anxiety inventory: manual. San Antonio: Psychological Corp.: Harcourt Brace Jovanovich. iv.
23. Posner K, Brown GK, Stanley B, Brent DA, Yershova KV, et al. (2011) The Columbia-Suicide Severity Rating Scale: initial validity and internal consistency findings from three multisite studies with adolescents and adults. Am J Psychiatry 168: 1266–1277.
24. Patton JH, Stanford MS, Barratt ES (1995) Factor structure of the Barratt impulsiveness scale. J Clin Psychol 51: 768–774.
25. Bernstein DP, Fink L, Handelsman L, Foote J, Lovejoy M, et al. (1994) Initial reliability and validity of a new retrospective measure of child abuse and neglect. Am J Psychiatry 151: 1132–1136.
26. de Jong GM, Timmerman IG, Emmelkamp PM (1996) The Survey of Recent Life Experiences: a psychometric evaluation. J Behav Med 19: 529–542.
27. Benjamini Y, Hochberg Y (1995) Controlling the False Discovery Rate - a Practical and Powerful Approach to Multiple Testing. Journal of the Royal Statistical Society Series B-Methodological 57: 289–300.
28. Chaudhuri A, Paichayontvijit T, Shen LF (2013) Gender differences in trust and trustworthiness: Individuals, single sex and mixed sex groups. Journal of Economic Psychology 34: 181–194.
29. Croson R, Buchan N (1999) Gender and culture: International experimental evidence from trust games. American Economic Review 89: 386–391.
30. Buchan NR, Croson RTA, Solnick S (2008) Trust and gender: An examination of behavior and beliefs in the Investment Game. Journal of Economic Behavior & Organization 68: 466–476.
31. Skuse DH (2005) X-linked genes and mental functioning. Human Molecular Genetics 14: R27–R32.
32. Brambilla F, Speca A, Pacchiarotti I, Biondi M (2010) Hormonal background of physiological aggressiveness in psychologically healthy women. Int J Psychophysiol 75: 291–294.
33. Bradford JM (1983) Research on sex offenders. Recent trends. Psychiatr Clin North Am 6: 715–731.
34. Kyomen HH, Nobel KW, Wei JY (1991) The Use of Estrogen to Decrease Aggressive Physical Behavior in Elderly Men with Dementia. Journal of the American Geriatrics Society 39: 1110–1112.
35. King-Casas B, Chiu PH (2012) Understanding interpersonal function in psychiatric illness through multiplayer economic games. Biol Psychiatry 72: 119–125.
36. Burnham TC (2007) High-testosterone men reject low ultimatum game offers. Proceedings of the Royal Society B-Biological Sciences 274: 2327–2330.
37. Harris JA, Rushton JP, Hampson E, Jackson DN (1996) Salivary testosterone and self-report aggressive and pro-social personality characteristics in men and women. Aggressive Behavior 22: 321–331.
38. Yamasue H, Abe O, Suga M, Yamada H, Rogers MA, et al. (2008) Sex-linked neuroanatomical basis of human altruistic cooperativeness. Cereb Cortex 18: 2331–2340.
39. Sanfey AG, Rilling JK, Aronson JA, Nystrom LE, Cohen JD (2003) The neural basis of economic decision-making in the Ultimatum Game. Science 300: 1755–1758.
40. Scheele D, Mihov Y, Kendrick KM, Feinstein JS, Reich H, et al. (2012) Amygdala Lesion Profoundly Alters Altruistic Punishment. Biol Psychiatry 72: E5–E7
41. de Quervain DJF, Fischbacher U, Treyer V, Schelthammer M, Schnyder U, et al. (2004) The neural basis of altruistic punishment. Science 305: 1254–1258.
42. Sacher J, Neumann J, Funfstuck T, Soliman A, Villringer A, et al. (2012) Mapping the depressed brain: A meta-analysis of structural and functional alterations in major depressive disorder. J Affect Disord 140: 142–148.
43. Diener C, Kuehner C, Brusniak W, Ubl B, Wessa M, et al. (2012) A meta-analysis of neurofunctional imaging studies of emotion and cognition in major depression. Neuroimage 61: 677–685.
44. Zhang HJ, Sun D, Lee TM (2012) Impaired social decision making in patients with major depressive disorder. Brain Behav 2: 415–423.
45. Harle KM, Allen JJ, Sanfey AG (2010) The impact of depression on social economic decision making. J Abnorm Psychol 119: 440–446.
46. Scheele D, Mihov Y, Schwederski O, Maier W, Hurlemann R (2013) A negative emotional and economic judgment bias in major depression. Eur Arch Psychiatry Clin Neurosci 263: 67–83.
47. Destoop M, Schrijvers D, De Grave C, Sabbe B, De Bruijn ER (2012) Better to give than to take? Interactive social decision-making in severe major depressive disorder. J Affect Disord 137: 98–105.
48. Elliott R, Zahn R, Deakin JF, Anderson IM (2011) Affective cognition and its disruption in mood disorders. Neuropsychopharmacology 36: 153–182.
49. Pizzagalli DA, Holmes AJ, Dillon DG, Goetz EL, Birk JL, et al. (2009) Reduced caudate and nucleus accumbens response to rewards in unmedicated individuals with major depressive disorder. Am J Psychiatry 166: 702–710.
50. Keedwell PA, Andrew C, Williams SC, Brammer MJ, Phillips ML (2005) A double dissociation of ventromedial prefrontal cortical responses to sad and happy stimuli in depressed and healthy individuals. Biol Psychiatry 58: 495–503.
51. Carlsmith JM, Gross AE (1969) Some effects of guilt on compliance. J Pers Soc Psychol 11: 232–239.
52. Zarrouf FA, Artz S, Griffith J, Sirbu C, Kommor M (2009) Testosterone and depression: systematic review and meta-analysis. J Psychiatr Pract 15: 289–305.
53. Heuser I (2002) Depression, endocrinologically a syndrome of premature aging? Maturitas 41 Suppl 1: S19–23.

54. Toren P, Dor J, Mester R, Mozes T, Blumensohn R, et al. (1996) Depression in women treated with a gonadotropin-releasing hormone agonist. Biol Psychiatry 39: 378–382.
55. Dekker J, Koelen JA, Peen J, Schoevers RA, Gijsbers-van Wijk C (2007) Gender differences in clinical features of depressed outpatients: preliminary evidence for subtyping of depression? Women Health 46: 19–38.
56. Frank E, Carpenter LL, Kupfer DJ (1988) Sex differences in recurrent depression: are there any that are significant? Am J Psychiatry 145: 41–45.
57. Szadoczky E, Rihmer Z, Papp ZS, Vitrai J, Furedi J (2002) Gender differences in major depressive disorder in a Hungarian community survey. International Journal of Psychiatry in Clinical Practice 6: 31–37.
58. Uebelacker LA, Strong D, Weinstock LM, Miller IW (2009) Use of item response theory to understand differential functioning of DSM-IV major depression symptoms by race, ethnicity and gender. Psychol Med 39: 591–601.
59. Lai CH (2011) Major depressive disorder: gender differences in symptoms, life quality, and sexual function. J Clin Psychopharmacol 31: 39–44.
60. Nolen-Hoeksema S (1990) Sex Differences in Depression. Palo Alto: Stanford University Press.
61. Barnett RC, Biener GK, Baruch GK (1987) Gender and Stress. New York: The Free Press.
62. Gustavsson G, Traskman-Bendz L, Higley JD, Westrin A (2003) CSF testosterone in 43 male suicide attempters. European Neuropsychopharmacology 13: 105–109.
63. Tripodianakis J, Markianos M, Rouvali O, Istikoglou C (2007) Gonadal axis hormones in psychiatric male patients after a suicide attempt. Eur Arch Psychiatry Clin Neurosci 257: 135–139.
64. Markianos M, Tripodianakis J, Istikoglou C, Rouvali O, Christopoulos M, et al. (2009) Suicide attempt by jumping: a study of gonadal axis hormones in male suicide attempters versus men who fell by accident. Psychiatry Res 170: 82–85.
65. Westheide J, Quednow BB, Kuhn KU, Hoppe C, Cooper-Mahkorn D, et al. (2008) Executive performance of depressed suicide attempters: the role of suicidal ideation. Eur Arch Psychiatry Clin Neurosci 258: 414–421.
66. Cáceda R, Durand D, Cortes E, Prendes S, Moskovciak TN, et al. (2014) Impulsive choice and psychological pain in acutely suicidal depressed patients. Psychosomatic Medicine 76: 445–451.
67. Soga T, Wong DW, Clarke IJ, Parhar IS (2010) Citalopram (antidepressant) administration causes sexual dysfunction in male mice through RF-amide related peptide in the dorsomedial hypothalamus. Neuropharmacology 59: 77–85.
68. Giltay EJ, Enter D, Zitman FG, Penninx BW, van Pelt J, et al. (2012) Salivary testosterone: associations with depression, anxiety disorders, and antidepressant use in a large cohort study. J Psychosom Res 72: 205–213.
69. Seelig BJ, Rosof LS (2001) Normal and pathological altruism. Journal of the American Psychoanalytic Association 49: 933–959.
70. Fujiwara T (2009) Is altruistic behavior associated with major depression onset? PLoS One 4: e4557.
71. Johnson ND, Mislin AA (2011) Trust games: A meta-analysis. Journal of Economic Psychology 32: 865–889.
72. Yen ST (2002) An econometric analysis of household donations in the USA. Applied Economics Letters 9: 837–841.

Overexpression of Human GATA-1 and GATA-2 Interferes with Spine Formation and Produces Depressive Behavior in Rats

Miyeon Choi[1]¶, Sung Eun Wang[2]¶, Seung Yeon Ko[2]¶, Hyo Jung Kang[3]¶, Seung Yeun Chae[2], Seung Hoon Lee[2], Yong-Seok Kim[1,2], Ronald S. Duman[4], Hyeon Son[1,2]*

1 Department of Biochemistry and Molecular Biology, College of Medicine, Hanyang University, Seoul, Korea, **2** Graduate School of Biomedical Science and Engineering, Hanyang University, Seoul, Korea, **3** Department of Life Science, Chung-Ang University, Seoul, Korea, **4** Laboratory of Molecular Psychiatry, Center for Genes and Behavior, Departments of Psychiatry, Neurobiology, and Laboratory Medicine, Yale University School of Medicine, New Haven, Connecticut, United States of America

Abstract

Functional consequences to which vertebrate GATA transcription factors contribute in the adult brain remain largely an open question. The present study examines how human GATA-1 and GATA-2 (hGATA-1 and hGATA-2) are linked to neuronal differentiation and depressive behaviors in rats. We investigated the effects of adeno-associated viral expression of hGATA-1 and hGATA-2 (AAV-hGATA1 and AAV-hGATA2) in the dentate gyrus (DG) of the dorsal hippocampus on dendrite branching and spine number. We also examined the influence of AAV-hGATA1 and AAV-hGATA2 infusions into the dorsal hippocampus on rodent behavior in models of depression. Viral expression of hGATA-1 and hGATA-2 cDNA in rat hippocampal neurons impaired dendritic outgrowth and spine formation. Moreover, viral-mediated expression of hGATA-1 and hGATA-2 in the dorsal hippocampus caused depressive-like deficits in the forced swim test and learned helplessness models of depression, and decreased the expression of several synapse-related genes as well as spine number in hippocampal neurons. Conversely, shRNA knockdown of GATA-2 increased synapse-related gene expression, spine number, and dendrite branching. The results demonstrate that hGATA-1 and hGATA-2 expression in hippocampus is sufficient to cause depressive like behaviors that are associated with reduction in spine synapse density and expression of synapse-related genes.

Editor: Shashank M. Dravid, Creighton University, United States of America

Funding: This research was supported by National Research Foundation grant of Korea (No. 2011-0028317) funded by Korea government awarded to HS. The funders had no role in study design, data collection and analysis, decision to publish, or preparation of the manuscript.

Competing Interests: The authors have declared that no competing interests exist.

* Email: hyeonson@hanyang.ac.kr

¶ These authors contributed equally to this work.

Introduction

There is a rich cross-talk between transcription factors and signaling pathways that regulate neuronal growth and synapse formation [1,2], and there is extensive evidence that changes in spine morphology couple with synaptic function in neurons [3]. These functional and structural changes in dendritic spines are thought to be the basis for learning and memory in the brain [4,5]. Consistent with this idea, changes in spine density are seen in several psychiatric disorders that are associated with deficits in social interaction, cognition and memory function [6]. However, how transcriptional regulation ultimately leads to specific alteration of brain function is not fully understood.

GATA-1 is a member of a family of six zinc-finger proteins, which bind to the (T/A)GATA(G/A) consensus sequence and play important roles in cellular differentiation and proliferation [7]. GATA transcription factors were first described for their role in the proliferation of progenitors and in lineage specification during early hematopoiesis [8,9]. Recently, GATA-1 was shown to exert repressive effects on spine formation in rat cortical neurons [10] and has been implicated in major depressive disorder (MDD) based on evidence that GATA-1 levels are increased postmortem prefrontal cortex and hippocampus of MDD subjects [11].

GATA-1 is expressed at relatively low levels in brain, but another member of the family GATA-2 is expressed at higher levels in mature neurons in mouse and rats [12–14]. GATA-2 plays a role in development of the mouse brain [15,16]. Phylogenic comparison reveals that GATA-1 protein and two of the DNA binding zinc finger domains are fully conserved between human, mouse and rat [17,18] (see also www.ihop-net.org/UniPub/iHOP). Human GATA-2 shares 98% amino acid sequence similarity to rats and mouse [7,19,20] and has identical zinc finger homology among these species. The zinc finger domains of hGATA-1 and hGATA-2 also have high sequence homology of ~98% (www.ihop-net.org/UniPub/iHOP). These findings indicate that the GATA-1 and GATA-2 are conserved in vertebrates. However, the influence of GATA transcription factors on adult brain, particularly the hippocampus, remains unclear. In addition, the role of GATA-2 in the actions of stress and in depression-like behaviors has not been examined.

In the current study we examined the influence of stress on the expression of GATA-2, and investigated and compared the effects of hGATA-1 and hGATA-2 transcription factors on neurite outgrowth, spine formation, and synapse-related genes that are regulated by these GATA transcription factor members in rat hippocampal neurons. We also examined the influence of hGATA-1 and hGATA-2 on depressive behaviors in rodent models. The studies aim to elucidate the functional relevance of the GATA transcription factors in hippocampal neurons and how these synaptic changes translate to alterations of depressive behaviors.

Materials and Methods

Culture of hippocampal primary neurons

Primary hippocampal neurons were prepared and processed as described previously [21]. Hippocampi from embryo day 16.5 Sprague–Dawley rat (Harlan Sprague Dawley, Indianapolis, IN, USA) embryos were used.

Construction of adeno-associated viral plasmids and viral production

To construct human GATA expression vector, human GATA cDNA was cloned from human cDNA library (Human Fetus Marathon-Ready cDNA, Clontech, Mountain View, CA, USA) by PCR. The following primer pairs were used for GATA cDNA cloning: for GATA-1 cloning, 5′-GCCACCATGGAGTTCCCT-GGCCTG-3′, which includes underlined Kozak sequence and spans nucleotides 1–18 of the human GATA-1 cDNA coding sequence (NM002049.3 GI: 183227689); and 5′-TCATGAGCT-GAGCGGAGC-3′, which is complementary to nucleotides 1225–1242 of the human GATA-1 cDNA coding sequence. For GATA-2 cloning, 5′-GCCACCATGGAGGTGGCGCCC-3′, which includes underlined Kozak sequence and spans nucleotides 1–15 of the human GATA-2 cDNA coding sequence (NM001145661.1 GI: 224611698); and 5′-CTAGCCCATGGCGGTCA-3′, which is complementary to nucleotides 1427–1443 of the human GATA-2 cDNA coding sequence.

PCR amplifications were performed in 50 μl reaction volumes with 1 μl (10–100 ng fetal cDNA), 4 U Pyrobest DNA polymerase (TAKARA, Tokyo, Japan), 200 μM each dNTP, 0.6 μM each primer, and 1.3 M betaine on a Thermal cycler (TECHNE, Staffordshire, UK). PCR reactions began with a denaturation step at 94°C for 5 min and 10 cycles of Touchdown (TD) PCR followed by 30 cycles of standard PCR were performed. TD PCR conditions were as follows: 10 s at 98°C, 30 s at annealing temperature stepdowns every cycles of 0.5°C (from +68°C to + 63°C), and 2 min at 72°C. The annealing temperature for the final 30 cycles of standard PCR was 62°C with denaturation and extension phases as above. Human GATA cDNA obtained from human fetus cDNA library (Clontech, Mountain View, CA, USA) by PCR was subcloned into pGEM-T-Easy vector (Promega, Madison, WI, USA). After confirmation of its sequence by DNA sequencing, cDNA clone was digested by *Eco*RI. The *Eco*RI fragments were blunt-ended with Klenow DNA polymerase (New England Biolabs, Ipswich, MA, USA) and ligated into the *Eco*RV site of modified adeno-associated viral vector encoding enhanced GFP (AAV-eGFP), generating AAV-eGFP-hGATA1 and AAV-eGFP-hGATA2. The virus was generated using a triple-transfection, helper-free method and was purified with a modified version of a published protocol [22].

Transfection with small hairpin RNA (shRNA)

Rat shRNAs of GATA2 and a control vector were purchased from GeneCopoeia (Rockville, MD, USA). Transfection of shRNAs (100 nM; target sequence, GGATGGCGTCAAGTAT-CAA) was performed using a Lipofectamine 2000 reagent according to the manufacturer's instructions (Invitrogen, Carlsbad, CA, USA).

RT-PCR analysis

Total RNA was prepared from cells with Trizol reagent (Life-technologies, Rockville, MD, USA). Reverse-transcription was conducted as previously described [21]. For quantitative real-time PCR (qRT-PCR), PCR was performed on an iCycler iQ Multi-Color Real-Time PCR Detection System (Bio-Rad Laboratories, Hercules, CA, USA). The housekeeping gene GAPDH was used as a control. Expression of each gene was normalized to the amount of GAPDH to calculate relative transcript levels. Normalized expression values were averaged, and average fold changes were calculated. The primer sequences are as follows: GAPDH, forward: 5′- CTCGTCCCATAGACAAAATGGT-GAAG-3′, reverse: 5′- AGACTCCACGACATACTCAG-CACC-3′; hGATA-1, forward: 5′-CTTGTAGTAGAGGCCG-CAGG-3′, reverse: 5′-GCTCTACCCTGCCTCAACTG-3′; hGATA-2, forward: 5′-TACCACAAGATGAATGGGCA-3′, reverse: 5′-TCTCCTGCATGCACTTTGAC-3′; rGATA1, forward: 5′- GATGGAATCCAGACGAGGAA -3′, reverse: 5′-CTCTCCGCAATTCCCACTAC -3′; rGATA2, forward: 5′-CAG CCT CCA GCT TCA CCC CT-3′ reverse 5′-TGA TGA GCG GCC GAT TCT GT-3′; PSD-95, forward: 5′-GACAAC-CAAGAAATACCGCT-3′, reverse: 5′-GCTTCTAGGGTGTC-CGTGTT-3′; GAP-43, forward: 5′-GGCTCTGCTACTACC-GATGC-3′, reverse: 5′-CTGTCGGGCACTTTCCTTAG-3′; RAB4B, forward: 5′-AGCCGGGAGACATACAACTC-3′, reverse: 5′-CCATCCTCTCCGGATCTAGT-3′; MAP2, forward: 5′-GCAAAGTAAGCCTGGTGA-3′, reverse, 5′-ATCTAAGG-GAAGAGTGAAAC-3′. GAD1, forward: 5′-CAGAAGTGAA-AACAAAAGGC-3′, reverse: 5′-AAACGCTCCATAAACAG-TCG-3′; vGluT1, forward: 5′-GGCAGTTTCCAGGACCTC-CACTC-3′, reverse: 5′-GCAAGAGGCAGTTGAGAAGGAGA-GAG-3′.

Immunocytochemistry and Immunohistochemistry

Cells were fixed as described before [23]. The following primary antibodies were used: mouse monoclonal anti-green fluorescent protein (GFP) (1:400, Roche Applied Sciences, Mannheim, Germany) and mouse monoclonal microtubule-associated protein-2 (MAP2) (1:500, Sigma-Aldrich, Saint Louis, MO, USA) antibodies. Cells were placed in goat anti-mouse secondary antibody conjugated to Alexa488 (1:400, Invitrogen, Carlsbad, CA, USA) or Cy3 (1:400, Roche Applied Sciences, Mannheim, Germany). Cells were photographed with a confocal microscope (Leica Microsystems, Wetzlar, Germany). Immunohistochemistry in rat brain was conducted as described previously [21].

Western blot analysis

Protein extracts were prepared as described previously [23]. The blot was probed with mouse monoclonal β-actin (1:1000, Santa Cruz, CA, USA), rabbit monoclonal anti-GATA-1 (1:500, Cell Signaling, Danvers, MA, USA), rabbit monoclonal anti-GATA-2 (1:500, Abcam, Cambridge, UK), rabbit polyclonal anti-postsynaptic density protein 95 (PSD-95) (1:1000, Abcam, Cambridge, UK), rabbit polyclonal anti-GAP43 (1:1000, Abcam, Cambridge, UK), mouse monoclonal anti-Tuj1 (1:1000, Covance,

Berkeley, CA, USA), rabbit polyclonal anti-lamin B1 (1:1000, Abcam, Cambridge, UK), mouse monoclonal anti-GFP (1:500, Santa Cruz, CA, USA) followed by treatment goat with anti-mouse or anti-rabbit IgG conjugated with peroxidase (1:1000, Santa Cruz, CA, USA). Bands were visualized with an ECL detection kit (GenDEPOT, TX, USA).

Spine density and dendritic arborization analysis

Images were acquired through Z-stacks, which typically consisted of 10 scans at high zoom at 1-μm steps in the z axis. For analysis of spine density in cultured hippocampal neurons, dendrite segments 40 μm in length, from 3 to 5 dendrites per neuron, were sampled from the cell body (proximal) and from end of dendrites (distal). In the hippocampal DG, we focused on second- or third-order dendrites from cells localized in one half of outer molecular layer. For each cell, 3 or more dendritic segments were used for spine analysis. Spine counting was conducted with a 60× objective using the Leica TCS SP5 (Leica Microsystems, Wetzlar, Germany). The number of spines was counted in a 10 μm segment. The final value was averaged from three rats per group and expressed as the number of spines/10 μm. Dendritic branching was investigated by Sholl analysis [24]. A transparent grid showing concentric circles was placed over the dendritic image, the smallest circle was centered in the soma and the distance between each circle was equivalent to 10 μm. Total dendritic length was estimated by counting the total number of circle intersections, and the density of dendrites was defined by counting the number of intersections on each circle. The confocal images of neurons were analyzed using Image J software (http://rsbweb.nih.gov/ij/) and the Sholl analysis plug-in.

Transcription factor binding motif search

The TFSEARCH (http://www.cbrc.jp/research/db/TFSEARCH.html) was used for the binding motif search in the promoter regions of candidate genes. The transcription factor binding sites were determined in the set of promoters with the parameter of exact matches of core sequences (threshold score = 90.0 as default value cut off) in the vertebrate matrix.

Animals, stereotaxic surgery and infusions

Male Sprague-Dawley rats (175–250 g) were pair-housed and maintained in standard conditions with a 12-hour light-dark cycle and ad libitum access to food and water. All animal experiments were approved by the Institutional Animal Care and Use Committee of Hanyang University and were performed in accordance with relevant guidelines and regulations. Stereotaxic surgery and infusions were conducted as previously described [21]. Rats were anesthetized with xylazine (6 mg/kg, i.m., Lloyd laboratories, Shenandoar, IA) and ketamine (80 mg/kg i.m., Fort Dodge Animal Health, Overland Park, KS). Bilateral viral injections were performed with coordinates −4.1 mm (anterior/posterior), ±2.4 mm (lateral), and −4.1 mm (dorsal/ventral) relative to the bregma.

Acute and chronic unpredictable stress (CUS) procedure

For acute stress, rats were individually restrained for a 2 h session in hemicylindrical (20.5×9×6 cm), well-ventilated, Plexiglas tubes. Animals were subsequently killed by rapid decapitation at 2 h after the onset of stress [25]. Ketamine was injected 30 min prior to the onset of stress. Control animals were decapitated immediately after removal from their home cages (total time lapse from removal from cage to decapitation: 1–3 min). CUS is an experimental procedure in which animals are exposed to a variable sequence of mild and unpredictable stressors. Our CUS procedure has been successfully used in the laboratory to produce behavioral changes. The CUS animals were subjected to the same 10 stressors (2 per day) described in Li *et al* [26], for a total of 21 days. Rats were then were treated with vehicle or ketamine (10 mg/kg, i.p.) on day 21 of CUS treatment 24 prior to sacrifice.

Forced swim test

A forced swim test (FST) was conducted as previously described [21]. Behavioral tests were analyzed by an experimenter blinded to the study code.

Learned helplessness paradigm

The learned helplessness procedure was performed in commercial shuttle boxes divided into two equal compartments by a central barrier (Gemini Avoidance System, San Diego Instruments, San Diego, CA, USA), as previously described [27]. A computer-operated guillotine door built into the central barrier allowed passage between compartments. On day 1, inescapable footshock (IES) was administered at one side of the shuttle box with the guillotine door closed (60 footshocks, 0.85 mA intensity, 15 sec average duration, 60 sec average intershock interval). Active avoidance testing consisted of 30 trials of escapable footshock (0.65 mA intensity, 35 sec maximum duration, 90 sec average intertribal interval) with the guillotine door open. Each trial used a fixed-ratio 1 schedule, during which one shuttle crossing by rats terminated the shock. Shock was terminated automatically if rats did not escape after 35 sec. A computer automatically recorded the number of escape failures.

Novelty suppressed feeding test and sucrose preference test

A novelty suppressed feeding test (NSFT) and sucrose preference test (SPT) were conducted as previously described [21].

Locomotor activity test (LMA)

The general locomotor activity of the rats in the open field test was measured by an automatic video tracking system (SmarTrack, Smartech, Madison, WI, USA). Rats were placed in the central part of the square-shaped arena (77 cm×77 cm×25 cm) and allowed to explore it for 10 min. Total distance traveled (locomotion activity) were recorded for 10 min.

Statistical analysis

Statistical significance was determined by Student's *t*-test. For behavioral results, statistical differences were determined by analysis of the variance (ANOVA; StatView 5, SAS Software). The *F* values and experimental degrees of freedom are included in the legends of the figures. All data were expressed as mean ± s.e.m.

Results

Expression of hGATA-1 and hGATA-2 in cultured rat hippocampal neurons

We first analyzed expression of rat GATA-1 and -2 (rGATA-1 and -2) in hippocampus. Figure 1a shows mRNA expression of rGATA-2. In contrast, rGATA-1 was not expressed at detectable levels in the hippocampus. Since the involvement of GATA-2 in cellular and behavioral abnormalities related to stress and depression remains an open question, we investigated the influence of acute and chronic stress on the expression levels of rGATA-2 mRNA in the hippocampus. Rats were exposed to acute restraint stress or chronic unpredictable stress (CUS), which results in anhedonic behavior that is reversed with antidepressant treatment, including the rapid acting agent ketamine [27]. While acute restraint had no effect, CUS exposure significantly increased levels of rGATA-2 mRNA in the hippocampus (Fig. 1b, c; $P<0.01$ compared with the nonstressed control). A single dose of ketamine (10 mg/kg) significantly decreased GATA-2 mRNA in acutely stressed rats, and completely reversed the effects of CUS (Fig. 1b, c; $P<0.05$).

Infection of cultured rat hippocampal neurons with AAV-hGATA1-eGFP or AAV-hGATA2-eGFP (Fig. 1a) induced an increase in the expression of hGATA-1 and hGATA-2 by RT-PCR, respectively, compared to control virus (vector only) as expected (Fig. 1b). Western blot analysis of nuclear extracts of the hippocampal neurons demonstrated that levels of hGATA-1 and hGATA-2 protein levels were also increased in response to AAV-hGATA1 and AAV-hGATA2 infection, respectively, compared to control virus (Fig. 1c). The majority of the cells transfected by AAV (with or without hGATA-1 and hGATA-2) differentiate into neurons as determined by the neuronal marker MAP2 (Fig. 1d, e). These experiments show that the hGATA proteins were produced in hippocampal neuronal cells. Infection of cells with AAV-hGATA1 or AAV-hGATA2 resulted in a similar total cell number compared to control virus (Fig. 1e), suggesting that cell survival was not affected by hGATA overexpression.

Dendritic length and spine density in rat hippocampal neurons

Viral expression of rat GATA1 significantly decreases the number of dendrite intersections in cultured rat cortical neurons, indicating decreased complexity (Kang et al., 2012). To investigate whether hGATA-1 and hGATA-2 can alter complexity of rat hippocampal neurons, we analyzed dendrite morphology by fixing and labeling neurons with a GFP-specific antibody (Fig. 2a), and

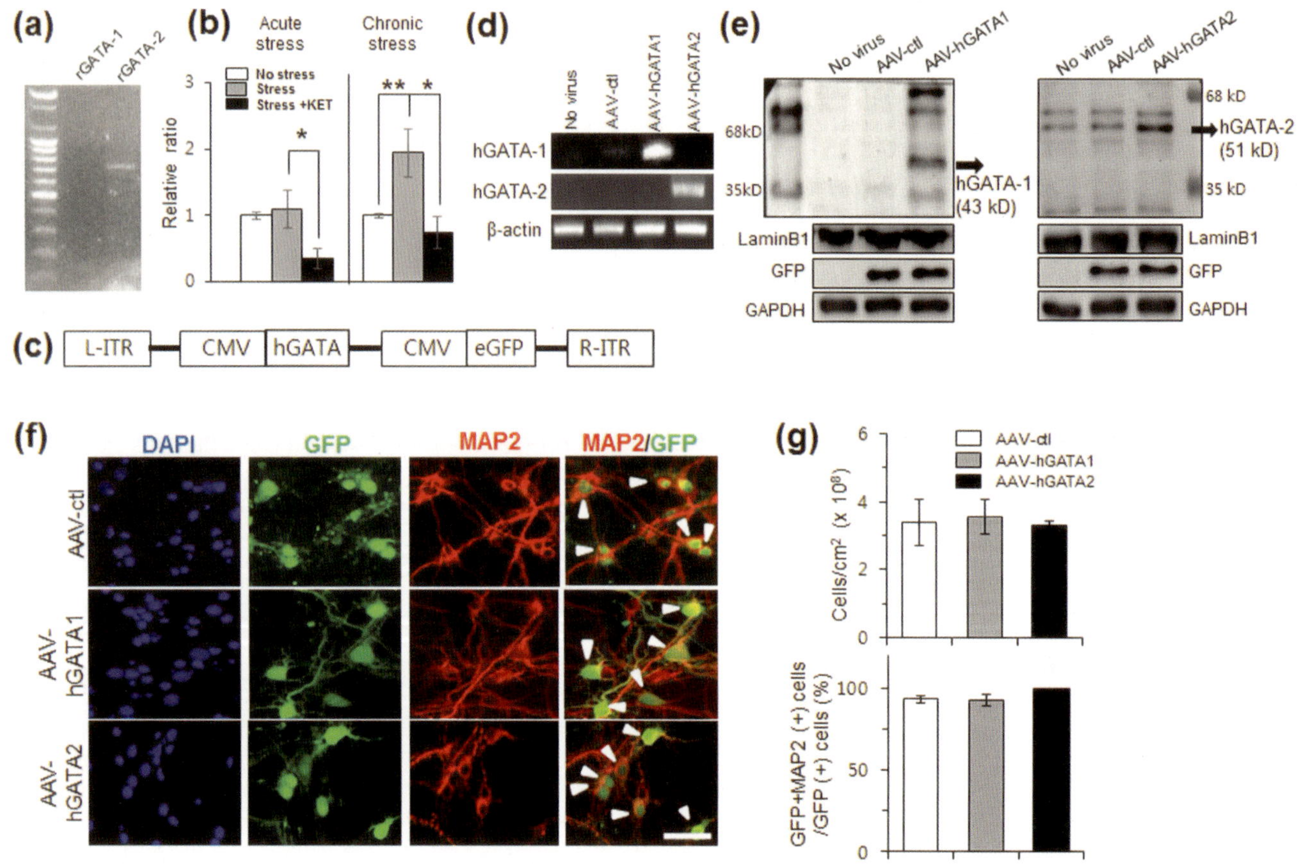

Figure 1. AAV-hGATA-enhanced GFP (eGFP) vector construction and expression in the hippocampal neurons. (a) RT-PCR analysis demonstrating expression of rGATA-2, but not r-GATA-1 in hippocampus. (b) Quantitative RT-PCR analysis of rGATA-2 in the rat hippocampus exposed to acute stress or CUS in the presence or absence of ketamine treatment. Rats were exposed to acute restraint stress for 2 h or CUS for 21 d and received either saline or ketamine (Stress+KET), and sections were subjected to quantitative RT-PCR. Results are expressed as a ratio of nonstressed controls and are the mean ± SEM, each analyzed in triplicate brain sections. rGATA-2 mRNA was increased in acute and CUS animals compared with nonstressed animals ($P<0.01$). CUS animals injected with KET showed a decrease in rGATA-2 mRNA compared with CUS animals ($P<0.05$; $n=6$ animals in each group). (c) L-ITR and R-ITR, left and right inverted terminal repeats, respectively; CMV, cytomegalovirus promoter. (d) RT-PCR of cDNA isolated from cultured hippocampal neurons transfected with AAV-hGATA1 and AAV-hGATA2. (e) Western blotting analysis was conducted to examine the expression of hGATA transcription factors, and representative blots were shown. The abundance of hGATA-1 (43 kD) and hGATA-2 (51 kD) protein in the nuclear extracts is increased in response to infection with AAV-hGATA1 or AAV-hGATA2. Nuclear extracts were determined by lamin B1, a nuclear marker. (f) Images of hippocampal neurons infected with AAV and stained with antibodies to GFP and MAP2. (g) The total number of cells was revealed by nuclear staining with DAPI. Transfection with AAV-hGATA1 or AAV-hGATA2 showed the same fraction of GFP(+) cells colabeled with MAP2 compared with transduction with AAV-ctl ($P>0.05$). The percentage of MAP2(+) cells among GFP(+) cells is shown as a fraction of the total GFP number of cells. Total MAP2(+) and GFP(+) cells (arrowheads) were counted with a microscope in 10 non-overlapping fields per well. Values represent mean ± s.e.m. from five independent experiments. Scale bar, 50 μm.

then measured the number of dendrite intersections using Sholl analysis [28]. Consistent with previous results in cortical neurons, viral expression of hGATA1 decreased the complexity of the dendritic arbor of hippocampal neurons (Fig. 2a). When dendritic length was plotted against the shell distances 10–100 µm, differences between AAV-ctl and AAV-hGATA1 were most marked for the middle 20–80 µm range (Fig. 2b; $P<0.05$). Decreased complexity in processes of GFP(+) cells that were infected with AAV-hGAT2 was greatest in the 20–50 µm range (Fig. 2b; $P<0.05$).

Since we observed a morphological change in the rat primary hippocampal neuronal cells that were transfected with AAV-hGATA1 and AAV-hGATA2, we then measured the spine density of those cells to further characterize the morphological changes. Spines protruding from second order dendrites were assessed separately for the proximal and distal dendrites, and results expressed as the number of spines per µm dendritic length (Fig. 2c, d). Infection of cells with AAV-hGATA1 significantly decreased spine density of proximal and distal dendrites compared to AAV-ctl (Fig. 2d; $P<0.001$). Spines of dendrites in cells transfected with AAV-hGATA2 also showed significant decreases in the proximal and distal segments (Fig. 2d; $P<0.01$). Alterations of spine-synapses are accompanied by regulation of postsynaptic proteins, including PSD-95 [27,29]. Consistent with this idea, the expression of PSD-95 was decreased in neurons transfected with AAV-hGAT1 and AAV-hGATA2 (Fig. 2e).

We then investigated protein levels of β-tubulin type III (Tuj1) and GAP-43, which are known to play an important role in

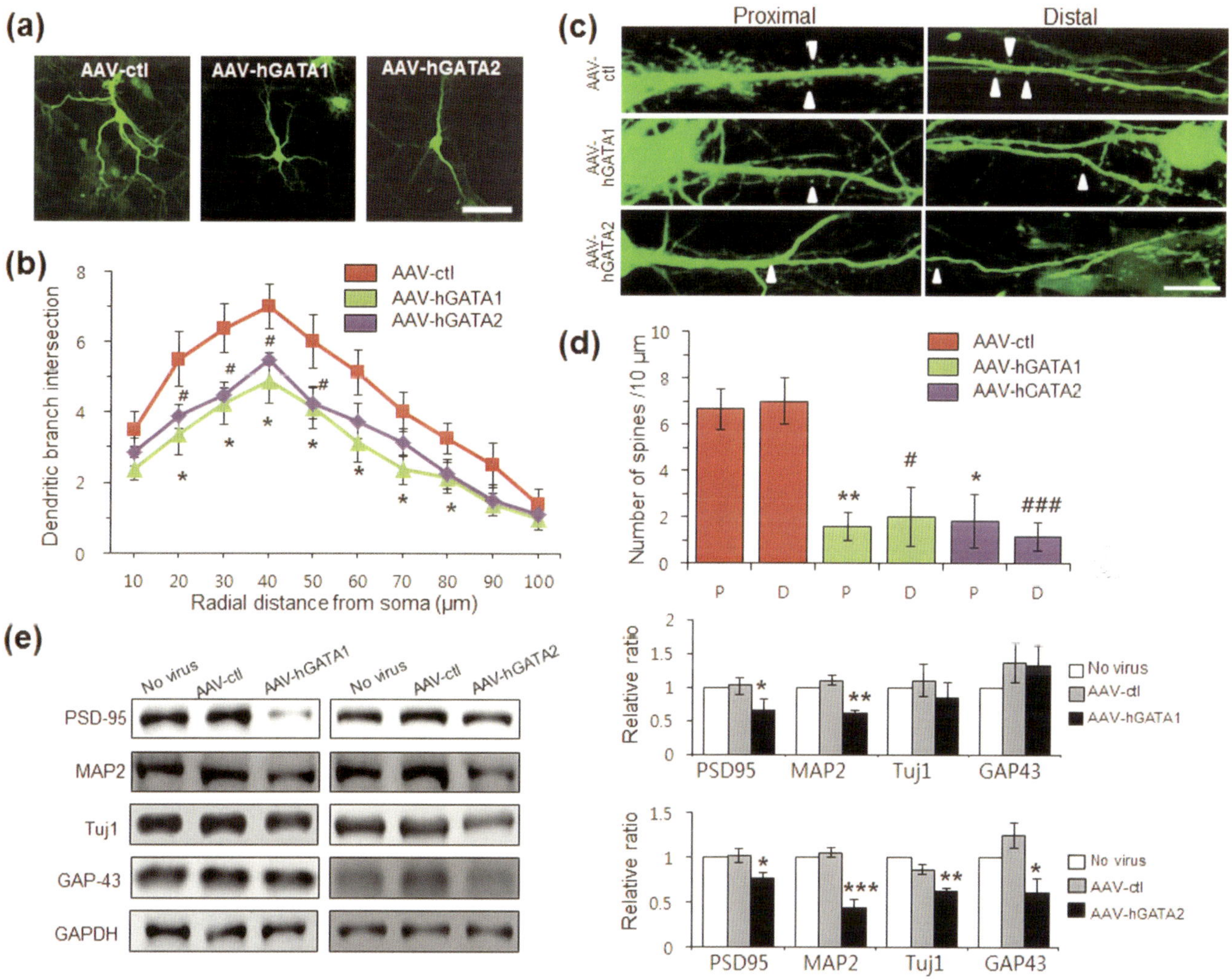

Figure 2. hGATA1 and hGATA-2 decreases dendritic arborization and spine density. Neuronal complexity in the hippocampal neurons transfected with AAV-hGATA1 or AAV-hGATA2 was analyzed based on three-dimensional projections of confocal stack images through complete neuritic extension of GFP(+) process. The neurons were transfected with AAV on 4 DIV and analyzed on 24 DIV. (a) An averaged image of multiple confocal planes across GFP(+) cells. (b) Sholl analysis of GFP(+) cells. Cells transfected with AAV-ctl presented neuritis with an increased ramification compared with cells transfected with AAV-hGAT1 and AAV-hGATA2 ($^{*}P<0.05$). (c) Representative images are shown of high-magnification Z-stack projections of dendrites of GFP(+) cells from AAV-ctl- and AAV-hGATA-transfected cells. A continuous stretch of dendritic processes was imaged. (d) The spine density (arrowheads) of proximal (P) and distal (D) segments was significantly decreased in AAV-hGATA-transfected cells compared to AAV-ctl-transfected rats ($^{*}P<0.05$, $^{**}P<0.01$ compared to proximal region of AAV-ctl; $^{\#}P<0.05$, $^{\#\#\#}P<0.001$ compared to distal region of AAV-ctl; $n=9$–12 neurons in each group). The data were expressed as the number of spines per 10 µm. (e) MAP2, PSD-95, Tuj1 and GAP-43 expression in the cells described in (a) determined by Western blot analysis. Expression levels are depicted relative to the level of cells that were not exposed to virus (: no virus) for comparison. ($n=3$–4 biological replicates per group). $^{*}P<0.05$, $^{**}P<0.01$, $^{***}P<0.001$ compared to control vector. Scale bars: *a*, 30 µm; *c*, 10 µm. Student's *t*-test.

neuronal differentiation, especially in neurite outgrowth [30]. Western blotting analyses showed a significant reduction in the protein levels of Tuj1 and GAP-43 in neurons transfected with AAV-hGATA2, but not AAV-hGATA1 (Fig. 2e). Protein levels of MAP2, which plays a role in neuronal maturation [23], were decreased by overexpression of hGATA1 or hGATA-2 (Fig. 2e).

hGATA-1 and hGATA-2 produces depressive behaviors

Given the negative effects of hGATA-1 and hGATA-2 on spine formation and dendritic arborization, we then examined the effects of hGATA-1 and hGATA-2 expression on behaviors in rat models of depression. The AAV vectors were bilaterally injected into the DG of adult rat hippocampus and behavioral testing was conducted 5 weeks after viral infusion (Fig. 3a). This resulted in widespread gene expression in the DG granule cell layer, as shown by viral expression of EGFP (Fig. 3b). Infusions of AAV-hGATA1 and AAV-hGATA2 into the hippocampus also increased levels of hGATA1 and hGATA2 mRNA, respectively, in microdissections of the infused DG area (Fig. 3c). Three models of depression/antidepressant response were tested, including the forced swim test (FST) and learned helplessness (LH), two behavioral despair models, and the sucrose preference test (SPT), a measure of anhedonia, a core symptom of depression [31]. These models are responsive to acute, subchronic, chronic antidepressants, respectively [31–33]. Both AAV-hGATA1 and AAV-hGATA2 infusions increased immobility in FST, a pro-depressive response during the initial period (300 sec) of testing (Fig. 3a; $P<0.05$, $P<0.001$, respectively). The depressant response was sustained in rats infused with AAV-hGATA2, but not AAV-hGATA1, during whole testing session (900 sec) ($P>0.1$, $P<0.05$, respectively). Spontaneous locomotor activity (LMA) was not different between these two groups, indicating that the effect observed in FST is not due to general ambulatory differences (Fig. 3e).

In the learned helplessness model, exposing animals to inescapable stress causes escape deficits. In the rats we studied here, infusion of both AAV-hGATA1 and AAV-hGATA2 increased the number of escape failures during the active avoidance testing, without exposure to an inescapable stressor (trials 1–30) (Fig. 3g, $P<0.05$). There were no significant differences in sucrose preference by AAV-hGATA-1 and AAV-hGATA2 compared to AAV-ctl groups (Fig. 3f, $P>0.05$). In addition, both AAV-hGATA1 and hGATA2 had no effect on the latency to feed NSFT, an animal model of anxiety that is responsive to chronic, but not acute antidepressant treatments [34] (Fig. 3h, $P>0.05$ compared to AAV-ctl). Home cage feeding and total fluid consumption were not different between the two groups (Fig. 3i, j). These results show that infusion of AAV-hGATA1 or AAV-hGATA2 produced depressive-like behaviors in two established rat models, the FST and LH.

hGATA-1 and hGATA-2 repress synapse-related genes

Previous chromatin immunoprecipitation studies have demonstrated that GATA-1 binds to the promoter elements of synapse-related genes, including Rab4b, indicating transcriptional control of these genes [10]. To investigate whether hGATA-1 and hGATA-2 could also regulate the expression of synapse-associated genes in hippocampus, mRNA levels were quantified by RT-PCR. Overexpression of hGATA1 or hGATA-2 in hippocampal DG results in down-regulation of Rab4b mRNA (Fig. 4a, b), a gene implicated in dendritic spine formation, consistent with previous results that elevated GATA-1 underlies the decreased transcription of Rab4b [10]. Given that AAV-hGATA1 and AAV-hGATA2 decrease levels of PSD-95 in cultured hippocampal neurons (Fig. 1a), we examined whether a similar effect is observed in DG transfected by AAV-hGATA1 and AAV-hGATA2. RT-PCR analysis demonstrated that PSD-95 and GAP-43 mRNA levels were decreased in response to AAV-hGATA1 or AAV-hGATA2 infusions into DG (Fig. 4). In addition, overexpression of hGATA-1 or hGATA-2 downregulated the levels of MAP2 mRNA, along with the glutamatergic neuronal marker vesicular glutamate transporter 1 (vGluT1) mRNA (Fig. 4d, e). However, overexpression of hGATA-1 or hGATA-2 had no effects on the differentiation of inhibitory neurons, as determined by quantitative RT-PCR analyzing glutamic acid decarboxylase 1 (GAD1) mRNA, the inhibitory neuronal marker (Fig. 4f). These results indicate that overexpressing hGATA might affect differentiation of glutamatergic neuron subpopulations, although it is possible that altered expression of vGluT1 is related to reduced spine formation. AAV-hGATA1 and AAV-hGATA2 infusion significantly decreased spine density by ~86% and ~50%, respectively (Fig. 4g, h, $P<0.001$, $P<0.05$, respectively, compared with the AAV-ctl group).

To directly test if synapse-related genes are regulated by GATA, we knocked down endogeneous GATA-2 with small hairpin RNAs (shRNAs) targeted against rat GATA-2 (shGATA-2) in hippocampal neuronal cultures; we did not examine knockdown of GATA-1 due to its low level of endogenous expression under baseline, non stress conditions [10], The transfection of shGATA-2 resulted in approximately 60% knockdown, as shown by real time RT-PCR and Western blot analysis (Fig. 5a, b). When compared to control neurons transfected with control vector alone, significant increases in the expression of Rab4b, PSD-95, GAP-43, MAP2 mRNAs were observed (Fig. 5c, d, e, f) in cells transfected with shGATA-2. The shGATA-2 incubation also significantly increased the spine density (Fig. 5g, h, $P<0.001$, compared with the control group). Regarding dendritic branch points in the MAP2(+) and GFP(+) neurons, we found that cultures differentiated with shGATA-2 contained neurons that had many more local secondary dendritic arborizations than the neurons in the control cultures (Fig. 5i, j, $P<0.001$ and $P<0.01$ compared to no transfection and control vectors, respectively). The shGATA-2 treatment significantly increased the length of spines (Figure S1 in File S1, $P<0.001$, compared with the control group). Together, these results suggest that hGATA-1 and hGATA-2 are involved in transcription of these synapse- and neurite-related genes, and in turn spine-synapse formation.

Discussion

Here we show that viral expression of hGATA-1 or hGATA-2 transcription factors suppress the expression of genes that are involved in spine formation and neurite outgrowth in the rat hippocampal cells. We also extend our previous studies and demonstrate that chronic stress exposure increases GATA-2 expression in the hippocampus and that this effect is reversed by the rapid acting antidepressant ketamine, supporting a role for GATA-2 in stress related behavioral alterations. Moreover, the results demonstrate that viral expression of hGATA-1 or hGAT-2 in the hippocampus of rat brain decrease in the expression of synapse related genes and cause depressive-like behaviors.

The results of behavioral testing indicate that expression of hGATA-1 and hGATA-2 increases vulnerability to developing 'depressive-like' behaviors. Notably, increased hGATA-1 and hGATA-2 levels in the hippocampal DG is sufficient to produce depressive-like effects in the FST and LH, models of behavioral despair and helplessness that are responsive to acute and subchronic antidepressant treatment, respectively. Expression of hGATA-1 or hGATA-2 had no effects on behavior in the SPT and NSFT, models of anhedonia and anxiety. The reasons for the

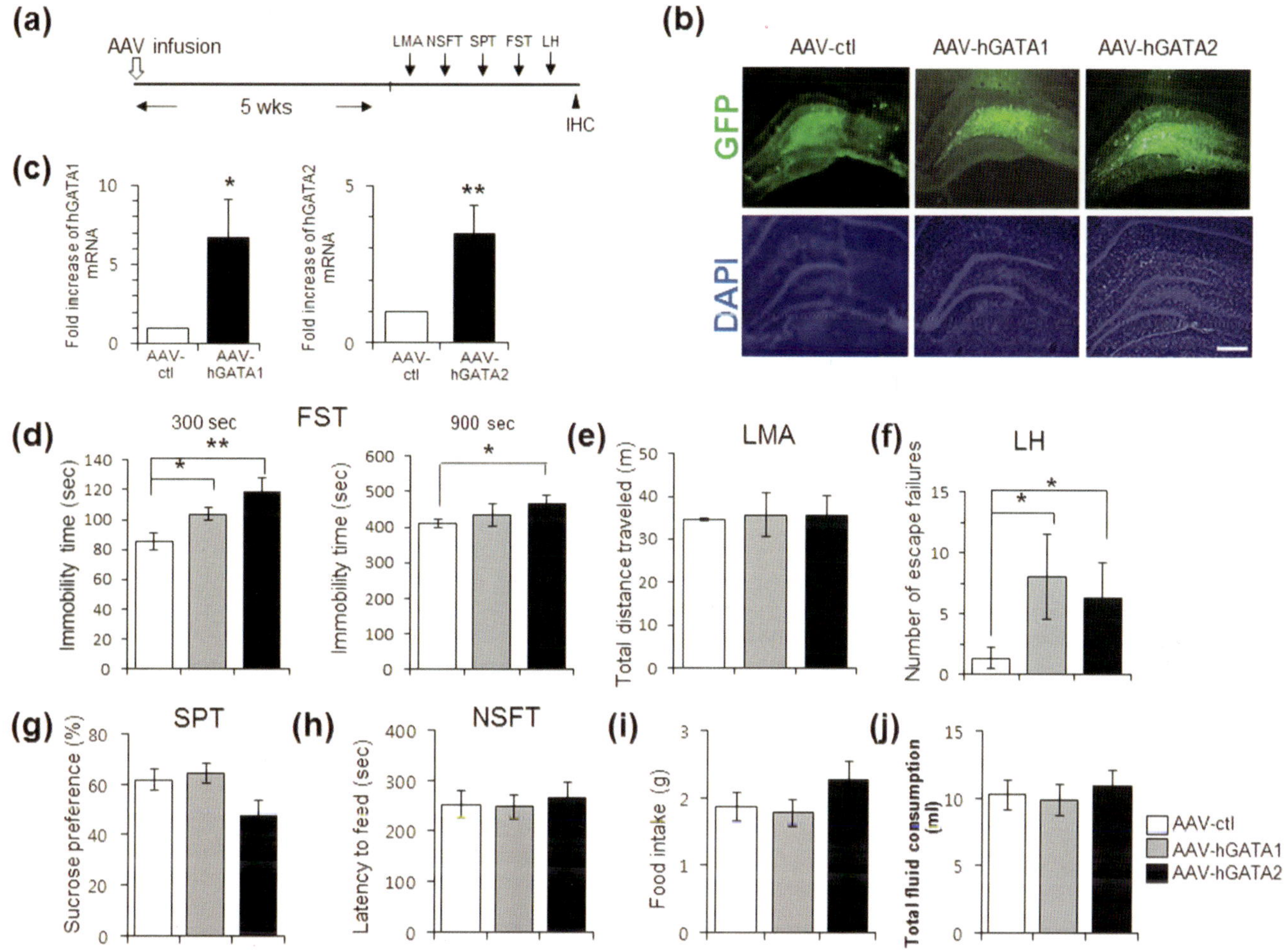

Figure 3. AAV-GATA infusions into hippocampus produce depression-like behavioral actions. (a) Experimental design. Animals were injected with AAV-ctl, AAV-hGATA1 or AAV-hGATA2 and 5 weeks later were tested in behavioral paradigms, and then hippocampal sections were harvested for and immunohistochemistry (IHC) and biochemistry. (b) Representative images of GFP(+) cells in DG from AAV-ctl-eGFP, AAV-hGATA1-eGFP and AAV-hGATA2-eGFP injected animals. (c) Quantitative RT-PCR analysis was conducted to examine the expression of hGATA1 and hGATA-2 mRNA ($^{**}P<0.01$). (d) FST. AAV-hGATA2 rats had a longer immobility score (time in seconds) than AAV-ctl-injected rats during the initial testing for 300 sec ($F_{1,12}=11.04$, $P=0.005$) and whole testing session for 900 sec ($F_{1,12}=5.12$, $P=0.042$). AAV-hGATA1 rats had a longer immobility score than AAV-ctl-injected rats during the initial testing for 300 sec ($F_{1,12}=5.79$, $P=0.034$; 900 sec: $F_{1,12}=0.52$, $P=0.48$). (e) Locomoter activity. The total distance moved in the box was similar between groups ($F_{1,10}=0.03$, $P=0.84$). (f) LH. AAV-hGATA1 or AAV-hGATA2 transduced rats had more escape failures than AAV-ctl animals (AAV-hGATA1: $F_{1,20}=7.09$, $P=0.028$; AAV-hGATA2: $F_{1,19}=5.85$, $P=0.038$). (g) SPT. Sucrose preference was not different both in AAV-hGATA1- or AAV-hGATA2-injected animals compared to AAV-ctl-injected animals (AAV-hGATA1: $F_{1,19}=0.08$, $P=0.67$; AAV-hGATA2: $F_{1,19}=0.19$, $P=0.78$). (h) NSFT. No differences in the latency to feed were shown between AAV-hGATA-injected animals and AAV-ctl-injected animals (AAV-hGATA1: $F_{1,19}=0.01$, $P=0.92$; AAV-hGATA2: $F_{1,19}=0.09$, $P=0.76$). (i-j) Home cage feeding and total fluid consumption. There was no difference in the home cage food intake (AAV-hGATA1: $F_{1,19}=0.08$, $P=0.76$; AAV-hGATA2: $F_{1,19}=0.79$, $P=0.38$) and total fluid consumption (AAV-hGATA1: $F_{1,19}=0.079$, $P=0.78$; AAV-hGATA2: $F_{1,19}=0.19$, $P=0.66$) between AAV-ctl-injected and AAV-hGATA-injected rats. Values represent mean ± s.e.m. from AAV-ctl ($n=10$), AAV-hGATA1 ($n=9$–11) and AAV-hGATA2 ($n=8$–11). Student's *t*-test (c). ANOVA test (d-j). $^{*}P<0.05$, $^{**}P<0.01$ compared to control vector. Scale bar: 200 μm.

lack of effects in SPT and NSFT are not clear but could be due to the responsiveness of these models to acute (FST), subchronic (LH), or chronic (SPT, NSFT) antidepressant treatments. Alternatively, the differential responses could be related to the role of hippocampus in these behaviors. It would be interesting in future studies to examine the influence of hGATA-1 and hGATA-2 expression in other brain regions, including the prefrontal cortex and amygdala on these behaviors. Nevertheless, the results demonstrate that hGATA-1 and hGATA-2 in the DG of hippocampus produces changes in neuronal morphology that contribute to the expression of depressive-like deficits in tests that assess despair and helplessness, but not anhedonia and anxiety.

Overexpression of GATA-1 in rat cortex has previously been shown to cause depressive behaviors that are associated with alterations of neuronal morphology [10]. Further evidence for a role of GATA1 in depression was provided by a recent genome microarray study of postmortem MDD subjects, which showed that levels of GATA1 mRNA were increased in the DG, but not CA1 subregion of the hippocampus [11]. Accordingly, we examined the influence of GATA transcription factors on the morphology of hippocampal neurons and depressive behaviors. This strategy allows analysis of the overall effects of these transcription factors on synapse related target genes that may occur via conserved GATA promoter sequences. An advantage of this approach is that we are examining the endogenous target

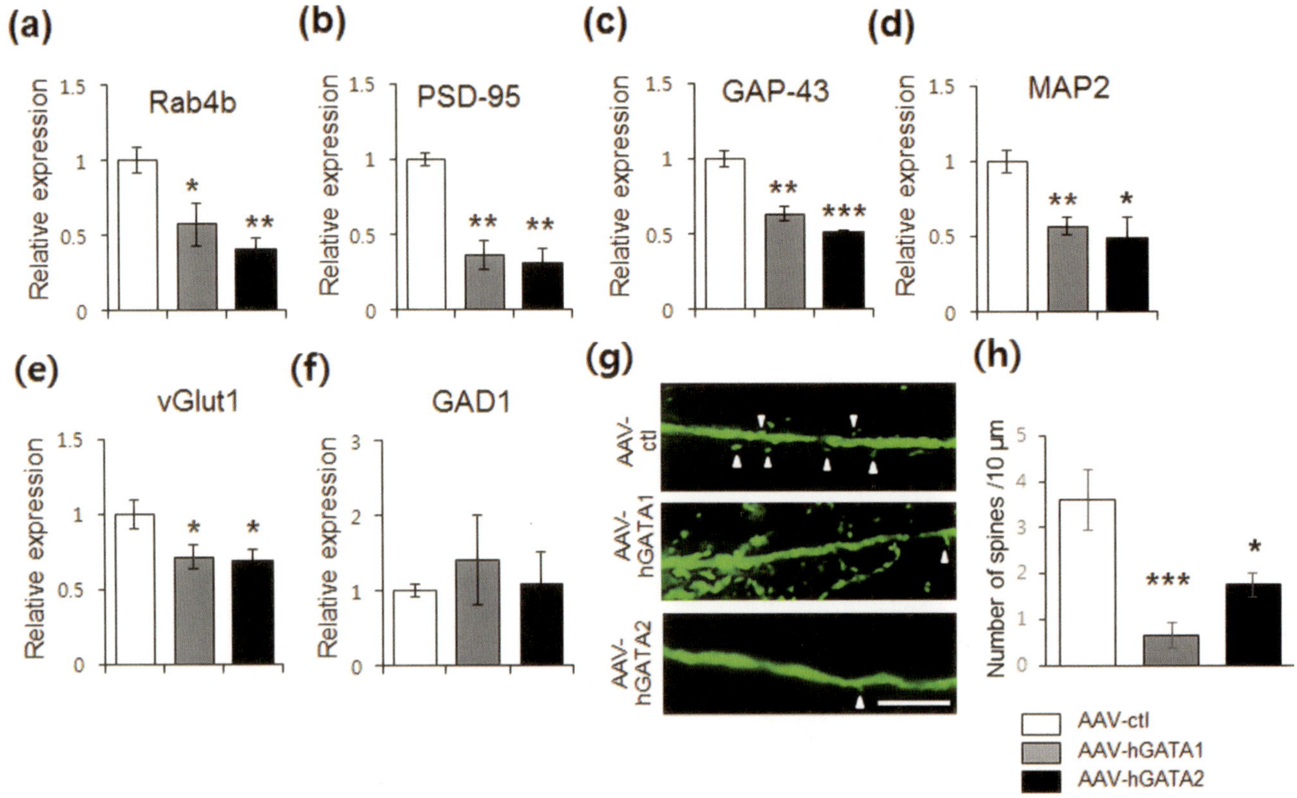

Figure 4. Transcriptional repression of synapse-related genes and a decrease in spine density by AAV-hGATA1 and AAV-hGATA2 in DG of the rat hippocampus. (a–d) Quantitative analysis of synapse-related genes in DG microdissected from rat hippocampus transfected with AAV-hGATA1 or AAV-hGATA2. Rab4b, AAV-hGATA1: $F_{1,4}=10.78$, $P=0.03$; AAV-hGATA2: $F_{1,4}=46.2$, $P=0.002$; PSD95, AAV-hGATA1: $F_{1,4}=31.73$, $P=0.004$; AAV-hGATA2: $F_{1,4}=42.8$, $P=0.002$; GAP43, AAV-hGATA1: $F_{1,4}=49.8$, $P=0.002$; AAV-hGATA2: $F_{1,4}=755.17$, $P=0.00001$; MAP2, AAV-hGATA1: $F_{1,4}=46.1$, $P=0.002$; AAV-hGATA2: $F_{1,4}=8.3$, $P=0.04$; vGlut1, AAV-hGATA1: $F_{1,4}=16.6$, $P=0.015$; AAV-hGATA2: $F_{1,4}=24.09$, $P=0.02$; GAD1, AAV-hGATA1: $F_{1,4}=0.004$, $P=0.95$; AAV-hGATA2: $F_{1,4}=1.59$, $P=0.27$. (g) Representative images are shown of high-magnification Z-stack projections of apical tuft segments of GFP(+) DG granule cells from AAV-ctl, AAV-hGATA1 and AAV-hGATA2-injected rats. (h) Density of dendritic spines (arrowheads) was significantly decreased in AAV-hGATA1- and AAV-hGATA2-injected rats compared with AAV-ctl-injected rats (a main effect of virus, $F_{2,13}=12.9$, $P<0.0001$; AAV-hGATA1: $F_{1,10}=21.15$, $P=0.0009$; AAV-hGATA2: $F_{1,7}=5.63$, $P=0.04$). The data were expressed as the number of spines per 10 μm. ANOVA test. $^{*}P<0.05$, $^{**}P<0.01$, $^{***}P<0.001$ compared to control vector. Values represent mean ± s.e.m. of 5–7 cells from three animals per group. Scale bar: 10 μm.

genes in their normal chromatin environment in rat hippocampal cells, which express GATA-2, and low levels of GATA-1 [14]. Based on low endogenous levels, viral expression of hGATA-1 may produce a distinct effect on the transactivation of genes. In contrast, because levels of endogenous GATA-2 are relatively high, viral expression of hGATA-2 may produce less physiological changes. However, hGATA-2 protein appears to exhibit a broader binding sequence specificity compared with that of mouse GATA-1 and hGATA-3 [35]. Thus even small changes in the level of hGATA-2 proteins might affect transactivation of GATA-2 responsive genes and in turn produces depressive-like deficits. Our results together with the previous finding [10] indicate that GATA1 induces depressive-like behaviors and a decrease in spine density when it is overexpressed either in the prefrontal cortex or hippocampus. Accordingly, hGATA-2, which produces similar depressive-like behaviors when expressed in hippocampal neurons, might have depressive effects on animal behaviors when it is overexpressed in the prefrontal cortex as well. Given that hGATA-1 and -2 control depressive-like behaviors in rats, one might assume there is a link between hGATA transcription factors and adult hippocampal neurogenesis, a form of neural plasticity that is increased by antidepressant treatments [36]. However, there have been no reports that GATA transcription factors regulate adult hippocampal neurogenesis, and further studies will be needed to address this question.

The results show that some of the synaptic plasticity-related genes normally expressed in neuronal cells respond to hGATA-1 and hGATA-2 transcription factor expression. Interestingly, besides previously known GATA-1 responding genes, PSD-95, GAP-43 and MAP2 showed a response to changes in levels of the hGATA-1/hGATA-2 *in vivo*. Our scans for canonical GATA sites throughout the locus based on aligned DNA sequences indicate that PSD-95, GAP-43 and MAP2 have potential GATA-1 and GATA-2 binding sites (http://www.cbrc.jp/research/db/TFSEARCH.html). Therefore, it appears that genes having conserved GATA sites showed a response to changes in levels of the GATA proteins. Indeed many genes have GATA promoter elements (conserved or not) because of the short recognition sequence (6 to 8 bp), which are frequently represented in genomic DNA (e.g. >50 sites in MAP2 gene) [35,37]. However, the functional regulation of GATA transcription factor binding *in vivo* is controlled by many different factors. The primary determinants of transcriptional outcome would be the context in which a potential binding site is embedded, local chromatin structure, and synergistic interactions with other transcription factors recognizing neighboring sites. Thus, the repressive effects of hGATA-1 and

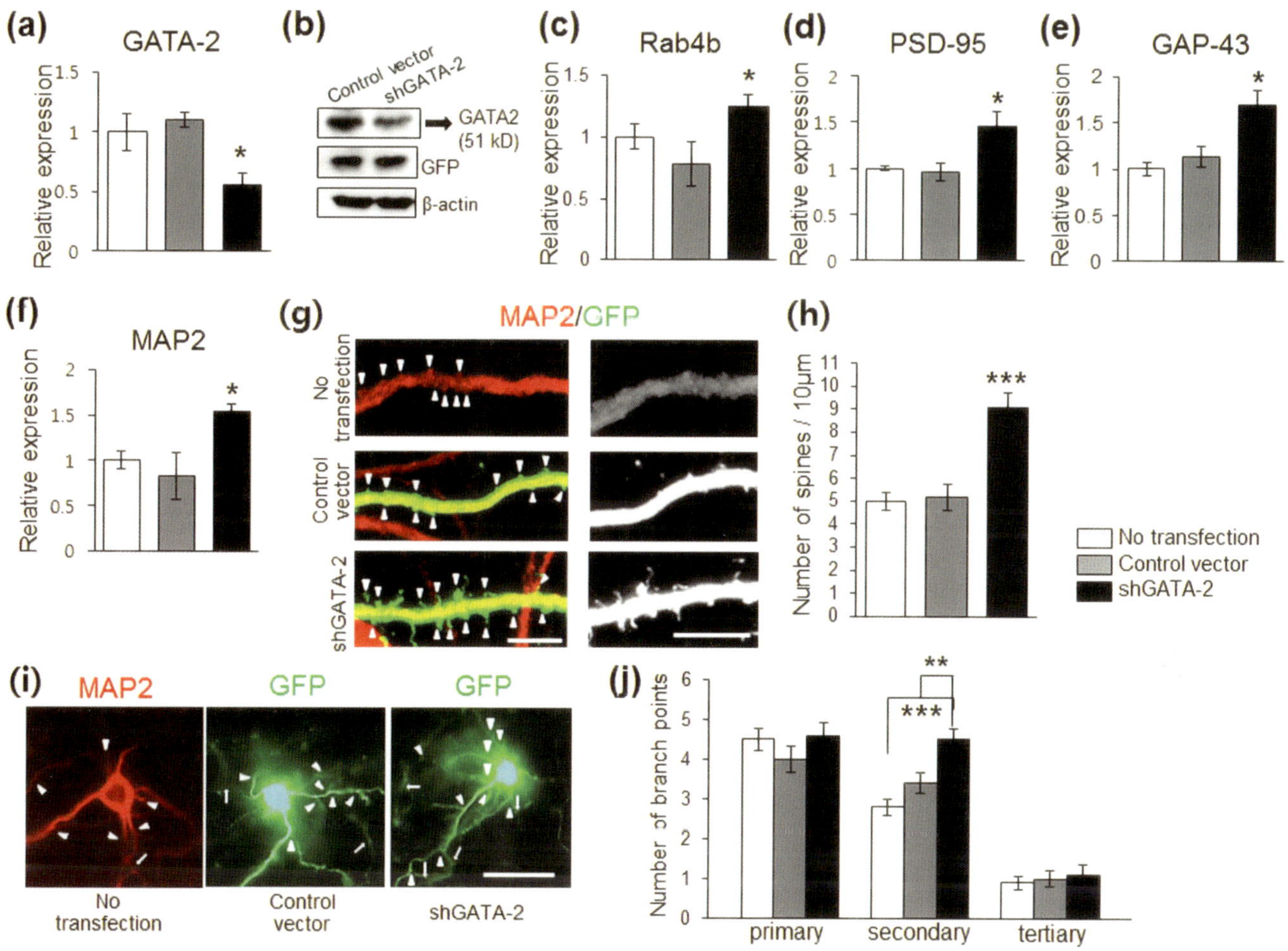

Figure 5. shGATA-2 increases synapse-related genes and spine density. (a–b) Transfection with shGATA-2 caused ~60% knockdown of GATA2 mRNA and protein expression in rat hippocampal cells. Western blotting analysis was conducted to examine the expression of endogeneous rat GATA-2, and representative blots were shown. The GATA-2 (51 kD) protein in the nuclear extracts is downregulated in response to transfection with shGATA-2 compared to control vector. (c–f) Quantitative analysis of synapse-related genes in rat hippocampal neurons transfected with shGATA-2. Rab4b, $P<0.05$, PSD95, $P<0.01$; GAP43, $P<0.05$; MAP2, $P<0.05$) (g) Representative images are shown of Z-stack projections of dendrites of MAP2(+) and GFP(+) cells from ctl- and shGATA2-transfected cells. A continuous stretch of dendritic processes was imaged. (right panel) high magnification. (h) Density of dendritic spines (arrowheads) was significantly increased in shGATA2-transfected cells compared with controls ($^{***}P<0.001$ compared to controls). The data were expressed as the number of spines per 10 μm. $n=5$–7 cells. (i) The number of dendritic branches exiting the soma (1′ dendrites), dendritic branches arborizing from 1′ dendrites (2′ dendrites, arrowheads) and dendritic branches arborizing from 2′ dendrites (3′ dendrites, arrows) were counted in neurons immunostained for MAP2 and GFP ($n=10$–15 cells per treatment). Student's *t* test. $^{*}P<0.05$, $^{**}P<0.01$, $^{***}P<0.001$ compared to control vector. Values represent mean ± s.e.m. Scale bar: 10 μm.

hGATA-2 on the synapse-related genes might not be solely due to the presence or number of DNA binding sites, but rather is related to the transcriptome environment of genes, which is also influenced by experiential and behavioral factors. Given the high degree of similarity of DNA binding zinc finger sequences between hGATA-1 and hGATA-2, hGATA-2 might be the primary repressor *in vivo* until hGATA-1 is induced by stimuli such as chronic stress. Further studies will be required to address how the mammalian GATA proteins regulate the transcription of synapse-related genes via different binding specificities at different sites *in vivo*.

Given that hGATA-1 and hGATA-2 may regulate spine morphology and synaptic function in hippocampal neurons and depressive behaviors in rats, further studies will be warranted to investigate whether hGATA-1 and hGATA-2 play distinct roles in neurons of the adult brain including hippocampus. Full evaluation of the expression and role of the hGATA-1 and hGATA-2 on the transcription of target genes in rodents, as well as the localization in different populations of neurons in human brain will further elucidate the molecular mechanisms that underlie the pathophysiology and eventually the treatment of stress related illnesses such as depression and related psychiatric disorders.

Supporting Information

File S1 Supporting Materials and Methods and Figure S1.

Author Contributions

Conceived and designed the experiments: HS. Performed the experiments: MC SEW SYK HJK SYC SHL YSK. Analyzed the data: HJK YSK HS. Contributed reagents/materials/analysis tools: RSD HS. Wrote the paper: RSD HS.

References

1. Gutierrez H, Davies AM (2011) Regulation of neural process growth, elaboration and structural plasticity by NF-kappaB. Trends Neurosci 34: 316–325.
2. Eyre H, Baune BT (2012) Neuroplastic changes in depression: a role for the immune system. Psychoneuroendocrinology 37: 1397–1416.
3. Kasai H, Matsuzaki M, Noguchi J, Yasumatsu N, Nakahara H (2003) Structure-stability-function relationships of dendritic spines. Trends Neurosci 26: 360–368.
4. Holtmaat A, Svoboda K (2009) Experience-dependent structural synaptic plasticity in the mammalian brain. Nat Rev Neurosci 10: 647–658.
5. Kasai H, Fukuda M, Watanabe S, Hayashi-Takagi A, Noguchi J (2010) Structural dynamics of dendritic spines in memory and cognition. Trends Neurosci 33: 121–129.
6. Glantz LA, Lewis DA (2000) Decreased dendritic spine density on prefrontal cortical pyramidal neurons in schizophrenia. Arch Gen Psychiatry 57: 65–73.
7. Pan X, Minegishi N, Harigae H, Yamagiwa H, Minegishi M, et al. (2000) Identification of human GATA-2 gene distal IS exon and its expression in hematopoietic stem cell fractions. J Biochem 127: 105–112.
8. Begley CG, Green AR (1999) The SCL gene: from case report to critical hematopoietic regulator. Blood 93: 2760–2770.
9. Shivdasani RA, Orkin SH (1996) The transcriptional control of hematopoiesis. Blood 87: 4025–4039.
10. Kang HJ, Voleti B, Hajszan T, Rajkowska G, Stockmeier CA, et al. (2012) Decreased expression of synapse-related genes and loss of synapses in major depressive disorder. Nat Med 18: 1413–1417.
11. Duric V, Banasr M, Licznerski P, Schmidt HD, Stockmeier CA, et al. (2010) A negative regulator of MAP kinase causes depressive behavior. Nat Med 16: 1328–1332.
12. Zhou Y, Yamamoto M, Engel JD (2000) GATA2 is required for the generation of V2 interneurons. Development 127: 3829–3838.
13. Craven SE, Lim KC, Ye W, Engel JD, de Sauvage F, et al. (2004) Gata2 specifies serotonergic neurons downstream of sonic hedgehog. Development 131: 1165–1173.
14. Wallach I, Zhang J, Hartmann A, van Landeghem FK, Ivanova A, et al. (2009) Erythropoietin-receptor gene regulation in neuronal cells. Pediatr Res 65: 619–624.
15. El Wakil A, Francius C, Wolff A, Pleau-Varet J, Nardelli J (2006) The GATA2 transcription factor negatively regulates the proliferation of neuronal progenitors. Development 133: 2155–2165.
16. Nardelli J, Thiesson D, Fujiwara Y, Tsai FY, Orkin SH (1999) Expression and genetic interaction of transcription factors GATA-2 and GATA-3 during development of the mouse central nervous system. Dev Biol 210: 305–321.
17. Morceau F, Schnekenburger M, Dicato M, Diederich M (2004) GATA-1: friends, brothers, and coworkers. Ann N Y Acad Sci 1030: 537–554.
18. Gong QH, Stern J, Dean A (1991) Transcriptional role of a conserved GATA-1 site in the human epsilon-globin gene promoter. Mol Cell Biol 11: 2558–2566.
19. Minegishi N, Ohta J, Suwabe N, Nakauchi H, Ishihara H, et al. (1998) Alternative promoters regulate transcription of the mouse GATA-2 gene. J Biol Chem 273: 3625–3634.
20. Kumari J, Bogwald J, Dalmo RA (2009) Transcription factor GATA-3 in Atlantic salmon (Salmo salar): molecular characterization, promoter activity and expression analysis. Mol Immunol 46: 3099–3107.
21. Son H, Banasr M, Choi M, Chae SY, Licznerski P, et al. (2012) Neuritin produces antidepressant actions and blocks the neuronal and behavioral deficits caused by chronic stress. Proc Natl Acad Sci U S A 109: 11378–11383.
22. Hommel JD, Sears RM, Georgescu D, Simmons DL, DiLeone RJ (2003) Local gene knockdown in the brain using viral-mediated RNA interference. Nat Med 9: 1539–1544.
23. Kim JS, Chang MY, Yu IT, Kim JH, Lee SH, et al. (2004) Lithium selectively increases neuronal differentiation of hippocampal neural progenitor cells both in vitro and in vivo. J Neurochem 89: 324–336.
24. Sholl DA (1953) Dendritic organization in the neurons of the visual and motor cortices of the cat. J Anat 87: 387–406.
25. Melia KR, Ryabinin AE, Schroeder R, Bloom FE, Wilson MC (1994) Induction and habituation of immediate early gene expression in rat brain by acute and repeated restraint stress. J Neurosci 14: 5929–5938.
26. Li N, Liu RJ, Dwyer JM, Banasr M, Lee B, et al. (2011) Glutamate N-methyl-D-aspartate receptor antagonists rapidly reverse behavioral and synaptic deficits caused by chronic stress exposure. Biol Psychiatry 69: 754–761.
27. Li N, Lee B, Liu RJ, Banasr M, Dwyer JM, et al. (2010) mTOR-dependent synapse formation underlies the rapid antidepressant effects of NMDA antagonists. Science 329: 959–964.
28. Beauquis J, Roig P, De Nicola AF, Saravia F (2010) Short-term environmental enrichment enhances adult neurogenesis, vascular network and dendritic complexity in the hippocampus of type 1 diabetic mice. PLoS One 5: e13993.
29. Keith D, El-Husseini A (2008) Excitation Control: Balancing PSD-95 Function at the Synapse. Front Mol Neurosci 1: 4.
30. Denny JB (2006) Molecular mechanisms, biological actions, and neuropharmacology of the growth-associated protein GAP-43. Curr Neuropharmacol 4: 293–304.
31. Banasr M, Duman RS (2008) Glial loss in the prefrontal cortex is sufficient to induce depressive-like behaviors. Biol Psychiatry 64: 863–870.
32. Hunsberger JG, Newton SS, Bennett AH, Duman CH, Russell DS, et al. (2007) Antidepressant actions of the exercise-regulated gene VGF. Nat Med 13: 1476–1482.
33. Banasr M, Chowdhury GM, Terwilliger R, Newton SS, Duman RS, et al. (2010) Glial pathology in an animal model of depression: reversal of stress-induced cellular, metabolic and behavioral deficits by the glutamate-modulating drug riluzole. Mol Psychiatry 15: 501–511.
34. Santarelli L, Gobbi G, Debs PC, Sibille ET, Blier P, et al. (2001) Genetic and pharmacological disruption of neurokinin 1 receptor function decreases anxiety-related behaviors and increases serotonergic function. Proc Natl Acad Sci U S A 98: 1912–1917.
35. Merika M, Orkin SH (1993) DNA-binding specificity of GATA family transcription factors. Mol Cell Biol 13: 3999–4010.
36. Malberg JE, Eisch AJ, Nestler EJ, Duman RS (2000) Chronic antidepressant treatment increases neurogenesis in adult rat hippocampus. J Neurosci 20: 9104–9110.
37. Gumina RJ, Kirschbaum NE, Piotrowski K, Newman PJ (1997) Characterization of the human platelet/endothelial cell adhesion molecule-1 promoter: identification of a GATA-2 binding element required for optimal transcriptional activity. Blood 89: 1260–1269.

8

No Evidence for the Association between a Polymorphism in the *PCLO* Depression Candidate Gene with Memory Bias in Remitted Depressed Patients and Healthy Individuals

Janna N. Vrijsen[1]*, Anne Speckens[1], Alejandro Arias-Vásquez[1,2,3,4], Barbara Franke[1,2,4], Eni S. Becker[5], Iris van Oostrom[1]

1 Department of Psychiatry, Radboud University Medical Centre, Nijmegen, the Netherlands, **2** Donders Institute for Brain, Cognition and Behaviour, Radboud University Medical Centre, Nijmegen, the Netherlands, **3** Department of Cognitive Neuroscience, Radboud University Medical Centre, Nijmegen, The Netherlands, **4** Department of Human Genetics, Radboud University Medical Centre, Nijmegen, The Netherlands, **5** Behavioural Science Institute, Radboud University Nijmegen, Nijmegen, The Netherlands

Abstract

The *PCLO* rs2522833 candidate polymorphism for depression has been associated to monoaminergic neurotransmission. In healthy and currently depressed individuals, the polymorphism has been found to affect activation of brain areas during memory processing, but no direct association of *PCLO* with memory bias was found. We hypothesized that the absence of this association might have been obscured by current depressive symptoms or genetically driven individual differences in reactivity to stressful events. Experiencing stressful childhood events fosters dysfunctional assumptions that are related to cognitive biases, and may modulate the predisposition for depression via epigenetic effects. The association between *PCLO* and memory bias, as well as interaction between *PCLO* and childhood events was studied in patients remitted from depression (N = 299), as well as a sample of healthy individuals (N = 157). The participants performed an emotional verbal memory task after a sad mood induction. Childhood trauma and adversity were measured with a questionnaire. The Genotype main effect, and Genotype by Childhood Events interaction were analyzed for memory bias in both samples. *PCLO* risk allele carrying remitted depressed patients did not show more negatively biased memory than non-risk allele carriers, not even patients with stressful childhood events. A similar pattern of results was found in healthy individuals. Memory bias may not be strongly associated with the *PCLO* rs2522833 polymorphism. We did not find any support for the *PCLO*-childhood events interaction, but the power of our study was insufficient to exclude this possibility.

Editor: Ulrike Schmidt, Max Planck Institute of Psychiatry, Germany

Funding: The study was funded by the department of Psychiatry of the Radboud University Medical Centre. The funders had no role in study design, data collection and analysis, decision to publish, or preparation of the manuscript.

Competing Interests: The authors have declared that no competing interests exist.

* Email: Janna.Vrijsen@radboudumc.nl

Introduction

Depression results in a high disease burden as well as increased mortality risk due to important impairments in social, emotional and physical functioning. Twin studies found that the genetic contribution to depression is up to 40% [1]. The SNP rs2522833 in the piccolo (*PCLO*) gene has been associated with current depression [2–5]. The *PCLO* gene encodes a presynaptic cytomatrix protein called piccolo. Specifically, the rs2522833 polymorphism leads to a serine to alanine substitution in the C2A calcium sensor domain of the protein and may affect protein stability [6,7]. Monoaminergic modulation of the hypothalamic pituitary adrenal system (involved in stress responses) may be a route through which *PCLO* affects depression vulnerability [4,8,9]. The C 'risk' allele is more frequent in depressed individuals than in healthy individuals and has been associated with heritable personality traits that predispose to depression in healthy individuals, such as 'harm avoidance' [4], as well as with changes in HPA responsiveness after treatment [9]. Other studies, however, were not able to replicate the association with clinical depression [7], or did not find an association with sub-clinical levels of depression [3].

Depression is a complex multifactorial condition and genetic studies so far have yielded mixed results [1]. Cognitive information processing styles associated with depression could be more closely related to genetic factors than the complex and heterogeneous phenotype of major depressive disorder and hence provide another way to study the association between candidate genes and depression [10,11]. Biased processing of emotional information is considered to be a strong contributor to the development as well as the recurrence of depression, and has also been associated with other forms of psychopathology such as anxiety, eating disorders, and addiction [12–17]. Negatively biased *memory*, however, seems particularly robust in depression [18–22]. Depressed individuals are inclined to have better memory for negative than positive information, compared to healthy individuals who tend to preferentially recall positive information [18,19,23]. Upon remission, sad mood state activates biased processing [24–27]. Biased memory in depression is strongest if the information is self-relevant [16], and is generally studied using explicit memory tasks [28–30].

Emotional processing biases have been associated with several depression candidate genes, such as the 5-HTTLPR polymorphism in the *SLC6A4* gene, and the *BDNF, COMT* and *NR3C2* genes (e.g. [31–36]). In addition to being related to depression, the risk ('C') allele in the *PCLO* rs2522833 polymorphism has also been associated with neural correlates of biased processing of emotional faces and memory bias [37–39]. Schott and colleagues [27] reported that C allele carriers had lower (non-emotional) memory performance, which was associated with reduced hippocampal activation. Woudstra and colleagues [39] found the *PCLO* polymorphism to affect activation of relevant brain regions (i.e. the anterior cingulate circuit, inferior frontal gyrus, and insula) during emotional memory processing in 89 currently depressed and 29 healthy individuals. However, no direct association between the *PCLO* genotype and emotional memory processing was found.

The complex interplay between genetic susceptibility and stressful life events is considered to be an important mechanism in the development of depression [40–42]. Especially stressful childhood events may be of importance [43]. Experiencing negative events in childhood can lead to dysfunctional basic assumptions about the self and the world [44]. These assumptions may induce cognitive biases, as information is processed in accordance with the (dysfunctional) assumptions. Subsequent stressful events may trigger biased processing, such as negatively biased attention and memory, and may contribute to vulnerability for developing symptoms of depression or to relapse (see cognitive models of depression, [44,45]). This process may be strongest in genetically susceptible individuals. Indeed, studies have found that depression risk allele carriers who experienced stressful life events generally show stronger negative memory bias and/or less positive memory bias [33,34,46]. Hence, stressful events may modulate the genetic risk effect on depressotypic information processing.

The fact that the interaction between genetic susceptibility and stressful events has not been examined so far may have contributed to the null-findings regarding the association of *PCLO* and memory bias. Furthermore, most of the participants in the Woudstra and colleagues [39] study were depressed at the time of testing. Participants'depressed mood [16], as well as concentration and memory problems associated with depression probably had a strong effect on emotional memory processing in the Woudstra and colleagues [39] study. This may have overshadowed the small effect of *PCLO* on memory bias. The aim of the current study was to examine the effect of *PCLO* on memory bias as well as the gene-childhood stress interaction in a group of patients remitted from depression and a group of healthy participants. We included a sample of remitted patients because this offers the possibility to study cognitive processes in individuals highly at risk for a (recurrent) depressive episode [47,48], while minimizing depressive symptoms or concomitants affecting cognitive biases [49]. The analyses were repeated in a sample of healthy individuals to confirm the pattern of results. We hypothesized to find an association between *PCLO* rs2522833 variation and memory bias in remitted depressed patients as well as healthy individuals. We expected this effect to be more pronounced in individuals who experienced stressful childhood events than in individuals who did not.

Methods and Materials

Participants

This study is part of a larger study, which aims to link cognitive biases to genetic susceptibility to depression in two independent samples of 360 undergraduate female students of the Radboud University Nijmegen (healthy individuals) and 327 individuals who were remitted from depression (remitted patients). Complete genotype data were available for a total of 351 healthy individuals. Half of the healthy individuals underwent the same sad mood induction procedure as the remitted depressed patients and were therefore selected for the current study. Two of the healthy individuals did not complete the memory task, resulting in a sample of N = 157 for the further analyses. The remitted depressed patients underwent the same sad mood induction. Complete genotype data were available for a total of 320 remitted patients, and complete genotype and memory bias data for a total of 299 remitted patients for further analyses. The remitted patients were recruited at the Department of Psychiatry of the Radboud University Medical Centre and other outpatient psychiatric services in the region. The participants were invited for the study by means of an information letter. Before the onset of the experiment, participants were given the opportunity to ask questions and they were instructed that they could stop at any time, without specification of a reason. Subsequently, they gave written informed consent. Participants were included in the remitted depressed patient group if they met the criteria of the DSM-IV [50] for a previous depressive episode. Exclusion criteria for both groups were: current depressive episode, current or lifetime bipolar disorder, current psychotic symptoms, alcohol or substance abuse within the past 6 months, deafness, blindness, neurological disorder, sensorimotor handicaps and intellectual disability. In order to assess in- and exclusion criteria, trained professionals interviewed eligible participants with the Structured Clinical Interview for the DSM-IV Axis-I disorders (SCID-I) [51]. The SCID-I has been demonstrated to have a good reliability [52,53]. State depressive symptoms were measured with the Beck Depression Inventory (BDI-II) [54]. Participants received course credit or a gift certificate in return for their participation. Participants were debriefed before they were rewarded for their participation. The study was approved by the Dutch Central Committee on Research involving Human Subjects (CCMO) and we complied with the Code of Ethics of the World Medical Association (Declaration of Helsinki) in the treatment of our participants.

Stressful childhood events

Stressful childhood events were assessed with an adapted version of the Life Events Questionnaire [55]. This version has previously been used in comparable studies [33,34,56]. Participants were asked to indicate whether they had experienced a set of life events before the age 16 of years, after the age of 16, and within the last year. A childhood traumatic events variable was calculated indicating whether or not participants experienced traumatic events (i.e. physical or sexual abuse) involving a family member or a non-family member before the age of 16 years. Because the prevalence of aggression and/or abuse was rather low in the sample of healthy individuals (16% of all participants) and we expect a similar effect of non-traumatic but highly stressful events, the effect of traumatic as well as stressful adverse childhood events was studied in this sample. This variable indicated whether or not participants experienced traumatic events (aggression and/or abuse) involving a family member or a non-family member and/or adverse events (parental loss, divorce of parents and/or prolonged separation of parents) before the age of 16 [33].

Sad mood induction

Prior to the memory task, participants were presented with a highly emotional sad film segment from the movie "Sophie's choice" [57]. They were instructed to let the emotionality of the film influence their mood as much as possible and to maintain the sad mood state. Participants rated their mood state using a computerized visual analog scale that ranged from −10 (indicating saddest mood) to 10 (indicating happiest mood) after the mood induction. Remitted patients also rated their mood state before the mood induction.

Memory bias

This memory task has been previously used and described [35,58]. Participants were presented with 12 depression-specific negative and 12 positive words in fixed order, with no more than two words of the same valence being presented consecutively. Words were selected from two databases (Dutch translation of the Affective Norms for English Words database; [59, and 60]). Each word was presented for 10 seconds in capital black letters against a white background. To make encoding self-referential, participants were instructed to vividly imagine themselves in a scene with the presented word [61]. After completion of this rating, the next word would appear on the screen. This task was followed by a short paper-and-pencil distraction task (Raven matrices) [62]. After that, participants were instructed to return to the computer for an unannounced free recall of the words from the previous computer task. Participants were instructed to type in all the words they could remember within three minutes. A difference-score representing memory bias was calculated by subtracting the number of correctly recalled negative words from the number of correctly recalled positive words. A negative score represented negative memory bias.

Genotyping

In healthy individuals, saliva samples were collecting using Oragene kit (DNA Genotek, Inc. Ottawa, Ontario, Canada). In remitted patients, blood was taken by venipuncture and DNA was isolated using standard protocols. Molecular analyses were performed in a CCKL-accredited laboratory at the Department of Human Genetics of the Radboud University Medical Centre. The *PCLO* rs2522833 polymorphism was genotyped using TaqMan analysis [63]. Genotyping failed for two remitted patients and nine healthy individuals, resulting in a call rate of 99.4% for remitted patients and 97.5% for healthy individuals, respectively. The *PCLO* allele frequency distribution in healthy individuals and remitted patients is presented in Table 1. Testing for Hardy-Weinberg equilibrium did not show deviation from the expected distribution of genotypes in healthy individuals, N = 351, $\chi^2 = .10$, df = 1, $p = .75$, nor in remitted patients, N = 320, $\chi^2 = .03$, df = 1, $p = .85$. Genotype groups were created in line with Woudstra and colleagues [39] and the association with depression: 'C' risk allele carriers (homozygous and heterozygous for C allele) versus 'A' non-risk allele carriers (homozygous for A allele).

Statistical analyses

The effects of *PCLO* genotype ('C' risk allele carriers, 'A' non-risk allele homozygotes), childhood trauma/adversity (no, yes) and their interaction on memory bias in remitted patients and healthy individuals were examined using analysis of co-variance (ANCOVA). In line with the Woudstra and colleagues [39] study, we also examined the two samples together. Because of their known effect on cognitive functioning and emotional processing, age and sex were included as covariates in the analyses.

Results

Sample descriptive and mood induction

Descriptives of the two independent samples are presented in Table 2. Pre mood induction mood ratings of 14 remitted patients were missing due to a programming error. The mood induction was successful in remitted patients as mood state decreased significantly from pre (M = 3.47 S.D.3.62) to post (M = .27 S.D. = 4.52), $F(1,284) = 236.91$, $p < .001$, Cohen's $f = .91$. The effect in healthy participants could not be evaluated because we did not have a baseline mood measure.

PCLO genotype main effect

Neither in remitted patients, $F(1,293) = 1.89$, $p = .170$, $f = .08$, nor in healthy individuals, $F(1,152) = .83$, $p = .363$, $f = .07$. *PCLO* a main effect of *PCLO* genotype on memory bias was found. The analysis of the whole two samples together did not yield an effect on memory bias either , $F(1,450) = 2.15$, $p = .144$, $f = .06$.

PCLO genotype x stressful childhood events interaction

The mean memory bias difference scores (# correctly recalled positive words - # correctly recalled negative words) are presented in Table 3. In remitted patients, genotype did not significantly interact with childhood trauma on memory bias, $F(1,293) = 1.18$, $p = .184$, $f = .08$. The results are similar when examining the interaction between genotype and childhood adversity (as in healthy individuals) instead of childhood trauma in remitted patients, $F(1,293) = .14$, $p = .713$, $f = .00$. The interaction between genotype and childhood adversity was not significant in healthy individuals either, $F(1,152) = 3.09$, $p = .081$, $f = .14$.

Restricting the analyses to female patients with remitted depression (N = 193) did not make any difference in terms of *PCLO* main effect, $F(1,188) = .93$, $p = .336$, $f = .07$, or interaction with childhood trauma, $F(1,188) = .42$, $p = .520$, $f = .04$.

No significant effect was found when examining the genotype by childhood adversity interaction in the two samples together, $F(1,450) = .57$, $p = .451$, $f = .03$. To check whether our non-significant results were due to a lack of statistical power, we conducted post hoc power analyses using Quanto power calculator (http://hydra.usc.edu/gxe/). The power analyses revealed that in order for a *PCLO* main effect of this size to be detected (80% chance) as significant at the 5% level, a sample of 134 participants would be required, and 2153 participants for an interaction effect.

Discussion

Previous studies have found an association between the *PCLO* rs2522833 polymorphism and neural correlates of biased processing in healthy and currently depressed individuals, but no direct effect of the *PCLO* genotype on memory bias [38,39]. Memory bias has been associated with other depression candidate genes, specifically in individuals who experienced stressful life events (e.g. [33,34]). Therefore, we hypothesized that the absence of the association between the *PCLO* genotype and memory bias in previous studies might have been due to genetically driven individual differences in reactivity to environmental stress [41], as well as to current depressive symptoms. The association

Table 1. The PCLO allele frequency distribution presented by number of participants and percentage of participants in remitted patients and healthy individuals.

	Remitted patients (N = 320)	Healthy individuals (N = 351)
Genotype	**N (%)**	**N (%)**
C/C	57 (18%)	67 (19%)
C/A	158 (49%)	176 (50%)
A/A	105 (33%)	108 (31%)

between the *PCLO* rs2522833 polymorphism, memory bias and the modulating effect of stressful childhood events was examined in a sample of remitted depressed patients and a healthy sample. We found no evidence for an association between the *PCLO* rs2522833 polymorphism and memory bias, nor for an interaction effect of the polymorphism with stressful childhood events. Our findings add to the current knowledge and suggest that the absence of an association between *PCLO* and memory bias may not be explained by current depressive symptoms, or by a gene-childhood stress interaction. However, the current study did not have sufficient power to detect the *PCLO*-childhood stress interaction and may have resulted in false negative findings. Therefore, we cannot rule out the possibility that the interaction effect exists, but was not detected due to a lack of power. A larger sample is required to confirm these results. Taken together, results from our study and the recent study by Woudstra and colleagues [39] indicate that verbal emotional memory bias may not be strongly associated with the *PCLO* rs2522833 polymorphism - unlike other genes that have been associated with both memory bias and depression (e.g. *BDNF*, *NR3C2*) - and may be implicated in other routes towards the susceptibility for depression.

It has been proposed that the *PCLO* rs2522833 polymorphism may be one of the genetic variants that increase the risk for depression by affecting the stress regulation capacity of the brain, possibly by altering monoaminergic neurotransmission, especially serotonin [39]. The imaging studies offer support for this [38,39]. Variation in the *PCLO* rs2522833 polymorphism was associated with amygdala activation during emotion processing, as well as lower striatum activation during emotional memory processing in depressed individuals. Altered activation in these neuronal circuits is related to depression and emotional information processes [64]. Based on the endophenotype model [10], the path from gene to brain activation is shorter and the link stronger, compared to the path from gene to cognitive measures, such as memory bias. Hence, the effects of *PCLO* may be too subtle to show up on a cognitive measure, while effects can be found on neural correlates of biased processing. We included, however, a larger sample than the previous study to examine the association of *PCLO* with memory bias [39] and we had sufficient power to detect a main effect of the *PCLO* polymorphism. The null-findings may therefore imply that the *PCLO* rs2522833 polymorphism is not related to emotional information processing that is associated with the susceptibility for depression.

Previous studies found an association between depression and the *PCLO* rs2522833 polymorphism when studying current major depressive disorder, but not for sub-clinical levels of depression [3,7,65]. To illustrate, in the study by Hek and colleagues [3], evidence for the association with depression was found in a well-diagnosed clinical subsample, but not in a sample of individuals with minor depression, self-reported depression, depression diagnosed by a general practitioner, or individuals using antidepressant medication. Sullivan and colleagues [7] also only found an association between *PCLO* and depression in a homogeneous clinically depressed subsample. Patients included in our study fulfilled the clinical criteria of one or more depressive episodes in the past. Our null-findings can therefore not be attributed to the selection of a too heterogeneous sample with subclinical levels of depression. However, it is important to note that we studied *PCLO* in relation to information processing styles that are associated with depression and the susceptibility for depression only, and not the association between *PCLO* and depressive disorder, as in the studies presented above.

Our results should be viewed in the context of some strengths and limitations. Strengths of our study are that we used two samples and that studying gene-bias associations in an affected sample is rather novel. Another strength of the study is that we avoided current symptoms overruling subtle cognitive effects by testing groups that are currently not depressed. A limitation is the

Table 2. Demographic and childhood events variables of the two independent samples. Childhood trauma refers to physical or sexual abuse before the age of 16 years and childhood adversity refers to childhood trauma and parental loss, divorce of parents and/or prolonged separation of parents before the age of 16. SD refers to standard deviation.

	Remitted patients (N = 299)	Healthy individuals (N = 157)
Variable	**Mean (SD)/%**	**Mean (SD)/%**
Age (years)	47.6 (11.9)	21.1 (3.7)
Sex (% female)	65%	100%
Childhood trauma (yes/no)	38%	15%
Childhood adversity (yes/no)	55%	48%

Table 3. Mean memory bias difference scores (# correctly recalled positive words - # correctly recalled negative words) and standard deviations (SD) for the PCLO genotype (risk allele 'C' carriers vs. non-risk allele 'A'-homozygotes) x childhood trauma interaction in remitted depressed individuals, and for the PCLO genotype x childhood adversity interaction in healthy individuals.

Genotype	Childhood trauma	Memory bias Mean (SD)
Remitted patients		
Risk allele carriers	No	1.24 (1.79)
	Yes	1.06 (2.01)
Non-risk allele carriers	No	1.24 (1.64)
	Yes	1.68 (1.99)
Healthy individuals	**Childhood adversity**	**Memory bias Mean (SD)**
Risk allele carriers	No	.88 (1.69)
	Yes	.94 (1.99)
Non-risk allele carriers	No	1.74 (1.97)
	Yes	.68 (2.18)

A higher score represents more positive relative to negative memory bias.

difference in sex distribution between the two samples, as SNPs within the *PCLO* gene have been associated with depression in females and not in males [66]. The fact that only female healthy individuals were included, limits the generalizability of these results. Another limitation may be the measurement method of the childhood events, as negative bias may have affected the participants' recall. The Life Events Questionnaire assesses the occurrence of several factual events during pre-determined periods of life. Because such specific events were assessed and generally adults' recall of specific childhood events is fairly accurate [67], it is in our opinion unlikely that recall had been distorted.

In conclusion, the presence of the *PCLO* risk allele may increase vulnerability for depression, but we found no indication for an association with memory bias. Memory bias may not be strongly associated with the *PCLO* rs2522833 polymorphism, unlike other genes that have been associated with depression (e.g. *BDNF*, *NR3C2*). Due to the insufficient power to detect a *PLCO*-childhood trauma interaction effect, we however cannot rule out that *PLCO* is associated with memory bias in individuals with stressful childhood events.

Acknowledgments

We would like to thank the participants for their time and effort.

Author Contributions

Conceived and designed the experiments: JV AS EB IVO. Performed the experiments: JV. Analyzed the data: JV AAV IVO. Contributed reagents/materials/analysis tools: JV. Wrote the paper: JV AS AAV BF IVO.

References

1. Sullivan PF, Neale MC, Kendler KS (2000) Genetic epidemiology of major depression: review and metaanalysis. Am J Psychiat 157: 1552–1562.
2. Bochdanovits Z, Verhage M, Smit AB, de Geus EJ, Posthuma D, et al. (2009) Joint reanalysis of 29 correlated SNPs supports the role of *PCLO*/Piccolo as a causal risk factor for major depressive disorder. Mol Psychiatr 14: 650–652.
3. Hek K, Mulder CL, Luijendijk HJ, van Duijn CM, Hofman A, et al. (2010) The *PCLO* gene and depressive disorders: replication in a population-based study. Hum Mol Genet 19: 731–734.
4. Minelli A, Scassellati C, Cloninger CR, Tessari E, Bortolomasi M, et al. (2012) *PCLO* gene: its role in vulnerability to major depressive disorder. J Affect Disord 139: 250–255.
5. Verbeek EC, Bevova MR, Bochdanovits Z, Rizzu P, Bakker IM, et al. (2013) Resequencing three candidate genes for major depressive disorder in a dutch cohort. PLoS One 8: e79921.
6. Betts MJ, Russell RB (2007) Amino-Acid Properties and Consequences of Substitutions, in Bioinformatics for Geneticists: A Bioinformatics Primer for the Analysis of Genetic Data, 2nd ed. John Wiley & Sons, Ltd, Chichester, UK. In: Barnes MR, editors. Bioinformatics for Geneticists: A Bioinformatics Primer for the Analysis of Genetic Data. Chichester, UK, Ltd, John Wiley & Sons 289–316.
7. Sullivan PF, de Geus EJ, Willemsen G, James MR, Smit JH, et al. (2009) Genome-wide association for major depressive disorder: a possible role for the presynaptic protein piccolo. Mol Psychiatry 14:359–375.
8. Kuehner C, Huffziger S, Witt SH, Rietschel M (2011) PCLO rs 2522833 impacts HPA system activity in healthy young adults. Transl. Psychiatry 1: e10.
9. Schuhmacher A, Mössner R, Höfels S, Pfeiffer U, Guttenthaler V, et al. (2011) *PCLO* rs2522833 modulates HPA system response to antidepressant treatment in major depressive disorder. Int J Neuropsychoph 14: 237–245.
10. Franke B, Neale BM, Faraone SV (2009) Genome-wide association studies in ADHD. Human Genetics 126:13–50.
11. Kendler KS, Neale MC (2010) Endophenotype: a conceptual analysis. Mol Psychiatr 15: 789–797.
12. De Raedt R, Koster EH (2010) Understanding vulnerability for depression from a cognitive neuroscience perspective: a reappraisal of attentional factors and a new conceptual framework. Cogn Affect Behav Neurosci 10: 50–70.
13. Klein AA, Nelson LM, Anker JJ (2013) Attention and recognition memory bias for alcohol-related stimuli among alcohol-dependent patients attending residential treatment. Addict Behav 38: 1687–1690.
14. LeMoult J, Joormann J (2012) Attention and memory biases in social anxiety disorder: The role of comorbid depression. Cognitive Ther Res 36: 47–57.
15. Mathews A, MacLeod C (2005) Cognitive vulnerability to emotional disorders. Annu Rev Clin Psycho 1: 167–95.
16. Gotlib IH, Joormann J (2010) Cognition and depression: Current status and future directions. Annu Rev Clin Psycho 6: 285–312.
17. Wingenfeld K, Terfehr K, Meyer B, Löwe B, Spitzer C (2013) Memory bias for emotional and illness-related words in patients with depression, anxiety and somatization disorders: an investigation with the directed forgetting task. Psychopathology 46: 22–27.
18. Matt GE, Vazquez C, Campbell WK (1992) Mood-congruent recall of affectively toned stimuli: A meta-analytic review. Clin Psychol Rev 12: 227–255.
19. Ridout N, Noreen A, Johal J (2009) Memory for emotional faces in naturally occurring dysphoria and induced sadness. Behav Res Ther 47: 851–860.
20. Vrijsen JN, Becker ES, Arias-Vásquez A, van Dijk MK, Speckens A, et al. (2014a) What is the contribution of different cognitive biases and stressful childhood events to the presence and number of previous depressive episodes? Psychiat Res 217: 134–42.
21. Williams JMG (1996) Depression and the specificity of autobiographical memory. Remembering our past: Studies in autobiographical memory. New York, NY, Cambridge University Press.

22. Williams JMG, Barnhofer T, Crane C, Hermans D, Raes F, et al. (2007) Autobiographical memory specificity and emotional disorder. Psychol Bull 133: 122–148.
23. Gotlib IH, Kasch KL, Traill S, Joormann J, Arnow BA, et al. (2004) Coherence and specificity of information processing biases in depression and social phobia. J Abnorm Psychol113;386–398.
24. Gupta R, Kar BR (2012) Attention and memory biases as stable abnormalities among currently depressed and currently remitted individuals with unipolar depression. Front Psychiatry 3: 99.
25. Joormann J, Gotlib IH (2007) Selective attention to emotional faces following recovery from depression. J Abnorm Psychol 116: 80–85.
26. McCabe SB, Gotlib IH, Martin RA (2000) Cognitive vulnerability for depression: Deployment of attention as a function of history of depression and current mood state. Cognitive Ther Res 24: 427–444.
27. Teasdale JD (1988) Cognitive vulnerability to persistent depression. Cognition and Emotion 2: 247–274.
28. Denny EB, Hunt RR (1992) Affective valence and memory in depression: dissociation of recall and fragment completion. J Abnorm Psychol 101: 575–580.
29. Ellwart T, Rinck M, Becker ES (2003) Selective memory and memory deficits in depressed inpatients. Depress Anxiety 17: 197–206.
30. Watkins PC, Mathews A, Williamson DA, Fuller RD (1992) Mood-congruent memory in depression: emotional priming or elaboration? J Abnorm Psychol 101: 581–586.
31. Fox E, Ridgewell A, Ashwin C (2009) Looking on the bright side: Biased attention and the human serotonin transporter gene. Proceedings in Biological Science 276: 1747–1751.
32. Pergamin-Hight L, Bakermans-Kranenburg MJ, van Ijzendoorn MH, Bar-Haim Y (2012) Variations in the promoter region of the serotonin transporter gene and biased attention for emotional information: a meta-analysis. Biol Psychiat 71: 373–379.
33. van Oostrom I, Franke B, Rijpkema M, Gerritsen L, Arias-Vasquez A, et al. (2012) Interaction between BDNF Val66Met and childhood stressful life events is associated to affective memory bias in men but not women. Biol Psychol 89: 214–219.
34. Vogel S, Gerritsen L, van Oostrom I, Arias-Vásquez A, Rijpkema M, et al. (2014) Linking genetic variants of the mineralocorticoid receptor and negative memory bias: interaction with prior life adversity. Psychoneuroendocrino 40: 181–190.
35. Vrijsen JN, van Oostrom I, Arias-Vásquez A, Franke B, Becker ES, et al. (2014 b) Association between genes, stressful childhood events and processing bias in depression vulnerable individuals. Genes Brain Behav 13: 508–516.
36. Williams LM, Gatt JM, Grieve SM, Dobson-Stone C, Paul RH, et al. (2010) COMT Val(108/158)Met polymorphism effects on emotional brain function and negativity bias. Neuroimage 53: 918–925.
37. Schott BH, Assmann A, Schmierer P, Soch J, Erk A, et al. (2014) Epistatic interaction of genetic depression risk variants in the human subgenual cingulate cortex during memory encoding. Tansl Psychiatry 4: e372.
38. Woudstra S, Bochdanovits Z, van Tol MJ, Veltman DJ, Zitman FG, et al. (2012) Piccolo genotype modulates neural correlates of emotion processing but not executive functioning. Translational Psychiatry 2: e99.
39. Woudstra S, van Tol MJ, Bochdanovits Z, van der Wee NJ, Zitman FG, et al. (2013) Modulatory Effects of the Piccolo Genotype on Emotional Memory in Health and Depression. PLoS One 8: e61494.
40. Caspi A, Sugden K, Moffitt TE, Taylor A, Craig IW, et al. (2003) Influence of life stress on depression: moderation by a polymorphism in the 5-HTT gene. Science 301: 386–389.
41. Caspi A, Hariri AR, Holmes A, Uher R, Moffitt TE (2010) Genetic sensitivity to the environment: the case of the serotonin transporter gene and its implications for studying complex diseases and traits. Am J Psychiat 167: 509–527.
42. Caspi A, Moffitt TE (2006) Gene-environment interactions in psychiatry: joining forces with neuroscience. Nature Review in Neuroscience 7: 583–590.
43. Perry B, Pollard R, Blakley T, Baker W, Vigilante D (1995) Childhood trauma, the neurobiology of adaptation, and "use-dependent" development of the brain: how "states" become "traits." Infant Ment Health J 16: 271–91.
44. Beck AT (2008) The evolution of the cognitive model of depression and its neurobiological correlates. Am J Psychiatry 165: 969–977.
45. Bower GH (1981) Mood and memory. American Psychologist 36: 129–148.
46. Firk C, Markus CR (2007) Review: Serotonin by stress interaction: A susceptibility factor for the development of depression? J Psychopharmacol 21: 538–544.
47. Bockting C, Spinhoven P, Koeter M, Wouters L, Schene A, for the Depression Evaluation Longitudinal Therapy Assessment (DELTA) Study Group (2006) Prediction of recurrence in recurrent depression and the influence of consecutive episodes on vulnerability for depression: a 2-year prospective study. J Clin Psychiat 67: 747–755.
48. Kanai T, Takeuchi H, Furukawa TA, Yoshimura R, Imaizumi T, et al. (2003) Time to recurrence after recovery from major depressive episodes and its predictors. Psychol Med 33: 839–845.
49. Bhagwagar Z, Cowen PJ (2007) It's not over when it's over: Persistent neurobiological abnomalities in recovered depressed patients. Psychol Med 38: 307–313.
50. American Psychiatric Association (1994) Diagnostic and statistical manual of mental disorders. 4th ed. American Psychiatric Association, Washington, DC.
51. First MB, Spitzer RL, Gibbon M, Williams JBW (1996) Structured Clinical Interview for DSM–IV Axis I Disorders-Clinician Version (SCID-CV) American Psychiatric Press, Washington, DC.
52. Skre I, Onstad S, Torgersen S, Kringlen E (1991) High interrater reliability for the Structured Clinical Interview for DSM–III–R Axis I (SCID-I) Acta Psychiat Scand 84: 167–173.
53. Williams JB, Gibbon M, First MB, Spitzer RL, Davis M, et al. (1992) The Structured Clinical Interview for DSM–III–R (SCID): Multisite test–retest reliability. Arch Gen Psychiat 49: 630–636.
54. Beck AT, Steer RA, Brown GK (1996) Beck Depression Inventory manual. 2nd ed. Psychological Corporation, San Antonio, TX.
55. Brugha TS, Cragg D (1990) The list of threatening experiences-the reliability and validity of a brief life events questionnaire. Acta Psychiat Scand 82: 77–81.
56. Gerritsen L, Tendolkar I, Franke B, Vasquez AA, Kooijman S, et al. (2011) BDNF Val66Met genotype modulates the effect of childhood adversity on subgenual anterior cingulate cortex volume in healthy subjects. Mol Psychiat 17: 597–603.
57. Fitzgerald DA, Arnold JF, Becker ES, Speckens AE, Rinck M, et al. (2011) How mood challenges emotional memory formation: an fMRI investigation. Neuroimage 56: 1783–1790.
58. Vrijsen JN, van Oostrom I, Isaac L, Becker ES, Speckens A (2014 c) Coherence between attentional and memory biases in sad and formerly depressed individuals. Cognitive Therapy and Research 38: 334–342.
59. Bradley MM, Lang PJ (1999) Affective norms for English words (ANEW): Instruction manual and affective ratings. Technical Report C-1, The Center for Research in Psychophysiology, University of Florida.
60. Phaf RH, van der Leij AR, Stienen BMC, Bierman D (2006) Positieve, neutrale en negatieve woorden bij minimale aanbieding: Een ordening door perceptuele clarificatie [Positive, neutral and negative words at minimal presentation levels: Ordering by perceptual clarification]. Technical Report, Universiteit van Amsterdam, Amsterdam, The Netherlands.
61. Rogers T, Kuiper N, Kirker W (1977) Self-reference and the encoding of personal information. Journal of Personality and Social Psychology 35: 677–688.
62. Raven JC (1958) Standard progressive matrices. H. K. Lewis, London.
63. Watson DE, Li B (2005) TaqMan applications in genetic and molecular toxicology. Int J Toxicol 24: 139–145.
64. van Tol MJ, Demenescu LR, van der Wee NJA, Kortekaas R, Marjan MA, et al. (2012) Functional magnetic resonance imaging correlates of emotional word encoding and recognition in depression and anxiety disorders. Biol Psychiatry 71: 593–602.
65. Shyn SI, Hamilton SP (2010) The genetics of major depression: moving beyond the monoamine hypothesis. Psychiatr Clin North Am 33: 125–140.
66. Aragam N, Wang KS, Pan Y (2011) Genome-wide association analysis of gender differences in major depressive disorder in the Netherlands NESDA and NTR population-based samples. J Affect Disord 133: 516–521.
67. Brewin CR, Andrews B, Gotlib IH (1993) Psychopathology and early experiences: A reappraisal of retrospective reports. Psychological Bulletin 113: 82–98.

Tracking Functional Brain Changes in Patients with Depression under Psychodynamic Psychotherapy Using Individualized Stimuli

Daniel Wiswede[1,8*], Svenja Taubner[2,8], Anna Buchheim[3,8], Thomas F. Münte[1], Michael Stasch[4], Manfred Cierpka[4], Horst Kächele[5,8], Gerhard Roth[6,8], Peter Erhard[6], Henrik Kessler[7,8]

1 Department of Neurology, University of Lübeck, Lübeck, Germany, **2** Department of Psychology, Alpen-Adria-University of Klagenfurt, Klagenfurt, Austria, **3** Institute of Psychology, University of Innsbruck, Innsbruck, Austria, **4** Institute of Psychosomatic Cooperation Research and Family Therapy, University of Heidelberg, Heidelberg, Germany, **5** Department of Psychosomatic Medicine and Psychotherapy, University of Ulm, Ulm, Germany, **6** Brain Research Institute, University of Bremen, Bremen, Germany, **7** Department of Psychosomatic Medicine and Psychotherapy, LWL University Hospital, Ruhr-University Bochum, Bochum, Germany, **8** Hanse Institute for Advanced Study, Delmenhorst, Germany

Abstract

Objective: Neurobiological models of depression posit limbic hyperactivity that should normalize after successful treatment. For psychotherapy, though, brain changes in patients with depression show substantial variability. Two critical issues in relevant studies concern the use of unspecific stimulation experiments and relatively short treatment protocols. Therefore changes in brain reactions to individualized stimuli were studied in patients with depression after eight months of psychodynamic psychotherapy.

Methods: 18 unmedicated patients with recurrent major depressive disorder were confronted with individualized and clinically derived content in a functional MRI experiment before (T1) and after eight months (T2) of psychodynamic therapy. A control group of 17 healthy subjects was also tested twice without intervention. The experimental stimuli were sentences describing each participant's dysfunctional interpersonal relationship patterns derived from clinical interviews based on Operationalized Psychodynamic Diagnostics (OPD).

Results: At T1 patients showed enhanced activation compared to controls in several limbic and subcortical regions, including amygdala and basal ganglia, when confronted with OPD sentences. At T2 the differences in brain activity between patients and controls were no longer apparent. Concurrently, patients had improved significantly in depression scores.

Conclusions: Using ecologically valid stimuli, this study supports the model of limbic hyperactivity in depression that normalizes after treatment. Without a control group of untreated patients measured twice, though, changes in patients' brain activity could also be attributed to other factors than psychodynamic therapy.

Editor: Huafu Chen, University of Electronic Science and Technology of China, China

Funding: The study was financially supported by the Hanse Institute for Advanced Study Delmenhorst (HWK), a non-profit foundation by the German federal states of Lower Saxony and Bremen and by the City of Delmenhorst. The authors DW, ST, AB, MC, H. Kächele, H. Kessler have been fellows of the HWK and used their fellowship to conduct this study. The authors also thank Matthias von der Tann, London, for his financial support. The funders had no role in study design, data collection and analysis, decision to publish, or preparation of the manuscript. The authors report no biomedical financial interests or potential conflicts of interest. DW, H. Kessler, and ST had full access to all of the data in the study and take responsibility for the integrity of the data and the accuracy of the data analysis.

Competing Interests: The authors have declared that no competing interests exist.

* Email: Daniel.wiswede@neuro.uni-luebeck.de

Introduction

In the search for neurobiological correlates of depression we have an increasingly clear picture of which brain areas typically show hyperactivity (e.g., amygdala, striatum and other limbic and subcortical regions) [1,2,3]. More recently, depression has been conceptualized in terms of network dysfunctions including cortico-limbic loops [3,4,5]. Consequently, those patterns of hyperactivity should normalize after treatment concurrently with clinical improvement [5,6]. For psychotherapy, though, the neural correlates of treatment effects in depression are less well understood [7,8,9,10,11]. Regarding changes in limbic and subcortical regions, for instance, increases as well as decreases have been reported after psychotherapy [8,11].

Two critical issues may contribute to this inconsistent picture [11,12]. First, many studies used unspecific resting state measurements before and after treatment or standardized emotional stimuli rather than specific symptom provocation. Second, psychotherapeutic treatments may have been too short (typically 6–16 weeks) to lead to psychological changes instantiated in either brain activity or structure. To address the first issue, we conducted a previously published initial study in patients with depression using individualized symptom-specific stimuli as described below [13]. The second point, assessing functional brain changes during long-term psychotherapy, is covered by the present communication.

To enhance the ecological validity of stimuli and thus increase the chance to detect treatment effects, we created sentences describing each patient's current dysfunctional interpersonal relations [13] derived from clinical interviews based on Operationalized Psychodynamic Diagnostics [14]. For control participants, sentences described major sources of personal distress without being attached to depression. These stimuli, compared to emotionally negative control sentences, led to activation in medial prefrontal cortex, anterior cingulate cortex and bilateral occipital cortex in patients and healthy controls. Compared to controls, patients showed enhanced activation in areas confirming the notion of limbic hyperactivity in depression [1,2,3] (amygdala, caudate nucleus and putamen) and other regions (parts of the inferior, medial and precentral/middle frontal gyrus, postcentral gyrus) [13].

Extending this earlier work, we conducted a longitudinal study with the subjects included in the previous publication [13] with repetition of the same experiment after eight months of psychodynamic therapy. For comparison, the group of healthy individuals from our previous study was also assessed with parallel tasks after eight months. The long observation period of eight months, the exclusive application of psychotherapy (no concurrent medication) and the application of an established diagnostic tool from depression therapy for stimulus generation constitute an advance over previous studies.

In addition to clinical improvement evidenced by a reduced score on the Beck Depression Inventory (BDI) we expected the treatment to lead to a reduction of the relative limbic hyperactivity found prior to therapy [13]. For the control group we neither expected a change in depression scores nor in brain activity.

Methods and Materials

Participants

Participants were the same as in our previous study [13] and comprised 18 unmedicated patients (age 39.8 years SD 12.8, 14 women) with recurrent major depressive disorder and 17 healthy controls (age 38.0, SD 11.6, 14 women). Patients were recruited from a psychoanalytic institute and diagnosed by two trained clinicians using the Structured Clinical Interviews I and II for DSM-IV (German version, [15]). They reported between 1 to 15 depressive episodes (M[SD] =5.6[5.5]), and their age at first occurrence of depression was between 8 and 40 years (M[SD] = 19.3[8.2]). Some patients had received various types of medication and psychotherapies during the course of their disease but had not received treatment within at least 6 months prior to inclusion in the study. Hence, the sample was completely free of psychotropic medication at the time of study. Exclusion criteria were other psychiatric conditions, substance abuse, significant medical or neurological conditions or eye problems. Control participants were matched for age, sex and education, and had no history of previous depressive episodes or other psychiatric conditions, including bipolar disorder (SCID). All participants were right-handed. In both groups, depression severity was assessed using the Beck Depression Inventory [16]. All participants were examined twice (mean time between first and second measurement in weeks: patients 33, range 29–34, controls 32.7, range 29–37). During this period, controls received no intervention while patients underwent psychotherapy by fully-trained, state-licensed and experienced therapists (n = 15) with a mean of 22.4 years (SD = 7.9) of experience in practicing psychotherapy in their respective private practice. A psychodynamic approach with a focus on intrapsychic conflicts and dysfunctional interpersonal relations represented in the OPD sentences used for stimulation (see below) was employed consistently for all patients. To foster adherence, the study therapists met monthly for group intervisions on a regular basis. Group intervision sessions were audiotaped for adherence control and assessing how therapies were affected by research [17]. All therapies were paid by the German health care system. The measuring time points will be referred to as T1 (first fMRI session, before therapeutic intervention for patients) and T2 (second fMRI session, after eight months of therapy for patients and eight months of waiting for controls). All participants gave written informed consent after complete description of the study and prior to their inclusion.

The study protocol had been approved by the ethical committee of the University of Ulm and was in compliance with national legislation, the principles expressed in the Declaration of Helsinki, and the Code of Ethical Principles for Medical Research Involving Human Subjects of the World Medical Association.

fMRI Stimuli

Individualized stimuli were generated based on an interview according to the system of Operationalized Psychodynamic Diagnostics (OPD) [14] conducted by a trained clinician (HeK). Videotaped material was rated independently by 2–3 expert raters (OPD-Trainers). Typical dysfunctional interpersonal relations were identified and served as basis for the stimuli ("OPD sentences"). For patients sentences described a current problematic interpersonal relation typical of their depressive cognitions. For controls, sentences represented a major source of interpersonal distress without being connected to clinical depression. Four sentences were selected representing the typical dysfunctional relationship theme of each person (e.g., "You wish to be accepted by others.", "Therefore you do a lot for them.", "That is often too close for them, so they retreat.", "Then you feel empty and lonesome."). These individual sentences served as stimuli during both fMRI-sessions (OPD condition). Word count and semantic structure of the stimulus sentences did not differ between patients and controls (average word count of the four sentences, Controls: 31 words, Patients: 33 words, T(33) = 1.1; n.s.). The control condition ("traffic") comprised four sentences, which described a stressful traffic situation ("The other driver makes a mistake.", "You are very upset about this.", "You react to the other driver.", "But he reacts inadequately."). Prior to testing, participants were asked to remember a recent and stressful situation they had experienced in traffic. The rationale behind this control condition was to induce negative emotions and recall autobiographical memories with a personally relevant situation including human interactions, but without engaging in specific depression-related, clinically relevant material. In order to separate the two conditions (OPD and traffic), and let subjects calm down after emotionally demanding sentences, "relaxation" sentences were inserted between conditions. Those sentences instructed participants to relax. Whereas the OPD sentences were derived individually for each person, "relaxation" and "traffic" were the same across all subjects and repetitions. OPD sentences were slightly but significantly longer (M[SD] =49.8 [9.1] characters) than "traffic" sentences (43.5 characters). The stimuli were exactly the same for T1 and T2.

fMRI Experiment

Sentences were presented by a projector onto a screen watched by the participants via a mirror while lying in the scanner. The four sentences of a condition (OPD, traffic, relaxation) were presented for 7.5 seconds each, resulting in 30 seconds blocks. During the OPD block participants were asked to mentally engage in situations with significant others, as described by the OPD sentences. They received no instruction to regulate their emotions, but should let spontaneous thoughts, emotions and memories come to mind. "Traffic" and "relaxation" conditions also comprised four sentences with each lasting 7.5 seconds. The instructions were to mentally engage either in the traffic situation or to relax. In total 12 "relaxation", 6 "traffic" and 6 "OPD" blocks were presented (white Arial font, size 16, black background). Blocks were separated by a 5-seconds fixation cross. The entire experiment lasted approximately 15 minutes.

Study Procedure

Four to six weeks prior to T1 fMRI assessment, all participants (patients and controls) were interviewed (SCID I+II, OPD) and filled out questionnaires (BDI) and informed consent forms. At the beginning of the fMRI session, they were briefed, saw their individual OPD sentences prior to actual scanning and were asked, whether the sentences fit and enticed them to think about their problematic relations. After scanning participants assessed the extent to which the OPD sentences were adequately describing their problematic relations and caused emotional arousal on a 7-point Likert scale. The scanning procedure and questionnaires were the same at T2.

Image Acquisition

Data were obtained using a 3T SIEMENS Magnetom Allegra head scanner (Siemens, Erlangen, Germany). Participants were positioned on the scanner couch and wore foam earplugs to reduce scanner noise. An experienced psychotherapist not involved in the therapy of the patients (ST or HeK) assisted with the setup procedure and coached the participants throughout the experiment. Data acquisition started with anatomical images (3D high resolution T1-weighted isotropic volume, MPRAGE-sequence (MPRAGE = Magnetization Prepared Rapid Gradient Echo); TR = 2.3 s, FOV = 256×256×176 mm^3, TE = 4.38 ms, TI = 900 ms, flip angle = 8°, 1 mm isovoxel, total acquisition time 14.45 min). Functional scans were performed using a single shot echo planar imaging sequence (EPI). A total of 365 T2*-weighted whole brain volumes were acquired (EPI-sequence; TR 2500 ms, TE 30 ms, flip angle 90°, FOV = 192 mm, matrix 64×64, 44 slices, slice thickness 3 mm, interleaved acquisition order, AC PC- Orientation, total acquisition time: 15.18 min).

Image Analysis

Data were analyzed and visualized using Brain Voyager QX 1.10 to 2.2 (Brain Innovation, Maastricht, Netherlands). Preprocessing: Functional data were slice-time corrected and motion was corrected relative to the first volume of the run. To remove low frequency drifts, data were high-pass filtered (3 cycles, three sine waves fall within the extent of the data). Structural and functional data were transformed into the standard space of Talairach and Tournoux [18], data points were labeled using Talairach Daemon [19]. The design matrix was modeled using the two gamma hemodynamic response function. Functional data were smoothed using an 8 mm full width at half maximum (FWHM) isotropic Gaussian Kernel. Group data were analyzed using random effects analyses based on z-transformed functional data. An ANOVA, including the within-factors CONDITION (OPD vs. traffic sentences), TIMEPOINT (T1 and T2) and between-factor GROUP (patient vs. control) was performed to identify differences in hemodynamic response. Motion-correction parameters were included in the GLM-Model as regressors of no interest.

Since we were interested in whether brain responses to individualized stimuli changed over time, we conducted a region-of-interest (ROI) analysis based on all clusters found to be significant in the GROUP × CONDITION interaction at T1 [13]. Those regions included parts of the right inferior frontal gyrus, the right amygdala, the medial frontal gyrus, the bilateral putamen, the precentral/middle frontal gyrus and the postcentral gyrus. In the ROI analyses, we tested the CONDITION × TIMEPOINT × GROUP interaction. To keep comparability with previous measurements at T1 [13], statistics were conducted and maps are shown with a threshold of $p<0.001$, uncorrected. A cluster size threshold of 16 voxels was consistently applied. Due to a lower risk of type I error, the ROI- analysis is reported with a threshold of $p<.05$ with correction for multiple comparisons based on False Discovery Rate (FDR) [20]. All active voxels are displayed in native resolution without interpolation and plotted on the Talairach-transformed brain; Talairach coordinates are reported as TAL x, y, z.

Results

Behavioral Results

Behavioral data are illustrated in figure 1. At T2 BDI scores had decreased in patients but not in controls (GROUP, $F(1,33) = 85.88$, $p<.001$; interaction GROUP × TIMEPOINT: $F(1,33) = 17.64$; $p<.001$).

At T2 OPD sentences were less adequate and less arousing (according to self-rating) to the patients compared to T1, whereas assessments did not change in controls (adequacy: GROUP ×

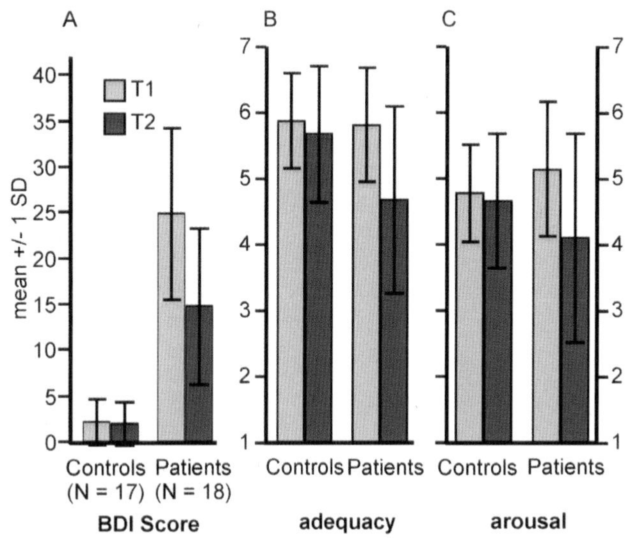

Figure 1. Depression and impact of OPD sentences at T1 and T2. A: BDI (Beck Depression Inventory) scores, B and C: rating of OPD sentences with respect to adequacy (B) and emotional arousal (C). Error bars show +/− 1 SD.

TIMEPOINT interaction, $F(1,33) = 8.39$; $p < .007$; arousal: interaction, $F(1,33) = 8.01$; $p < .008$).

BDI scores in the patient group were not correlated to either the OPD adequacy or arousal scores. The correlation between OPD adequacy and arousal was weak and not significant ($r = .39$, $p < .15$).

fMRI Results

Main effects of condition with stronger activations for OPD relative to traffic sentences were found in a large occipital cluster (center of gravity TAL −2, −71, 4), the anterior cingulate cortex (TAL −2, 42, 2), and superior frontal gyrus (TAL 18,35,45). There was also activation in two bilateral cluster comprising the putamen and the lateral globus pallidus and extending to the thalamus (TAL 23, −22, 4 and −25, −20, 1, respectively), and in the superior/medial frontal gyrus (TAL −11,48,39). This pattern was similar to that found at T1 [13]. As shown in figure 2, at T2, a group by condition interaction was found for a part of the medial frontal gyrus/Anterior Cingulate (TAL 1,46,4; BA 32,10,24). Although both groups showed increased activation to OPD relative to traffic sentences (see main effect of CONDITION), the difference between OPD and traffic sentences was less pronounced in patients at T2.

In the T1-restricted ROI analysis which examined regions that had shown a group by condition interaction at T1, a significant group by condition by time-point interaction was found in several regions as illustrated in figure 3. In all clusters stronger activations to OPD sentences in patients at T1 were no longer seen at T2.

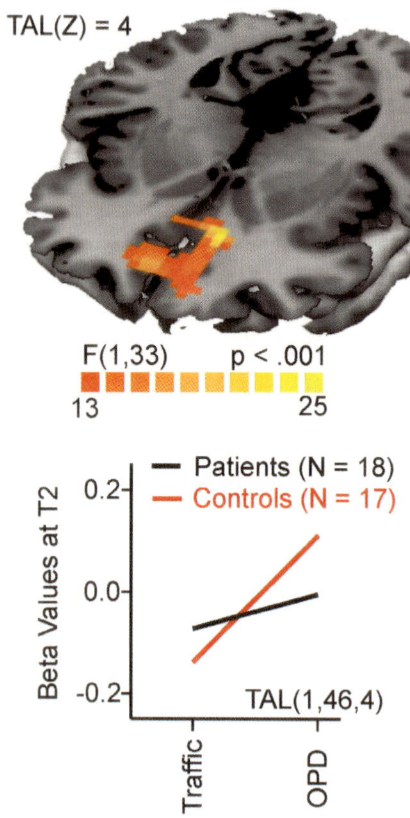

Figure 2. Interaction effect CONDITION × GROUP at T2. Interaction plots are given for the active cluster based on beta values for OPD and traffic sentences, $p < .001$, cluster threshold 16 voxels.

Discussion

Prior to psychotherapy, patients with depression of the current study had shown hyperactivity relative to healthy controls in limbic and subcortical regions (e.g. amygdala, basal ganglia) when they were confronted with their individual dysfunctional relations associated with their depression [13]. In the follow-up reported here this relative hyperactivity disappeared after eight months of psychodynamic therapy with a focus on current dysfunctional relationship patterns. The patients' brain activity before therapy is in line with a wealth of studies [1,2,3], supporting the validity of our novel experimental approach with individualized and clinically-derived OPD stimuli. The fact that the OPD sentences were derived from a structured clinical interview, rated by independent experts and approved by the patients as individual "sore spots" (self-rating of adequacy) backs their external, i.e. ecological, validity. The patients' brain activity after therapy is consistent with the results of a recent study on patients with recurrent major depression treated with psychodynamic therapy, which found decrease of limbic activity after 15 months of treatment during the presentation of personalized sentences concerning attachment related themes [21]. The current study demonstrated that changes in limbic reactivity in depression can already be traced after 8 months of psychodynamic psychotherapy if related to current dysfunctional relationship themes that have been shown to maintain depression. Patients' brain activation changes over time found in our study can be understood following a classical approach to "pathological" brain processes in depression [3,5,6]: Limbic hyperactivity is the neurobiological marker indicating dysfunctions in emotion processing systems that are intrinsically linked to depression. If the patients improve clinically (as indicated by significantly lower BDI scores in our sample after eight months of psychotherapy) the dysfunctions and consequently the limbic hyperactivity should no longer be apparent ("normalization"). While reviews of neural changes after psychotherapy have reported inconsistent results [8,11], our results support the proposed models of neurobiological effects of psychotherapy [3,5,6] and confirm studies showing normalization of limbic hyperactivity after psychotherapy [22].

We briefly focus on the functional significance of the limbic regions being differentially active at T1 but not T2 as revealed by our ANOVA interaction analysis. The amygdala has repeatedly been discussed as being hyperactive in depression [23,24,25, 26,27,28]. We speculate here that enhanced amygdala activity in depressed individuals at T1 reflects their higher emotional involvement in problematic relations. Hyperactivity in patients before psychotherapy in putamen and caudate nucleus is also plausible according to a recent meta-analysis, where the basal ganglia have consistently displayed increased activity in depression after induction of negative affect [24]. This is not surprising, since the basal ganglia have rich interconnections with limbic structures (including the amygdala) and prefrontal areas, and form part of many cortico-subcortical loops engaged in reward and punishment, affect and motivation [29,30,31]. The finding that at least two regions show hyperactivity before psychotherapy and are no longer hyperactive after seven months of psychotherapy supports the model of hyperactive limbic regions in depression and "normalization" thereof after psychotherapy [32]. The second main finding, revealed by whole-brain exploratory analysis of existing differences between patients and healthy controls at T2, may lead to an alternative approach to interpret brain activation. At T1, in both groups large areas of the medial prefrontal cortex were active when confronted with OPD sentences. At T2, there was still a major activity in those regions for the same contrast but

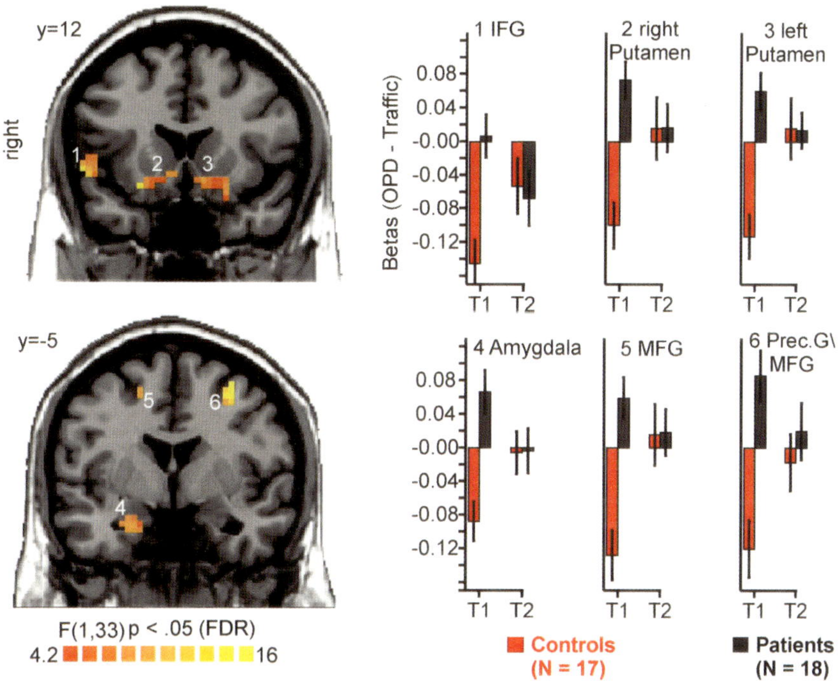

Figure 3. ROI-Analysis; GROUP × CONDITION × TIMEPOINT interaction. Clusters were defined by GROUP × CONDTION interaction at T1. The diagram depicts beta values at T1 and T2. p<.05 FDR corrected, Cluster-threshold 16 voxels.

less so for patients. Considering the involvement of the medial prefrontal cortex in self-referential processing in depression [33], this could signal a decreased self-focus – a cognitive bias associated with depression – in patients after therapy. In fact, recently Cognitive Behavioural Therapy has been shown to reduce medial prefrontal cortex activity associated with self-referential processing when viewing negative stimuli in patients with depression [34] and reduced activity in the medial prefrontal cortex has been demonstrated after 15 months of psychodynamic psychotherapy in patients with depression when dealing with attachment-related topics [21]. Alternatively, we speculate here that activity in medial prefrontal cortex reflects the regulation of emotions initially necessary to cope with the strongly emotional OPD sentences that is less pronounced (and necessary) in patients after eight months of psychotherapy dealing with the content covered by those sentences. As numerous studies have found, the medial prefrontal cortex is crucial for the down-regulation of limbic and subcortical regions when subjects are exposed to strong emotions [35]. This function is vital for patients with depression who are often overwhelmed by such strong negative emotions. In fact, it has been pointed out that brain alterations in depression might not only reflect the pathological process itself but also compensatory mechanisms [5,21,36,37]. One key aspect of psychodynamic therapy in depression is to help the patients gain insight into their dysfunctional relations (as described in the OPD sentences) such that they no longer represent a strong source of distress. Alternatively, patients could have "accepted" their interpersonal problems over the course of psychotherapy to the extent that confrontation with them does not call for such urgent attention and emotion regulation. At T2, patients were in fact significantly less emotionally aroused when confronted with the relationship patterns (self-rating of emotional arousal). For controls, the OPD sentences still provide comparable emotional arousal and lead to brain activity in medial prefrontal cortex, since they received no intervention helping them to cope with their stressful interpersonal situations. In this interpretation, activity in medial prefrontal cortex at T1 could reflect a compensatory mechanism to cope with strong emotional stimuli that is less needed when patients "worked" with the problematic content in psychotherapy over eight months leading to less self-rated arousal and consequently less need to regulate emotions. The interpretation that brain changes were induced by working through dysfunctional relations expressed in the OPD stimuli over the course of psychotherapy points to a limitation of the study design. Although study therapists met on a regular basis to foster adherence and aimed at considering their patients' dysfunctional relations, this could not provide full control over what exactly happened within each therapy session. The lack of an exact and standardized treatment protocol is common for psychodynamic therapy (as opposed to some forms of cognitive behavior therapy) and could not be changed without sacrificing individual therapists' degrees of freedom. Since this is among the first studies investigating neural correlates of psychodynamic therapy in depression, the focus is primarily on effectiveness in a "naturalistic" setting (as opposed to the strict criteria applied in randomized controlled trials). Future investigations building on this study should consider the application of manualized forms of psychodynamic therapy to increase coherence.

Considering the main limitation of our study, the major result – normalization of pre-treatment hyperactivity – could as well be explained by regression-to-the-mean effects. This is a known issue in the literature [38] and has also influenced the discussion of results similar to ours in the study by Fu and colleagues [22]. This possible confound is hard to tackle with statistical means, though, and could only be refuted with a control group of untreated patients with depression measured twice. Ethical considerations ruled out this change in study design for obvious reasons. With this limitation in mind, we cannot infer that patients' changes in brain activity measured over eight months are in fact a causal result of the psychotherapeutic intervention or due to a natural course of depression. Considering the relatively high placebo response rates in major depression [39], spontaneous remission from depressive symptoms is discussed as an important factor in the long-term view. Normalization of brain activity could therefore as well be an unspecific effect not related to treatment. Our patients have had a relatively long history of recurrent depressive episodes and unsuccessful treatments before inclusion in our study. Since for patients with comparable severity of depression remission rates under treatment are substantially lower [40], it is less likely that our study patients showed spontaneous remissions within the eight-month observation period. Arguing in favor of specific effects of our study intervention, the efficacy and effectiveness of psychodynamic therapy, which can best be compared to our approach and its superiority over waiting-list controls has been reported in two meta-analyses [41,42] (But see [43] for a critical discussion). Additionally, fMRI measurement times were scattered throughout the year to minimize seasonal effects in the course of depression. Finally, the differential pattern found for the interaction effect of condition × group at T1 (both groups with high MPFC activity) and T2 (less increase in MPFC activity for patients) cannot be due to a regression to the mean effect, which would affect both groups alike.

In summary, our results confirm the model of limbic hyperactivity in depression that normalizes after treatment in the case of psychodynamic therapy with novel stimuli that are individually tailored and reflect clinically relevant content. Moreover, less activity in presumably compensatory networks (medial prefrontal cortex) for patients after working with the relevant issues in psychotherapy points to exciting new ways of designing future studies with individualized stimuli.

Acknowledgments

We gratefully acknowledge the invaluable cooperation of patients and therapists. We are indebted to Gregor Szycik, Henk Jansma and Armin Heinecke for discussions regarding data analysis, to Manfred Herrmann for logistical support and to Anna Stumpe and Melanie Löbe for their help in data acquisition.

Author Contributions

Conceived and designed the experiments: DW ST H. Kessler MC MS AB TFM. Performed the experiments: DW ST H. Kessler PE. Analyzed the data: DW. Wrote the paper: DW ST H. Kessler TFM MS MC PE GR AB H. Kächele.

References

1. Drevets WC (2003) Neuroimaging abnormalities in the amygdala in mood disorders. Ann N Y Acad Sci 985: 420–444.
2. Fitzgerald PB, Laird AR, Maller J, Daskalakis ZJ (2008) A meta-analytic study of changes in brain activation in depression. Hum Brain Mapp 29: 683–695.
3. Mayberg HS (1997) Limbic-cortical dysregulation: a proposed model of depression. J Neuropsychiatry Clin Neurosci 9: 471–481.
4. Drevets WC, Price JL, Furey ML (2008) Brain structural and functional abnormalities in mood disorders: implications for neurocircuitry models of depression. Brain Struct Funct 213: 93–118.
5. Mayberg HS (2003) Modulating dysfunctional limbic-cortical circuits in depression: towards development of brain-based algorithms for diagnosis and optimised treatment. Br Med Bull 65: 193–207.
6. DeRubeis RJ, Siegle GJ, Hollon SD (2008) Cognitive therapy versus medication for depression: treatment outcomes and neural mechanisms. Nat Rev Neurosci 9: 788–796.
7. Beutel ME (2006) Functional neuroimaging in psychotherapy research. Bundesgesundheitsblatt Gesundheitsforschung Gesundheitsschutz 49: 749–758.
8. Frewen PA, Dozois DJ, Lanius RA (2008) Neuroimaging studies of psychological interventions for mood and anxiety disorders: empirical and methodological review. Clin Psychol Rev 28: 228–246.
9. Kumari V (2006) Do psychotherapies produce neurobiological effects? Acta Neuropsychiatrica 18: 61–70.
10. Linden DE (2006) How psychotherapy changes the brain - the contribution of functional neuroimaging. Mol Psychiatry 11: 528–538.
11. Roffman JL, Marci CD, Glick DM, Dougherty DD, Rauch SL (2005) Neuroimaging and the functional neuroanatomy of psychotherapy. Psychol Med 35: 1385–1398.
12. Linden DE (2008) Brain imaging and psychotherapy: methodological considerations and practical implications. Eur Arch Psychiatry Clin Neurosci 258 Suppl 5: 71–75.
13. Kessler H, Taubner S, Buchheim A, Münte TF, Stasch M, et al. (2011) Individualized and Clinically Derived Stimuli Activate Limbic Structures in Depression: An fMRI Study. PLoS One 6: e15712.
14. OPD-Task-Force (2008) Operationalized Psychodynamic Diagnosis OPD-2. Manual of Diagnosis and Treatment Planning. Kirkland: Hogrefe & Huber.
15. Wittchen HU, Wunderlich U, Gruschwitz S, Zaudig M (1997) SKID-I: Strukturiertes Klinisches Interview für DSM-IV. Achse I: Psychische Störungen. Göttingen, Bern, Toronto, Seattle: Hogrefe.
16. Hautzinger M, Bailer M, Worall H, Keller F (1994) Beck-Depressions-Inventar (BDI). Bern: Hans Huber.
17. Taubner S, Buchheim A, Rudyk R, Kachele H, Bruns G (2012) How does neurobiological research influence psychoanalytic treatments?-Clinical observations and reflections from a study on the interface of clinical psychoanalysis and neuroscience. Am J Psychoanal 72: 269–286.
18. Talairach J, Tournoux P (1988) Co-Planar Stereotaxic Atlas of the Human Brain: Three-Dimensional Proportional System. Stuttgart: Georg Thieme.
19. Lancaster JL, Woldorff MG, Parsons LM, Liotti M, Freitas CS, et al. (2000) Automated Talairach atlas labels for functional brain mapping. Hum Brain Mapp 10: 120–131.
20. Genovese CR, Lazar NA, Nichols T (2002) Thresholding of statistical maps in functional neuroimaging using the false discovery rate. Neuroimage 15: 870–878.
21. Buchheim A, Viviani R, Kessler H, Kächele H, Cierpka M, et al. (2012) Changes in prefrontal-limbic function in major depression after 15 months of long-term psychotherapy. PloS One 7: e33745.
22. Fu CH, Williams SC, Cleare AJ, Scott J, Mitterschiffthaler MT, et al. (2008) Neural responses to sad facial expressions in major depression following cognitive behavioral therapy. Biol Psychiatry 64: 505–512.
23. Drevets WC (2003) Neuroimaging abnormalities in the amygdala in mood disorders. Ann N Y Acad Sci 985: 420–444.
24. Fitzgerald PB, Laird AR, Maller J, Daskalakis ZJ (2008) A meta-analytic study of changes in brain activation in depression. Hum Brain Mapp 29: 683–695.
25. Mayberg HS (2003) Modulating dysfunctional limbic-cortical circuits in depression: towards development of brain-based algorithms for diagnosis and optimised treatment. Br Med Bull 65: 193–207.
26. Whalen PJ, Shin LM, Somerville LH, McLean AA, Kim H (2002) Functional neuroimaging studies of the amygdala in depression. Semin Clin Neuropsychiatry 7: 234–242.
27. Siegle GJ, Steinhauer SR, Thase ME, Stenger VA, Carter CS (2002) Can't shake that feeling: event-related fMRI assessment of sustained amygdala activity in response to emotional information in depressed individuals. Biol Psychiatry 51: 693–707.
28. Siegle GJ, Thompson W, Carter CS, Steinhauer SR, Thase ME (2007) Increased amygdala and decreased dorsolateral prefrontal BOLD responses in unipolar depression: related and independent features. Biol Psychiatry 61: 198–209.
29. Kopell BH, Greenberg BD (2008) Anatomy and physiology of the basal ganglia: implications for DBS in psychiatry. Neurosci Biobehav Rev 32: 408–422.
30. Kelley AE (2004) Memory and addiction: shared neural circuitry and molecular mechanisms. Neuron 44: 161–179.
31. Camara E, Rodriguez-Fornells A, Münte TF (2008) Functional connectivity of reward processing in the brain. Front Hum Neurosci 2: 19.
32. Mayberg HS (1997) Limbic-cortical dysregulation: a proposed model of depression. J Neuropsychiatry Clin Neurosci 9: 471–481.
33. Lemogne C, Delaveau P, Freton M, Guionnet S, Fossati P (2012) Medial prefrontal cortex and the self in major depression. J Affect Disord 136: e1–e11.
34. Yoshimura S, Okamoto Y, Onoda K, Matsunaga M, Okada G, et al. (2014) Cognitive behavioral therapy for depression changes medial prefrontal and ventral anterior cingulate cortex activity associated with self-referential processing. Soc Cogn Affect Neurosci 9: 487–493.
35. Ochsner KN, Gross JJ (2005) The cognitive control of emotion. Trends Cogn Sci 9: 242–249.
36. Kessler H, Traue H, Wiswede D (2011) Why we still don't understand the depressed brain - Not going beyond snapshots. Psychosoc Med 8.
37. Lewis DA (2000) Distributed disturbances in brain structure and function in schizophrenia. American Journal of Psychiatry 157: 1–2.
38. Barnett A, van der Pols J, Dobson A (2005) Regression to the mean: what it is and how to deal with it. International Journal of Epidemiology 34: 215–220.

39. Walsh BT, Seidman SN, Sysko R, Gould M (2002) Placebo response in studies of major depression - Variable, substantial, and growing. JAMA 287: 1840–1847.
40. Rush AJ, Trivedi MH, Wisniewski SR, Nierenberg AA, Stewart JW, et al. (2006) Acute and longer-term outcomes in depressed outpatients requiring one or several treatment steps: A STAR*D report. Am J Psychiatry 163: 1905–1917.
41. Leichsenring F, Rabung S (2008) Effectiveness of long-term psychodynamic psychotherapy: a meta-analysis. JAMA 300: 1551–1565.
42. Leichsenring F, Rabung S, Leibing E (2004) The efficacy of short-term psychodynamic psychotherapy in specific psychiatric disorders: a meta-analysis. Arch Gen Psychiatry 61: 1208–1216.
43. Bhar SS, Thombs BD, Pignotti M, Bassel M, Jewett L, et al. (2010) Is longer-term psychodynamic psychotherapy more effective than shorter-term therapies? Review and critique of the evidence. Psychother Psychosom 79: 208–216.

10

Might Depression, Psychosocial Adversity, and Limited Social Assets Explain Vulnerability to and Resistance against Violent Radicalisation?

Kamaldeep Bhui[1]*, Brian Everitt[2], Edgar Jones[3]

1 Wolfson Institute of Preventive Medicine, Barts and The London School of Medicine and Dentistry, Queen Mary University of London, London, United Kingdom, **2** Institute of Psychiatry King's College London, London, United Kingdom, **3** King's Centre for Military Health Research, Institute of Psychiatry, King's College London, London, United Kingdom

Abstract

Background: This study tests whether depression, psychosocial adversity, and limited social assets offer protection or suggest vulnerability to the process of radicalisation.

Methods: A population sample of 608 men and women of Pakistani or Bangladeshi origin, of Muslim heritage, and aged 18–45 were recruited by quota sampling. Radicalisation was measured by 16 questions asking about *sympathies for violent protest and terrorism*. Cluster analysis of the 16 items generated three groups: most sympathetic (or most vulnerable), most condemning (most resistant), and a large intermediary group that acted as a reference group. Associations were calculated with depression (PHQ9), anxiety (GAD7), poor health, and psychosocial adversity (adverse life events, perceived discrimination, unemployment). We also investigated protective factors such as the number social contacts, social capital (trust, satisfaction, feeling safe), political engagement and religiosity.

Results: Those showing the most sympathy for violent protest and terrorism were more likely to report depression (PHQ9 score of 5 or more; RR = 5.43, 1.35 to 21.84) and to report religion to be important (less often said religion was *fairly* rather than *very important*; RR = 0.08, 0.01 to 0.48). Resistance to radicalisation measured by condemnation of violent protest and terrorism was associated with larger number of social contacts (per contact: RR = 1.52, 1.26 to 1.83), less social capital (RR = 0.63, 0.50 to 0.80), unavailability for work due to housekeeping or disability (RR = 8.81, 1.06 to 37.46), and not being born in the UK (RR = 0.22, 0.08 to 0.65).

Conclusions: Vulnerability to radicalisation is characterised by depression but resistance to radicalisation shows a different profile of health and psychosocial variables. The paradoxical role of social capital warrants further investigation.

Editor: Ignacio Correa-Velez, Queensland University of Technology, Australia

Funding: The study received no grant funding. The data collection was commissioned from IPSOS-MORI and resourced by Professor Bhui. The statistical analyses were part funded by Careif, www.careif.org, an international mental health charity. Careif had no role in study design, data collection and analysis, decision to publish, or preparation of the manuscript.

Competing Interests: The data collection was commissioned from IPSOS-MORI. KB and EJ are trustees of Careif. KB is Director of MSc Psychological Therapies, MSc Transcultural Mental Healthcare, and co-Director of MSc Mental Health and Law. EJ is Director of MSc War and Psychiatry. There are no patents, products in development or marketed products to declare.

* Email: k.s.bhui@qmul.ac.uk

Background

A process termed 'radicalisation' is proposed by governments across the world to explain how ordinary people with no history of criminality commit aggressive and terrorist acts against innocent civilians in their own country [1]. Conceptualised in social and psychological terms, this theory of radicalisation proposes a pathway which begins with the development of sympathies towards violent protest and terrorism through to active participation in violent terrorist acts [2,3]. It is acknowledged that not all those with sympathies progress to become violent terrorists. Counter-terrorism efforts have been largely restricted to identifying high-risk individuals rather than understanding how to prevent radicalisation by intervening at an earlier stage of the process. Public health policies, research and interventions offer a different approach to health protection and intervene at the level of populations and *identify and reduce common risk* factors whilst *promoting protective factors and resistance* to rare diseases and damaging behaviour. Might this approach be applied to prevent radicalisation?

The recent waves of terrorism are sometimes understood as extreme religious movements with a particular focus on Islamic fundamentalism [4], but research into the propaganda spread by these groups suggests that it is political rhetoric disguised as religious ideology [5]. [6] Thus terrorism may be conceptualised as a powerful form of persuasion that induces fear and makes political gains by promoting dangerous and infectious ideas [6]. Taking this analogy further, Stares and Yacoubian propose that public health methods used to prevent the transmission of communicable diseases can also be deployed to inhibit the spread of terrorist philosophy [7,8]. In their model, terrorist organisations are akin to a host, militant ideologies are the infectious agents, and settings such as prisons or even the internet act as vectors or vehicles for transmission. In fact, population approaches in public health are already being used to combat bio-terrorism and war [9,10], homicide, violence, self-harm and suicide [11]. To advance this approach to prevent radicalisation we require a better understanding of risk and protective factors.

Among the conditions implicated in the radicalisation process are a sense of inequity and injustice, perceived discrimination, marginalisation, and a lack of integration in wider society [12] [13]. These narratives of adversity, alongside migration experiences, have also been proposed as causing depression and psychosis [14–19]. Social explanations and psychiatric opinions abound when known terrorists face conviction [20], yet there are few empirical population studies that investigate these possible explanations for radicalisation and terrorism [21,22]. One exception is an exploratory study of 52 teenage boys in Gaza that found depressive symptoms were common in supporters of 'religio-political aggression', whilst anxiety was heightened amongst Palestinian supporters of radical action [23]. Another interesting study used convergence of psychometric measures from 356 suicide-bombers, tapes of self-immolations of 15 terrorists, and 918 'zealots' in order to isolate risk factors [24]. The emergent profile implicated susceptibility to 'dogma-induced psychotic depression' amongst many other social and political characteristics. A risk-assessment instrument developed in Canada explored common characteristics of terrorists from diverse backgrounds [25,26]. This identified perceived grievances about victimization and injustice as risk factors, whilst contact with other extremists, social isolation, previous exposure to violence, commitment to acts of terrorism because of anger or because of sacred ideology about rewards of participating in terrorism were proposed as contextual factors. Strikingly, protective factors in this study included a change in attitudes and beliefs about the role of terrorism in their lives, condemnation of it, and a commitment to move away from such acts.

Social capital has been implicated in radicalisation and terrorism [27]. This concept captures the assets, resources or 'capital' available to individuals and groups; it has been defined as community cohesion and resilience resulting from a rich associational life based on a strong array of co-operative social networks [11,28–31]. Poor health and depressive symptoms can be a consequence of low social capital, isolation and inequalities, as well as experience of hardship, such as discrimination [32–34].

This study tests hypotheses about depression, psychosocial adversity and social assets as risk and resiliency factors in the early phases of radicalisation when preventive interventions might make the biggest impact [35]. In our previous paper we described a new way of assessing sympathies for violent protest and terrorism (SVPT) [36]. SVPT were rare (present in less than 3% of a population sample) so the study had limited power to detect effects. And we had not considered degrees of condemnation of violent protest and terrorism (CVPT) as a marker of resistance or as protective factors. Furthermore, whilst developing an outcome based on factor analysis, we removed items relating to international relations and government policy. In this paper, we use all the outcome data and methods to refine and improve our measure of radicalisation including all the items originally generated by focus groups and refined by testing.

In this paper we identify modifiable protective and risk factors that might be used to address vulnerabilities. We hypothesise that depressive symptoms, psychosocial adversity and limited social assets are positively correlated with SVPT and negatively correlated with CVPT. Furthermore, in our previous paper, we found that continuous measures of depressive and of anxiety symptoms did not correlate with SVPT, but we did not test non-linear associations across different levels of SVPT and CVPT, and nor did we test different validated thresholds used for screening for depression.

In this paper we address these limitations and ask the following research questions:

Are depression, psychosocial adversity and limited social assets risk (associated with SVPT) or protective (associated with CVPT) factors?

What demographic and psychosocial characteristics confer protection by showing associations with CVPT?

Are there risk and protective factors that show trends, akin to dose response relationships, for differing levels of condemnation to sympathies for violent protest and terrorism?

Methods Section

Sample

We surveyed 608 people of Pakistani or Bangladeshi family origins, aged 18–45, of Muslim heritage and living in East London and Bradford. The study sample methods have previously been reported (http://www.plosone.org/article/info%3Adoi%2F10.1371%2Fjournal.pone.0090718) [36]. Bradford was chosen because a significant proportion of the Muslim population live in traditional and relatively isolated areas characterised by poverty and deprivation. These factors are often thought to generate dissatisfaction and grievances, for example, when expressed through conflict between gangs and during riots [30,34]. East London with a substantial Muslim population offers a contrast, having greater cultural diversity and wider opportunities for employment. Individuals were recruited to the study by quota samples, a standard method for opinion polls that entails setting quotas for participation on a range of demographic factors [37]. The expected number of Muslim households in each output area was estimated using the 2001 Census and mid-year 2010 estimates, and then classified into high, medium or low concentration areas. A disproportionately stratified sample of 70 sampling points was drawn; the sample over-represented areas with high and medium concentrates of Muslim households to improve the efficiency of recruitment. Within each sampling point, a representative population of Muslims aged 18–45 was interviewed: quotas were set on age, gender, working status, and whether Bangladeshi or Pakistani origin.

Data Collection

The data were collected by IPSOS-MORI Social Research Institute. All questions were piloted and refined following two sets of four interviews to check wording, sensitivity, and questioning styles. Interviewers from IPSOS-MORI have significant experience of research into sensitive topics including religion and terrorism. IPSOS-MORI employs a workforce of trained interviewers resident in the communities where the survey took place so they could frame questions sensitively about social, lifestyle, health and safety issues for young Muslims. The pilot work did not indicate difficulties. Although the option of language and gender specific interviews was available, it did not prove necessary.

Questions were asked in a computer-assisted format with prompts and cues so that sensitive questions could be answered anonymously.

Survey Questions

A measure of risks for and resilience against violent radicalization. There is currently no well-established measure of radicalisation at a population level. Therefore, as reported in our previous paper [36], we developed survey questions by a series of interactive focus groups with young people of Muslim heritage and with members of a community panel of religious and non-religious organisations. This preceded the survey. The focus group generated a spectrum of 16 acts of protest ranging from non-violent (one item) through to more and more extreme acts, and culminating in acts of terrorism; for example, use of suicide bombs to fight injustice or commit terrorist acts (see Tables S1 and S2). In the survey, subjects were asked to rate their sympathies or condemnation of these acts. All except two of these items were scored on a 7-point Likert scale from -3 (completely condemn) to + 3 (completely sympathise). Thus the higher the score, the greater were the sympathies for violent protest and terrorism. Two questions asked about sympathies for or condemnation of the British government's decision to send British troops to Afghanistan and to Iraq. These were reverse-scored as, according to our focus group discussions during item generation, condemnation rather than sympathies would be consistent with a more radicalised perspective [4].

Risk and protective factors. Social capital can be measured in many ways and is known to be associated with violence [30,31], suicide [38] and mental health [39]. To measure social capital, we asked about satisfaction with living in the area (very satisfied, fairly satisfied, neither satisfied or dissatisfied, fairly dissatisfied, very dissatisfied), number of years living in a particular area (<1 year, 1 to <2 years, 2 to <5 years, 5 to <10 years, > or = 10 years), how many people in local area can be trusted (many, some, a few or none), and feelings of safety when alone in the area after dark (very safe, fairly safe, fairly unsafe, very unsafe). Answers were scored and summed so that a *higher* score reflected *higher social capital* (0–18). As a measure of social isolation and support, we asked about the number of contacts by telephone, email, or visit in the preceding two weeks by friends or relatives.

Understanding of political processes or ready access to political institutions might serve as protective factors as they offer a democratic and non-violent method to address perceived injustices. We assessed political engagement by asking about participation in 12 types of activity in the preceding three years. These questions were from the Department of Communities and Citizenship Survey [40]. These questions addressed voting in local council elections, political discussions, signing a petition, donations to a charity or campaigning organisation, payment of membership fees to a charity or campaigning organisation, voluntary work, a boycott for political, ethical, environmental or religious reasons, political views expressed online, attendance at a political meeting, donations to or membership of a political party, and participation in a demonstration or march. The total number of activities formed a measure of political engagement (scores from 0–12) [40].

We assessed perceived discrimination by asking four questions from the EMPIRIC study [33]; these asked about physical assault, damage to property and insults in the preceding 12 months, and any instance of unfair treatment at work where these events were thought to be related to race, skin colour, religion or ethnic background insults. The measure of threatening life events included injury, bereavement, separations, loss of job, financial crisis, problems with the police or courts, theft and major stressful events in the preceding 12 months (score 0–12) [41].

Given the emphasis on religiosity as an explanation, questions on religiosity were included. These questions asked about the importance of religion in everyday life (very important versus fairly important/not important/don't know) and frequency of attending a mosque (weekly or more, monthly or less frequently, or never). We also asked about a number of demographic characteristics (age, employment), place of birth.

Health Outcomes. To measure general functioning related to poor health, four Likert questions were adapted from the SF12 [42]. These self-report measures assessed general health, reduced activities because of physical or emotional problems, being limited by physical or emotional problems, and not being able to undertake any vigorous activities. They were each recoded to binary variables and summed so that a higher total score indicated poorer health (scores range from 0–4). Anxiety was measured by the Generalised Anxiety Disorder Assessment (GAD-7) [43] and depression by the Patient Health Questionnaire (PHQ-9) as total scores and as non-linear scores using validated thresholds [44].

Statistical Analyses. We calculated the number of people showing sympathies for or condemnation of violent protest and terrorism (Table S1: for each of the Likert items we show weighted and unweighted estimates). The weighting was for combined design effect and response weights to ensure the estimates were reflective of population level findings. Weighted calculations were undertaken in STATA 11.0 using the 'pw' command to provide robust standard errors and the procedure does not inflate the sample bases [45].

To explore whether there was evidence of distinct groups of respondents who exhibited varying degrees of radicalisation, a particular method of *cluster analysis* was applied to the data for the 16 radicalisation items [46]. In this study a *classification likelihood method* was used [46,47]. The Bayesian Information Criterion was used to determine the number of cluster in the data. The clustering was carried out on the principal component scores from a principal components analysis of the original 16 item scores. The clustering was carried out using different numbers of principal component scores and the most stable solution found was the one with the three groups described in this papers. The cluster analysis was implemented in the *mclust* package in R. All other analyses were conducted in STATA (11.0).

A cluster analysis of the 16-item measure of sympathies for violent protest and terrorism produced a three-group solution: a group that was most sympathetic (group 3, n = 92), least sympathetic (group 1, n = 93), and a large intermediary group (group 2, n = 423). The values of the mean score for each group suggest the cluster labels reflect an ordinal variable for radicalisation, so the study has potential to identify dose-response relationships. (Table S2: the mean scores for each cluster are shown overall and for each of the 16 items).

For each of the proposed risk and protective factors, we calculated the total sample size for each response category, and show the total weighted prevalence (%) and standard error (se) for categorical variables; for continuous variables we provided and weighted mean and standard error (se).

After defining the three groups derived from cluster analysis, univariable weighted distributions health measures and potential risk and resiliency factors were calculated and charted for each of the three *cluster derived groups*. The three-group cluster derived variable was used as a three level outcome in multinomial logistic regression models (univariable and multivariable); the largest group, group 2 served as the reference category.

For the weighted multivariable model, all the variables were included in order to provide the most conservative model that would take account of potential residual confounding. The findings are shown as Risk Ratios, and 95% confidence intervals and probability values (RR, 95% CI, p). Religious practice and importance were included to test whether the findings were sustained independent of religiosity. A gender interaction term with depressive symptoms was considered given depression is more common in women. Model fit with and without the interaction term was assessed using the likelihood ratio test.

Our 'a priori' framework for interpreting the results proposed that any variable more commonly found in group 3 compared to 2 was associated with sympathies for violent protest and terrorism, and was therefore a risk factor for violent radicalisation; in contrast variables less common in group 3 compared with 2 would offer resistance or be like resiliency factors. Any variables that were more common in group 1 compared with 2 would be implicated as a correlate of condemnation of violent protest and terrorism and therefore would be interpreted as a offering resistance or resiliency; any variable less common in group 1 compared to 2 would then be implicated as undermining resistance.

Ethical approval. Ethical approval was from Queen Mary, University of London Research Ethics Committee (REC); additional legal advice influenced the wording of questions. The REC reviewed and approved all the questions, and the information sheets and consent forms. The study was subject to an independent monitoring committee chaired by a professor of ethics in the law department at Queen Mary University of London. No adverse incidents or issues were reported during data collection. Data were collected by individual interviews, administered on a laptop computer by interviewers. Consent was recorded by checking an appropriate box before proceeding with the computer-based survey.

Results

Demographic, psychosocial, and health characteristics

Table 1 shows weighted response rates for each of the demographic, psychosocial and health characteristics. The weighted data representative of the population show a sample composed mostly of the 26–35 year age group, who are mostly employed and born in the UK, living in London; for the majority, religion was reported as *very important* in their daily lives, a point supported at least weekly mosque attendance.

Weighted (unadjusted) population prevalence estimates of risk and protective factors were charted by the three groups derived by cluster analysis. The data for demographic characteristics are charted in Figure 1 as percentages and standard errors. Figure 2 shows the psychosocial and health characteristics.

In comparison with group 2, unemployment was less common in group 1 (RR = 0.23, 95%CI: 0.07–0.77, p = 0.02); social capital was poorer in group 1 (RR = 0.76, 95%CI: 0.63–0.92, p = 0.004; people in group 1 were less likely to be born in the UK (RR = 0.22, 95%CI: 0.08–0.65, p = 0.006). Among migrants, the number of years of residence in the UK did not show any relationship with cluster membership (unreported data).

In comparison with group 2, political engagement was poorer for group 3 (RR = 0.63, 95%CI: 0.44 to 0.9, p = 0.01) and depressive symptoms appear to be more prevalent for group 3 (weighted mean 5.00, 95%CI: 2.95 to 7.06) (weighted mean 3.14, 95%CI: 1.38 to 4.90). Psychosocial adversity and poor health appeared not to be relevant.

In order to address potential confounders, adjusted logistic regression models were built. This approach addresses potential confounding influences that might show associations in unadjusted analyses that are not sustained in multivariable analyses; or negative confounders may mask true associations in unadjusted analyses for these only to be revealed in multivariable analyses.

Multivariable analyses (weighted)

Table 2 sets out the estimated risk ratios and associated confidence intervals for associations between cluster derived groups and demographic characteristics, psychosocial adversity, social capital and health measures, adjusted for ethnicity and religiosity. The comparisons are of group 3 with group 2, and of group 1 with group 2. Overall there was good model fit ($R2 = 25.38$, $X2 = 85.51$, $df = 44$, $p = 0.0002$),

Compared with the group 2, people in the group showing most sympathies for violent protest and terrorism (group 3) were more likely to report depressive symptoms, less likely to include people of Bangladeshi ethnic origin, and less likely to include people reporting religion as fairly rather than very important in their lives. Low levels of political engagement were no longer associated with membership of group 3. Contrary to popular views about radicalisation, unemployment, educational achievements, discrimination, and stressful life events did not show associations with sympathies towards violent protest and terrorism.

Group 1 showed the most condemnation of violent protest and terrorism. Group 1 was more likely (compared with group 2) to include people unavailable for work (mostly women who were looking after the home) and migrants born outside of the UK who would therefore have migrated to the UK; Group 1 compared with 2, reported a greater number of social contacts, lower social capital, and marginally more depressive symptoms. In univariable analyses, fewer people in groups 1 were unemployed, compared with group 2. Theis findings were not sustained in multivariable analyses.

The PHQ score was entered as a continuous score of depressive symptoms. The PHQ score does not indicate clinically significant depressive symptoms and there may be threshold effects. In order to investigate the relationship between depression and cluster derived group membership further, we applied validated clinical thresholds used to screen for mild (5 or more) and moderate (10 or more) depression. On repeating the analyses, mild depression was associated with membership of group 3 but moderate depression was not (see Table 3). If depression was entered as a binary variable using a threshold of 5 or more to indicate mild and moderate depressive symptoms, depression was still more prevalent in group 3. A log likelihood ratio test indicated no difference in model fit between a 3 (none, mild, moderate) or 2 category (none, mild and more severe) measure of depression ($X2 = 2.91$, $df = 2$, $p = 0.23$). Although gender was not associated with cluster membership, the point estimates indicate women were less likely to be in group 1 and more likely to be in group 3; and given depression is more common in women, this model was repeated with an interaction term between gender and depression. This model did not show a better fit (likelihood ratio test $X2 = 4.44$, $df = 2$, $p = 0.11$); the findings overall remained identical with a non-significant interaction term. In order to assess whether the suicide item in the PHQ9 was driving the associations with depression, we repeated these models without this item and found the same overall findings.

Discussion

Principal findings

Depressive symptoms (PHQ score of 5 or more indicating at least mild depression) were more common among those showing

Table 1. Demographic, psychosocial & health characteristics.

			Weighted
DEMOGRAPHICS			
Age group	18–25	%	25.98
(N = 599)	26–35	%	48.91
	36–45	%	25.11
Gender	Men	%	54.45
(n = 608)	Women	%	45.55
Single	Yes	%	54.45
(N = 608)	No	%	45.55
Employment status	Employed	%	50.26
(N = 608)	Full time education	%	11.05
	Unemployed	%	9.92
	Permanent disability/retired	%	0.64
	Look after house		28.14
City	London	%	80.62
(N = 608)	Bradford	%	19.38
ETHNICITY AND RELGIOSITY			
Ethnic Group	Pakistani	%	46.65
(n = 608)	Bangladeshi	%	53.35
Born in UK	Yes	%	70.93
(n = 608)	No		29.07
Importance of Religion to way of life	Very	%	71.99
(N = 608)	Fairly, not or don't know	%	28.1
Attending a place of worship: mosque	Never	%	28.47
(N = 604)	Monthly or less	%	13.86
	Weekly or more	%	57.68
PSYCHOSOCAL ADVERSITY AND SOCIAL CAPITAL			
Social capital score		mean	7.61
(N = 608)		se	0.21
Total social contacts		mean	4.64
(N = 608)		se	0.21
Political engagement		mean	1.98
(N = 608)		se	0.12
Discrimination		mean	0.2
(N = 608)		se	0.04
Life events		mean	0.58
(N = 608)		se	0.07
HEALTH MEASURES			
Generalised anxiety on GAD score		mean	2.95
(N = 562)		se	0.47
Depressive symptom on PHQ9 score		mean	3.34
(N = 527)		se	0.5
Poor Health Total Score		mean	0.74
(greater score = poorer health)		se	0.11
(N = 608)			

the most sympathy towards violent protest and terrorism. Although previous studies of terrorists have not shown significantly greater levels of severe mental illness (for example, psychoses with delusions and hallucinations), small studies of convicted terrorists and of teenagers in Palestine have suggested depressive and anxiety symptoms are important [23] [13]. One study seeking to define religious terrorism proposed the presence of 'dogma induced psychotic depression' but this investigation was not based

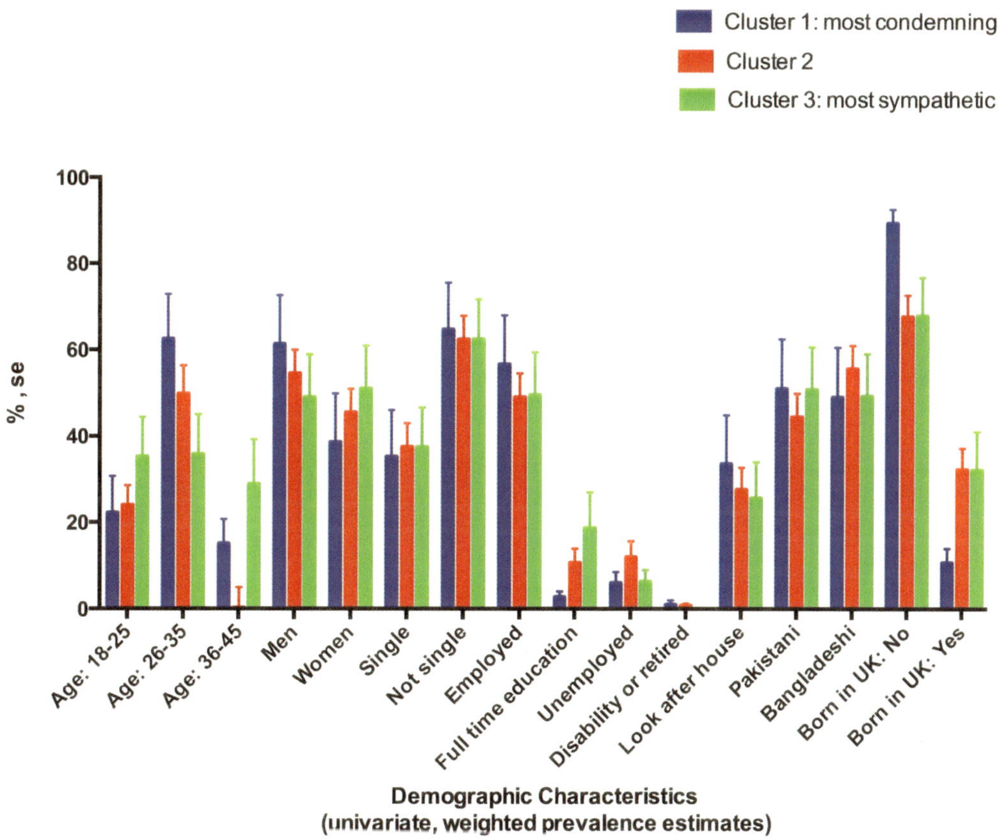

Figure 1. Demographic characteristics by clusters (univariable, weighted data).

on a structured diagnostic or screening instrument. The place of psychological distress in terrorism is controversial [48]. It is known that low mood is associated with hopelessness about the future, and suicidal feelings, perhaps mediated through feelings of low self-esteem, cognitive distortions in weighing up everyday events and experiences as more negative [38]. These cognitive biases may be seen as adaptive if they reflect social and economic injustices, and experiences of structural violence; or these may reflect depressive illness if there is not a history of such adversity. Our findings suggest the latter, that depressive symptoms independent of psychosocial adversity were associated with sympathies towards violent protest and terrorism.

More generally, depression has been implicated in acts of aggression [49,50]. Although depression and aggression can be present from an early age and have genetic and neurochemical origins [50,51], depression can also be a consequence of chronic adversity, and can lead to maladaptive behaviour, social strain [33] or abnormal personality development [51]. Personality disorder is often implicated in crime, but is an unlikely explanation of our finding as the majority of our sample were in employment and reported active social networks (and additionally did not report frequent hospital attendance due to accidents and injuries; unreported data).

Social isolation has been proposed as a risk factor for radicalization [52], and is also implicated as a link between biological mechanisms of aggression and depression when tested in animal models [53]. Consistent with this perspective, we found that the group showing the strongest condemnation appeared to have more social contacts. Isolation from the wider community, together with feelings of identification and cohesion within terrorist organisations, are a proposed mechanism by which people are persuaded to take up violence, under the influence of newly formed radical affiliations [12,19]. In multivariate analyses, women seemed more likely to be in the most sympathetic group, indicating greatest risk; this finding did not reach statistical significance. A higher risk for women has previously been reported but only where social isolation, powerlessness and oppression limited alternative opportunities or lifestyles [54]. More in-depth qualitative work exploring Muslim women's experiences of disadvantage and oppression may offer useful insights into the place of gender politics and gender disadvantage as mechanism of radicalisation.

A surprising finding was that low levels of social capital were not related to sympathies towards terrorism but were associated with greater condemnation of terrorist acts. In our study, social capital was measured by satisfaction with residential area, trust in neighbours and feelings of safety. As expected in accord with the wider literature, poor social capital was associated with depression (unreported data), suggesting that the survey questions seem to tap the appropriate concepts [55]. A low score, therefore, reflected fears associated with the neighbourhood, including violence in the community, and explains condemnation of perceived threats. This finding is also consistent with a recent analysis suggesting that higher social capital can actually foster the formation of terrorist groups through greater opportunities for co-operation and by the exploitation of altruistic aspirations in a open democratic political system [27]. However, a study of social capital and terrorism, conducted over 12 years in 150 countries, showed that as well as fostering more terrorist organisations, higher social capital actually correlated with fewer terrorist attacks. So the influence of social

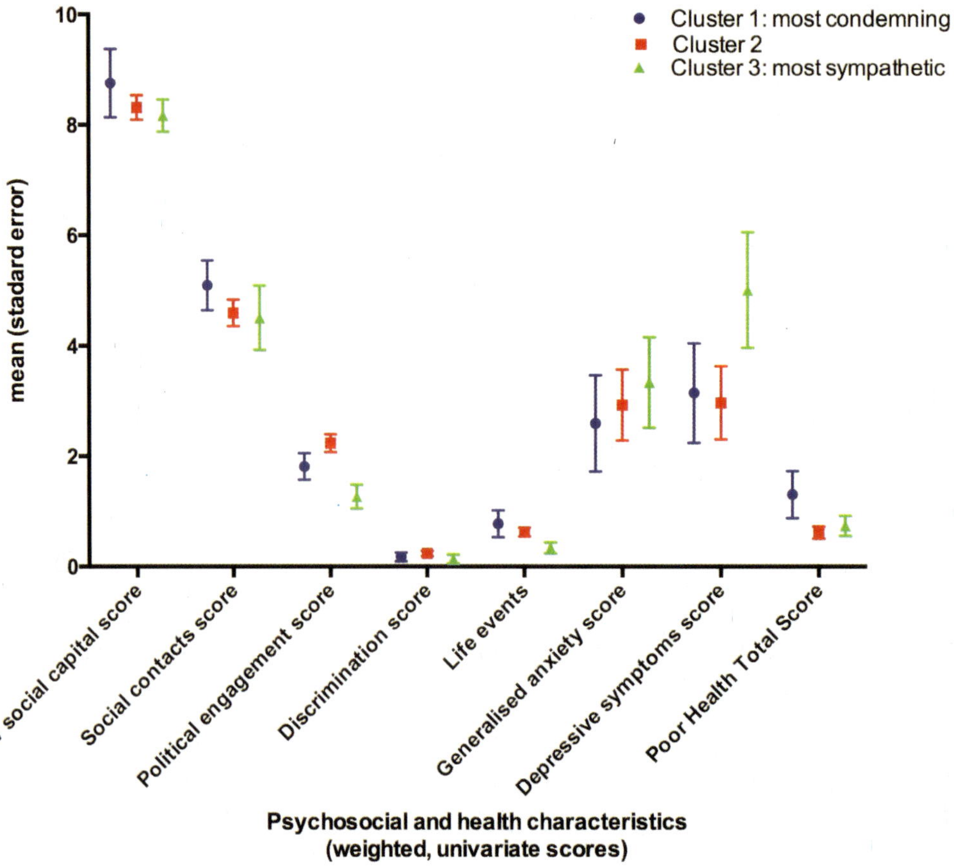

Figure 2. Psychosocial and health characteristics by clusters (multivariable, weighted data).

capital is complex and it does not seem to be easily modified for predictable preventive effects.

Strengths and Weaknesses

Although the three-group solution was selected by a statistically acceptable method of cluster analysis using a variety of sensible criteria to indicate the 'correct' number of groups, the clusters derived should be regarded as a preliminary and useful basis for understanding and describing the survey responses. Replication is recommended as one study does not provide definitive conclusions on which to base policy.

As a cross-sectional study, causality cannot be directly inferred but the three groups derived from cluster analysis are akin to an ordinal variable permitting the comparison of specific characteristics across the three groups. However, no single variable showed linear trends across all three clusters. This suggests protective factors associated with condemnation are different to those associated with the development of sympathies for violent protest and terrorism. Alternatively, we may have not included other factors that might be linearly related with developing sympathies for radicalisation.

Importantly, this study does not show which people who are sympathisers are likely to progress to terrorist acts. However, there is a sequence of events consistent with the stages of radicalization [35], each with specific contexts and risk of progression [7]. This model of public health epidemiology recommends that those 'infected' with radical ideology, or already radicalised, need to be isolated so that they cannot influence those around them. The criminal justice system fulfils this function. Those who are vulnerable require inoculation through a wider set of ideas, including orthodox religious texts that decry homicide and terrorism. Furthermore, social networks promote resistance by offering a range of cultural identities and opportunities and this in itself may be protective; for example, integrated cultural identities protect against psychological distress in young people by offering bridging social capital across contrasting identity groups [56]. Studies of resilience to such radicalising ideas, where resilience consists of resistance despite exposure to radicalising ideas in the presence of SVPT, are needed.

Another reason for studying and preventing SVPT in the population is that these become part of the political rhetoric of terrorists and are used to justify their actions. Through encouraging SVPT, terrorists and extremists can seek resources for their cause. There may be communalities with other extremist movements, for example, animal rights protesters, or in situations of war and conflict, or where extreme right wing parties target particular ethnic, racial or religious groups [57,58]. Indeed, the boundaries between protest movements and terrorism require further investigation.

We had interpreted condemnation of sending British troops to conflict zones as consistent with radicalisation because terrorists have reported such actions as justification for their acts [4]. We generated our items to measure radicalisation by reference to such literature and by focus groups assuring us of face and content validity. However, such condemnation could also indicate a position of conscientious objection. In people of Muslim heritage, this stance might be misunderstood to indicate radicalisation rather than an anti-war or pacifist political position. Future studies

Table 2. Multivariable Multinomial Logistic Regression comparing clusters three (most sympathetic) and cluster one (most condemning) with cluster two as the reference category (weighted).

		Cluster 1				Cluster 3			
		RR	**LCI**	**UCI**	**P**	**RR**	**LCI**	**UCI**	**P**
DEMOGRAPHICS									
Age groups	18–25	1				1			
	26–35	1.56	0.35	6.96	0.56	0.54	0.15	1.97	0.35
	36–45	1.4	0.33	5.87	0.65	0.72	0.14	3.64	0.69
Gender	Male	1				1			
	Female	0.26	0.06	1.15	0.08	2.92	0.78	10.98	0.11
Single	No	1				1			
	Yes	2.19	0.46	10.37	0.33	0.62	0.17	2.3	0.48
Employment	Employed	1				1			
	FT student	0.75	0.17	3.33	0.71	2.22	0.31	15.77	0.43
	Unemployed	0.94	0.25	3.51	0.93	0.43	0.09	2.06	0.29
	Retired, ill or housewife	8.81	2.06	37.64	**0.003**	0.27	0.06	1.21	0.09
ETHNICITY & RELIGIOSITY									
Ethnicity	Pakistani	1				1			
	Bangladeshi	1.24	0.46	3.29	0.67	0.32	0.11	0.94	**0.04**
Born in UK	No	1				1			
	Yes	0.22	0.08	0.65	**0.006**	0.52	0.14	1.91	0.33
Importance of religion in your life	Very	1				1			
	Fairly	0.67	0.18	2.48	0.54	0.08	0.01	0.48	**0.006**
	Not/don't know	0.36	0.04	2.89	0.33	0.07	0.01	0.81	**0.03**
Frequency of attending place of worship	Never	1				1			
	Monthly or less	1.42	0.37	5.52	0.41	0.65	0.16	2.6	0.54
	weekly or more	2.83	0.7	11.48	0.14	0.56	0.11	2.8	0.48
PSYCHOSOCIAL ADVERSITY AND SOCIAL CAPITAL									
Social capital score		0.63	0.5	0.8	**<0.001**	1	0.8	1.26	0.97
Total contacts in previous week		1.52	1.26	1.83	**<0.001**	0.95	0.73	1.24	0.7
Political Engagement Score		0.98	0.77	1.25	0.89	0.77	0.55	1.07	0.12
Threatening Life Events Score		1.13	0.67	1.9	0.64	0.47	0.2	1.12	0.09
Discrimination score		0.61	0.31	1.19	0.64	0.66	0.23	1.92	0.45
HEALTH MEASURES									
Anxiety score on GAD7		0.79	0.61	1.03	0.09	0.94	0.75	1.19	0.61
Depression score on PHQ9		1.22	1	1.48	**0.04**	1.33	1.03	1.72	**0.03**
Total Health Score		0.89	0.56	1.39	0.6	0.7	0.43	1.11	0.13

Table 3. Association of Depression category with cluster membership (fully adjusted model).

	Cluster 1			Cluster 3		
Depression Category	**RR**	**95%CI**	**P value**	**RR**	**95%CI**	**p value**
None (PHQ score 0–4)	1			1		
Mild (PHQ score 5–9)	1.53	0.34 to 6.87	0.58	5.22	1.33 to 20.54	**0.02**
Moderate (PHQ score > or =10)	9.54	0.43 to 210.34	0.15	6.52	0.35 to 121.78	0.21
None (PHQ score 0–4)	1			1		
Mild or moderate (PHQ score 5 or more)	2.03	0.47 to 8.76	0.34	5.43	1.35 to 21.84	**0.02**

Cluster 2 is reference.
Repeating the analysis after removing the suicide item from the PHQ9 measure of depression produces the same overall findings.

will need to carefully discern whether such political objections are separate from beliefs that are on the pathway to radicalisation. We did not find political engagement to be associated with radicalisation suggesting that our findings are unlikely to reflect political activism or conscientious objection.

Terrorist organisations in the past and in other cultures were motivated by different social and political factors. As a result, our findings relate to the current priorities of counter-terrorism in Europe and North America, namely of understanding and preventing the radicalisation of home-grown youth. It would not be prudent to generalise the findings to other contexts and types of terrorism, although similar research is feasible in other contexts. For example, although 'psychotic depression' was implicated in a study undertaken in a conflict zone [24], our findings indicate a modest effect of depressive symptoms; we did not measure clinical symptoms of psychosis directly. The attribution of psychosis defined on the basis of delusions is subject to criticism, as delusions are culturally shaped and can be seen as psychopathological only if the beliefs held are culturally inappropriate. Fear of the enemy, paranoia and depressive symptoms may be seen as ordinary responses to war and conflict. Thus the study of psychological distress in future studies must consider context: the influence of conflict, culture and war on SVPT. Furthermore, our finding suggest that depressive symptoms may be both protective and risk factors, but it was only depressive symptoms meeting a screening threshold for mild depressive illness that were risk factors. The place of depressive symptoms clearly warrants further investigations.

Implications

Terrorist acts not only result in death, illness, and severe injury to members of the public and emergency services, they also impact adversely on social cohesion, accentuating divisions between different racial and religious groups [59–61]. They raise legitimate fears about safety and security [61,62]. Trauma, multiple bereavements, and fear can have long-term consequences for psychological health [63]. A preventive approach to radicalisation is not part of current UK counter-terrorism policy, which focuses on those likely to commit terrorist acts. Our study shows that there are modifiable risk and protective factors for the earliest stage on the pathway to violent protest. The potential benefits of disrupting the pathways to radicalisation go beyond security issues and have implications for preventing significant depressive symptoms, promoting wellbeing and perhaps social capital [64]. More research is needed into the causes of depressive thinking implicated in our study. Future studies must investigate the place of different types of social assets, depressive symptoms, and psychosocial adversity in the process of radicalisation in different heritage groups and in different country and regional contexts. Our methods do offer an alternative paradigm for testing interventions aimed at preventing or reversing the early stages of violent radicalisation.

Key Messages

- Studies of sympathies for terrorism and violent radicalisation are needed and feasible to undertake in a Muslim minority country.
- Mild depressive symptoms as assessed on the PHQ9 are associated with sympathies for violent protest and terrorism.
- A greater number of social contacts and being a migrant were associated with more condemnation. Poorer social capital and being unavailable for work because of housewife roles and disability were associated with condemnation.
- Future work needs to investigate whether standardised measures of social capital to replicate this unexpected finding and to help understand the mechanisms.

Supporting Information

Table S1 Proportion (as %) of respondents endorsing each Likert response of the 16 Radicalization items.

Table S2 Means scores for each item and all items by clusters.

Author Contributions

Conceived and designed the experiments: KB. Performed the experiments: EJ KB. Analyzed the data: KB BE. Contributed to the writing of the manuscript: KB. Managed the study: KB. Reviewed the questionnaires: EJ KB. Secured ethical permissions: EJ KB. Oversaw the data collection by a survey company, IPSOS-MORI: EJ KB. Performed statistical analyses: KB BE. Provided comments to manuscript: EJ BE. Prepared first draft: KB. Edited subsequent drafts: KB. Had full access to all the data and final responsibility for the decision to submit: KB.

References

1. Stroink M (2007) Processes and preconditions underlying terrorism in second-generation immigrants. Journal of Peace Psychology 13: 19.
2. Horgan J (2009) Walkng away from terrorism: accounts of disengagement from radical and extremist movements. New York: Routledge. 186 p.
3. Levy BS, Sidel VW (2008) War and Public Health: An Overview. In: Levy BS, Sidel V, editors. War & Public Health. New York: Oxford University Press. pp. 3–18.
4. HomeAffairsCommittee (2012) The roots of violent radicalisation. London: House of Commons.
5. Allgulander C (1994) Suicide and mortality patterns in anxiety neurosis and depressive neurosis. Arch Gen Psychiatry 51: 708–712.
6. O'Shaughnessy N, Baines R (2009) Selling terror: The symbolisation and positioning of jihad. Marketing Theory 9(2). 14.
7. Stares PB, Yacoubian M (2007) Terrorism as a Disease: An Epidemiological Model for Countering Islamist Extremism. Mathew B Ridgeway Centre for international Security Studies. Pittsburgh. United States.
8. Stares P, Yacoubian M (2008) Rethinking the war on terror: new approaches to conflict prevention and management in the post 9/11 world. Washington DC, United States.
9. Levy BS, Sidel VW (2008) War and Public Health. New York: Oxford University Press.
10. Levy BS, Sidel VW (2011) Terrorism and Public Health: A Balanced Approach to Strengthening Systems and Protecting People. Oxford, United Kingdom: Oxford University Press. 416 p.
11. Bhui K, Hicks M, Lashely M, Jones E (2012) Public Health Approaches to Prevent Violent Radicalization. BMC Medicine 10: 16–24.
12. Radicalisation ECEGoV (2008) Radicalisation Processes leading to acts of terrorism: European Commission.
13. Victoroff J (2005) The Mind of the Terrorist: A Review and Critique of Psychological Approaches. The Journal of Conflict Resolution 49: 39.
14. Li M (2013) Discrimination and Psychiatric Disorder Among Asian American Immigrants: A National Analysis by Subgroups. J Immigr Minor Health.
15. Berg AO, Melle I, Rossberg JI, Romm KL, Larsson S, et al. (2011) Perceived discrimination is associated with severity of positive and depression/anxiety symptoms in immigrants with psychosis: a cross-sectional study. BMC Psychiatry 11: 77.
16. Veling W, Selten JP, Susser E, Laan W, Mackenbach JP, et al. (2007) Discrimination and the incidence of psychotic disorders among ethnic minorities in The Netherlands. Int J Epidemiol 36: 761–768.
17. Tunnard C, Rane LJ, Wooderson SC, Markopoulou K, Poon L, et al. (2014) The impact of childhood adversity on suicidality and clinical course in treatment-resistant depression. J Affect Disord 152–154: 122–130.
18. Levecque K, Van Rossem R (2014) Depression in Europe: does migrant integration have mental health payoffs? A cross-national comparison of 20 European countries. Ethn Health.
19. Christmann K (2012) Preventing religious radicaliasation and violent extremism. London: Youth Justice Board.
20. Stoddard FJ Jr., Gold J, Henderson SW, Merlino JP, Norwood A, et al. (2011) Psychiatry and terrorism. J Nerv Ment Dis 199: 537–543.
21. Neuman P (2008) Recruitment and Mobilisation for Islamist Militant Movements in Europe. Brussels: European Commission.
22. Alderdice JT (2009) Sacred values: psychological and anthropological perspectives on fairness, fundamentalism, and terrorism. Ann N Y Acad Sci 1167: 158–173.
23. Victoroff J, Quota S, Adelman JR, Celinska B, Stern N, et al. (2010) Support for religio-political aggression among teenaged boys in Gaza: Part I: psychological findings. Aggress Behav 36: 219–231.
24. Schbley A (2003) Defining Religious Terrorism: A Causal and Anthological Profile. Studies in Conflict & Terrorism 26: 105–134.
25. Pressman DE, Flockton J (2012) Calibrating risk for violent political extremists and terrorists: the VERA2 structured assessment. The British Journal of Forensic Practice 14: 15.
26. Beardsley NL, Beech AR (2013) Applying violent extremist risk assessment (VERA) to a sample of terrorist case studies. Journal of Aggression, Conflict and Peace Research 5: 12.
27. Helfstein S (2013) Social Capital and Terrorism. Defence and Peace Economics: 1–18.
28. Alino JJ, Jimenez JL, Flores SC, Alcocer MI (2010) Efficacy of transcranial magnetic stimulation (TMS) in depression: naturalistic study. Actas Esp Psiquiatr 38: 87–93.
29. Jayaweera J, Choudhury T (2008) Immigration, faith and cohesion. York Joseph Rowntree Fondation.
30. Galea S, Karpati A, Kennedy B (2002) Social capital and violence in the United States, 1974–1993. Soc Sci Med 55: 1373–1383.
31. El Hajj T, Afifi RA, Khawaja M, Harpham T (2011) Violence and social capital among young men in Beirut. Inj Prev 17: 401–406.
32. Marmot M (2005) Social determinants of health inequalities. Lancet 365: 1099–1104.
33. Bhui K, Stansfeld S, McKenzie K, Karlsen S, Nazroo J, et al. (2005) Racial/ethnic discrimination and common mental disorders among workers: findings from the EMPIRIC Study of Ethnic Minority Groups in the United Kingdom. Am J Public Health 95: 496–501.
34. Kenway P, Palmer G (2007) Poverty among ethnic groups: how and why does it matter? York.
35. Silber M, Bhatt A (2007) Radicalization in the West: the Homegrown Threat. New York New York City Police Department.
36. Bhui K, Warfa N, Jones E (2014) Is violent radicalisation associated with poverty, migration, poor self-reported health and common mental disorders? PLoS One 9: e90718.
37. Rubin GJ, Brewin CR, Greenberg N, Simpson J, Wessely S (2005) Psychological and behavioural reactions to the bombings in London on 7 July 2005: cross sectional survey of a representative sample of Londoners. BMJ 331: 606.
38. Patel V (2010) Building social capital and improving mental health care to prevent suicide. Int J Epidemiol 39: 1411–1412.
39. Henderson S, Whiteford H (2003) Social capital and mental health. Lancet 362: 505–506.
40. Service. Esd (2011) Local Goverment and Communities Citizenship Survey. UK.
41. Brugha T, Bebbington P, Tennant C, Hurry J (1985) The List of Threatening Experiences: a subset of 12 life event categories with considerable long-term contextual threat. Psychol Med 15: 189–194.
42. Ware J Jr., Kosinski M, Keller SD (1996) A 12-Item Short-Form Health Survey: construction of scales and preliminary tests of reliability and validity. Med Care 34: 220–233.
43. Swinson RP (2006) The GAD-7 scale was accurate for diagnosing generalised anxiety disorder. Evid Based Med 11: 184.
44. Kroenke K, Spitzer RL, Williams JB (2001) The PHQ-9: validity of a brief depression severity measure. J Gen Intern Med 16: 606–613.
45. StataCorpLP (2011) STATA 11.0. Texas USA: StataCorp LP 4905 Lakeway Drive, College Station, Texas 77845–4512. USA.
46. Everitt BS, Landau S, Leese M, Stahl M (2011) Cluster Analysis Shewhard W, Wilks S, editors. Chichester, West Sussex, UK.: John Wiley & Sons Ltd.
47. Banfield JD, RafertyAE (1993) Model-Based Gaussian and Non-Gaussian Clustering. Biometrics 49: 18.
48. Brym R, Araj B (2012) Are suicide bombers suicidal? Studies in Conflict & Terrorism 35: 10.
49. Benezech M, Bourgeois M (1992) [Homicide is strongly correlated to depression and not to mania]. Encephale 18 Spec No 1: 89–90.
50. Osipova DV, Kulikov AV, Popova NK (2009) C1473G polymorphism in mouse tph2 gene is linked to tryptophan hydroxylase-2 activity in the brain, intermale aggression, and depressive-like behavior in the forced swim test. J Neurosci Res 87: 1168–1174.
51. Bradvik L, Berglund M (2011) Repetition of suicide attempts across episodes of severe depression. Behavioural sensitisation found in suicide group but not in controls. BMC Psychiatry 11: 5.
52. McCauley C, Moskalenko M (2011) How Radicalization Happens to Them and Us: How Radicalization Happens to Them and Us: Oxford University Press. 240 p.
53. Matsumoto T, Matsushita S, Okudaira K, Naruse N, Cho T, et al. (2011) Depression and suicide risk of outpatients at specialized hospitals for substance use disorder: comparison with depressive disorder patients at general psychiatric clinics. Nihon Arukoru Yakubutsu Igakkai Zasshi 46: 554–559.
54. Berko A (2012) The smarter bomb. women and children as suicide bombers. Plymouth, UK.: Rowland & Littlefield.
55. De Silva MJ, McKenzie K, Harpham T, Huttly SR (2005) Social capital and mental illness: a systematic review. J Epidemiol Community Health 59: 619–627.
56. Bhui KS, Lenguerrand E, Maynard MJ, Stansfeld SA, Harding S (2012) Does cultural integration explain a mental health advantage for adolescents? Int J Epidemiol 41: 791–802.
57. Collins JG (1990) Terrorism and animal rights. Science 249: 345.
58. Levy B, Sidel V (2008) War and Public Health. New York: Oxford University Press.
59. Kosashvili Y, Loebenberg MI, Lin G, Peleg K, Zvi F, et al. (2009) Medical consequences of suicide bombing mass casualty incidents: the impact of explosion setting on injury patterns. Injury 40: 698–702.
60. Kerridge BT, Khan MR, Sapkota A (2012) Terrorism, civil war, one-sided violence and global burden of disease. Med Confl Surviv 28: 199–218.
61. Feeney JM, Wallack MK (2011) Taking the terror out of terrorism: mortality data after 9/11. Lancet 378: 851–852.
62. Jordan HT, Brackbill RM, Cone JE, Debchoudhury I, Farfel MR, et al. (2011) Mortality among survivors of the Sept 11, 2001, World Trade Center disaster: results from the World Trade Center Health Registry cohort. Lancet 378: 879–887.
63. Berninger A, Webber MP, Cohen HW, Gustave J, Lee R, et al. (2010) Trends of elevated PTSD risk in firefighters exposed to the World Trade Center disaster: 2001–2005. Public Health Rep 125: 556–566.
64. Post JM (2010) "When hatred is bred in the bone:" the social psychology of terrorism. Ann N Y Acad Sci 1208: 15–23.

11

Hippocampal and Left Subcallosal Anterior Cingulate Atrophy in Psychotic Depression

Kelly Rowe Bijanki*, Brendan Hodis, Michael C. Brumm, Emily L. Harlynn, Laurie M. McCormick

Department of Psychiatry, University of Iowa Roy J. and Lucille A. Carver College of Medicine, Iowa City, Iowa, United States of America

Abstract

Background: Psychotic depression is arguably the most diagnostically stable subtype of major depressive disorder, and an attractive target of study in a famously heterogeneous mental illness. Previous imaging studies have identified abnormal volumes of the hippocampus, amygdala, and subcallosal region of the anterior cingulate cortex (scACC) in psychotic depression, though studies have not yet examined the role of family history of depression in these relationships.

Methods: 20 participants with psychotic depression preparing to undergo electroconvulsive therapy and 20 healthy comparison participants (13 women and 7 men in each group) underwent structural brain imaging in a 1.5 T MRI scanner. 15 of the psychotic depression group had a first-degree relative with diagnosed affective disorders, while the healthy control group had no first-degree relatives with affective disorders. Depression severity was assessed with the Hamilton Depression Rating Scale and duration of illness was assessed in all patients. Automated neural nets were used to isolate the hippocampi and amygdalae in each scan, and an established manual method was used to parcellate the anterior cingulate cortex into dorsal, rostral, subcallosal, and subgenual regions. The volumes of these regions were compared between groups. Effects of laterality and family history of affective disorders were examined as well.

Results: Patients with psychotic depression had significantly smaller left scACC and bilateral hippocampal volumes, while no group differences in other anterior cingulate cortex subregions or amygdala volumes were present. Hippocampal atrophy was found in all patients with psychotic depression, but reduced left scACC volume was found only in the patients with a family history of depression.

Conclusions: Patients with psychotic depression showed significant reduction in hippocampal volume bilaterally, perhaps due to high cortisol states associated with this illness. Reduced left scACC volume may be a vulnerability factor related to family history of depression.

Editor: Kewei Chen, Banner Alzheimer's Institute, United States of America

Funding: Funding for this study was provided by a Collaborative Interdisciplinary Project Grant from the University of Iowa College of Medicine (LM) (http://obermann.uiowa.edu/programs/interdisciplinary-research-grants) and a Nellie Ball Trust Foundation Grant (LM) (https://research.uiowa.edu/grantbulletin/show.php/25137). The funders had no role in study design, data collection and analysis, decision to publish, or preparation of the manuscript.

Competing Interests: The authors have declared that no competing interests exist.

* Email: kelly-rowe@uiowa.edu

Introduction

Depression is the highest contributor to disease burden in middle- and high-income countries [1], and among all of its subtypes, psychotic depression is the most severe variant [2,3]. Psychotic depression represents a mood disorder distinct from non-psychotic major depression based on differences in symptomatology, disease course, treatment response, cognitive dysfunction, and biological features [4]. Approximately 20% of people with major depression are thought to experience psychosis, though this number rises to 50–60% in groups of patients with treatment-refractory major depression [5]. Patients with psychotic depression can be sensitively (84%) and specifically (99%) discerned from their non-psychotically depressed counterparts on the basis of their endorsements of unusual thought content, an item on the Brief Psychiatric Rating Scale [6,7]. Patients with psychotic depression are reported to show greater cognitive deficits, have previous episodes with psychosis, longer duration of episodes, and a greater likelihood of recurrence [7]. In addition, they show greater hypothalamo-pituitary-adrenal axis activation and have higher cortisol levels than their non-psychotically depressed counterparts [8]. Psychotic depression has been advanced as the most diagnostically stable presentation of major depressive disorder [9]; in one study, 92.3% of patients with psychotic depression experienced previous and/or subsequent psychotic episodes [10]. From a research perspective, this diagnostic stability makes patients with psychotic depression an ideal group to study. Kronmuller and colleagues have elegantly articulated the importance of reducing variability in chronicity and severity of depressive illness for the purposes of research [11].

Reports of volumetric brain abnormalities in major depressive disorder have been mixed, likely owing to the heterogeneity of depressive symptoms and etiologies, as well as demographic differences among samples. Many studies report abnormalities of the hippocampus, amygdala, ventral anterior cingulate and prefrontal cortex in depressive illness [12–14]. Overall, it appears that there are significant effects of illness chronicity on hippocampus and amygdala atrophy in major depressive disorder, where longer illness duration correlates with more severe tissue loss [13,15,16]. One previous study [4] has examined hippocampus and amygdala volumes in three groups: psychotic major depression, non-psychotic major depression, and healthy controls. Results indicated that patients with psychotic depression had significant amygdala atrophy compared with the other two groups, and there were no significant group differences in hippocampal volumes. In contrast, a more recent study [50] examined virtually identical participant groups and found no significant differences between psychotic and non-psychotic major depressive disorder patients in amygdala or hippocampus volumes. However, they did observe that patients with major depression (regardless of the presence of psychosis) tended to have larger amygdala volumes than controls.

In recent years, research on depression has turned toward the ventral anterior cingulate cortex and the two sub-regions that comprise it; the subcallosal and subgenual regions (scACC and sgACC respectively). Decreased activity has been noted in these areas in response to antidepressant medication, placebo treatment, and electroconvulsive therapy (ECT). Increased activity in these regions is noted in treatment non-responders, the currently depressed and transiently sad people compared to healthy controls [17]. One recent study [50] examined group-wise differences in the volume of this brain region in patients with psychotic depression as compared with non-psychotic major depression and healthy controls, reporting no significant differences between depression groups, but significant atrophy in the left subgenual region compared with controls.

An important terminological shift must be acknowledged in the literature on the ventral anterior cingulate. Early research on the anatomy and function of the area used the term "subgenual" to define the entirety of the ventral anterior cingulate cortex underlying the genu of the corpus callosum. In recent years, the term "subgenual" has been revised to include only a small volume of the posterior ventral ACC, also frequently termed "Brodmann Area 25" (Figure 1, yellow region). The anterior section of the ventral ACC, or ventral Brodmann Area 24 has since been termed "subcallosal" (Figure 1, green region). For example, decreased activity has been shown in the "subgenual cingulate" (identical to the subcallosal + subgenual cingulate as defined in the current study) in patients with familial unipolar major depressive disorder and that this decrease in activity corresponded with a 48% reduction in volume of the structure [18].

In the current study we aimed to examine the neural correlates of psychotic depression using structural MRI volumetric techniques. Based on findings reported across the depression literature, we defined six regions of interest for the current study: the hippocampus, the amygdala, and four parcellations of the anterior cingulate cortex (dorsal, rostral, subcallosal, and subgenual). Two previous reports from our lab [19,20] have suggested the left subcallosal cingulate and the hippocampus as major mediators of treatment response in ECT for psychotic depression. We anticipated seeing group differences in volumes in these regions, especially on the left side. In contrast with the previous study by Vassilopoulou and colleagues, we also aimed to examine the role of family history of affective disorders in any observed volumetric abnormality of these structures. Furthermore, the current study expands on previous findings [4] by including measures of the anterior cingulate cortex and by examining patients whose depression may have been more homogeneous (in that all participants in the current study experienced very severe psychotic depression and were being treated with ECT at the time of neuroimaging). The current study additionally expands on the findings of Drevets et al. [18] by examining patients with psychotic depression and including measures of medial temporal lobe structures.

Methods

Participants

The current study included 20 participants with psychotic unipolar major depression (here termed "psychotic depression") and 20 age- and sex-matched healthy comparison participants (see Table 1 for demographics). Healthy comparisons were recruited from the community through newspaper advertisements and were screened using an abbreviated version of the Comprehensive Assessment of Symptoms and History. Comparison participants were excluded if they had current or past major medical, neurological, or psychiatric illnesses, or if they had a family history of schizophrenia or affective disorders.

The participants in the psychotic depression group took part in a larger study that reported neuroimaging findings before and after ECT [19,20]. All participants met DSM-IV criteria for major depression with psychotic features and completed an MRI scan prior to or early in treatment with ECT (scans gathered after an average of 3.5 ECT doses). Eighteen participants (90%) underwent inpatient hospitalization at the University of Iowa Hospitals and Clinics and were referred for ECT by their psychiatrist on clinical grounds; the other two participants (10%) had been referred for ECT treatment on an outpatient basis. Data on the duration of depressive episode, as well as family histories of affective disorders and information on medication usage (Table 1) were taken from interviews conducted by trained psychiatrists during the course of treatment and documented in the participants' medical records. Participants had a range of current episode duration: 55% had been depressed for less than 6 months; 20% had been depressed for between 6 and 12 months; 5% had been depressed for between 12 and 24 months, 20% had been depressed for greater than 24 months at the time of data collection. Participants were rated as having a family history of affective disorder if there was unequivocal documentation of a first-degree relative (i.e. parent, sibling, or child) with diagnosed depression, bipolar disorder and/or suicide attempt based upon review of their medical records. Medications were assessed an average of 8 days prior to MRI scan and excluded "pro re nata" medications given for acute care of psychotic depression during hospitalization.

All participants in the psychotic depression group had a pre-ECT score of at least 30 on the 28-item Hamilton Depression Rating Scale (indicating severe depression) and had at least one psychotic symptom. Participants were excluded if they had a diagnosis of bipolar disorder or schizophrenia, met criteria for alcohol or illicit drug abuse or dependence within the past three months, or had been treated with a previous course of ECT within the past three months. After complete description of the study to the participants, written informed consent was obtained. This study was approved by The University of Iowa Institutional Review Board (200402013).

Measures

All participants in the psychotic depression group completed clinical interviews using the Scales for the Assessment of Negative and Positive Symptoms (SANS/SAPS) [21,22]. Scores from the

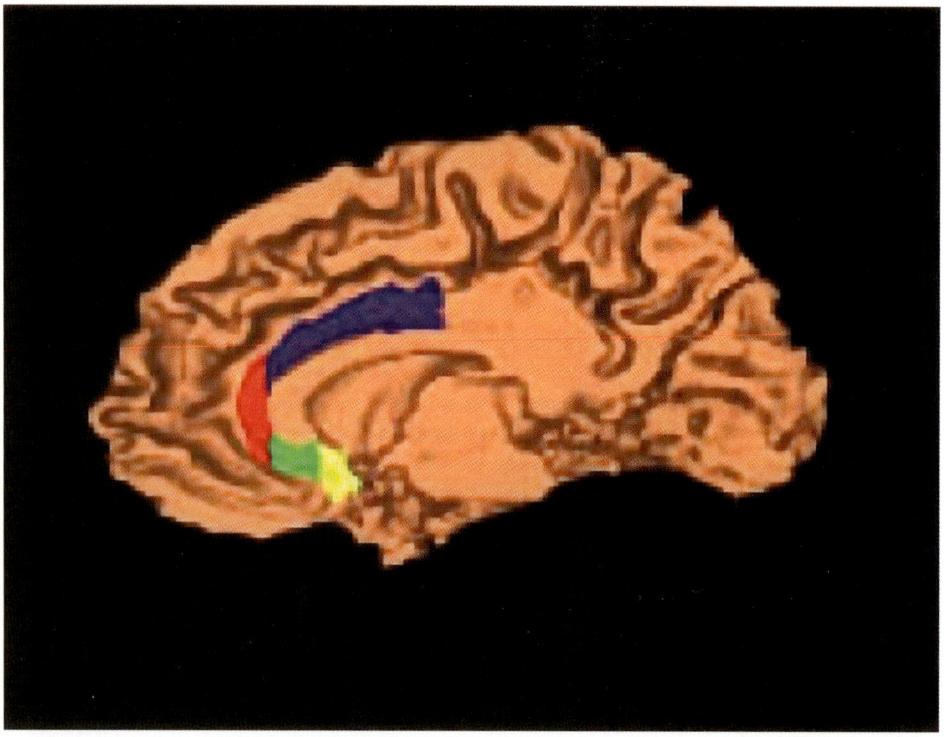

Figure 1. Parcellations of the anterior cingulate cortex. Dorsal anterior cingulate cortex (ACC) shown in blue, rostral ACC in red, subcallosal ACC in green, subgenual ACC in yellow. Figure reprinted with permission from John Wiley and Sons, from McCormick et al., (2008).

SANS/SAPS were divided into three dimensions: (1) psychoticism (scale 0–10), based on global ratings of delusions and hallucinations; (2) disorganization (scale 0–15), based on global ratings of bizarre (disorganized) behavior, positive formal thought disorder, and inappropriate affect; and (3) negative symptoms (scale 0–25), based on global ratings of alogia, anhedonia-asociality, avolition-apathy, affective flattening, and attention. The most common psychotic symptom in the current sample was delusional guilt.

In addition, all psychotic depression participants completed the 28-item Hamilton Depression Rating Scale (HAM-D) [23], as well as the Hamilton Anxiety Rating Scale (HAM-A) [24]. Both are clinician-administered instruments that assess symptoms and

Table 1. Demographic Comparison between Psychotic Depression and Healthy Control groups.

	Psychotic Depression Mean (SD) [n = 20]	HC Mean (SD) [n = 20]	DF	Statistic	*p*-value
Age	46.0 (9.5)	45.4 (9.9)	38	$t = -0.201$	$p = 0.841$
Education	13.3 (2.8)	14.5 (1.6)	38	$t = 1.737$	$p = 0.090$
Sex	65% F (13 f: 7 m)	65% F (13 f: 7 m)	1	$X^2 = 0.000$	$p > 0.999$
HAM-D	38.5 (5.4)	–	–	–	–
HAM-A	28.8 (7.9)	–	–	–	–
Family History of Affective Disorders	75%	–	–	–	–
Medication Use					
Antidepressant	95%	–	–	–	–
Anxiolytic	25%	–	–	–	–
Antipsychotic	40%	–	–	–	–
Lithium	5%	–	–	–	–

Note: Age and education reported in years. HAM-D = Hamilton Depression Rating Scale, HAM-A = Hamilton Anxiety Rating Scale, HC = healthy control, DF = degrees of freedom, SD = standard deviation. Family history of affective disorders included evidence of depression, bipolar disorder, or suicide attempt in a first degree relative. Data on family histories of affective disorders and medication usage were taken from interviews conducted by trained psychiatrists during the course of treatment and documented in the participants' medical records. Medications were assessed an average of 8 days prior to MRI scan and excluded "pro re nata" medications given for acute care of psychotic depression during hospitalization.

severity of a patient's depressive and anxious symptoms, with higher scores indicating increasing severity of symptoms. Scores above 30 on the HAM-D and HAM-A are generally taken to indicate "very severe" anxiety and depression.

Neuroimaging

Multimodal magnetic resonance imaging (MRI) scans were obtained using either a 1.5-T GE Signa scanner (10 psychotic depression participants and 20 healthy controls; GE Medical Systems, Milwaukee, WI) or on a 1.5-T Siemens Avanto scanner (10 psychotic depression participants; Erlangen, Germany). The sequences collected included a standard T1-weighted three-dimensional spoiled gradient recall acquisition (TE = 5 ms; TR = 24 ms; flip angle = 30°–50°; two excitations; FOV = 26 cm; matrix = 256×256; slice thickness = 1.5–1.7 mm). Two-dimensional T2 sequences were also acquired (TE = 24–98 ms; TR = 3000–9500 ms; flip angle = 90°–180°; one excitation; FOV = 26 cm; matrix = 256×256; slice thickness = 3.0 mm). All scans were visually assessed for quality and for motion artifacts.

Automated processing of the structural images was performed using BRAINS2 (Brain Research: Analysis of Images, Networks, and Systems) software [25], which includes automated AC-PC alignment, image alignment, image intensity standardization, tissue classification, and brain extraction. Then, automated neural nets were used to parcellate the hippocampi and amygdalae bilaterally [26,27]. These neural nets were then reviewed by human raters following procedures as outlined by [28] and, when necessary, hand-corrected following procedures as outlined by [29].

The hand-tracing methods for parcellating the ACC (Figure 1) have been described at length elsewhere [30], and the previous methods were strictly followed for the identification of the dorsal, rostral, and subgenual ACC. For the current study, the previous parcellation method for the subcallosal ACC was modified slightly; the subcallosal region includes only the continuation of the rostral cingulate gyrus as it wraps around the genu of the corpus callosum, rather than additionally including paracingulate gyrus. The anterior boundary of the subcallosal ACC is defined by the anteriormost slice where the forceps major of the corpus callosum is no longer connected through the genu on the coronal view. The posterior boundary is placed one slice anterior to where the putamen first is visible within the basal ganglia. The superior boundary is formed by the ventral continuation of the callosal sulcus. The inferior boundary of this region is defined by the termination of the primary cingulate sulcus (whether or not a secondary sulcus is evident) [31].

Twenty-one psychotic depression participants and 20 HC participants received structural neuroimaging scans. One psychotic depression participant was excluded from the study due to profound damage from a traumatic brain injury. Two other psychotic depression participants' scans failed the amygdala and hippocampus neural net application and were excluded from those analyses, though their ACC regions were parcellated satisfactorily. One HC participant's scan failed the amygdala ANN but his or her data were usable for hippocampal and ACC measures. Therefore, the following samples were available for analysis: amygdala (18 psychotic depression, 19 HC), hippocampus (18 psychotic depression, 20 HC), ACC subregions (20 psychotic depression, 20 HC). Of the two psychotic depression participants whose amygdala and hippocampus neural nets failed, one had a positive family history of affective disorders.

Statistical Analyses

All data underlying the current manuscript are presented as Supplementary Files (Dataset S1, Dataset S2, Variable Definitions S1), including raw numerical data and variable descriptions. Statistical analyses used the standard alpha level of .05 for statistical significance and used two-tailed tests. Demographic data were examined to demonstrate that there were no significant differences between the experimental and control groups, using independent samples t-tests (age, education) and chi-squared tests (sex) (Table 1). For methodological reasons, half of the psychotic depression group received their neuroimaging scans on a different scanner (Siemens) than the rest of the participants (GE). For this reason, we used a multivariate general linear model to confirm that there were no effects of scanner on the imaging measures used in the study.

Next, independent samples t-tests were used to examine the volumetric differences in the regions of interest (hippocampus, amygdala, dorsal ACC, rostral ACC, subcallosal ACC, subgenual ACC, and total intracranial volume) between the experimental and control groups. The hippocampus test precluded an assumption of equal variances, so the degrees of freedom for that test were adjusted accordingly. After the initial hypothesis testing, these group-wise comparisons were re-calculated using a multivariate model adjusting for total intracranial volume (indicated with asterisks in Table 2). Finally, the results of these comparisons were further adjusted for the false discovery rate [32], and results remaining significant after that adjustment are indicated with pluses (Table 2).

A more detailed examination of laterality effects in the hippocampus and subcallosal ACC was conducted using independent samples t-tests and repeating the statistical adjustments for total intracranial volume and false discovery rate. Finally, we examined the psychotic depression group to see if there was an effect of family history of affective disorders on hippocampal and subcallosal ACC volumes, again using independent samples t-tests.

Results

There were no significant differences between participants with psychotic depression and healthy comparisons in terms of sample size, age, education, or sex (see Table 1). Patients with psychotic depression additionally completed the Hamilton Depression and Anxiety Rating Scales (HAM-D and HAM-A) (Table 1), as well as Scales for the Assessment of Negative and Positive Symptoms of Schizophrenia (SANS: mean = 12.9, SD = 3.4; SAPS-Psychoticism: mean = 3.3, SD = 1.8; SAPS-Disorganization: mean = 0.5, SD = 0.8). The psychotic depression group was further characterized in terms of family history of affective disorders, where fifteen of the twenty participants with psychotic depression had a family history of a first-degree relative with an affective disorder. There were no differences between psychotic depression patients with and without family histories in terms of baseline HAM-D score ($t = -.065$, $DF = 19$, $p = .949$). Psychotic depression patients had an average duration of current episode of less than six months (55%), and the majority used antidepressant medications (Table 1). Because of the possibility of confounding due to the use of two different scanners in the neuroimaging acquisition, we used a multivariate general linear model to confirm that there were no effects of scanner on the imaging measures used in the study. This analysis confirmed that there was a non-significant effect of scanner on the brain regions examined in the current study (Pillai's Trace = 0.315, $F = .880$, $p = .577$).

Group-wise comparisons examined regional brain volumetric differences between psychotic depression and HC participants in

Table 2. Comparison of psychotic depression group with healthy controls on brain volumetrics.

	Psychotic Depression Mean (SD)	HC Mean (SD)	DF	Statistic	*p*-value
Total ICV	1345.74 (170.18)	1388.78 (160.59)	38	t = 0.823	$p=0.416$
Hippocampus[a]	4.12 (0.37)	4.58 (0.52)	34.33	t = 3.166	$p=0.003^{*+}$
Amygdala[b]	2.18 (0.30)	2.28 (0.36)	36	t = 0.948	$p=0.349$
Subcallosal ACC	0.71 (0.23)	0.93 (0.22)	38	t = 3.036	$p=0.004^{*+}$
Subgenual ACC	1.02 (0.28)	1.04 (0.29)	38	t = −0.196	$p=0.845$
Dorsal ACC	7.39 (1.26)	7.00 (0.88)	38	t = −1.139	$p=0.262$
Rostral ACC	4.32 (1.66)	4.20 (1.04)	38	t = −0.263	$p=0.794$

Note: Raw means and standard deviations presented (reported in cubic centimeters).
*comparisons that remain significant after adjustment for total ICV.
+comparisons that remain significant after adjustment for false discovery rate.
[a]sample included 18 psychotic depression and 20 HC participants with no significant differences between groups on demographic variables (age $p=0.772$, education $p=0.114$, sex $p=0.804$).
[b]sample included 19 psychotic depression and 19 HC participants. Hippocampal t-test adjusted because of violation of the assumption of equal variances.
ICV = intracranial volume, reported in cubic centimeters. ACC = anterior cingulate cortex.

raw volumes of the hippocampus, amygdala, dorsal ACC, rostral ACC, subcallosal ACC, and subgenual ACC. These analyses showed that the only significant differences between groups were in the hippocampus and the subcallosal ACC (see Table 2). These comparisons were calculated twice; once uncorrected, and once controlled for total intracranial volume and adjusted for false discovery rate.

Laterality effects were then assessed. While both sides of the hippocampus were found to be significantly smaller in psychotic depression participants than healthy comparisons, the reduction in subcallosal ACC volume was driven primarily by left-sided atrophy (Table 3). Hippocampal volume in the psychotic depression group averaged 10.1% smaller than healthy controls, while the left subcallosal ACC was 31.4% smaller than controls. Furthermore, it was found that within the psychotic depression group, those with a positive family history of affective disorders (15 of the 20 participants) had significant atrophy of the left subcallosal ACC ($t=3.809$, $df=24.590$, $p=.001$) when compared with healthy controls, while the five without family history showed normal volume of the structure ($t=.497$, $df=23$, $p=.624$). On average, psychotic depression patients with a family history of affective disorders had left scACC volumes 38.5% smaller than healthy controls. By comparison, there was no effect of family history of affective disorder on the finding of hippocampal atrophy ($t=.531$, $df=16$, $p=.603$). Both subgroups of depressed patients had significantly smaller hippocampal volumes than healthy comparison subjects (positive family history: $t=2.350$, $df=10.888$, $p=.039$; negative family history: $t=2.972$, $df=32$, $p=.006$).

Discussion

Participants with psychotic depression were compared with healthy controls on measures of the hippocampus, amygdala, dorsal ACC, rostral ACC, subcallosal ACC, and subgenual ACC. As hypothesized, this study demonstrates a pattern of significantly smaller bilateral hippocampus and left-sided subcallosal cingulate volumes in patients with psychotic depression when compared to age-matched healthy control participants. Left subcallosal ACC atrophy was highly significant only in the group of psychotic depression subjects with a family history of affective disorders, while hippocampal atrophy was found bilaterally and was not dependent on whether there was a family history of affective disorders.

Left scACC atrophy in patients with depression who also have a family history of affective disorders is consistent with three previous studies, all of which examined the undifferentiated "subgenual" region, which included what are now termed the subcallosal and subgenual subregions [18,33,34]. The current finding is consistent with that of [18], which reported a 48% reduction in left "subgenual" cingulate volume in a group of patients with familial unipolar depression compared with healthy controls. The second study [33] showed a 20% reduction in left "subgenual" cingulate volumes in patients with affective disorders compared with healthy controls, and a 24% reduction in patients with familial affective disorders compared to patients with non-familial affective disorders. The third study [34] further showed that women with MDD had significantly smaller left "subgenual" ACC volumes than controls, with no reduction on the right. Another study has shown a 23.8% reduction in the volume of the subgenual cingulate bilaterally in familial major depressive disorder [35]. Histological analysis showed that this volume reduction was related to decreased numbers of glia in the region while the number of neurons remained unchanged [35]. It is unclear why only the left sided atrophy of the subcallosal cingulate cortex appears to be driven by genetics in the current sample, in that it was only observed in those psychotic depression patients with a family history of affective disorders. However, one previous study [50] in patients with psychotic depression reported a similar finding, and similarly constrained to the left subgenual cingulate.

Several previous studies have identified the presence of bilateral hippocampal atrophy in MDD patients, which was supported by the findings of the current study [12,13,15,16]. We did not confirm the previous finding from Keller et al. [4], who reported amygdala atrophy rather than hippocampal atrophy specifically in psychotic depression. This discrepancy could be related to the use in the current study of a new, automated method for measuring amygdala and hippocampus volumes, rather than the manual method used in the previous study, which was originally developed for use in a pediatric population [36]. The current study also used a 1.5 T MRI (3T in Keller et al.), as well as older (mean age 45 in the current study; 36 in Keller et al.), and more depressed participants (mean HAM-D = 38 current study; mean HAM-D = 30 in Keller et al.).

Table 3. Laterality effects on hippocampus and subcallosal ACC volumes in psychotic depression compared to age-matched healthy comparisons.

	Psychotic Depression Mean (SD) [n = 20]	HC Mean (SD) [n = 20]	DF	Statistic	*p*-value
Left Hippocampus[a]	2.05 (0.181)	2.30 (0.276)	33.08	t = 3.303	$p = 0.002$ *+
Right Hippocampus[a]	2.07 (0.214)	2.28 (0.262)	36	t = 2.797	$p = 0.008$ *+
Left subcallosal ACC	0.289 (0.087)	0.421 (0.174)	38	t = 3.035	$p = 0.004$ *+
Right subcallosal ACC	0.425 (0.213)	0.507 (0.143)	33.25	t = 1.420	$p = 0.165$

Note: Raw means and standard deviations presented (reported in cubic centimeters).
*comparisons that remain significant after adjustment for total ICV.
+comparisons that remain significant after adjustment for false discovery rate.
[a]sample included 18 participants with psychotic depression and 20 HC participants with no significant differences between groups on demographic variables (age $p = 0.772$, education $p = 0.114$, sex $p = 0.804$). Left hippocampal and right subcallosal ACC t-tests adjusted because of violation of the assumption of equal variances. ICV = intracranial volume, reported in cubic centimeters. ACC = subcallosal anterior cingulate cortex.

The exact neurobiological underpinnings of depression and psychotic depression remain to be completely elucidated, though there are hints at the mechanisms, one of which is related to glucocorticoid toxicity of the hippocampus following prolonged exposure to the stress hormone cortisol. Intense stress, such as that experienced during severe depression, can cause reduced expression of brain-derived neurotrophic factor (BDNF) in the hippocampus and elevated expression of cortisol, leading to decreased hippocampal neurogenesis and overall atrophy of the structure [37,38]. Patients with psychotic depression may be especially vulnerable to decreased hippocampal neurogenesis and overall atrophy because they (more so than their non-psychotic depressed counterparts) experience elevated cortisol expression [4,39] ECT, and to a lesser extent antidepressant medications, have been shown to promote synaptogenesis and neurogenesis in the hippocampus [40–42]. Psychotic depression is highly responsive to ECT treatment, with a 95% response rate [43] and the mechanism of this response may be linked to increased neurogenesis in the hippocampus [42]. It is possible that in psychotic depression, ECT is the most effective treatment because it most strongly promotes neurogenesis in the hippocampus, perhaps even to such an extent that it can overcome the stress-induced atrophy of the structure.

The ACC and the hippocampus are connected through the limbic system and may function as pacemakers for theta oscillations in the brain [44–46]. Previous studies have shown that theta activity in the ACC could predict treatment response to antidepressants, and that ECT could change theta activity in the scACC in depressed patients [47,19]. The scACC is also the primary brain target for deep brain stimulation (DBS) for treatment-resistant depression in a large multi-site study [48]. Resolution of depressive symptoms with DBS of the scACC has also been associated with changes in theta activity and pre-treatment theta activity may even predict response to DBS [49].

The current study included a sample of patients with psychotic depression that was so severe and treatment resistant to necessitate treatment with ECT. The current study was limited by a relatively small sample, a lower-powered MR scanner, and included only cross-sectional data. In order to remedy the limitations of the current study, future studies with this population should include both pre- and post-ECT MRI with a higher resolution 3T scanner and with diffusion weighted imaging to allow tractography studies to specifically look at hippocampal-ACC connections. It will also be important to further assess whether these findings are specific to psychotic depression or high cortisol states, and whether they exist in other subtypes of MDD severe enough to require ECT. However, the current study has shown for the first time that the volume of the hippocampus is significantly smaller in patients with psychotic depression than in controls, and that there are significant effects of family history on atrophy of the scACC specifically. These findings may provide further insight into the pathophysiology of psychotic depression, and highlight the importance of consideration of family history and brain structural changes over the course of the illness.

Supporting Information

Dataset S1 All data underlying the current manuscript are presented here in comma-separated variable format for easy access.

Dataset S2 All data underlying the current manuscript are presented here in IBM SPSS software file format with variable definitions and other descriptive information embedded.

Variable Definitions S1 Definitions for each variable heading in Dataset S1 and Dataset S2.

Acknowledgments

The authors thank the participants of the current study for the time and energy they contributed to the project. Without their support, this study would never have been possible.

Author Contributions

Conceived and designed the experiments: LM MB. Performed the experiments: LM MB. Analyzed the data: KB BH MB EH LM. Contributed reagents/materials/analysis tools: BH KB. Contributed to the writing of the manuscript: KB BH MB EH LM.

References

1. WHO (2008) The global burden of disease: 2004 update. Geneva: World Health Organization.
2. Lykouras E, Malliaras D, Christodoulou GN, Papakostas Y, Voulgari A, et al. (1986) Delusional depression: phenomenology and response to treatment: a prospective study. Acta Psychiatr Scand 73: 324–329.

3. Rothschild AJ, Benes F, Hebben N, Woods B, Luciana M, et al. (1989) Relationships between brain CT scan findings and cortisol in psychotic and nonpsychotic depressed patients. Biol Psychiatry 26: 565–575.
4. Keller J, Shen L, Gomez RG, Garrett A, Solvason HB, et al. (2008) Hippocampal and amygdalar volumes in psychotic and nonpsychotic unipolar depression. Am J Psychiatry 165: 872–880.
5. Dubovsky SL (1991) What we don't know about psychotic depression. Biol Psychiatry 30: 533–536.
6. Overall JE, Gorham DE (1961) The brief psychiatric rating scale. Psychol Rep. 10: 799–812.
7. Keller J, Schatzberg AF, Maj M (2007) Current issues in the classification of psychotic major depression. Schizophr Bull 33: 877–885.
8. Hill SK, Keshavan MS, Thase ME, Sweeney JA (2004) Neuropsychological dysfunction in antipsychotic-naïve first-episode unipolar psychotic depression. Am J Psychiatry 161: 996–1003.
9. Charney DS, Nelson JC (1981) Delusional and nondelusional unipolar depression: further evidence for distinct subtypes. Am J Psychiatry 138: 328–333.
10. Helms PM, Smith RE (1983) Recurrent psychotic depression: Evidence of diagnostic stability. J Affect Disord. 5: 51–54.
11. Kronmuller KT, Schroder J, Kohler S, Gotz B, Victor D, et al. (2009) Hippocampal volume in first episode and recurrent depression. Psychiatry Res. 174: 62–66.
12. Videbech P, Ravnkilde B (2004) Hippocampal volume and depression: a meta-analysis of MRI studies. Am J Psychiatry 161: 1957–1966.
13. Campbell S, MacQueen G (2006) An update on regional brain volume differences associated with mood disorders. Curr Opin Psychiatry 19: 25–33.
14. Drevets WC, Price JL, Furey ML (2008) Brain structural and functional abnormalities in mood disorders: implications for neurocircuitry models of depression. Brain Struct Funct 213: 93–118.
15. MacQueen GM, Campbell S, McEwen BS, Macdonald K, Amano S, et al. (2003) Course of illness, hippocampal function, and hippocampal volume in major depression. Proc Natl Acad Sci U S A 100: 1387–1392.
16. Sheline YI, Sanghavi M, Mintun MA, Gado MH (1999) Depression duration but not age predicts hippocampal volume loss in medically healthy women with recurrent major depression. J Neurosci. 19: 5034–5043.
17. Mayberg HS (2009) Targeted electrode-based modulation of neural circuits for depression. J Clin Invest. 119: 717–725.
18. Drevets WC, Price JL, Simpson JR, Todd RD, Reich T, et al. (1997) Subgenual prefrontal cortex abnormalities in mood disorders. Nature. 386: 824–827.
19. McCormick LM, Boles Ponto LL, Pierson RK, Pierson RK, Johnson HJ, et al. (2007) Metabolic correlates of antidepressant and antipsychotic response in patients with psychotic depression undergoing electroconvulsive therapy. J ECT 23: 265–273.
20. McCormick LM, Yamada T, Yeh M, Brumm MC, Thatcher RW (2009) Antipsychotic effect of electroconvulsive therapy is related to normalization of subgenual cingulate theta activity in psychotic depression. J Psychiatr Res 43: 553–560.
21. Andreasen NC (1984) Scale for the assessment of positive symptoms. Iowa City: University of Iowa.
22. Andreasen NC (1982) Negative symptoms in schizophrenia: definition and reliability. Arch Gen Psychiatry 39: 784–788.
23. Hamilton M (1960) A rating scale for depression. J Neurol Neurosurg Psychiatry. 23: 56–63.
24. Hamilton M (1959) The assessment of anxiety states by rating. Br J Med Psychol. 32: 50–55.
25. Magnotta VA, Harris G, Andreasen NC, O'Leary DS, Yuh WTC, et al. (2002) Structural MR image processing using the BRAINS2 toolbox. Comput Med Imaging Graph. 26: 251–264.
26. Powell HWR, Richardson MP, Symms MR, Boulby PA, Thompson PJ, et al. (2008) Preoperative fMRI predicts memory decline following anterior temporal lobe resection. J Neurol Neurosurg Psychiatry 79: 686–693.
27. Schumann CM, Hamstra J, Goodlin-Jones BL, Lotspeich LJ, Kwon H, et al. (2004) The amygdala is enlarged in children but not adolescents with autism; the hippocampus is enlarged at all ages. Neurobiol Disease 24: 6392–6401.
28. Aylward EH, Liu D, Nopoulos PC, Ross CA, Pierson RK, et al. (2012) Striatal volume contributes to the prediction of onset of Huntington disease in incident cases. Biol Psychiatry 71: 822–828.
29. Pantel J, O'Leary DS, Cretsinger K, Bockhold HJ, Keefe H, et al. (2000) A new method for the in vivo volumetric measurement of the human hippocampus with high neuroanatomical accuracy. Hippocampus 10: 752–758.
30. McCormick LM, Ziebell S, Nopoulos P, Cassell M, Andreasen NC, et al. (2006) Anterior cingulate cortex: an MRI-based parcellation method. Neuroimage 32: 1167–1175.
31. Coryell W, Nopoulos P, Drevets W, Wilson T, Andreasen NC (2005) Subgenual prefrontal cortex volumes in major depressive disorder and schizophrenia: Diagnostic specificity and prognostic implications. Am J Psychiatry 162: 1706–1712.
32. Benjamini Y, Hochberg Y (1995) Controlling the false discovery rate: a practical and powerful approach to multiple testing. J R Stat Soc Series B Stat Methodol 57: 289–300.
33. Hirayasu Y, Shenton ME, Salisbury DF, Kwon JS, Wible CG, et al. (1999) Subgenual cingulate cortex volume in first-episode psychosis. Am J Psychiatry 156: 1091–1093.
34. Botterton KN, Raichle ME, Drevets WC, Heath AC, Todd RD (2002) Volumetric reduction in left subgenual prefrontal cortex in early onset depression. Biol Psychiatry 51: 342–344.
35. Ongur D, Drevets WC, Price JL (1998) Glial reduction in the subgenual prefrontal cortex in mood disorders. Proc Natl Acad Sci U S A 95: 13290–13295.
36. Kates WR, Abrams MT, Kaufmann WE, Breiter SN, Reiss AL (1997) Reliability and validity of MRI measurement of the amygdala and hippocampus in children with fragile X syndrome. Psychiatry Res 75: 31–48.
37. Nestler EJ, Barrot M, DiLeone RJ, Eisch AJ, Gold SJ, et al. (2002) Neurobiology of Depression. Neuron 34: 13–25.
38. Sheline YI (2003) Neuroimaging studies of mood disorder effects on the brain. Biol Psychiatry 54: 338–352.
39. Hill SC, Keshavan MS, Thase ME, Sweeney JA (2004) Neuropsychological dysfunction in antipsychotic-naïve first-episode unipolar psychotic depression. Am J Psychiatry 161: 996–1003.
40. Malberg JE, Eisch AJ, Nestler EJ, Duman RS (2000) Chronic antidepressant treatment increases neurogenesis in adult rat hippocampus. J Neurosci. 20: 9104–9110.
41. Scott BW, Wojtowicz TJ, McIntyre Burnham W (2000) Neurogenesis in the dentate gyrus of the rat following electroconvulsive shock seizures. Exp Neurol 165: 231–236.
42. Nordanskog P, Dahlstrand U, Larsson MR, Larsson EM, Knutsson L, et al. (2010) Increase in hippocampal volume after electroconvulsive therapy in patients with depression: a volumetric magnetic resonance imaging study. J ECT 26, 62–67.
43. Petrides G, Fink M, Husain MM (2001) ECT remission rates in psychotic versus nonpsychotic depressed patients: a report from CORE. J ECT. 17: 244–253.
44. Buzsaki G (2002) Theta oscillations in the hippocampus. Neuron, 33: 325–340.
45. Ishii R, Shinosaki K, Inouye T (1999) Medial prefrontal cortex generates frontal midline theta rhythm. Neuroreport, 10: 675–679.
46. Asada H, Fukuda Y, Tsunoda S, Yamaguchi M, Tonoike M (1999) Frontal midline theta rhythms reflect alternative activation of prefrontal cortex and anterior cingulate cortex in humans. Neurosci Lett, 274: 29–32.
47. Pizzagalli DA (2011) Frontocingulate dysfunction in depression: toward biomarkers of treatment response. Neuropsychopharmacology Rev. 36: 183–206.
48. Lozano AM, Giacobbe P, Hamani C, Rizvi SJ, Kennedy SH, et al. (2012) A multicenter pilot study of subcallosal cingulate area deep brain stimulation for treatment-resistant depression. J Neurosurg 116(2): 315–322.
49. Broadway JM, Holtzheimer PE, Hilimire MR (2012) Frontal theta cordance predicts 6-month antidepressant response to subcallosal cingulate deep brain stimulation for treatment-resistant depression: a pilot study. Neuropsychopharmacology. 37: 1764–1772.
50. Vassilopoulou K, Papathanasiou M, Michopoulos I, Boufidou F, Oulis P, et al. (2013) A magnetic resonance imaging study of hippocampal, amygdala and subgenual prefrontal cortex volumes in major depression subtypes: melancholic versus psychotic depression. J Affect Disord. 146: 197–204.

Rheumatoid Arthritis and the Risk of Bipolar Disorder: A Nationwide Population-Based Study

Chih-Chao Hsu[1]¶, San-Chi Chen[2]¶, Chia-Jen Liu[2,3], Ti Lu[1], Cheng-Che Shen[4], Yu-Wen Hu[3,5], Chiu-Mei Yeh[6], Pan-Ming Chen[7], Tzeng-Ji Chen[6,8], Li-Yu Hu[1,3]*

1 Department of Psychiatry, Kaohsiung Veterans General Hospital, Kaohsiung, Taiwan, **2** Division of Hematology and Oncology, Department of Medicine, Taipei Veterans General Hospital, Taipei, Taiwan, **3** Institute of Public Health & School of Medicine, National Yang-Ming University, Taipei, Taiwan, **4** Department of Psychiatry, Chiayi Branch, Taichung Veterans General Hospital, Chiayi, Taiwan, **5** Cancer Center, Taipei Veterans General Hospital, Taipei, Taiwan, **6** Department of Family Medicine, Taipei Veterans General Hospital, Taipei, Taiwan, **7** Department of Psychiatry, Yuanshan Branch, Taipei Veterans General Hospital, Yilan, Taiwan, **8** School of Medicine, National Yang-Ming University, Taipei, Taiwan

Abstract

Background: Studies have suggested that chronic inflammation plays an essential role in the pathophysiology of both rheumatoid arthritis (RA) and bipolar disorder. The most common clinical features associated with RA are anxiety and depression. The risk of bipolar disorder among patients with RA has not been characterized adequately.

Objective: To determine the association between RA and the subsequent development of bipolar disorder and examine the risk factors for bipolar disorder among patients with RA.

Methods: We identified patients who were diagnosed with RA in the Taiwan National Health Insurance Research Database. A comparison cohort was created by matching patients without RA with those with RA according to age, sex, and comorbidities. The occurrence of bipolar disorder was evaluated in both cohorts.

Results: The RA cohort consisted of 2,570 patients, and the comparison cohort consisted of 2,570 matched control patients without RA. The incidence of bipolar disorder (incidence rate ratio =2.13, 95% confidence interval [CI] =1.12–4.24, $P = .013$) was higher among patients with RA than among control patients. Multivariate, matched regression models revealed that asthma (hazard ratio [HR] =2.76, 95% CI 1.27–5.96, $P = .010$), liver cirrhosis (HR =3.81, 95% CI =1.04–14.02, $P = .044$), and alcohol use disorders (HR =5.29, 95% CI =1.71–16.37, $P = .004$) were independent risk factors for the development of bipolar disorder among patients with RA.

Conclusion: RA might increase the incidence of bipolar disorder development. Based on our data, we suggest that, following RA diagnosis, greater attention be focused on women with asthma, liver cirrhosis, and alcohol use disorder. Prospective clinical studies of the relationship between RA and bipolar disorder are warranted.

Editor: Anil Kumar, University of Missouri-Kansas City, United States of America

Funding: This study was supported by a grant from Taipei Veterans General Hospital (V103B-022 and V103E10-001). The funders had no role in study design, data collection and analysis, decision to publish, or preparation of the manuscript.

Competing Interests: The authors have declared that no competing interests exist.

* Email: chrishuly@gmail.com

¶ These authors contributed equally to this work.

Introduction

Rheumatoid arthritis (RA), an autoimmune disease, impairs patient health and has wider implications regarding health policy and costs. RA primarily affects the joints, but can also affect the entire body, causing systemic symptoms [1]. Several studies have compared patients with RA and healthy controls and have demonstrated that the mechanism involved in the pathogenesis of RA symptoms is related to chronic inflammation and associated with various cytokines [2].

Interest has grown in the psychiatric aspects of autoimmune diseases characterized by chronic inflammation, which might induce psychiatric illnesses through neuroinflammation and neurotransmitter abnormalities. Autoimmune diseases have been proved to be associated with psychiatric disorders, particularly schizophrenia, major depressive disorder, and bipolar disorder [3]. Studies have identified an association between RA and psychiatric disorders, particularly depressive disorder and schizophrenia [4–6]. However, the existence of this association remains uncertain. Moreover, few studies have investigated the association between RA and bipolar disorder.

Studies have shown that numerous cytokines circulating in plasma might impair the function of the blood-brain barrier [7],

Table 1. Baseline characteristics of patients with rheumatoid arthritis (RA) and the matched cohort.

Characteristics	Patients with RA n = 2,570 (%)		Matched cohort n = 2,570 (%)		*p* value
Median age, years (interquartile range)	51(41–60)		51(41–60)		
Age, years					
≥50	1,358	52.8	1,358	52.8	1.000
<50	1,212	47.2	1,212	47.2	
Sex					
Male	639	24.9	639	24.9	1.000
Female	1,931	75.1	1,931	75.1	
Comorbidities					
Hypertension	790	30.7	793	30.9	1.000
Dyslipidemia	739	28.8	739	28.8	0.157
COPD	582	22.6	583	22.7	0.973
Diabetes mellitus	497	19.3	497	19.3	1.000
Asthma	408	15.9	406	15.8	0.939
Chronic kidney disease	329	12.8	329	12.8	0.235
Cerebrovascular disease	310	12.1	309	12.1	1.000
Alcohol use disorder	65	2.5	53	2.1	<0.001
Liver cirrhosis	64	2.5	47	1.8	0.103
Malignancies	58	2.3	46	2.1	0.264
Coronary artery disease	27	1.1	24	0.9	0.928
Median follow-up years (interquartile range)	6.1(3.4–8.6)		6.1(3.4–8.6)		0.673

COPD, chronic obstructive pulmonary disease.

indicating that peripheral inflammation is associated with the upregulation of central nervous system (CNS) inflammation. Several studies have shown that chronic inflammation plays a vital role in the pathophysiology of common mental disorders [8], including bipolar disorder [9]. Therefore, we hypothesized that a history of RA increases the risk of the subsequent onset of bipolar disorder.

To test our hypothesis, we designed a nationwide population-based study to investigate the incidence of bipolar disorder among patients with RA.

Patients and Methods

Data Sources

The Taiwan National Health Insurance (NHI) program offers comprehensive, universal health insurance to all residents of Taiwan. The NHI program covers more than 96% of the residents of Taiwan and is contracted with 99% of all hospitals and clinics in Taiwan [10]. The program provides coverage for outpatient, inpatient, emergency, and traditional Chinese medicine services as well as prescription drugs. Multiple NHI databases, including NHI enrollment files, claims data, and a prescription drug registry, are managed and publicly released by the National Health Research Institutes (NHRI) of Taiwan. The Institutional Review Board of Taipei Veterans General Hospital approved this study (2013-03-035AC). Written consent from the study patients was not obtained because the NHI dataset consists of deidentified secondary data used for research purposes; the Institutional Review Board of Taipei Veterans General Hospital issued a formal written waiver for the need for consent. The National Health Insurance Research Database (NHIRD) is publicly released by the NHRI for research purposes only. Although confidentiality is guaranteed according to the data regulations of the NHRI, studies using this database still must be approved by the ethics committee. Detailed information on data requests is provided on the NHRI Web site (http://nhird.nhri.org.tw). Comments, problems, or requests regarding data application can be sent to the following NHRI email address: nhird@nhri.org.tw.

Study Design and Patients

We conducted a retrospective cohort study of patients who were newly diagnosed with RA between January 1, 2000, and December 31, 2010. We identified RA cases in the Taiwan National Health Insurance Research Database (NHIRD) based on International Classification of Diseases, Ninth Revision, Clinical Modification (ICD-9-CM) Code 714.0 and included only patients with RA who received a catastrophic illness certificate. The NHI program has specified 30 categories of catastrophic illness (e.g., cancers, hemophilia, autoimmune diseases including RA, and chronic renal failure). Eligible patients can apply for catastrophic illness certificates, and if approved, they are exempted from copayment of related medical costs. In this study, we relied on physicians' ability to make accurate diagnoses. However, RA diagnosis involves multiple criteria and ruling out diseases with RA-like symptoms. The possibility that RA diagnoses were misclassified was a concern. The issuance of certificates is validated based on a careful review of medical records, laboratory studies, and imaging studies conducted by at least 2 specialists. Therefore, we included only patients with RA who received a catastrophic illness certificate to ensure that RA diagnoses were valid. Several studies that have examined the epidemiology of systemic autoimmune diseases, particularly RA, by using the NHIRD have been published [11,12].

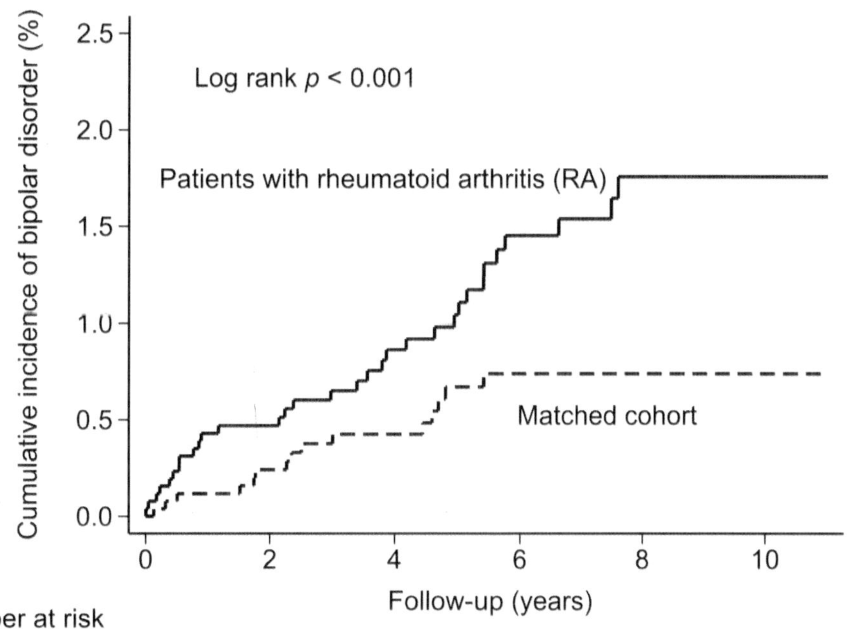

Number at risk

Patients with RA	2,570	2,313	1,790	1,310	781	271
Matched cohort	2,570	2,313	1,794	1,319	786	263

Figure 1. Cumulative incidence of bipolar disorder among patients with rheumatoid arthritis (RA) and the matched cohort.

Patients with bipolar disorder between January 1, 2000 and December 31, 2010 were identified based on the ICD-9-CM codes for bipolar disorder (296.0X, 296.1X, 296.4X, 296.5X, 296.6X, 296.7X, 296.80, or 296.89). However, to ensure that the bipolar disorder diagnoses in the database were reliable, we collected data on prescriptions of psychotropic agents for these patients. The role of medication in bipolar disorder treatment is firmly established. Therefore, we excluded patients who were diagnosed with bipolar disorder (according to ICD-9-CM codes) but did not receive any medication. We collected information on the use of drugs approved by the Food and Drug Administration of Taiwan for treating one (or more) phases of bipolar disorder, including acute mania/mixed episodes, bipolar depression, and bipolar maintenance. In addition to mood stabilizers, atypical antipsychotics such as aripiprazole, olanzapine, quetiapine, risperidone, and ziprasidone were included. These drugs were classified according to the World Health Organization Anatomical Therapeutic Chemical classification. Only patients who were prescribed these drugs for at least one month were included in our study. Furthermore, patients with mood disorders resulting from a general medical condition (ICD-9-CM Code 293.83) and patients with a history of mood disorders before the enrollment date were excluded from our study.

For each patient with RA in the NHIRD, one patient without RA matched according to age, sex, comorbidities [13], and enrollment date was selected. Although numerous studies have identified several comorbidities as risk factors for RA, based on the inflammation hypothesis proposed in this study, other inflammation-associated comorbidities were considered potential confounders. The exclusion criteria applied to the case cohort were applied to the matched comparison cohort. Both the patients with RA and comparison patients were followed until the development of bipolar disorder, death, or the end of the study period.

Statistical Analysis

The diagnosis of bipolar disorder served as the primary dependent variable. We calculated the bipolar disorder incidence rates (per 10 000 person-y) and the incidence rate ratios (IRRs). The study groups were compared using the χ^2 test for categorical variables. The Kaplan-Meier method was used to estimate the cumulative incidence of bipolar disorders, and a Cox proportional hazard model was used to identify risk factors for bipolar disorder in patients with RA. The qualifying criterion for inclusion in the multivariate analysis was a result in the univariate analysis with a P value of less than .1. The Perl programming language (Version 5.12.2) was used to extract data from the databases. Microsoft SQL Server 2005 (Microsoft Corp., Redmond, WA, USA) was used for data linkage, processing, and control sampling. The SPSS, Version 19.0 for Windows (IBM, Armonk, NY, USA) and the SAS, Version 9.2 (SAS Institute, Cary, NC, USA) computer software programs were used to perform all statistical analyses. Comparison results with a P value less than .05 were considered statistically significant.

Results

Patient Characteristics

Table 1 shows demographic and comorbidity data on the patients with RA and control patients. The median age of the patients was 51 years (interquartile range =41–60 y). The majority of patients in both cohorts were women (75.1%). Diabetes mellitus, chronic obstructive pulmonary disease, asthma, liver cirrhosis, alcohol use disorder, malignancy, chronic kidney disease, cerebral vascular disease, dyslipidemia, hypertension, and coronary artery disease were the most common comorbidities. No statistically significant differences were observed in baseline comorbidity data between the study groups.

Table 2. Incidence of bipolar disorder among patients with rheumatoid arthritis (RA) and the matched cohort.

	Patients with RA		Matched cohort			
	No. of bipolar disorder	**Per 10,000 person-years**	**No. of bipolar disorder**	**Per 10,000 person-years**	**Risk ratio (95% CI)**	***p* value**
Total	32	20.7	15	9.7	2.13(1.12–4.24)	0.013
Age						
≥50	14	18.5	7	9.3	1.99(0.75–5.84)	0.136
<50	18	22.8	8	10.1	2.26(0.93–6.00)	0.051
Sex						
Male	5	13.0	3	7.8	1.67(0.33–10.76)	0.505
Female	27	23.2	12	10.3	2.25(1.10–4.87)	0.017
Follow-up						
0–1 y	11	43.1	3	11.7	3.67(0.97–20.50)	0.035
1–5 y	12	14.6	11	13.4	1.09(0.44–2.73)	0.839
≥5 y	9	19.0	1	2.1	8.99(1.25–394.20)	0.012

CI, confidence interval.

Incidence of Bipolar Disorder

The cumulative incidence rates of bipolar disorder are shown in Figure 1. As shown in Table 2, the risk of developing bipolar disorder was significantly higher among patients with RA than among patients in the matched cohort (IRR = 2.13; 95% confidence interval [CI] = 1.12–4.24; *P* = .013). After stratifying patients according to age and sex, we observed that patients with RA under 50 years old exhibited an increased incidence of subsequent bipolar disorder (IRR = 2.26; 95% CI = 0.93–6.00; *P* = .051), even when no obvious statistical difference was observed. Moreover, women with RA exhibited a higher risk of developing subsequent bipolar disorder than did men (IRR = 2.25; 95% CI = 1.10–4.87; *P* = .017). Furthermore, we stratified patients according to follow-up duration and observed that the risk of subsequent bipolar disorder was significantly higher in the first year (IRR = 3.67; 95% CI = 0.97–20.5; *P* = .035) and more than 5 years (IRR = 8.99; 95% CI = 1.25–394.20; *P* = .012) after RA diagnosis. Overall, our study indicated that the incidence of the development of bipolar disorder following RA diagnosis was 20.7 per 10 000 person-years.

Risks Factors for Bipolar Disorder Among Patients with Rheumatoid Arthritis

The results of the univariate and multivariate analyses revealed that asthma (hazard ratio [HR] = 2.76; 95% CI = 1.27–5.96; *P* = .010), liver cirrhosis (HR = 3.81; 95% CI = 1.04–14.02; *P* = .044), alcohol use disorders (HR = 5.29; 95% CI = 1.71–16.37; *P* = .004), and substance abuse (HR = 37.42; 95% CI = 10.31–135.82; *P* < .001) were independent risk factors for the development of bipolar disorder among patients with RA (Table 3).

Discussion

This is the first population-based study to examine RA as a risk factor for bipolar disorder by using a matched cohort and a maximal follow-up period of 10 years. The major finding of our study was the discovery of a higher incidence of subsequent bipolar disorder among patients with RA. Furthermore, women with RA had a higher risk of developing subsequent bipolar disorder than did men, and asthma, liver cirrhosis, and alcohol use disorder are potential risk factors for developing bipolar disorder.

This study revealed that patients with RA were at a higher risk of subsequent bipolar disorder. We hypothesized that this risk is linked to the mechanisms of immune dysfunction. Bipolar disorder development after RA might result from the inflammatory process activated by RA. In 2012, Lampa et al [14] investigated the influence of peripheral chronic joint inflammatory disease in RA on CNS inflammation and revealed that the chronic peripheral inflammatory process activated by RA might cause the upregulation of CNS inflammation. Studies have evidenced that chronic and mild inflammation in the periphery are key contributors to the pathophysiology of CNS inflammation in bipolar disorder [15,16] and that dysregulation of the inflammatory process in the brain triggers and exacerbates atherosclerosis, hypertension, diabetes, obesity, and hyperthyroidism [17–20]. Animal models have indicated that peripheral cytokines reach the brain through various mechanisms, including a leaky brain barrier, active transport, activation of endothelial cells, and binding to cytokine receptors [21]. In short, cytokines created through infectious and inflammatory processes play a vital role in mediating the cross-talk between the immune system and the brain and are therefore possible contributors to the development of several psychiatric diseases, including bipolar disorder [22,23].

Table 3. Risk factors for bipolar disorder among patients with rheumatoid arthritis.

Variables	Univariate analysis		Multivariate analysis[a]	
	HR (95% CI)	*p* value	HR (95% CI)	*p* value
Age ≥50 years	1.28(0.63–2.57)	0.493		
Female	1.77(0.68–4.58)	0.243		
Comorbidities				
Hypertension	1.17(0.55–2.48)	0.680		
Dyslipidemia	0.66(0.27–1.60)	0.356		
COPD	1.79(0.85–3.79)	0.127		
Diabetes mellitus	1.26(0.55–2.92)	0.587		
Asthma	3.12(1.50–6.48)	0.002	2.76(1.27–5.96)	0.010
Chronic kidney disease	0.50(0.12–2.09)	0.340		
Cerebrovascular disease	1.91(0.79–4.65)	0.153		
Alcohol use disorder	9.87(3.78–25.80)	<0.001	5.29(1.71–16.37)	0.004
Liver cirrhosis	4.87(1.48–16.01)	0.009	3.81(1.04–14.02)	0.044
Malignancies	1.78(0.24–13.03)	0.572		
Coronary artery disease	3.43(0.47–25.11)	0.226		

HR, hazard ratio; CI, confidence interval; COPD, chronic obstructive pulmonary disease.
[a]All factors with $p<0.1$ in univariate analyses and age were included in the Cox multivariate analysis, and age, sex was enter in the Cox multivariate analysis.

Epidemiological studies have indicated that men and women are equally likely to develop bipolar disorder [24]. However, certain studies have revealed that sex steroid hormones play an essential role in immune response; specifically immune-stimulating effects caused by estrogen might trigger the inflammatory process. In other words, women are more vulnerable to immune dysfunction than men [25–27]. These findings might explain why women with RA had a higher risk of developing bipolar disorder than did women without RA.

When the patients were stratified according to follow-up duration, the incidence of bipolar disorder was significantly higher in the first year and more than 5 years after RA diagnosis. The first result might have been caused by detection bias; patients with symptoms of bipolar disorder might have been diagnosed shortly after RA diagnosis. The second result was compatible with our inflammation hypothesis regarding the association between RA and bipolar disorder. In contrast to acute inflammation, chronic inflammation persists for a prolonged period of time. We hypothesized that, in the long term, the chronic inflammatory process becomes a pathophysiology for the development of bipolar disorder [28].

Our analysis revealed that asthma, liver cirrhosis, and alcohol use disorder were independent risk factors associated with subsequent bipolar disorder in patients with RA. Evidence has indicated that chronic inflammatory processes in asthma and liver cirrhosis, like the pathophysiology of RA, involve cytokine interactions [29–31], and this combined and augmented chronic inflammatory effect might subsequently induce bipolar disorder. Moreover, cytokines that potentially cause depression and anxiety in liver cirrhosis [32] might also be associated with the development of bipolar disorder [33]. In addition, alcohol use disorder was associated with subsequent bipolar disorder in patients with RA. Several studies have indicated that alcohol consumption is associated with a lower incidence of disease and an improved quality of life among female patients with RA [34,35]. However, other studies have revealed that alcohol use disorders and bipolar disorder share certain genetic characteristics and are similar according to neuroimaging and biochemical findings [36,37]. Thus, alcohol use disorder might be an independent risk factor for the development of bipolar disorder among patients with RA.

Our study is the first retrospective study to examine RA as a risk factor for the development of bipolar disorder. A matched cohort study design comprising a population-based cohort of patients with RA and adequate controls for comorbidity constitute the strengths of our study. However, several limitations that are inherent to the use of claims databases should be considered. First, the diagnosis of RA in the NHIRD was based on the ICD-9 CM code and the issuance of a catastrophic illness certificate. Thus, the severity of RA as a risk factor for subsequent bipolar disorder was not explored. Second, the causal relationship was assessed mainly according to the chronological order in which the 2 conditions were diagnosed. However, both conditions might require long-term treatment, and the possibility that bipolar disorder causes RA cannot be excluded entirely. Third, information was unavailable on several demographic variables such as socioeconomic status, lifestyle, and family history, which might have provided useful information regarding factors that are potentially associated with RA and bipolar disorder [38,39]. Finally, this epidemiologic study was based on an observational design rather than an experimental design. Data on the relationship between the exacerbation of RA and the severity of bipolar disorder in patients with RA were unavailable. Therefore, the direction of causality in the association between the aforementioned possible risk factors and bipolar disorder development among patients with RA could not be determined.

In conclusion, this study revealed that RA increases the incidence of bipolar disorder development, suggesting that the RA-related inflammatory process is associated with increased expression of neuropsychiatric disturbances. Based on our data, we suggest that greater attention be focused on women, particularly those with asthma, liver cirrhosis, and alcohol use disorder. Additional prospective clinical studies on the relationship between RA and bipolar disorder are warranted.

Acknowledgments

We thank Huei-Sing Chang and Cheng-Fang Hong for their technical assistance. The study was based in part on data from the National Health Insurance Research Database provided by the Bureau of National Health Insurance, Department of Health, Taiwan and managed by the National Health Research Institutes. The interpretation and conclusion contained herein do not represent the views of the Bureau of National Health Insurance, the Department of Health, or the National Health Research Institutes.

Author Contributions

Conceived and designed the experiments: C-CH L-YH S-CC. Performed the experiments: C-JL C-CS Y-WH C-MY. Analyzed the data: C-CH L-YH C-JL TL. Contributed reagents/materials/analysis tools: C-JL P-MC T-JC. Contributed to the writing of the manuscript: S-CC C-CH L-YH.

References

1. Wasserman AM (2011) Diagnosis and management of rheumatoid arthritis. Am Fam Physician 84: 1245–1252.
2. Calabrese LH (1999) Rheumatoid arthritis and primary care: the case for early diagnosis and treatment. J Am Osteopath Assoc 99: 313–321.
3. Najjar S, Pearlman DM, Alper K, Najjar A, Devinsky O (2013) Neuroinflammation and psychiatric illness. J Neuroinflammation 10: 43.
4. Dickens C, McGowan L, Clark-Carter D, Creed F (2002) Depression in rheumatoid arthritis: a systematic review of the literature with meta-analysis. Psychosom Med 64: 52–60.
5. Torrey EF, Yolken RH (2001) The schizophrenia-rheumatoid arthritis connection: infectious, immune, or both? Brain Behav Immun 15: 401–410.
6. Nicassio PM (2010) Arthritis and psychiatric disorders: disentangling the relationship. J Psychosom Res 68: 183–185.
7. Abbott NJ, Ronnback L, Hansson E (2006) Astrocyte-endothelial interactions at the blood-brain barrier. Nat Rev Neurosci 7: 41–53.
8. Kivimaki M, Shipley MJ, Batty GD, Hamer M, Akbaraly TN, et al. (2013) Long-term inflammation increases risk of common mental disorder: a cohort study. Mol Psychiatry.
9. Stertz L, Magalhaes PV, Kapczinski F (2013) Is bipolar disorder an inflammatory condition? The relevance of microglial activation. Curr Opin Psychiatry 26: 19–26.
10. Wu CY, Chen YJ, Ho HJ, Hsu YC, Kuo KN, et al. (2012) Association between nucleoside analogues and risk of hepatitis B virus-related hepatocellular carcinoma recurrence following liver resection. JAMA 308: 1906–1914.
11. Lai NS, Tsai TY, Li CY, Koo M, Yu CL, et al. (2013) Increased frequency and costs of ambulatory medical care utilization prior to the diagnosis of rheumatoid arthritis: A national population-based study. Arthritis Care Res 27: 22146.
12. Lai CH, Lai MS, Lai KL, Chen HH, Chiu YM (2012) Nationwide population-based epidemiologic study of rheumatoid arthritis in Taiwan. Clin Exp Rheumatol 30: 358–363. Epub 2012 Jun 2026.
13. Khan NF, Perera R, Harper S, Rose PW (2010) Adaptation and validation of the Charlson Index for Read/OXMIS coded databases. BMC Fam Pract 11: 1.
14. Lampa J, Westman M, Kadetoff D, Agreus AN, Le Maitre E, et al. (2012) Peripheral inflammatory disease associated with centrally activated IL-1 system in humans and mice. Proc Natl Acad Sci U S A 109: 12728–12733.
15. Goldstein BI, Kemp DE, Soczynska JK, McIntyre RS (2009) Inflammation and the phenomenology, pathophysiology, comorbidity, and treatment of bipolar disorder: a systematic review of the literature. J Clin Psychiatry 70: 1078–1090.
16. Hamdani N, Tamouza R, Leboyer M (2012) Immuno- inflammatory markers of bipolar disorder: a review of evidence. Front Biosci (Elite Ed) 4: 2170–2182.
17. Drake C, Boutin H, Jones MS, Denes A, McColl BW, et al. (2011) Brain inflammation is induced by co-morbidities and risk factors for stroke. Brain Behav Immun 25: 1113–1122.
18. Ross R (1999) Atherosclerosis is an inflammatory disease. Am Heart J 138: S419–420.
19. Hu LY, Shen CC, Hu YW, Chen MH, Tsai CF, et al. (2013) Hyperthyroidism and risk for bipolar disorders: a nationwide population-based study. PLoS One 8: e73057.
20. Thomsen AF, Kessing LV (2005) Increased risk of hyperthyroidism among patients hospitalized with bipolar disorder. Bipolar Disord 7: 351–357.
21. Miller AH, Maletic V, Raison CL (2009) Inflammation and its discontents: the role of cytokines in the pathophysiology of major depression. Biol Psychiatry 65: 732–741.
22. Brietzke E, Stertz L, Fernandes BS, Kauer-Sant'anna M, Mascarenhas M, et al. (2009) Comparison of cytokine levels in depressed, manic and euthymic patients with bipolar disorder. J Affect Disord 116: 214–217.
23. Rege S, Hodgkinson SJ (2013) Immune dysregulation and autoimmunity in bipolar disorder: Synthesis of the evidence and its clinical application. Aust N Z J Psychiatry 47: 1136–1151.
24. Price AL, Marzani-Nissen GR (2012) Bipolar disorders: a review. Am Fam Physician 85: 483–493.
25. Cutolo M, Sulli A, Straub RH (2012) Estrogen metabolism and autoimmunity. Autoimmun Rev 11: A460–464.
26. Cutolo M, Villaggio B, Seriolo B, Montagna P, Capellino S, et al. (2004) Synovial fluid estrogens in rheumatoid arthritis. Autoimmun Rev 3: 193–198.
27. Cutolo M, Sulli A, Capellino S, Villaggio B, Montagna P, et al. (2004) Sex hormones influence on the immune system: basic and clinical aspects in autoimmunity. Lupus 13: 635–638.
28. Berk M, Williams LJ, Jacka FN, O'Neil A, Pasco JA, et al. (2013) So depression is an inflammatory disease, but where does the inflammation come from? BMC Med 11: 200.
29. Naik SR, Wala SM (2013) Inflammation, allergy and asthma, complex immune origin diseases: mechanisms and therapeutic agents. Recent Pat Inflamm Allergy Drug Discov 7: 62–95.
30. Shukla S, Shukla H, Kumar S, Aharwal RP, Gupta VK, et al. (2013) Allergy and inflammation: an immunological and therapeutic approach. Recent Pat Inflamm Allergy Drug Discov 7: 135–150.
31. Kocabayoglu P, Friedman SL (2013) Cellular basis of hepatic fibrosis and its role in inflammation and cancer. Front Biosci (Schol Ed) 5: 217–230.
32. Ko FY, Tsai SJ, Yang AC, Zhou Y, Xu LM (2013) Association of CD8 T cells with depression and anxiety in patients with liver cirrhosis. Int J Psychiatry Med 45: 15–29.
33. Liu HC, Yang YY, Chou YM, Chen KP, Shen WW, et al. (2004) Immunologic variables in acute mania of bipolar disorder. J Neuroimmunol 150: 116–122.
34. Bergman S, Symeonidou S, Andersson ML, Soderlin MK (2013) Alcohol consumption is associated with lower self-reported disease activity and better health-related quality of life in female rheumatoid arthritis patients in Sweden: data from BARFOT, a multicenter study on early RA. BMC Musculoskelet Disord 14: 218.
35. Lu B, Rho YH, Cui J, Iannaccone CK, Frits ML, et al. (2013) Associations of Smoking and Alcohol Consumption with Disease Activity and Functional Status in Rheumatoid Arthritis. J Rheumatol.
36. Farren CK, Hill KP, Weiss RD (2012) Bipolar disorder and alcohol use disorder: a review. Curr Psychiatry Rep 14: 659–666.
37. Pettinati HM, O'Brien CP, Dundon WD (2013) Current status of co-occurring mood and substance use disorders: a new therapeutic target. Am J Psychiatry 170: 23–30.
38. Waxmonsky JA, Thomas MR, Miklowitz DJ, Allen MH, Wisniewski SR, et al. (2005) Prevalence and correlates of tobacco use in bipolar disorder: data from the first 2000 participants in the Systematic Treatment Enhancement Program. Gen Hosp Psychiatry 27: 321–328.
39. Schoeyen HK, Birkenaes AB, Vaaler AE, Auestad BH, Malt UF, et al. (2011) Bipolar disorder patients have similar levels of education but lower socio-economic status than the general population. J Affect Disord 129: 68–74.

13

Saccadic Eye Movements in Depressed Elderly Patients

Nicolas Carvalho[1,2]*, Nicolas Noiret[1,4], Pierre Vandel[1,2,3], Julie Monnin[1,2,3], Gilles Chopard[1,2], Eric Laurent[4,5]*

1 Department of Clinical Psychiatry, University Hospital, Besançon, France, **2** E.A. 481, Laboratory of Neurosciences, University of Franche-Comté, Besançon, France, **3** CIC-IT 808 Inserm, Besançon University Hospital, Besançon, France, **4** E.A. 3188, Laboratory of Psychology, University of Franche-Comté, Besançon, France, **5** UMSR 3124/FED 4209 MSHE Ledoux, CNRS and University of Franche-Comté, Besançon, France

Abstract

The primary aim of this study was to characterize oculomotor performances in elderly depressed patients. The second aim was to investigate whether cognitive inhibition measured by the antisaccade task was associated with a psychomotor retardation or rather with a more specific cognitive-motor inhibition deficit. Twenty patients with a major depressive disorder and forty-seven healthy subjects performed two eye movement tasks. Saccadic reaction time and error rates were analyzed in the prosaccade task to obtain basic parameters of eye movements. Saccade latency, error rates and correction rates were evaluated in the antisaccade task to investigate inhibition capacities. Performances were impaired in patients, who exhibited a higher reaction time and error rates compared to controls. The higher time cost of inhibition suggested that the reaction time was not related to global psychomotor retardation alone. The higher time cost of inhibition could be explained by a specific alteration of inhibition processes evaluated by the antisaccade task. These changes were associated with the severity of depression. These findings provide a new perspective on cognitive inhibition in elderly depressed patients and could have important clinical implications for our understanding of critical behaviors involving deficits in inhibitory processes in the elderly.

Editor: Jan Kassubek, University of Ulm, Germany

Funding: This study was supported by a grant from the French Ministry of Health (Programme Hospitalier de Recherche Clinique: PHRC n°2009-A00942-55). The funders had no role in study design, data collection and analysis, decision to publish, or preparation of the manuscript.

Competing Interests: The authors have declared that no competing interests exist.

* Email: nic.carvalh@gmail.com (NC); eric.laurent@univ-fcomte.fr (EL)

Introduction

Cognitive inhibition, a major component of executive functioning, has been found to be impaired in depressed patients [1,2]. This function has been defined as a deletion of an automated response by the deliberate control of this response based on changes in background characteristics [3] or previously activated processes [4]. Cognitive inhibition would affect the characteristics of inputs and outputs of distracter elements to make the analysis and response processes for relevant elements available and more effective [5]. Houghton and Tipper [6] have shown that inhibition processes correspond to the cognitive function applied to the content that should be deleted.

An effective way to assess cognitive inhibition is based on oculomotor measurements particularly through the prosaccade and the antisaccade tasks [7–9]. Prosaccades are usually conceived as reflexive eye movements towards a peripherally appearing target. The prosaccade task has been used to evaluate basic characteristics of speed, latency and accuracy of saccadic eye movements. In contrast, the antisaccade task probes the ability to inhibit the automatic orientation of the eye in the direction of a peripherally appearing target in the vision fields [10]. Antisaccades are conceived as highly voluntary eye movements in the opposite direction to a peripherally appearing target. The antisaccade task is more reliable for assessing the inhibition function compared to many other tasks [11]. Antisaccade latency and error rates (ER) reflect critical cognitive abilities and can help us quantify an inhibition deficit [12].

A few reported studies have examined cognitive inhibition in depression. Sweeney *et al.* [13] showed that patients with depression - compared with healthy subjects - have greater difficulty in suppressing saccades towards a peripheral target in the antisaccade task. However, no difference in latency or speed was found. The study of Mahlberg *et al.* [14] showed that patients with depression had longer reaction times (RT) than controls in prosaccade tasks, suggesting that a psychomotor retardation affecting reflexive eye movement could characterize some depressive symptoms. The study conducted by De Lissnyder *et al.* [15] reported that dysphoric subjects had longer RT than controls in the antisaccade task. Globally, these results highlight the need to distinguish between basic reflexive components evaluated by prosaccade tasks and more elaborated executive processes involved in the inhibition required by the antisaccade task. A systematic distinction between these processes is critical to better characterize the kind of cognitive-motor processes that are altered in depression (i.e., global eye movement retardation *vs.* specific inhibitory disorder).

Moreover, all these studies only included young depressed patients. No information is available concerning oculomotor abilities in depressed elderly patients. Nevertheless, elderly depression differs from younger adult depression with a higher sadness, a psychomotor retardation, a difficulty to express their pain [16], a deficit in motor response and in response selection [17]. Depression in the elderly remains under-diagnosed [18] due to many co-morbidities such as somatic disorders [19], cerebrovascular pathologies [20] or Alzheimer's disease [21].

The main objective of our research was to characterize oculomotor performances in elderly depressed patients. We hypothesized that depressed elderly patients would have a higher reaction time in both prosaccade and antisaccade tasks, because of global psychomotor retardation, which was previously reported in these patients. The second objective of this study was to determine whether higher antisaccade reaction time is only related to psychomotor retardation or if it is also due to a specific inhibitory problem. This is in accordance with the above mentioned alteration of response selection problems known in these patients.

Methods

1. Participants

Elderly depressed patients were recruited from the psychiatric wards of Besançon University Hospital. Non-depressed controls were mainly recruited from the open University, which welcomes many older adults. Twenty depressed patients and forty-seven controls were included and matched for age (±5 years), sex, and education level. All patients had a major depressive disorder (MDD) according to the DSM-IV criteria [22], and a Montgomery-Asberg Depression Rating Scale (MADRS) [23] score higher than 25. Exclusion criteria for both groups were progressive psychiatric illness (e.g. schizophrenia, bipolar disorders), acute or chronic neurological pathologies (e.g. traumatic brain injury, brain tumors, stroke, and dementia) and presence of ophthalmic illnesses. Patients were all on stable medication at least for 4 weeks before inclusion screening. All patients were on antidepressants, 92% on anxiolytics, 80% benzodiazepines, 48% antipsychotics and 44% hypnotics. All participants gave their written informed consent to participate in the study. The research protocol was approved by the Committee for the Protection of Persons (CPP-Est-II), and was conducted in accordance with the principles laid down by the Declaration of Helsinki.

All participants underwent a complete neuropsychological battery of tests and eye movement tasks as described below. These assessments were performed within a maximum period of one month.

2. Neuropsychological assessment

The RAPID neuropsychological battery [24] was designed to ensure that no participant had cognitive impairments associated with early dementia. This battery included pencil and paper tasks assessing six cognitive domains: *(1) Global cognitive function*: Mini-Mental State Examination (MMSE) [25]; *(2) Attention/processing speed*: Trail Making Test Part A (TMT A) [26] and Crossing-Off Test (COT) [27]; *(3) Constructional praxis*: part of the Signoret's battery of cognitive efficacy (BEC 96) [28]; *(4) Executive function*: Trail Making Test Part B (TMT B) [26] and Isaacs Set Test (IST) [29]; *(5) Verbal Memory*: Memory Impairment Screen (MIS) [30] and Free and Cued Selective Recall Test (FCSRT) [31,32]; *(6) Language:* Picture naming task (DO 30) [24]. In addition to the RAPID battery, each participant completed the Stroop test [33] in order to measure inhibitory processing.

3. Eye movement tasks

All participants were seated in a quiet room. Eye movements were recorded using video-oculography techniques based on the corneal reflection of infra-red light. We used an ASL EYE-TRAC 6 system (ASL - Bedford, MA.) with a H6 optic camera mounted in a chin rest for stabilizing the head position. This system permits to capture data with good temporal (sampling at 120 Hz) and spatial resolution (accuracy of 0.1° of the visual angle). The device was calibrated for each participant at the beginning of the experimental sessions. The standard calibration of Eye-Track 6 User Interface Program (Version 1.62.1.0) with 3×3 calibration points was initially used. This was followed by an auto-calibration procedure, the 9 green points appearing one after another when the device automatically detected the subject's eye. Each participant performed a prosaccade task and then an antisaccade task. These tasks were presented in two separate blocks, the prosaccade task before the antisaccade task. In the prosaccade task, participants were instructed to fix their gaze, as quickly and accurately as possible, on the red dot appearing in the periphery of the screen. In the antisaccade task, participants were instructed to fix their gaze, as quickly and accurately as possible, on the opposite side relative to the red dot appearing in periphery of the screen, [34]. Between the two tasks, an auto-calibration was then performed again.

For both tasks, each trial began with a 2-s presentation of a central fixation dot. After this time, the peripheral red target appeared horizontally (H), on the right or left, or vertically (V), on the top or bottom, at different eccentricity levels (4°; 6°; 8°; 10°) in a randomized order (Figure 1) and for 2-s. The number of target eccentricity levels for the antisaccade task was limited in order to reduce its duration (4°; 8°). There were 4 trials in each condition of dot presentation. The central dot and the peripheral dot diameters each subtended a visual angle of 0.6°.

Pictures were presented on a 21-in. LCD screen (ASUS LCD Monitor VH 196, 32 bits color, 1024 by 768 pixels screen resolution, refresh rate of 70 Hz) at a distance of 70 cm from the participants. The images subtended a visual angle of 32.6°. Inquisit software (Millisecond Software, Version 3.0.3.2, Seattle, WA) was used to create the different tasks.

4. Eye Movement data analysis

Analyses were performed using the ASL-Result software. Fixations, total duration of fixation, and RT were computed on the basis of fixation detection criteria. Periods during which the eye did not vary from more than 1° of visual angle during at least 100 ms were considered as fixations. Accuracy zones around the red dot measured 1.8°.

Prosaccade. Recorded data were the RT (i.e., the time between the appearance of the peripheral target and the start of the correct subsequent saccade), the gain corresponding to the ratio of the saccade amplitude divided by the target step amplitude. A gain of <1 indicated that the saccade was hypometric and a gain of >1 indicated that the saccade was hypermetric.

Antisaccade. The RT, the ER (i.e., percentage of trials with initial incorrect saccade corresponding to a saccade toward the peripheral target), and the correction factor (CF) (i.e., sequence made of a first saccade toward the peripheral dot position and a second saccade in the opposite direction) were recorded.

When the saccade RT was lower than 80 ms (typically anticipatory saccade response) [35] or higher than 600 ms (typically delayed response), trials were excluded from data analysis [36].

5. Statistical analyses

A Shapiro-Wilk test was performed to assess the normality of data. The equality of variance was controlled by a Fisher-Snedecor

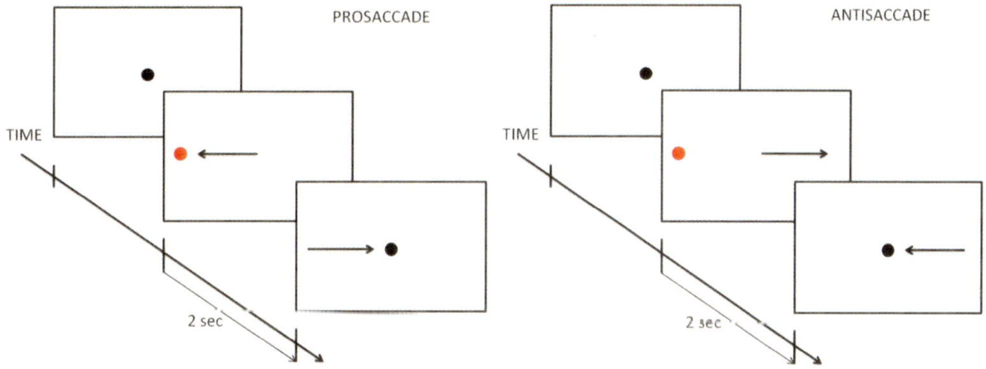

Figure 1. Eye movement tasks.
doi:10.1371/journal.pone.0105355.g001

test. Categorical variables were compared using the chi-square test or the Fisher's exact test (if the sample size was less than 5). Mixed ANOVAs including the factor group (depressed patients *vs.* controls), direction (horizontal *vs.* vertical) and eccentricity (4°; 6°; 8°; 10°) were performed. Newman–Keuls post-hoc tests were applied when appropriate. The Greenhouse-Geisser correction was used when sphericity was not assumed.

Differences between both groups in the prosaccade and antisaccade tasks were evaluated using ANCOVAs including group (depressed, control) as a factor, and neuropsychological [All RAPID neuropsychological battery scores, MMSE, memory scores (free and total recall score of the FCSRT), information processing speed scores (Stroop M and C, TMT A, COT), executive functions scores (TMT B-A, IST, Stroop INT)] and psychiatric (MADRS) scores, as covariates.

The significance alpha level was fixed to 0.05. Effect sizes were measured by partial Eta squared (η^2_p), with small, medium and large effects defined as 0.01, 0.06 and 0.14 respectively [37]. All computations were performed using Stata Software release 10.1 (StataCorp, College Station, TX).

Results

Demographic, psychiatric and neuropsychological data of the two groups are presented in table 1. There was no significant differences in age (depressed mean = 70.4, SD = 9.62; control mean = 66.72, SD = 5.48; $W_{67} = 0.81$, $p = 0.41$), gender ($\chi^2_{(1)} = 1.10$, $p = 0.29$) or educational level ($\chi^2_{(3)} = 5.25$, $p = 0.21$) between patients and controls. Scores on the MADRS were significantly higher in the patient group (MADRS: $W_{67} = 6.36$, $p < 0.001$). Though patients with depression performed significantly worse than controls on most neuropsychological tests (Table 1), none of them had cognitive impairment sufficiently severe to constitute early dementia. As mentioned earlier, ANCOVAs were applied in order to control potential effects of neuropsychological performances on eye movements.

1. Differences in parameters of saccadic eye movements

1.1. Prosaccade reaction time. Depressed patients had a significantly higher RT than controls [$F(1,65) = 24.71$, $p < 0.001$, $\eta^2_p = 0.27$, d = 1.3] (Table 2). There was no effect of direction [$F(1,65) = 2.27$, p = 0.14, $d_s < 0.76$], eccentricity [$F(1,65) = 2.5$, p = 0.11, $d_s < 0.77$] and no interaction between direction and eccentricity [$F(1,65) = 0.91$, p = 0.34, $d_s < 0.43$].

1.2. Prosaccade gain. The accuracy of prosaccade was not reduced in depressed group in comparison with the control group [$F(1,65) = 0.02$, p = 0.89, $\eta^2_p < 0.001$, d = 0.04] (Table 2).

1.3. Antisaccade reaction time. Depressed subjects had longer mean reaction times than controls [$F(1,65) = 22.11$, $p < 0.001$, $\eta^2_p = 0.26$, d = 1.33] (Table 2). There was a significant effect of direction [$F(1,65) = 10.98$, $p < 0.01$, $d_s > 0.28$]. Horizontal RT was significantly higher for depressed patients (M = 420 ms, SD = 152) than healthy controls (M = 272 ms, SD = 52) ($p < 0.05$; d = 1.30) but there was no difference in vertical direction ($M_{depressed} = 326$ ms, $SD_{depressed} = 138$; $M_{controls}$ mean = 296 ms, $SD_{controls} = 63$; p = 0.22; d = 0.27). There was no effect of eccentricity [$F(1,65) = 0.59$, p = 0.44, $d_s < 0.99$] and no interaction between direction and eccentricity [$F(1,65) = 0.05$, p = 0.82, $d_s < 0.04$].

1.4. Antisaccade error rate. Depressed patients had higher ER than controls [$F(1,65) = 23.68$, $p < 0.001$, $\eta^2_p = 0.27$, d = 1.22] (Table2). There was no significant effect of direction [$F(1,65) = 0$, p = 1, $d_s < 1.15$], eccentricity [$F(1,65) = 0.001$, p = 0.97, $d_s < 0.99$] and no interaction between direction and eccentricity [$F(1,65) = 0.02$, p = 0.87, $d_s < 0.85$].

1.5. Antisaccade correction factor. Depressed patients and controls had a similar correction rate of antisaccade errors [$F(1,65) = 0.99$, p = 0.32, $\eta^2_p = 0.01$, d<0.001] (Table 2).

2. Time cost of inhibition

In addition to direct measures of RT, the time cost of inhibition (antisaccade RT minus prosaccade RT) was calculated in order to control global eye movement retardation and provide a more reliable evaluation of the cognitive inhibition function (required in the antisaccade task). The time cost of inhibition was significantly higher in depressed patients (M = 114 ms, SD = 89) than in controls (M = 53 ms, SD = 42) [$F(1,65) = 30.69$; $p < 0.001$].

3. Analysis of confounding variables (ANCOVA)

Due to the significant disparity in cognitive performances of the depressed patients and controls, we reanalyzed the eye movement performances explored in the two tasks using neuropsychological tests as predictor variables. All RAPID neuropsychological scores, MMSE, memory scores, information processing scores and executive function scores were not found to be significant predictors for eye movement performance differences ($F_s > 0.01$; $p_s > 0.05$).

With a MADRS score of 31.7 for the depressed patients and 2.3 for the healthy controls, our data were reanalyzed using MADRS as a predictor variable of eye movement differences. As reported above, a mixed ANOVA had indicated that depressed patients had significantly lower eye movements performances than controls except for prosaccade gain and antisaccade CF. After adjustment

Table 1. Demographic and clinical data.

Characteristic	MDD(N = 20)	HC(N = 47)	p
Age	70.4±9.6	66.7±5.5	N.S.
Female	15(75)	29(61.7)	N.S.
Education (%)			N.S.
Low	25	21	N.S.
Medium	30	32	N.S.
High	45	47	N.S.
MADRS, (range 0–60)	31.7±5.6	2.3±2.3	<0.001
MIS Score, (range 0–8)	7.4±0.6	7.8±0.5	<0.001
IST Score,	31.3±5.3	43.3±5.8	<0.001
MMSE score, (range 0–30)	26.1±3.2	29.1±0.9	<0.001
FCSRT score, (range 0–48)			
Free recall	20.4±7.1	26.3±4.4	0.02
Total recall	43.4±6.8	45.7±2.5	N.S.
COT score,	145.6±48.4	213.7±42.1	<0.001
TMT score,			
Part A (range 0–150)	73.1±49.3	34.6±9.1	<0.001
Part B (range 0–300)	236.7±133.8	105.6±47.2	<0.001
BEC 96, (range 0–6)	5.6±1.1	6±0.2	0.03
DO 30, (range 0–30)	29.5±0.8	29.8±0.5	N.S.
Stroop Task score,			
Word	100±22.2	110.9±13.7	N.S.
Color	71.1±11.5	82.1±11.3	<0.001
Incompatible color-word	33.8±12.5	44±9	0.006
Interference	-8.3±9.5	-3.2±7.4	0.02

Legend: MDD, Major Depressive Disorder; HC, Healthy Controls; MADRS, Montgomery Asberg Depression Rating Scale; MIS, Memory Screen Impairment; IST, Isaacs Set Test; MMSE, Mini Mental State Examination; FCSRT, Free and Cued Selective Recall Test; COT, Crossing Off Test; TMT, Trail Making Test; BEC 96, Bec 96 figure Copy; DO 30, Picture naming task with 30 items; N.S., not significant.
Values given as *n* (%) or mean ± SD.

by the MADRS, the oculomotor performances between the two groups did not differ significantly except for prosaccade gain and antisaccade CF. These results confirmed an effect of MADRS score on eye movements (Table 3).

Discussion

In this study, oculomotor impairments were found in elderly depressed patients. In the prosaccade and antisaccade tasks, depressed patients had higher RT and ER than controls.

Table 2. Means and standard deviations for the saccadic reaction time, gain, error and correction rates.

Oculomotor parameter	MDD(N = 20)	HC(N = 47)	p	η^2_p
Prosaccades				
RT (ms)	291±59	231±28	<0.001	0.27
Gain	0.97±0.3	0.98±0.03	N.S.	<0.001
Antisaccades				
RT (ms)	405±116	284±54	<0.001	0.26
ER (%)	62±28.6	31±21.5	<0.001	0.27
CF (%)	83±17.6	83±24.9	N.S.	0.01

Legend: MDD, Major Depressive Disorder; HC, Healthy Controls; RT, Reaction time; ER, Error Rates; CF, Correction Factor; N.S., not significant.
Values given as mean ± SD.

Table 3. Eye movement performances×MADRS interaction between the 2 groups.

		Group		
Covariable	**Dependent variable**	$F_{1,65}$	p	η^2_p
MADRS	Pro RT	3.68	N.S.	0.05
	Pro gain	7.97	<0.01	0.11
	Anti RT	0.02	N.S.	<0.001
	Anti ER	0.5	N.S.	<0.01
	Anti CF	2.79	N.S.	<0.01
	Anti - Pro RT	0.96	N.S.	0.06

Legend: MADRS, Montgomery Asberg Depression Rating Scale; Pro, Prosaccade; Anti, Antisaccade; RT, Reaction time; ER, Error Rates; CF, Correction Factor; η^2_p: effect size; N.S., not significant.

For both groups, the RT was longer in the antisaccade task than in the prosaccade task due to the incompatibility between the target position and the target-directed movement. This result was consistent with those found in other studies [38,39]. Moreover, patients with depression had higher RT in both prosaccade and antisaccade task compared to controls.

We cannot deny the effect of global eye movement retardation, since we found significant differences in RT even in the prosaccade task. Many studies have shown altered cortical structures such as the cerebellum [40,41], the dorsolateral prefrontal cortex [42,43] and frontal eye fields [44] in depression that could play a role in the RT of eye saccade [45–47]. In our study, depressed patients also had higher ER in the antisaccade task. Alteration of motor adjustment could have played a role in the antisaccade task as well as in the prosaccade task [48].

However, we ensured that differences found in the antisaccade task were not only due to psychomotor retardation. First, we controlled neuropsychological performances. Second, we computed the time cost of inhibitory processes. Inhibitory processing is altered in patients with depression, which affects saccade latency. Inhibitory processing may be changed at the selection stage of the motor response [49] that is sent to the oculomotor system. Indeed, it has been suggested that an alteration of this function could be related to attentional biases observed in depression through its involvement in the selective attention process. It is also noteworthy that all differences that were reported concerning RT, gain and ER, in prosaccades, antisaccades, and in the differential measures specific to inhibition cost, were dependent on the MADRS scores, but globally not predicted by classic neuropsychological tests. Therefore, depression seems to be at the heart of the changes in eye movements, and not the result of more generic neuropsychological alterations. The relative independency of neuropsychological scores and eye movement performances in elderly depression constitutes eye tracking as a complementary tool for inhibitory capacity evaluation in depressive disorders.

However, our analyses suggest that psychomotor retardation was not the major cause of patients' worse performances in the antisaccade task. The depressed elderly also exhibited reduced performances on the interference score of the Stroop test. These results suggest an inhibition deficit in depressed patients affecting interference performance. However, it may be questioned whether this is the same deficit that causes impairment on the antisaccade task. Indeed, the lack of correlation between the Stroop interference score and antisaccade minus prosaccade RT ($rho = -0.34$, $p = 0.16$), prosaccade gain ($rho = 0.35$, $p = 0.15$) or antisaccade error rates ($rho = 0.32$, $p = 0.19$) suggests that there could be an additional specific alteration of the inhibition mechanism at the level of the movement planning process [50]. The antisaccade task requires a motor response at the opposite of the target whereas the Stroop test requires an incongruent motor response [51]. In the Stroop test, inhibition corresponds to both the interference (the mechanism that prevents irrelevant information entered in memory) and inhibition (active suppression process). Several studies using different tasks to assess the inhibition showed that the correlations between the scores of these tasks were low or nonexistent [52,53]. Several studies have reported a link between cognitive impairment and an inhibition deficit in depression [54–56] associated with pre-frontal cortex dysfunctions [57,58], especially when executive functions were scrutinized [59,60]. Other cognitive functions may also be linked to inhibition such as working memory [61,62]. However, these results remain controversial [54]. Methodological differences regarding the sample size and the heterogeneity of inclusion criteria could explain these disparities. Generally, the involvement of executive functions and inhibition mechanisms would be most important but this not only depends on the different types of depression [63–65], but also on their severity [56] and the age at the first depressive episode [66,67]. Additional efforts are needed to identify precise processes than underlie the changes in inhibitory capacities. For example, Crawford *et al.* [68] found that the RT in prosaccade and antisaccade tasks did not differ between patients with Alzheimer disease (AD) and control subjects. However, patients with AD had more ER in the antisaccade task. Moreover, these performances were correlated with the severity of cognitive impairment in AD patients [68,69]. In our study, elderly depressed patients had an inhibition deficit characterized by an higher ER in the antisaccade task, although the difference between depressed patients and controls in prosaccade and antisaccade RT seems to be related both to the effect of inhibition impairment and psychomotor retardation. These results were correlated with severity of the depression but not with cognitive impairment. Therefore, the current results may open new windows on specific moderation of the prefrontal cortex by affective circuits, possibly through amygdala-prefrontal cortex connections [70], even when stimuli are not emotional in nature. Current research also provides us with information about the specificity of motor inhibition impairment in elderly depressive patients, since this impairment is relatively independent from more cognitive-verbal processes measured by classic neuropsychological tests (e.g., Stroop test).

Inhibition deficit has been shown to be related to suicide risk in elderly depressed patients [71]. Cognitive inhibition is involved in decision-making and could help the depressed patient in preventing late-life suicide [72]. Cognitive inhibition could also reduce the intrusion of suicidal ideation and rumination [71]. Alexopoulos [73] suggested that the presence of cognitive inhibition alteration could be predictive of a lack of therapeutic response to antidepressants in the depressed elderly. Moreover, Malsert *et al.* [74] reported that the RT and ER performances in antisaccade task were associated with the severity of depression and could predict response to transcranial magnetic stimulation over the dorsolateral prefrontal cortex. Our results suggest that the oculomotor performances evaluated by the RT and the ER could be useful measurements of cognitive inhibition in elderly depressed patients. These performances are *complementary* to classical neuropsychological measurements since they seem to be at least partially independent. Further research would be required in order to confirm the interest of using eye movement measurements to predict treatment response or suicidal risks in elderly patients.

A possible limitation of this study, which is common to many experiments in the field, is related to the effect of drugs. Various studies have shown that drugs can affect eye movements [75]. Fafrowicz *et al.* [76] have highlighted an increase in saccadic RT in healthy volunteers treated by anxiolytic drugs. Green *et al.* [77] have also demonstrated an increase in antisaccade errors in schizophrenic patients treated by benzodiazepine. However, other series did not show any treatment effects on eye movements [78] or latency and ER for antisaccade in schizophrenic and depressed patients [79]. To reduce intervening effects, we ensured that all patients were in a stable phase of their disease and were not showing any clinical signs of drug side effects.

In conclusion, the results of this study have offered a new insight into the cognitive-motor inhibition impairment of elderly depressed patients. We used two simple eye movement tasks and additional data analysis focusing on the cost of inhibitory processes. Elderly depression was never previously studied based on this methodology. From a theoretical point of view, this questions the validity of a monolithic approach to cognitive inhibition.More specific conceptual categories are needed in order to account for the multiplicity of inhibitory processes and behaviors. From a clinical point of view, implications may include a more precise evaluation of inhibitory capacities in patients. Complementary research is needed in order to measure the predictive power of the manipulated variables on ecologically-relevant behaviors (i.e., suicidal risk, therapeutic response to treatment).

Acknowledgments

The authors are grateful to Richard Medeiros, Medical Editor of Medical Editing International for editing the manuscript, Emmanuel Haffen, Djamila Bennabi, Laurianne Vuillez for psychiatric assessments and Gregory Tio for their useful suggestions.

Author Contributions

Conceived and designed the experiments: EL PV JM. Performed the experiments: NC NN PV GC. Analyzed the data: NC NN. Contributed reagents/materials/analysis tools: NC EL PV GC NN JM. Contributed to the writing of the manuscript: NC EL PV GC JM NN.

References

1. Austin MP, Ross M, Murray C, O'Carroll RE, Ebmeier KP, et al. (1992) Cognitive function in major depression. Journal of Affective Disorders 25: 21–29.
2. Foster SM, Davis HP, Kisley MA (2013) Brain responses to emotional images related to cognitive ability in older adults. Psychology and Aging 28: 179–190.
3. Nigg JT (2000) On inhibition/disinhibition in developmental psychopathology: views from cognitive and personality psychology and a working inhibition taxonomy. Psychol Bull 126: 220–246.
4. Harnishfeger KK (1995) The development of cognitive inhibition : theories, definitions and research evidence. In: Dempster FN, Brainerd CJ, editors. Interference and inhibition in cognition. San Diego: Academic Press. pp. 175–204.
5. Harnishfeger KK, Bjorklund DF (1994) A developmental perspective on individual differences in inhibition. Learning and Individual Differences 6: 331–355.
6. Houghton G, Tipper SP (1994) A model of inhibitory mechanisms in selective attention. Inhibitory processes in attention, memory, and language. In: Dagenbach D, Carr TH, editors. Inhibitory processes in attention, memory, and language. San Diego, CA, US: Academic Press. pp. 53–112.
7. Everling S, Munoz DP (2000) Neuronal correlates for preparatory set associated with pro-saccades and anti-saccades in the primate frontal eye field. The Journal of Neuroscience 20: 387–400.
8. Leigh RJ, Kennard C (2004) Using saccades as a research tool in the clinical neurosciences. Brain 127: 460–477.
9. Hutton SB (2008) Cognitive control of saccadic eye movements. Brain and Cognition 68: 327–340.
10. Rafal R, Henik A (1994) The neurology of inhibition: Integrating controlled and automatic processes. In: Dagenbach D, Carr TH, editors. Inhibitory processes in attention, memory, and language. San Diego: Academic Press. pp. 1–51.
11. Currie J, Ramsden B (1991) Validation of a clinical antisaccadic eye movements test in the assessment of dementia. Archive Neurology 48: 949.
12. Miyake A, Friedman NP, Emerson MJ, Witzki AH, Howerter A, et al. (2000) The unity and diversity of executive functions and their contributions to complex "Frontal Lobe" tasks: a latent variable analysis. Cognitive Psychology 41: 49–100.
13. Sweeney JA, Strojwas MH, Mann JJ, Thase ME (1998) Prefrontal and cerebellar abnormalities in major depression: evidence from oculomotor studies. Biological Psychiatry 43: 584–594.
14. Mahlberg R, Steinacher B, Mackert A, Flechtner KM (2001) Basic parameters of saccadic eye movements–differences between unmedicated schizophrenia and affective disorder patients. European Archive of Psychiatry and Clinical Neuroscience 251: 205–210.
15. De Lissnyder E, Derakshan N, De Raedt R, Koster EH (2011) Depressive symptoms and cognitive control in a mixed antisaccade task: specific effects of depressive rumination. Cognition & Emotion 25: 886–897.
16. Fiske A, Wetherell JL, Gatz M (2009) Depression in older adults. Annual Review of Clinical Psychology 5: 363–389.
17. Joormann J, Yoon KL, Zetsche U (2007) Cognitive inhibition in depression. Applied and preventive psychology 12: 128–139.
18. Mecocci P, Cherubini A, Mariani E, Ruggiero C, Senin U (2004) Depression in the elderly: new concepts and therapeutic approaches. Aging Clinical and Experimental Research 16: 176–189.
19. Gallagher D, O'Regan C, Savva GM, Cronin H, Lawlor BA, et al. (2012) Depression, anxiety and cardiovascular disease: Which symptoms are associated with increased risk in community dwelling older adults? Journal of Affective Disorders.
20. Alexopoulos GS (2006) The vascular depression hypothesis: 10 years later. Biological Psychiatry 60: 1304–1305.
21. Thorpe L, Groulx B (2001) Depressive syndromes in dementia. Canadian Journal of Neurological Sciences 28: S83–95.
22. APA (2000) Diagnostic and Statistical Manual of Mental Disorders, Fourth Edition: DSM-IV®. Paris: American Psychiatric Association.
23. Montgomery SA, Asberg M (1979) A new depression scale designed to be sensitive to change. The British Journal of Psychiatry 134: 382–389.
24. Ferreira S, Vanholsbeeck G, Chopard G, Pitard A, Tio G, et al. (2010) [Comparative norms of RAPID neuropsychological battery tests for subjects aged between 50 and 89 years]. Revue Neurologique 166: 606–614.
25. Folstein MF, Folstein SE, McHugh PR (1975). "Mini-mental state". A practical method for grading the cognitive state of patients for the clinician. The Journal of Psychiatric Research 12: 189–198.
26. Reitan RM (1958) Validity of the Trail Making Test as an indicator of organic brain damage. Perceptual and Motor Skills 8: 271–276.
27. Goldman WP, Baty JD, Buckles VD, Sahrmann S, Morris JC (1999) Motor dysfunction in mildly demented AD individuals without extrapyramidal signs. Neurology 53: 956–962.
28. Signoret J-L (1989) Evaluation des troubles de la mémoire et des désordres cognitifs associés. Paris, France: Ipsen.
29. Isaacs B, Kennie AT (1973) The Set test as an aid to the detection of dementia in old people. The British Journal of Psychiatry 123: 467–470.
30. Buschke H, Kuslansky G, Katz M, Stewart WF, Sliwinski MJ, et al. (1999) Screening for dementia with the memory impairment screen. Neurology 52: 231–238.
31. Grober E, Buschke H (1987) Genuine memory deficits in dementia Developmental Neuropsychology 3: 13–36.

32. Van der Linden M, Coyette F, Poitrenaud J, Kalafat M, Calicis F, et al. (2004) L'épreuve de rappel libre/rappel indicé à 16 items (RL/RI-16). L'évaluation des troubles de la mémoire Présentation de quatre tests de mémoire épisodique (avec leur étalonnage). Marseille, France: Solal. pp. 25–44.
33. Stroop JR (1935) Studies of interference in serial verbal reactions. Journal of Experimental Psychology 18: 643–662.
34. Everling S, Fischer B (1998) The antisaccade: a review of basic research and clinical studies. Neuropsychologia 36: 885–899.
35. Fischer B, Weber H (1992) Characteristics of "anti" saccades in man. Experimental Brain Research 89: 415–424.
36. Nijboer T, Vree A, Dijkerman C, Van der Stigchel S (2010) Prism adaptation influences perception but not attention: evidence from antisaccades. Neuroreport 21: 386–389.
37. Cohen J (1988) Statistical power analysis for the behavioral sciences. Hillsdale, NJ: Erlbaum.
38. Godijn R, Kramer AF (2007) Antisaccade costs with static and dynamic targets. Perception & Psychophysics 69: 802–815.
39. Gooding DC, Mohapatra L, Shea HB (2004) Temporal stability of saccadic task performance in schizophrenia and bipolar patients. Psychological Medicine 34: 921–932.
40. Liu Z, Xu C, Xu Y, Wang Y, Zhao B, et al. (2010) Decreased regional homogeneity in insula and cerebellum: a resting-state fMRI study in patients with major depression and subjects at high risk for major depression. Psychiatry Research 182: 211–215.
41. Robinson FR, Fuchs AF (2001) The role of the cerebellum in voluntary eye movements. Annual Review of Neuroscience 24: 981–1004.
42. Baxter LR, Schwartz JM, Phelps ME, Mazziotta JC, Guze BH, et al. (1989) Reduction of prefrontal cortex glucose metabolism common to three types of depression. Archives of General Psychiatry 46: 243–250.
43. Crevits L, Van den Abbeele D, Audenaert K, Goethals M, Dierick M (2005) Effect of repetitive transcranial magnetic stimulation on saccades in depression: a pilot study. Psychiatry Research 135: 113–119.
44. Gaymard B, Ploner CJ, Rivaud S, Vermersch AI, Pierrot-Deseilligny C (1998) Cortical control of saccades. Experimental Brain Research 123: 159–163.
45. Pierrot-Deseilligny C, Muri RM, Ploner CJ, Gaymard B, Demeret S, et al. (2003) Decisional role of the dorsolateral prefrontal cortex in ocular motor behaviour. Brain 126: 1460–1473.
46. Pierrot-Deseilligny C, Muri RM, Ploner CJ, Gaymard B, Rivaud-Pechoux S (2003) Cortical control of ocular saccades in humans: a model for motricity. Progress in Brain Research 142: 3–17.
47. Pierrot-Deseilligny C, Milea D, Muri RM (2004) Eye movement control by the cerebral cortex. Current Opinion in Neurology 17: 17–25.
48. Munoz DP, Everling S (2004) Look away: the anti-saccade task and the voluntary control of eye movement. Nature Review Neuroscience 5: 218–228.
49. Bonin-Guillaume S, Hasbroucq T, Blin O (2008) [Psychomotor retardation associated to depression differs from that of normal aging]. Psychologie & Neuropsychiatrie du Vieillissement 6: 137–144.
50. Hamilton AC, Martin RC (2005) Dissociations among tasks involving inhibition: a single-case study. Cognitive, Affective & Behavioral Neuroscience 5: 1–13.
51. Unsworth N, Spillers GJ, Brewer GA, McMillan B (2011) Attention control and the antisaccade task: a response time distribution analysis. Acta Psychologica 137: 90–100.
52. Gallo JJ, Coyne JC (2000) The challenge of depression in late life: bridging science and service in primary care. JAMA 284: 1570–1572.
53. Kramer AF, Humphrey DG, Larish JF, Logan GD, Strayer DL (1994) Aging and inhibition: beyond a unitary view of inhibitory processing in attention. Psychol Aging 9: 491–512.
54. Austin MP, Mitchell P, Goodwin GM (2001) Cognitive deficits in depression: possible implications for functional neuropathology. The British Journal of Psychiatry 178: 200–206.
55. Baudic S, Tzortzis C, Barba GD, Traykov L (2004) Executive deficits in elderly patients with major unipolar depression. Journal of Geriatric Psychiatry and Neurology 17: 195–201.
56. Boone KB, Lesser IM, Miller BL, Wohl M, Berman N, et al. (1995) Cognitive functioning in older depressed outpatients: Relationship of presence and severity of depression to neuropsychological test scores. Neuropsychology 9: 390–398.
57. Funahashi S (2001) Neuronal mechanisms of executive control by the prefrontal cortex. Neuroscience Research 39: 147–165.
58. Naismith SL, Norrie LM, Mowszowski L, Hickie IB (2012) The neurobiology of depression in later-life: clinical, neuropsychological, neuroimaging and pathophysiological features. Progress in Neurobiology 98: 99–143.
59. Baudic S, Benisty S, Dalla Barba G, Traykov L (2007) [Impairment of executive function in elderly patients with major unipolar depression: influence of psychomotor retardation]. Psychologie & Neuropsychiatrie du Vieillissement 5: 65–71.
60. Marazziti D, Consoli G, Picchetti M, Carlini M, Faravelli L (2010) Cognitive impairment in major depression. European Journal of Pharmacology 626: 83–86.
61. Eenshuistra RM, Ridderinkhof KR, van der Molen MW (2004) Age-related changes in antisaccade task performance: inhibitory control or working-memory engagement? Brain and Cognition 56: 177–188.
62. Gohier B, Ferracci L, Surguladze SA, Lawrence E, El Hage W, et al. (2009) Cognitive inhibition and working memory in unipolar depression. Journal of Affective Disorders 116: 100–105.
63. Basso MR, Bornstein RA (1999) Neuropsychological deficits in psychotic versus nonpsychotic unipolar depression. Neuropsychology 13: 69–75.
64. Palmer BW, Boone KB, Lesser IM, Wohl MA, Berman N, et al. (1996) Neuropsychological deficits among older depressed patients with predominantly psychological or vegetative symptoms. Journal of Affective Disorders 41: 17–24.
65. Winograd-Gurvich C, Georgiou-Karistianis N, Fitzgerald PB, Millist L, White OB (2006) Ocular motor differences between melancholic and non-melancholic depression. Journal of Affective Disorders 93: 193–203.
66. Alexopoulos GS (2003) Role of executive function in late-life depression. Journal of Clinical Psychiatry 64: 18–23.
67. Lockwood KA, Alexopoulos GS, Kakuma T, Van Gorp WG (2000) Subtypes of cognitive impairment in depressed older adults. The American Journal of Geriatric Psychiatry 8: 201–208.
68. Crawford TJ, Higham S, Renvoize T, Patel J, Dale M, et al. (2005) Inhibitory control of saccadic eye movements and cognitive impairment in Alzheimer's disease. Biol Psychiatry 57: 1052–1060.
69. Shafiq-Antonacci R, Maruff P, Masters C, Currie J (2003) Spectrum of saccade system function in Alzheimer disease. Arch Neurol 60: 1272–1278.
70. Townsend JD, Torrisi SJ, Lieberman MD, Sugar CA, Bookheimer SY, et al. (2013) Frontal-amygdala connectivity alterations during emotion downregulation in bipolar I disorder. Biol Psychiatry 73: 127–135.
71. Richard-Devantoy S, Jollant F, Kefi Z, Turecki G, Olie JP, et al. (2012) Deficit of cognitive inhibition in depressed elderly: a neurocognitive marker of suicidal risk. Journal of Affective Disorders 140: 193–199.
72. Dombrovski AY, Butters MA, Reynolds CF, 3rd, Houck PR, Clark L, et al. (2008) Cognitive performance in suicidal depressed elderly: preliminary report. The American Journal of Geriatric Psychiatry 16: 109–115.
73. Alexopoulos GS (2005) Depression in the elderly. Lancet 365: 1961–1970.
74. Malsert J, Guyader N, Chauvin A, Polosan M, Poulet E, et al. (2012) Antisaccades as a follow-up tool in major depressive disorder therapies: a pilot study. Psychiatry Research 200: 1051–1053.
75. Ball DM, Glue P, Wilson S, Nutt DJ (1991) Pharmacology of saccadic eye movements in man. 1. Effects of the benzodiazepine receptor ligands midazolam and flumazenil. Psychopharmacology 105: 361–367.
76. Fafrowicz M, Unrug A, Marek T, van Luijtelaar G, Noworol C, et al. (1995) Effects of diazepam and buspirone on reaction time of saccadic eye movements. Neuropsychobiology 32: 156–160.
77. Green JF, King DJ (1998) The effects of chlorpromazine and lorazepam on abnormal antisaccade and no-saccade distractibility. Biological Psychiatry 44: 709–715.
78. Flechtner KM, Steinacher B, Sauer R, Mackert A (2002) Smooth pursuit eye movements of patients with schizophrenia and affective disorder during clinical treatment. European Archive of Psychiatry and Clinical Neuroscience 252: 49–53.
79. Katsanis J, Kortenkamp S, Iacono WG, Grove WM (1997) Antisaccade performance in patients with schizophrenia and affective disorder. Journal of Abnormal Psychology 106: 468–472.

14

Common and Rare Variant Analysis in Early-Onset Bipolar Disorder Vulnerability

Stéphane Jamain[1,2,3]*, Sven Cichon[4,5,6,7], Bruno Etain[1,2,3,8], Thomas W. Mühleisen[5,6], Alexander Georgi[9,10], Nora Zidane[1,2,3], Lucie Chevallier[1,2,3], Jasmine Deshommes[1,2,3,11,12], Aude Nicolas[1,2,3], Annabelle Henrion[1,2,3], Franziska Degenhardt[5,6], Manuel Mattheisen[5,6,13], Lutz Priebe[5,6], Flavie Mathieu[1,2,3], Jean-Pierre Kahn[3,14], Chantal Henry[1,2,3,8], Anne Boland[15], Diana Zelenika[15], Ivo Gut[15], Simon Heath[15], Mark Lathrop[15], Wolfgang Maier[10], Margot Albus[9], Marcella Rietschel[9,10], Thomas G. Schulze[9,16], Francis J. McMahon[17], John R. Kelsoe[18], Marian Hamshere[19], Nicholas Craddock[19], Markus M. Nöthen[5,6], Frank Bellivier[1,3,20,21], Marion Leboyer[1,2,3,8]

1 Institut National de la Santé et de la Recherche Médicale U955, Psychiatrie Génétique, Créteil, France, **2** Université Paris-Est, Faculté de Médecine, Créteil, France, **3** Fondation FondaMental, Créteil, France, **4** Institute of Neuroscience and Medicine (INM-1), Research Center Juelich, Juelich, Germany, **5** Institute of Human Genetics, University of Bonn, Bonn, Germany, **6** Department of Genomics, Life and Brain Center, University of Bonn, Bonn, Germany, **7** Division of Medical Genetics, University Hospital and Department of Biomedicine, University of Basel, Basel, Switzerland, **8** Assistance Publique - Hôpitaux de Paris, Hôpital Henri Mondor-Albert Chenevier, Pôle de Psychiatry, Créteil, France, **9** Department of Genetic Epidemiology in Psychiatry, Central Institute of Mental Health, Mannheim, Germany, **10** Department of Psychiatry, University of Bonn, Bonn, Germany, **11** Assistance Publique - Hôpitaux de Paris, Hôpital Henri Mondor-Albert Chenevier, Plate-forme de Resources Biologiques, Créteil, France, **12** Institut National de la Santé et de la Recherche Médicale Centre d'Investigation Clinique 006, Hôpital Henri Mondor-Albert Chenevier, Pôle Recherche Clinique Santé Publique, Créteil, France, **13** Department of Biomedicine and the Centre for Integrative Sequencing, Aarhus University, Aarhus, Denmark, **14** Département de Psychiatrie et de Psychologie Clinique, Centre Hospitalier Universitaire de Nancy, Hôpital Jeanne-d'Arc, Toul, France, **15** Commissariat à l'Energie Atomique, Institut Génomique, Centre National de Génotypage, Evry, France, **16** Department of Psychiatry and Psychotherapy, University Medical Center, Georg-August-Universität, Göttingen, Germany, **17** Unit on the Genetic Basis of Mood and Anxiety Disorders, National Institute of Mental Health, National Institutes of Health, US Department of Health and Human Services, Bethesda, MD, United States of America, **18** Department of Psychiatry, University of California San Diego, La Jolla, CA, United States of America, **19** MRC Centre for Neuropsychiatric Genetics and Genomics, School of Medicine, Cardiff University, Heath Park, Cardiff, United Kingdom, **20** Assistance Publique - Hôpitaux de Paris, Groupe Hospitalier Lariboisière-F. Widal, Pôle de Psychiatrie, Paris, France, **21** Université Paris Diderot, Paris, France

Abstract

Bipolar disorder is one of the most common and devastating psychiatric disorders whose mechanisms remain largely unknown. Despite a strong genetic contribution demonstrated by twin and adoption studies, a polygenic background influences this multifactorial and heterogeneous psychiatric disorder. To identify susceptibility genes on a severe and more familial sub-form of the disease, we conducted a genome-wide association study focused on 211 patients of French origin with an early age at onset and 1,719 controls, and then replicated our data on a German sample of 159 patients with early-onset bipolar disorder and 998 controls. Replication study and subsequent meta-analysis revealed two genes encoding proteins involved in phosphoinositide signalling pathway (*PLEKHA5* and *PLCXD3*). We performed additional replication studies in two datasets from the WTCCC (764 patients and 2,938 controls) and the GAIN-TGen cohorts (1,524 patients and 1,436 controls) and found nominal *P*-values both in the *PLCXD3* and *PLEKHA5* loci with the WTCCC sample. In addition, we identified in the French cohort one affected individual with a deletion at the *PLCXD3* locus and another one carrying a missense variation in *PLCXD3* (p.R93H), both supporting a role of the phosphatidylinositol pathway in early-onset bipolar disorder vulnerability. Although the current nominally significant findings should be interpreted with caution and need replication in independent cohorts, this study supports the strategy to combine genetic approaches to determine the molecular mechanisms underlying bipolar disorder.

Editor: Chunyu Liu, University of Illinois at Chicago, United States of America

Funding: This work was supported by INSERM (Poste d'Accueil INSERM to B.E.), Assistance Publique des Hôpitaux de Paris, the Agence Nationale pour la Recherche (ANR NEURO2006 – Project MANAGE_BPAD), the Centre National de Génotypage (Centre d'Energie Atomique, Evry, France) and the Réseau Thématique de Recherche et de Soins en Santé Mentale (Fondation FondaMental). The funders had no role in study design, data collection and analysis, decision to publish, or preparation of the manuscript.

Competing Interests: The authors have declared that no competing interests exist.

* Email: stephane.jamain@inserm.fr

Introduction

Numerous genome-wide association (GWA) studies have recently been performed on bipolar disorder (BD), but few signals were replicated and meta-analyses identified only a couple of associated genes, such as *CACNA1C*, *ODZ4* and *NCAN*, with a small effect size [1–4]. Although convergent evidences argue in favour of a role for these genes in vulnerability to BD [5–9], more extensive studies suggest it might be involved in other psychiatric disorders [3,10,11]. The difficulty to identify susceptibility genes specific to BD could be due to the ethnic heterogeneity, as a consequence of the huge number of patients and controls required to get genome-wide significant signals, or to the clinical and a genetic heterogeneity of the DSM-IV "bipolar disorder" entity.

In the current study, we focused on patients with BD selected with an early age at onset, a clinical characteristic known to identify a subgroup of patients with a higher morbid risk for BD in relatives [12–17]. We then compared these data to those observed in two previously published GWA studies of BD, conducted by the Wellcome Trust Case Control Consortium (WTCCC) [18] and the Genetic Association Information Network Bipolar Sample (GAIN-BP) [19]. Finally, we screened our regions of interest for rare variants, suspected to have a larger effect size, and suggested the importance of combined approaches in the identification of vulnerability genes to BD.

Materials and Methods

Ethics Statement

Protocols and procedures were approved by the research ethics board of the Pitié-Salpêtrière Hospital in Paris for the French sample and the ethics committees of the Faculties of Medicine at the Universities of Bonn and Mannheim/Heidelberg for the German sample. Written informed consent was obtained from all subjects prior to study participation.

Sample

French sample. Two hundred and twenty patients of French descent with at least three grandparents from mainland France were collected through a French national network for mental health (Fondation FondaMental) in three university-affiliated psychiatry departments (Paris-Créteil, Bordeaux and Nancy) as previously described [12]. All patients met DSM-IV criteria [20] for BD type I (N = 172), type II (N = 46) or BD not otherwise specified (N = 2) before the age of 22. The age at onset was defined by the first mood episode (depressive, manic or hypomanic) and was retrospectively assessed using medical case notes and information obtained with the Diagnostic Interview for Genetic Studies (DIGS) [21]. The threshold of 22 was chosen on the basis of previous admixture analyses [16,22–25].

German sample. One hundred and sixty-seven German patients were recruited from consecutive admissions to the psychiatric inpatient units of the Central Institute of Mental Health in Mannheim and the Department of Psychiatry and Psychotherapy of the University of Bonn (BOMA bipolar study). These patients received a lifetime diagnosis of BD type I based on DSM-IV criteria and had an age at onset lower than 22.

Control population. Genotyping data from 1,823 French controls and 629 German controls were provided by the *Centre National de Génotypage* (CNG, Evry, France). These samples were previously collected and were not screened for psychiatric disorders. They have been genotyped for association and population studies as described elsewhere [26] and permission to use them were obtained from the original investigators. DNA from 380 additional German controls were collected in the above mentioned German hospitals. An additional sample of 293 unaffected French controls screened for personal history of psychiatric disorders using the DIGS has been screened for mutation in the *PLCXD3* exon 2, in order to determine the specificity of the p.R93H mutation.

DNA extraction and genotyping

DNA was isolated from lymphocytes either directly from venous blood sample or after transformation by Epstein Barr virus. Isolation was performed by salting-out with saturated sodium chloride solution [27]. French and German cases were genotyped at the CNG, using HumanHap550 or Human 610-Quad BeadArrays and the Infinium II assay (Illumina, San Diego, CA, USA). Control samples were genotyped on HumanHap300 (N = 2,503) or on HumanHap550 BeadArrays (N = 380). In order to determine whether the use of multiple arrays might result in a population stratification, we performed a multidimensional scaling analysis based on pairwise identity-by-state distance between pairs of individuals. The good clustering of all individuals showed that there was no stratification due to the use of multiple arrays (Figure S1 in File S1).

Quality control criteria

All samples were passed through the standard quality-control procedures followed at the CNG for GWA studies, as described elsewhere [26]. For the French population, the quality control was performed using the PLINK toolset [28] on a total of 317,131 commons SNPs genotyped in 2,043 DNA samples (Table S1 in File S1). We removed monomorphic SNPs, as those with a minor allele frequency (MAF) lower than 0.01 and SNPs with a call rate lower than 0.97. We performed a missing chi-square test that compares, for each SNP, missingness between cases and controls and excluded SNPs with $P<10^{-3}$. Then, we removed SNPs that did not show Hardy-Weinberg proportions in controls, using a significant threshold at $P<10^{-3}$. In parallel, we removed male samples with more than 0.5% or female samples with less than 20% heterozygous markers on the X chromosome and individuals with a call rate lower than 0.97. We estimated the average genome-wide identity-by-state (IBS) sharing between individuals and analysed the clustering using a multidimensional scaling (MDS) plot. Hence, we excluded 15 individuals (3 cases and 12 controls) with a low level of identity. After pruning, the final data set consisted in 261,525 SNPs genotyped in 1,930 individuals (211 cases and 1,719 controls) that were used for association study. Identical quality control criteria were used for the replication sample from Germany (Table S1 in File S1) and MDS plot showed 6 controls to be removed. This led to a final data set of 288,167 SNPs and 1,157 individuals (159 patients and 998 controls).

Association analysis

Basic case/control association analyses were performed using the PLINK software v1.07 [28]. A haplotype analysis was performed on the two most associated regions using sliding windows of two to five SNPs shifting by one SNP at a time. We tested for case/control haplotype-based association using a chi-square test with one degree of freedom. Only window with best *P*-values are reported for each region. Imputation data were based on the 3,967,651 SNPs genotyped in 90 subjects of the CEU population of the HapMap project (http://www.hapmap.org). Imputation was performed using PLINK and consisted in estimating the allele frequencies of an ungenotyped SNP based on its surrounding haplotypic background.

Genotyping data from the WTCCC [18] and the GAIN-TGen collection [19] were provided for BD patients with an age at onset lower than 22 and for controls. In the WTCCC, BD was defined according to Research Diagnostic Criteria [29] and included BD type I, type II, schizoaffective disorders and manic disorders. The WTCCC sample was genotyped on Affymetrix 500K array, containing only few SNPs in common with the Illumina arrays used in other samples. Thus, the genotype correlation data were obtained for SNPs within a 1 Mbp window, based on individuals and SNPs in the CEU HapMap filtered set (http://www.hapmap.org) and the 2,938 WTCCC control sample combined [18]. An association test between 764 early-onset patients and 2,938 controls was performed, using SNPs with a genotyped correlation higher than 0.2 with associated SNPs at $P<5\times10^{-5}$ identified through the meta-analysis.

All patients from the GAIN-TGen cohort met DSM-IV criteria for BD type I. Imputed data from the GAIN-TGen bipolar case-control sample [30] were obtained, using the MACH software with phased haplotypes from the 60 HapMap-CEU founders (release 22). Allele frequencies of 15 SNPs out of the 16 associated SNPs at $P<5\times10^{-5}$, were compared between 1,524 patients with an early age at onset and 1,436 controls.

A flow chart summarizing all steps of the genetic analysis is shown on the Figure S2 in File S1.

Detection of copy number variations

Copy number variations were detected by fluorescence level comparison through the chromosome, using the SnipPeep software (R. Toro, Pasteur Institute, France). The deletion in *PLCXD3* was confirmed by quantitative PCR analysis using one internal and two external couples of primers and Mesa Green qPCR master mix plus (Eurogentec, Liege, Belgium). PCR were performed and run in a Mastercycler ep realplex2S (Eppendorf, Hamburg, Germany) for the deleted patient and two unaffected controls, known to have no deletion in the regions under study. Each real-time PCR was performed in triplicate and assessed by comparing Ct at a determined threshold between the three amplicons and the three individuals.

Mutation screening in PLCXD3

The *PLCXD3* coding regions were amplified for 334 French subjects with BD, sequenced by the Sanger's method using the BigDye terminator v3.1 cycle sequencing kit (Life Technologies, Carlsbad, CA, U.S.A.) and run on a 16-Capillary ABI PRISM 3130xl genetic analyzer. The *PLCXD3* exon 2 was sequenced for 293 unaffected French controls. All primers used for PCR amplifications and sequence analyses are available on request.

Results

Analysis of a French cohort

We carried out an association study on 211 patients with early-onset BD of French origin and 1,719 matched controls, who have been genotyped on an Illumina platform with 261,525 single nucleotide polymorphisms (SNPs) passing quality control. The estimation of an inflation factor [31] showed a good genetic homogeneity in our sample ($\lambda = 1.03$), suggesting that no correction for genomic control was needed. According to the genome-wide significance threshold of $P = 5\times10^{-8}$, no significant difference in allele frequencies was observed in our sample, but 17 SNPs showed a nominal $P<5\times10^{-5}$ (Table S2 in File S1), suggesting these loci may be associated with vulnerability to early-onset forms of BD. Interestingly, the lowest *P*-value (*rs10096683*, $P=4.11\times10^{-6}$, OR = 2.26), was observed for a SNP located on chromosome 8p22, a region that has previously been associated with schizophrenia [32–35] and suicide behaviour in patients with recurrent major depression [36].

Replication on a German cohort

Next, we selected 14,037 SNPs with a $P<0.05$ to perform a replication study on an independent sample of 159 German subjects with an early-onset BD and 998 matched controls (Table S1 in File S1). Again, a good genetic homogeneity ($\lambda = 1.04$) was observed after quality control for this sample. Out of the 14,037 SNPs previously selected, 13,734 were genotyped in the German sample, and 739 showed a $P<0.05$, showing a significant over-representation ($P<0.03$) of nominally significant *P*-values. The most associated SNP in the German sample was located on chromosome 12 upstream to the *PLEKHA5* gene (*rs2970836*, $P=5.3\times10^{-6}$, OR = 1.76).

Meta-analysis on the French and the German cohorts

We subsequently performed a meta-analysis, combining data from the French and the German cohorts, yielding a sample of 370 patients with early-onset BD and 2,717 controls. Again, no locus reaches the genome-wide significant threshold. The largest difference in allele frequencies between cases and controls was observed for chromosome 12 (*rs2961365*, $P_{meta}=1.6\times10^{-6}$, $OR_{meta}=1.57$) with no evidence of heterogeneity between the two cohorts ($Q=0.94$, 1 degree of freedom, $I^2=0$). In this region, 5 SNPs showed a difference in allele frequencies at $P<5\times10^{-5}$ in 355 Kbp (Figure 1, Table 1). These SNPs span two genes, *PLEKHA5* and *AEBP2*. The second strongest association with no heterogeneity ($Q=0.59$, 1 degree of freedom, $I^2=0$) was observed for chromosome 5p13 (*rs10512793*, $P_{meta}=2.7\times10^{-6}$, $OR_{meta}=1.61$), in which two SNPs, spaced by 196 Kbp, showed a difference in allele frequencies at $P<5\times10^{-5}$ (Figure 1, Table 1). These two SNPs were located in the *OXCT1* gene, and upstream to *PLCXD3*. In order to further explore the associated peak in these two regions, we used a three-SNP sliding window and performed a haplotype analysis. Whereas no further significant difference, as compared to single SNP analysis, was observed on chromosome 12p12, a more significant difference between patients and controls was observed on chromosome 5p13 for the combination of *rs624097-rs316762-rs10512793*, for which an overall $P_{meta}=2.6\times10^{-7}$ was observed (Figure 1).

Imputation data

In order to refine the association signal in these two regions, we imputed data for ungenotyped SNPs in the French and the German cohorts based on the 3.9 million SNPs genotyped in the CEU population of the HapMap project. The results of the two populations were then combined to perform an association study. After imputation, we observed an increased signal for chromosome 12 with the lowest estimated *P*-value for *rs10743315* ($P=2.1\times10^{-7}$, OR = 1.61) located in *PLEKHA5* (Figure 1). On the contrary for chromosome 5, the lowest *P*-value was observed for the genotyped SNP, *rs10512793*.

Replication studies on the WTCCC and the GAIN-TGen cohorts

We analysed the top-16 SNPs ($P<5\times10^{-5}$) out of the meta-analysis in two additional samples of early-onset bipolar patients, already genotyped on different platforms through the WTCCC and the GAIN and performed a mega-analysis including the four samples (Table S3 in File S2). Only 4 SNPs, genotyped in a subsample of 764 early-onset bipolar patients and 2,938 matched

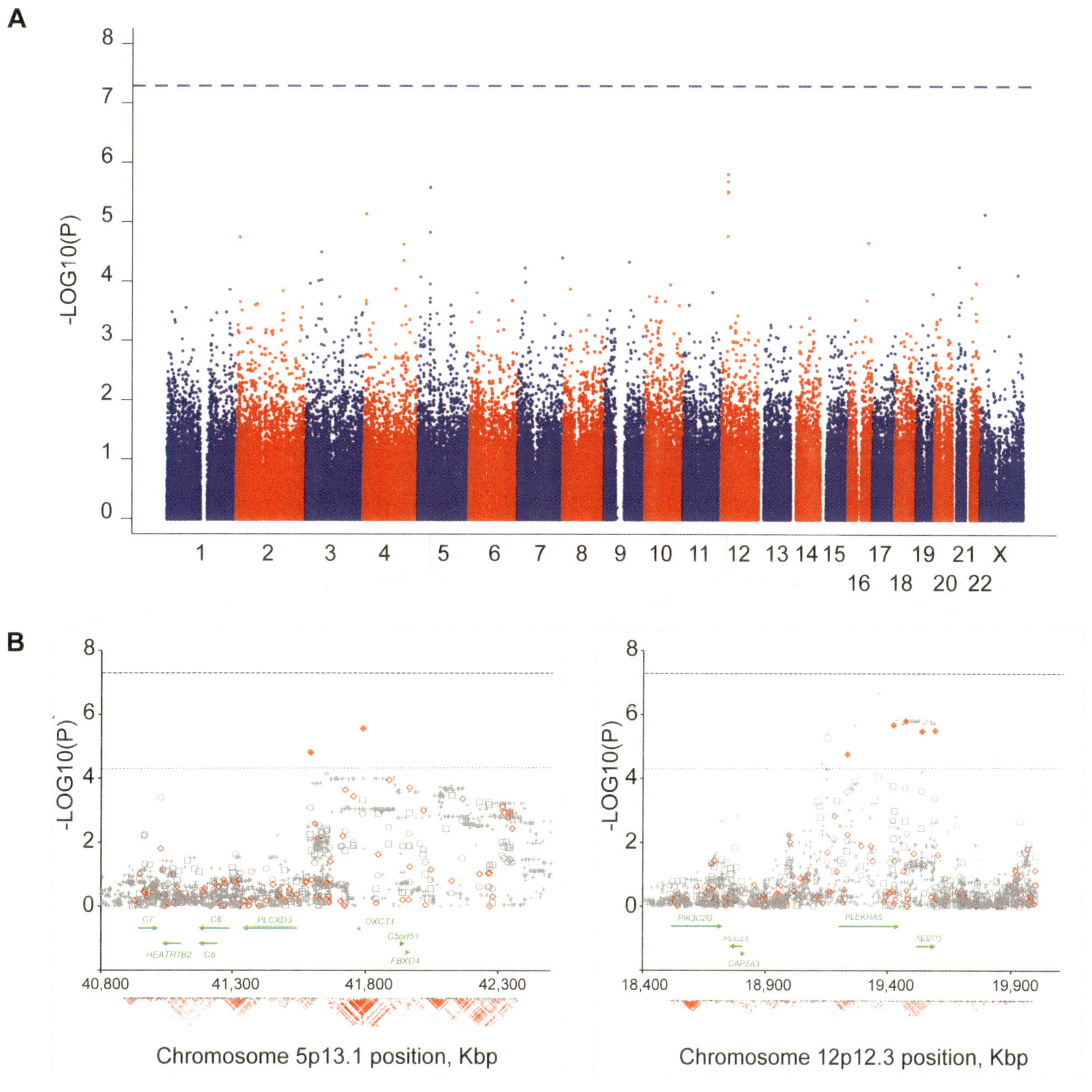

Figure 1. Genome-wide association results and detailed peak association regions. (**A**) Manhattan plot of the meta-analysis performed on early-onset bipolar patients and controls from France and Germany. Physical position is shown along the *x* axis and –log10(*P*-value) is shown along the *y* axis. (**B**) Detail of the two most associated regions on chromosomes 5p13 and 12p12. Allele frequency differences are represented by –log10(*P*-values) for the French (open grey circles), the German (open grey squares) and the meta- (open red diamonds) analyses. Grey crosses represent –log10(*P*-value) for imputed ungenotyped SNPs. The most associated SNP for each region is shown with orange circle. On chromosome 12p12, the lowest *P*-value ($P = 2.1 \times 10^{-7}$) was observed for an imputed SNP (*rs10743315*). On chromosome 5p13, the lowest *P*-value ($P = 2.6 \times 10^{-7}$) was observed for a three-SNPs window haplotype (light blue line) located downstream to *OXCT1* and upstream to *PLCXD3* (*rs624097-rs316762-rs10512793*). The genome-wide significant threshold ($P = 5 \times 10^{-8}$) is indicated by the blue dash line and the dot black line shows a threshold at $P = 5 \times 10^{-5}$. The largest differences in allele frequencies are represented with filled diamonds. Gene position and annotation (http://genome.ucsc.edu/) are symbolised by green arrows. Linkage disequilibrium (r^2) estimated according to HapMap CEU population SNPs (release 3) is symbolised in the bottom part of each figure. Darker red indicates higher values.

controls from the United Kingdom out of the WTCCC, were either directly or in strong linkage disequilibrium ($r^2 > 0.99$) with SNPs genotyped in the WTCCC sample. None of them showed a nominal *P*-value ($P < 0.05$). However, two SNPs on chromosome 5p13 in lower linkage disequilibrium ($r^2 = 0.65$) with *rs822135* showed a nominal *P*-value (*rs625487*, $P = 0.02$, OR = 1.15 and *rs633407*, $P = 0.02$, OR = 1.15) (data not shown). Both were located approximately 55 Kbp upstream to *PLCXD3* and 165 Kbp downstream to *OXCT1*. In addition, one SNP (*rs2565666*), located on chromosome 12p12, 21 Kbp downstream to *PLEKHA5* and 42 Kbp upstream to *AEBP2*, also showed a nominal *P*-value (*rs2565666*, $P = 0.03$, OR = 1.22) (data not shown). We

Table 1. Regions associated at $P<5\times10^{-5}$ with early-onset BD in meta-analysis.

				French sample				German sample				Meta-analysis			
CHR	SNP	Position[a] (bp)	Allele	Allele frequency in early-onset BD patients	Allele frequency in controls	*P*	OR	Allele frequency in early-onset BD patients	Allele frequency in controls	*P*	OR	P_{meta}	OR_{meta}	Q	I^2
12	*rs2961365*	19,469,374	T	0,23	0,16	$1,88\times10^{-04}$	1,58	0.23	0.16	2.12×10^{-03}	1.56	1.58×10^{-6}	1.57	0.94	0
12	*rs3752823*	19,419,905	A	0,15	0,10	$2,03\times10^{-03}$	1,58	0.16	0.09	1.70×10^{-04}	1.89	2.09×10^{-6}	1.71	0.43	0
5	*rs10512793*	41,787,459	C	0,19	0,13	$1,24\times10^{-03}$	1,54	0.20	0.13	4.64×10^{-04}	1.72	2.68×10^{-6}	1.61	0.59	0
12	*rs2900433*	19,588,898	T	0,23	0,16	$4,13\times10^{-04}$	1,55	0.23	0.16	2.01×10^{-03}	1.57	3.13×10^{-6}	1.56	0.96	0
12	*rs7305762*	19,535,793	G	0,23	0,16	$2,46\times10^{-04}$	1,57	0.23	0.16	3.53×10^{-03}	1.53	3.26×10^{-6}	1.55	0.89	0
4	*rs12500759*	7,760,780	T	0,21	0,29	$7,54\times10^{-04}$	0,66	0.23	0.32	2.76×10^{-03}	0.66	7.40×10^{-6}	0.66	1.00	0
X	*rs952076*	13,856,877	T	0,20	0,28	$2,61\times10^{-03}$	0,65	0.19	0.29	5.94×10^{-04}	0.56	7.48×10^{-6}	0.61	0.51	0
5	*rs822135*	41,590,915	A	0,25	0,33	$8,12\times10^{-04}$	0,68	0.26	0.34	5.54×10^{-03}	0.69	1.50×10^{-5}	0.68	0.94	0
12	*rs4764470*	19,233,420	A	0,27	0,20	$2,55\times10^{-04}$	1,53	0.25	0.20	1.84×10^{-02}	1.39	1.73×10^{-5}	1.47	0.60	0
2	*rs7608161*	9,668,060	G	0,34	0,27	$2,90\times10^{-03}$	1,38	0.33	0.25	1.68×10^{-03}	1.50	1.82×10^{-5}	1.43	0.64	0
16	*rs7185187*	69,315,056	T	0,11	0,06	$5,99\times10^{-04}$	1,80	0.12	0.07	9.63×10^{-03}	1.65	2.24×10^{-5}	1.73	0.74	0
4	*rs6857347*	139,528,195	G	0,43	0,50	$6,80\times10^{-03}$	0,75	0.41	0.51	7.62×10^{-04}	0.66	2.40×10^{-5}	0.71	0.41	0
3	*rs13091545*	52,352,334	G	0,25	0,18	$1,73\times10^{-04}$	1,57	0.20	0.16	4.64×10^{-02}	1.35	3.24×10^{-5}	1.48	0.44	0
7	*rs4716990*	155,616,697	G	0,37	0,29	$6,12\times10^{-04}$	1,45	0.36	0.29	1.99×10^{-02}	1.34	4.04×10^{-5}	1.40	0.66	0
4	*rs12505439*	139,521,194	A	0,35	0,29	$9,91\times10^{-03}$	1,32	0.40	0.30	1.05×10^{-03}	1.50	4.48×10^{-5}	1.40	0.44	0
9	*rs3739657*	85,177,755	C	0,28	0,36	$2,21\times10^{-03}$	0,71	0.31	0.39	6.87×10^{-03}	0.70	4.74×10^{-5}	0.71	0.98	0

OR, odds ratio; Q, *P*-value for Cochrane's Q statistic; I^2, heterogeneity index.
[a]position from the short arm telomere based on Hg18.

also compared a sample of 1,524 early-onset bipolar patients with 1,436 controls out of the combined GAIN-TGen cohorts. None out of the 15 tested SNPs showed a nominal P-value (Table S3 in File S2). The mega-analysis showed a high heterogeneity between the samples from France and Germany and the two samples from U.K. and U.S.A. This analysis resulted in a low signal on chromosomes 5p13 and 12p12 (*rs10512793*, $P_{mega} = 5.05 \times 10^{-2}$, $OR_{mega} = 1.38$ and *rs3752823*, $P_{mega} = 5.79 \times 10^{-2}$, $OR_{mega} = 1.43$, respectively). The strongest association observed in the mega-analysis for SNPs tested in at least three of the four populations was observed on chromosome 7q36.3 in a gene desert (*rs4716990*, $P_{mega} = 3.78 \times 10^{-2}$, $OR_{mega} = 1.25$).

Structural abnormalities in region of interest

Fluorescence level of genotyped SNPs was only available for a subsample of early-onset patients of French and German origin (N = 321). We analysed this fluorescence level in the two 1.5 Mbp regions of interest on chromosome 5p13 and 12p12. On chromosome 5p13, we identified, in a French patient who manifested a first mood episode by the age of 17, a 90-Kbp deletion removing the *PLCXD3* promoter region as well as the first coding exon of the gene (Figure 2), whereas no copy number variation has been previously reported in this region in the database of genomic variations (http://projects.tcag.ca/variation/). Although DNA was not available for first-degree relatives of this patient, the deletion was confirmed using quantitative PCR analysis (data not shown). In order to determine whether independent family specific mutations might be frequently found in bipolar patients, we screened all coding exons of *PLCXD3* in 334 French subjects (204 patients with early-onset BD and 130 patients with late-onset BD). Three synonymous variations (p.V58, p.A130 and p.P251) were found in these patients, and one amino acid change (p.R93H) was identified in one subject with early-onset BD type I and obsessive compulsive disorder. This variation was not found in 293 unaffected matched controls. This amino acid is highly conserved through evolution and, according to PolyPhen-2 [37], this variation is predicted to strongly affect the function of the protein. Further analysis of the available DNA sample in this family showed that this variation was transmitted from the father (Figure S3 in File S1). The patient manifested first mood symptoms by the age of 19. Although his father did not meet criteria for mood disorder according to DSM-IV, his first cousin manifested major depressive disorder by the age of 65. Unfortunately, no DNA was available for this subject.

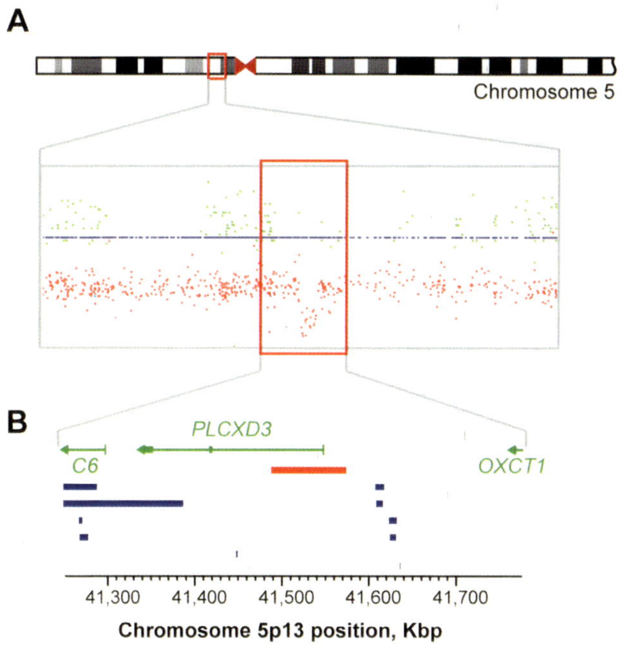

Figure 2. Copy number variation identified on chromosome 5p13. (**A**) Fluorescence level of SNPs of the region for the deleted patient visualized using SnipPeep. Red dots represent fluorescence level of SNPs and green dots correspond to the SNP heterozygocity. (**B**) Chromosomal position of the deletion. Gene position and annotation (http://genome.ucsc.edu/) are symbolised by green arrows. Deletions reported in the Database of Genomic Variants (http://projects.tcag.ca/variation/) are represented with blue bars. No duplication has been reported in this region. A red bar represents the deletion identified in the patient with early-onset BD.

Discussion

The important clinical heterogeneity of BD has probably hampered the identification of vulnerability genes so far. After tumultuous starts, GWA studies have enabled the identification of robust and replicable genetic findings of weak effect, in regions of *CACNA1C*, *ODZ4* and *NCAN*, but without disease specificity [4]. In this study, we conducted a genome-wide approach on a highly heritable phenotype, focusing on patients with an early age at onset. Based on the genotyping data of 261,525 SNPs, we did not identify SNPs that reached the genome-wide significant threshold in our patients and controls of French origin. This was most likely due to the small sample size of our cohort. We calculated the statistical power of our study, using the CaTS software [38] and estimated that we had 80% chance to detect only SNPs with a genetic risk factor higher than 1.7 (Figure S4 in File S1). However, recent data from larger cohort studies showed a polygenic component in BD [3,39], consistent with a combine vulnerability resulting from many variants of weak effect. We thus conducted a replication study on a German cohort of patients with early-onset BD and performed a subsequent meta-analysis. Although it did not reach the genome-wide significant threshold, the most associated region in our meta-analysis was located on chromosome 12p12. This region has been previously associated with bipolar disorder [40–42] and more specifically when patients had an early age at onset of mania [40]. Five SNPs in this region showed a difference in allele frequencies between patients and controls, spanning two genes, *PLEKHA5* and *AEBP2*. The genetic refinement using imputed data showed the lowest P-value for a SNP located in *PLEKHA5* (*rs10743315*, $P = 2.1 \times 10^{-7}$). *PLEKHA5* encodes a protein containing a pleckstrin homology domain, which interacts with phosphatidylinositol 3-phosphate [43]. Few elements are known about this gene except its ubiquitous pattern of expression, including foetal and adult brains. Nevertheless, there is compelling evidence for the implication of the phosphatidylinositol signalling pathway in the etiopathogeny of BD and the two most effective mood stabilisers for BD (lithium and valproate) directly inhibit this pathway [44]. Further exploration of response to mood stabilizer in regards to the *PLEKHA5* genotypes might help in understanding the difference observed according to the patients' age at onset [15].

The second most associated region in our meta-analysis was located on chromosome 5p13. In this region, the highest difference in allele frequencies between patients with early-onset BD and controls was observed for *rs10512793*. This SNP was located in *OXCT1*, which encodes a 3-oxoacid CoA transferase 1. This enzyme catalyzes the reversible transfer of CoA from succinyl-CoA to acetoacetate and is thus the first step of ketone body utilization, the main source of lipid-derived energy for the brain

[45]. Mutations in this gene are associated with succinyl CoA:3-oxoacid CoA transferase (SCOT) deficiency, characterised by episodes of severe ketoacidosis [46,47], which can also emerge during treatment with some atypical antipsychotics [48]. However, the haplotype analysis of this region suggested that the associated peak might be located more likely downstream to *OXCT1* and upstream to *PLCXD3*. This result is consistent with the 90 Kbp-deletion reported in one of the French patients and that removed the promoter region and the first coding exon of *PLCXD3*. Further exploration of this gene revealed a mutation predicting to change the amino acid sequence of the protein (p.R93H) and transmitted from his father, who had a first cousin with major depressive disorder. Interestingly, this gene encodes a phosphatidylinositol-specific phospholipase C, strengthening the involvement of the phosphoinositide-signalling pathway in vulnerability to BD. Note that tricyclic antidepressants (e.g. desipramine), which are known to induce rapid cycling or induce manic or hypomanic episodes in some patients with BD [49], stimulate phospholipase C activity and the production of the second messenger inositol 1,4,5-trisphosphate [50]. In addition, experiments performed using rat cultured hippocampal neurons revealed that desipramine rapidly enhanced the spontaneous SNAP25-dependent vesicular release of glutamate [51]. This Ca^{2+} dependent mechanism is consistent with our previously reported association between *SNAP25* and early-onset BD [12] and with the strong associations observed between SNPs located in *CACNA1C* and BD [1,3].

The main limitation of our study is not to reach the stringent genome-wide threshold. Although this might translate an absence of common genetic variations for a clinical subgroup based on an early age at onset, this is also a direct consequence of the small sample size and the loss of power inherent to the subphenotype analysis. Similar study on larger sample should be performed to confirm our data and valid the relevance of such approach. Nevertheless, results observed in our French subsample with an early age at onset have been replicated in a German sample and supported by the data from the WTCCC with similar phenotype criteria.

Another possible cause of the loss of power in our analysis is the categorical exploration of the age at onset. Despite a widely valid threshold for the age at onset [16,17,22–25], a continuous exploration of this variable would allow to determine whether specific loci might lead to various agé at onset, which would result, under multiplicative or additive models, in an overall early age-at-onset in patients. Such hypothesis is supported by the recent observation of the International Schizophrenia Consortium, which showed the molecular genetic evidence for a substantial polygenic component to the risk of BD involving thousands of common alleles of very small effect [39]. Similar analysis should thus be performed according to the patients' age at onset, but this should require larger samples for the study and the replication analysis.

In conclusion, although we did not reach the genome-wide significant threshold in our association study, we report here convergent data between our GWA study on early onset BD, the structural abnormality observed in one patient and a missense mutation reported in one family with early-onset BD. The difficulties to reach the stringent genome-wide significant threshold suggest that larger samples should be included, which will also help in better defining the most convenient strategy to take into account the age at onset of patients. Although the current nominally significant findings should be interpreted with caution and need replication in independent cohorts, our results displayed that the combined exploration of common and rare variants in BD can reveal identical pathways suggesting both approaches should be systematically used in further genetic exploration of this disorder. Using these approaches, we provided evidence that variations in phosphoinositide secondary messenger signalling pathway, and for the first time, that the *PLEKHA5* and *PLCXD3* genes, might confer vulnerability to early-onset BD. Further exploration of these mechanisms might be used to better identify markers of prognosis and help the development of innovative treatment for these severe forms of the disease.

Supporting Information

File S1 Contains Tables S1-S2 and Figures S1-S4.

File S2 Contains Table S3.

Acknowledgments

We thank bipolar patients and controls for their participation.

We acknowledge the Wellcome Trust Case Control Consortium (www.WTCCC.org.uk), the Genetic Association Information Network (www.fnih.org) and the Translational Genomics Research Institute (www.tgen.org), their memberships and funders, for generating and publishing data used for replication.

We thank E. Abadie, the Cochin Hospital cell library (Prof. J. Chelly), the Clinical Investigation Centre (Dr. O. Montagne) and the Biological Resources Centre (Prof. B. Ghaleh) of Mondor Hospital, and blood donor centre (Drs. J.L. Beaumont and B. Mignen, EFS, Créteil) for technical assistance.

We thank B. Cochet, R. Cohen, O. Elgrabli, A. Raust and L. Zanouy for their participation in the clinical evaluation of patients.

We thank Dr. R. Toro for the SnipPeep software and Prof. T. Bourgeron for helpful discussion and comments on the manuscript.

The team of M. Leboyer is part of the École des Neurosciences de Paris Ile-de-France network, member of the Bio-Psy Labex and member of the European Network of Bipolar Research Expert Centres (ENBREC).

Author Contributions

Conceived and designed the experiments: SJ M. Leboyer FB BE M. Lathrop. Performed the experiments: SJ LC JD AN AH FD LP AB. Analyzed the data: SJ SC BE TWM NZ LC FD MM LP FM DZ IG SH TGS MH. Contributed reagents/materials/analysis tools: BE AG JPK CH IG SH M. Lathrop WM MA MR TGS FJM JRK NC MMN FB M. Leboyer. Wrote the paper: SJ SC BE TWM TGS MH NC FB M. Leboyer.

References

1. Ferreira MA, O'Donovan MC, Meng YA, Jones IR, Ruderfer DM, et al. (2008) Collaborative genome-wide association analysis supports a role for ANK3 and CACNA1C in bipolar disorder. Nat Genet 40: 1056–1058.
2. Cichon S, Muhleisen TW, Degenhardt FA, Mattheisen M, Miro X, et al. (2011) Genome-wide association study identifies genetic variation in neurocan as a susceptibility factor for bipolar disorder. Am J Hum Genet 88: 372–381.
3. Psychiatric GWAS Consortium Bipolar Disorder Working Group (2011) Large-scale genome-wide association analysis of bipolar disorder identifies a new susceptibility locus near ODZ4. Nat Genet 43: 977–983.
4. Craddock N, Sklar P (2013) Genetics of bipolar disorder. Lancet 381: 1654–1662.
5. Kempton MJ, Ruberto G, Vassos E, Tatarelli R, Girardi P, et al. (2009) Effects of the CACNA1C risk allele for bipolar disorder on cerebral gray matter volume in healthy individuals. Am J Psychiatry 166: 1413–1414.
6. Wessa M, Linke J, Witt SH, Nieratschker V, Esslinger C, et al. (2010) The CACNA1C risk variant for bipolar disorder influences limbic activity. Mol Psychiatry 15: 1126–1127.
7. Roussos P, Giakoumaki SG, Georgakopoulos A, Robakis NK, Bitsios P (2011) The CACNA1C and ANK3 risk alleles impact on affective personality traits and startle reactivity but not on cognition or gating in healthy males. Bipolar Disord 13: 250–259.

8. Green EK, Hamshere M, Forty L, Gordon-Smith K, Fraser C, et al. (2013) Replication of bipolar disorder susceptibility alleles and identification of two novel genome-wide significant associations in a new bipolar disorder case-control sample. Mol Psychiatry 18: 1302–1307.
9. Heinrich A, Lourdusamy A, Tzschoppe J, Vollstadt-Klein S, Buhler M, et al. (2013) The risk variant in ODZ4 for bipolar disorder impacts on amygdala activation during reward processing. Bipolar Disord 15: 440–445.
10. Green EK, Grozeva D, Jones I, Jones L, Kirov G, et al. (2010) The bipolar disorder risk allele at CACNA1C also confers risk of recurrent major depression and of schizophrenia. Mol Psychiatry 15: 1016–1022.
11. Moskvina V, Craddock N, Holmans P, Nikolov I, Pahwa JS, et al. (2009) Gene-wide analyses of genome-wide association data sets: evidence for multiple common risk alleles for schizophrenia and bipolar disorder and for overlap in genetic risk. Mol Psychiatry 14: 252–260.
12. Etain B, Dumaine A, Mathieu F, Chevalier F, Henry C, et al. (2010) A SNAP25 promoter variant is associated with early-onset bipolar disorder and a high expression level in brain. Mol Psychiatry 15: 748–755.
13. Etain B, Mathieu F, Rietschel M, Maier W, Albus M, et al. (2006) Genome-wide scan for genes involved in bipolar affective disorder in 70 European families ascertained through a bipolar type I early-onset proband: supportive evidence for linkage at 3p14. Mol Psychiatry 11: 685–694.
14. Grigoroiu-Serbanescu M, Martinez M, Nothen MM, Grinberg M, Sima D, et al. (2001) Different familial transmission patterns in bipolar I disorder with onset before and after age 25. Am J Med Genet 105: 765–773.
15. Leboyer M, Henry C, Paillere-Martinot ML, Bellivier F (2005) Age at onset in bipolar affective disorders: a review. Bipolar Disord 7: 111–118.
16. Bellivier F, Etain B, Malafosse A, Henry C, Kahn JP, et al. (2014) Age at onset in bipolar I affective disorder in the USA and Europe. World J Biol Psychiatry 15: 369–376.
17. Geoffroy PA, Etain B, Scott J, Henry C, Jamain S, et al. (2013) Reconsideration of bipolar disorder as a developmental disorder: importance of the time of onset. J Physiol Paris 107: 278–285.
18. The Wellcome Trust Case Control Consortium (2007) Genome-wide association study of 14,000 cases of seven common diseases and 3,000 shared controls. Nature 447: 661–678.
19. Smith EN, Bloss CS, Badner JA, Barrett T, Belmonte PL, et al. (2009) Genome-wide association study of bipolar disorder in European American and African American individuals. Mol Psychiatry 14: 755–763.
20. American Psychiatric Association (1994) Diagnostic and Statistical Manual of Mental Disorders. Washington, DC: American Psychiatric Press.
21. Nurnberger JI Jr, Blehar MC, Kaufmann CA, York-Cooler C, Simpson SG, et al. (1994) Diagnostic interview for genetic studies. Rationale, unique features, and training. NIMH Genetics Initiative. Arch Gen Psychiatry 51: 849–859; discussion 863–844.
22. Bellivier F, Golmard JL, Henry C, Leboyer M, Schurhoff F (2001) Admixture analysis of age at onset in bipolar I affective disorder. Arch Gen Psychiatry 58: 510–512.
23. Bellivier F, Golmard JL, Rietschel M, Schulze TG, Malafosse A, et al. (2003) Age at onset in bipolar I affective disorder: further evidence for three subgroups. Am J Psychiatry 160: 999–1001.
24. Lin PI, McInnis MG, Potash JB, Willour V, MacKinnon DF, et al. (2006) Clinical correlates and familial aggregation of age at onset in bipolar disorder. Am J Psychiatry 163: 240–246.
25. Manchia M, Lampus S, Chillotti C, Sardu C, Ardau R, et al. (2008) Age at onset in Sardinian bipolar I patients: evidence for three subgroups. Bipolar Disord 10: 443–446.
26. Heath SC, Gut IG, Brennan P, McKay JD, Bencko V, et al. (2008) Investigation of the fine structure of European populations with applications to disease association studies. Eur J Hum Genet 16: 1413–1429.
27. Miller SA, Dykes DD, Polesky HF (1988) A simple salting out procedure for extracting DNA from human nucleated cells. Nucleic Acids Res 16: 1215.
28. Purcell S, Neale B, Todd-Brown K, Thomas L, Ferreira MA, et al. (2007) PLINK: a tool set for whole-genome association and population-based linkage analyses. Am J Hum Genet 81: 559–575.
29. Spitzer RL, Endicott J, Robins E (1978) Research diagnostic criteria: rationale and reliability. Arch Gen Psychiatry 35: 773–782.
30. Manolio TA, Rodriguez LL, Brooks L, Abecasis G, Ballinger D, et al. (2007) New models of collaboration in genome-wide association studies: the Genetic Association Information Network. Nat Genet 39: 1045–1051.
31. Devlin B, Roeder K (1999) Genomic control for association studies. Biometrics 55: 997–1004.
32. Pulver AE, Lasseter VK, Kasch L, Wolyniec P, Nestadt G, et al. (1995) Schizophrenia: a genome scan targets chromosomes 3p and 8p as potential sites of susceptibility genes. Am J Med Genet 60: 252–260.
33. Kendler KS, Myers JM, O'Neill FA, Martin R, Murphy B, et al. (2000) Clinical features of schizophrenia and linkage to chromosomes 5q, 6p, 8p, and 10p in the Irish Study of High-Density Schizophrenia Families. Am J Psychiatry 157: 402–408.
34. Gurling HM, Kalsi G, Brynjolfson J, Sigmundsson T, Sherrington R, et al. (2001) Genomewide genetic linkage analysis confirms the presence of susceptibility loci for schizophrenia, on chromosomes 1q32.2, 5q33.2, and 8p21–22 and provides support for linkage to schizophrenia, on chromosomes 11q23.3–24 and 20q12.1–11.23. Am J Hum Genet 68: 661–673.
35. Cheng R, Juo SH, Loth JE, Nee J, Iossifov I, et al. (2006) Genome-wide linkage scan in a large bipolar disorder sample from the National Institute of Mental Health genetics initiative suggests putative loci for bipolar disorder, psychosis, suicide, and panic disorder. Mol Psychiatry 11: 252–260.
36. Zubenko GS, Maher BS, Hughes HB 3rd, Zubenko WN, Scott Stiffler J, et al. (2004) Genome-wide linkage survey for genetic loci that affect the risk of suicide attempts in families with recurrent, early-onset, major depression. Am J Med Genet B Neuropsychiatr Genet 129B: 47–54.
37. Adzhubei IA, Schmidt S, Peshkin L, Ramensky VE, Gerasimova A, et al. (2010) A method and server for predicting damaging missense mutations. Nat Methods 7: 248–249.
38. Skol AD, Scott LJ, Abecasis GR, Boehnke M (2006) Joint analysis is more efficient than replication-based analysis for two-stage genome-wide association studies. Nat Genet 38: 209–213.
39. Purcell SM, Wray NR, Stone JL, Visscher PM, O'Donovan MC, et al. (2009) Common polygenic variation contributes to risk of schizophrenia and bipolar disorder. Nature 460: 748–752.
40. Faraone SV, Glatt SJ, Su J, Tsuang MT (2004) Three potential susceptibility loci shown by a genome-wide scan for regions influencing the age at onset of mania. Am J Psychiatry 161: 625–630.
41. Avramopoulos D, Lasseter VK, Fallin MD, Wolyniec PS, McGrath JA, et al. (2007) Stage II follow-up on a linkage scan for bipolar disorder in the Ashkenazim provides suggestive evidence for chromosome 12p and the GRIN2B gene. Genet Med 9: 745–751.
42. Lorenzi C, Delmonte D, Pirovano A, Marino E, Bongiorno F, et al. (2010) Searching susceptibility loci for bipolar disorder: a sib pair study on chromosome 12. Neuropsychobiology 61: 10–18.
43. Dowler S, Currie RA, Campbell DG, Deak M, Kular G, et al. (2000) Identification of pleckstrin-homology-domain-containing proteins with novel phosphoinositide-binding specificities. Biochem J 351: 19–31.
44. Schloesser RJ, Huang J, Klein PS, Manji HK (2008) Cellular plasticity cascades in the pathophysiology and treatment of bipolar disorder. Neuropsychopharmacology 33: 110–133.
45. Mitchell GA, Kassovska-Bratinova S, Boukaftane Y, Robert MF, Wang SP, et al. (1995) Medical aspects of ketone body metabolism. Clin Invest Med 18: 193–216.
46. Kassovska-Bratinova S, Fukao T, Song XQ, Duncan AM, Chen HS, et al. (1996) Succinyl CoA: 3-oxoacid CoA transferase (SCOT): human cDNA cloning, human chromosomal mapping to 5p13, and mutation detection in a SCOT-deficient patient. Am J Hum Genet 59: 519–528.
47. Fukao T, Mitchell GA, Song XQ, Nakamura H, Kassovska-Bratinova S, et al. (2000) Succinyl-CoA:3-ketoacid CoA transferase (SCOT): cloning of the human SCOT gene, tertiary structural modeling of the human SCOT monomer, and characterization of three pathogenic mutations. Genomics 68: 144–151.
48. Torrey EF, Swalwell CI (2003) Fatal olanzapine-induced ketoacidosis. Am J Psychiatry 160: 2241.
49. Goodwin GM, Anderson I, Arango C, Bowden CL, Henry C, et al. (2008) ECNP consensus meeting. Bipolar depression. Nice, March 2007. Eur Neuropsychopharmacol 18: 535–549.
50. Fukuda H, Nishida A, Saito H, Shimizu M, Yamawaki S (1994) Imipramine stimulates phospholipase C activity in rat brain. Neurochem Int 25: 567–571.
51. Bouron A, Chatton JY (1999) Acute application of the tricyclic antidepressant desipramine presynaptically stimulates the exocytosis of glutamate in the hippocampus. Neuroscience 90: 729–736.

15

The Serenity of the Meditating Mind: A Cross-Cultural Psychometric Study on a Two-Factor Higher Order Structure of Mindfulness, Its Effects, and Mechanisms Related to Mental Health among Experienced Meditators

Ulrich S. Tran[1]*, Ausiàs Cebolla[2,3], Tobias M. Glück[1], Joaquim Soler[4,5], Javier Garcia-Campayo[6], Theresa von Moy[1]

1 University of Vienna, Vienna, Austria, **2** University Jaume I, Castelló de la Plana, Spain, **3** Ciber Fisiopatologia de la obesidad y la nutrición (CIBEROBN), Santiago de Compostela, Spain, **4** Department of Psychiatry, Hospital de la Santa Creu i Sant Pau, Barcelona, Spain, **5** Universitat Autònoma de Barcelona (UAB), Centro de Investigación Biomédica en Red de Salud Mental (CIBERSAM), Institut d'Investigació Biomèdica-Sant Pau (IIB-SANT PAU), Barcelona, Spain, **6** University of Zaragoza, Instituto Aragones de Ciencias de la Salud, Red Investigación Atención Primaria (RD 12/005/006), Zaragoza, Spain

Abstract

Objective: To investigate the psychometric and structural properties of the Five Facets Mindfulness Questionnaire (FFMQ) among meditators, to develop a short form, and to examine associations of mindfulness with mental health and the mechanisms of mindfulness.

Methods: Two independent samples were used, a German ($n = 891$) and a Spanish ($n = 393$) meditator sample, practicing various meditation styles. Structural and psychometric properties of the FFMQ were investigated with multigroup confirmatory factor analysis and exploratory structural equation modeling. Associations with mental health and mechanisms of mindfulness were examined with path analysis.

Results: The derived short form broadly matched a previous item selection in samples of non-meditators. Self-regulated Attention and Orientation to Experience governed the facets of mindfulness on a higher-order level. Higher-order factors of mindfulness and meditation experience were negatively associated with symptoms of depression and anxiety, and perceived stress. Decentering and nonattachment were the most salient mechanisms of mindfulness. Aspects of emotion regulation, bodily awareness, and nonattachment explained the effects of mindfulness on depression and anxiety.

Conclusions: A two-component conceptualization for the FFMQ, and for the study of mindfulness as a psychological construct, is recommended for future research. Mechanisms of mindfulness need to be examined in intervention studies.

Editor: Susana Jiménez-Murcia, University Hospital of Bellvitge-IDIBELL; CIBER Fisiopatología Obesidad y Nutrición (CIBERObn), Instituto Salud Carlos III; Department of Clinical Sciences, School of Medicine, University of Barcelona, Spain

Funding: These authors have no support or funding to report.

Competing Interests: The authors have declared that no competing interests exist.

* Email: ulrich.tran@univie.ac.at

Introduction

Converging evidence shows that mindfulness-based interventions (MBIs) are efficacious in the treatment of psychological disorders, the reduction of stress, and for improving well-being [1]. MBIs assume that mindfulness is an intrinsic state that all humans can cultivate through a variety of techniques, including, but not limited to, meditation. It is further assumed that long-term meditation practice cultivates mindfulness skills and that these skills, in turn, promote psychological well-being [2]. Parallel to the development of, and research on, MBIs there has been a growing interest regarding theoretical models of mindfulness [3,4], its assessment [5], and its mechanisms of action [6].

Bishop et al. [3] proposed a two-component model of mindfulness that incorporates self-regulated attention (i.e., sustained attention on the present moment) and orientation to experience (i.e., the open, curious, and accepting attitude), which is one of the most widely-adopted in the field [7]. So far, however, only one of the many widely-used mindfulness questionnaires has been developed with direct reference to a two-component conceptualization, the Philadelphia Mindfulness Scale [8,9]. Other widely-used questionnaires, like the Mindfulness Attention Awareness Scale (MAAS [10]), were developed with reference to Self-Determinant theory [11] or, as in the case of the Kentucky

Inventory Mindfulness Skills (KIMS [12]), Dialectical Behavior Therapy [13].

One comprehensive and increasingly applied self-report measure of mindfulness, the Five Facets of Mindfulness Inventory (FFMQ [14]), was derived from scales that measure mindfulness as a trait in daily life. The FFMQ is composed of 39 items, stemming from the KIMS, the Freiburg Mindfulness Inventory [15], the Mindfulness Questionnaire [16], the MAAS, and the Cognitive and Affective Mindfulness Scale [17]. It has a five-facetted structure: Observe, Describe, Act with Awareness, Nonjudging of Inner Experience and Nonreactivity to Inner Experience. Besides in English, the FFMQ has been validated in a number of other languages (Chinese [18], Dutch [19], German [20], Spanish [21], and Swedish [22]), using patient, meditating, and non-meditating samples.

Even though conceptualized to represent a hierarchical factor structure, with mindfulness on top of the five facets, empirical research among non-meditators repeatedly showed that Observe fits only insufficiently into this structure, or is even unrelated to overall mindfulness [14,19,20,22–24]. Among non-meditators, Observe appeared to indicate ruminative tendencies with regard to symptoms of anxiety, while facets of mindfulness were otherwise negatively related with psychological symptoms and positively with well-being [14,20,25]. Nonreact was reported to show only weak measurement properties [14,20].

Recently [20], it was suggested that the FFMQ may be better represented by a two-factor higher-order structure, representing Self-regulated Attention and Orientation to Experience, as in the model of Bishop et al. [3]. It was predicted that these two factors, only modestly correlated among non-meditators [20], would be more strongly correlated among meditators, reflecting thus effects of meditation experience. Currently, data on two possible higher-order factors of mindfulness, their intercorrelation, and their associations with mental health among meditators are lacking. Moreover, various short forms of the FFMQ have been proposed [18,20,22,26], indicating that its scale composition may need improvement. Items of the FFMQ were reported to show different psychometric properties among meditators and non-meditators [27]. Currently, it is unclear which FFMQ items are best suited to measure mindfulness, its facets, and its higher-order factor(s) among meditators.

Investigating the specificity of facets and higher-order factors of the FFMQ with regard to the beneficial effects of mindfulness on psychopathological symptoms and disorders appears specifically interesting for clinical research. Facet specificity of beneficial effects has been observed for symptoms of PTSD [28] and of anxiety and depression [29], involving specifically Actaware and Nonjudge that were later found to load also on the same higher-order factor, Orientation to Experience [20]. Changes of mindfulness may be reliably measured with the FFMQ, and the increase of mindfulness has been shown to specifically precede the reduction of stress, related to chronic illness, chronic pain, and other life circumstances, in a mindfulness-based stress reduction program [30]. More generally, it is known that mindfulness exerts beneficial effects on psychological health in various contexts and for different disorders [31], for example, by improving emotion regulation [32] and decreasing tendencies of rumination [33,34], which play an important role in most psychopathologies [35,36]. The evaluation of existing interventions, the development of new interventions, but also psychopathological research may thus benefit from investigations into mindfulness and by conceptualizing mindfulness on both a facet and on a higher-order level, using the FFMQ.

As to the mechanisms of action that underlie mindfulness, Hölzel et al. [6] proposed four major components: Attention regulation, body awareness, emotion regulation (reappraisal/revalorization; exposure, extinction, and reconsolidation), and a change in perspective on the self. Reviewed in detail by [6], mindfulness fosters the ability to sustain attention on a chosen object and to return attention to the object, when there have been distractions; bodily awareness is raised, as usually the object of attention is one of internal experience: Breathing, emotions, or bodily sensations. There are two effects on emotion regulation: One regarding the fostering of a nonjudgmental, accepting stance towards ongoing emotional reactions ('reappraisal' in [6]; here termed 'revalorization'); the other regarding the fostering of a willingness to expose oneself to whatever is in the field of awareness, and to refrain from (automatic) internal reactivity. Lastly, mindfulness brings with it a change in perspective on the self: An adaptive detachment from identifying with a static self; instead, mindfulness fosters the awareness that the self is not permanent and unchanging.

Even though there is ample of empirical evidence with regard to these four mechanisms (see [6]; for more recent evidence see, e.g., [37,38]), there have been, to our best of knowledge, no comprehensive attempts to systematically investigate the associations of these mechanisms with the facets and higher-order factor(s) of mindfulness among meditators yet. Determining which of these mechanisms primarily effectuate the beneficial effects of meditation and mindfulness on mental health could inform the future development of MBIs and help explaining why MBIs actually do work.

Therefore, the objectives of the present study were (a) to investigate the psychometric and structural properties of the FFMQ among experienced meditators, (b) to develop an abridged form of the FFMQ, thereby testing whether the item selections of previous short forms were replicable among meditators, and (c) to examine whether a two-factor higher-order structure, apparent among non-meditators, could also be observed among meditators. Finally, we examined the associations of the higher-order factor(s) of mindfulness with (d) depression, anxiety, and perceived stress, and (e) the proposed mechanisms of mindfulness, and we investigated (f) which mechanisms of mindfulness explained uniquely the beneficial effects of mindfulness on mental health (i.e., depression and anxiety). All psychometric and structural analyses, and analyses on the associations of mindfulness on depression and anxiety, were based on multigroup analyses, using two large and independent meditator samples from German-speaking countries and Spain. Results were thus cross-validated and analyses allowed also for cross-cultural comparisons, further broadening the generalizability of our results.

We hypothesized that a two-factor higher-order structure of mindfulness can be reliably replicated among experienced meditators, regardless of country of origin. However, we expected that the two higher-order factors were higher intercorrelated among meditators than previously among non-meditators. Furthermore, we expected that meditation experience increased the effects of mechanisms through which mindfulness exerts its beneficial effects on mental health, and that mechanisms of mindfulness fully mediated the associations of meditation experience and of mindfulness on mental health.

Method

Participants

Two meditator samples were used in this study, a predominantly German sample and a Spanish sample. Sample characteristics are displayed in Table 1. The German sample comprised 81% Germans, 15% Austrians, 2% Swiss, and 2% participants with other nationalities. Participants in both samples came from a wide age range and had various educational backgrounds. A majority meditated more often than on a weekly basis, around 52% four or more times a week in the German sample and around 36% on a daily basis in the Spanish sample (assessment of meditation frequency differed between samples). Most participants had meditated for more than four years, but there was also a wide range of meditation experience in the two samples.

Concerning sample differences, the German meditators included more women and were on average older and less highly educated than the Spanish meditators. However, the German meditators meditated more often and had on average more meditation experience than the Spanish meditators. With regard to meditation type, there were more Zen and Vipassana practitioners among the Spanish meditators, whereas more Tibetan meditation, yoga, and 'other' meditation styles practitioners among the German meditators. The 'other' category subsumed among German meditators mind-and-body meditation styles (15.8%), e.g., combinations of yoga and Vipassana or Zen, Transcendental Meditation (11.1%), Naikan (8.2%), Qi Gong (7.5%), Tai Chi (5.4%), and autogenic training (2.9%). The relatively large remaining proportion (49.1%) included various individual styles. Based on an Internet research, we concluded that from a technical point of view that these individual styles (e.g., Christian repetitive prayer or Tantra meditation practice) appeared not to differ substantially from styles like Vipassana, Zen, Transcendental meditation or yoga. They could also be roughly categorized into either concentrative, open monitoring, or a mixture of these two meditation styles.

The study was approved by the Aragon Ethics Committee (Spanish sample) and the department of psychology (German-speaking sample) and performed in accordance with the ethical standards of the 1964 Declaration of Helsinki (both samples) and Austrian ethical regulations for clinical research (German-speaking sample). All participants gave written informed consent prior to inclusion in the study.

Procedure and measures

Participants in the German sample were recruited with help of (1) the German Buddhist Union (*Deutsche Buddhistische Union*, DBU), an umbrella organization of 63 member-groups comprising more than 600 German Buddhists groups and of individual Buddhists; (2) the professional institution for German Yoga teachers (*Berufsverband der Yogalehrenden in Deutschland*, BDY), numbering more than 3000 members; (3) the Austrian Buddhist Society (*Österreichische Buddhistische Religionsgemeinschaft*, ÖBR), an umbrella organization of around 30 Austrian Buddhist groups. DBU, BDY, and ÖBR disseminated detailed information on the study and the link to an online survey (www.sociosurvey.de) among their members and member-groups. Data collection itself took place between July and September 2011. Participation was entirely anonymous and participants received no remuneration. There were no exclusion criteria except that participants had to be over 18 years of age. As an incentive, participants could opt-in to take part in the drawing of six Amazon gift cards, worth € 50 each. Participants were also encouraged to disseminate the link to the online survey among meditating friends and acquaintances. Furthermore, the link was also disseminated among non-meditators; these data, however, were not of interest for the present study. The online survey was accessed 2099 times, and complete data of 984 persons (47%) were obtained, another

Table 1. Sample Characteristics.

	German Sample	Spanish Sample	Statistical test
n	891	393	
Women, *n* (%)	661 (74.2%)	220 (56.0%)	$\chi^2(1) = 41.98^{***}$
Age, *M* (*SD*)	48.65 (10.52)	43.97 (10.60)	$t(1280) = 7.30^{***}$, $d = 0.44$
Min–Max	20–82	18–75	
Education			
Primary or lower secondary	10 (1.1%)	7 (1.8%)	$\chi^2(2) = 54.26^{***}$
Upper secondary	363 (40.7%)	77 (19.6%)	
University/diploma	518 (58.1%)	309 (78.6%)	
Frequency meditating			
> Once a week	675 (75.8%)	256 (66.1%)[a]	$\chi^2(2) = 13.46^{***}$
Once a week	66 (7.4%)	46 (11.9%)[a]	
<Once a week	150 (16.8%)	85 (22.0%)[a]	
Meditation experience in years (*Md*)[b]	8.00	4.00	*U* test, $z = 7.90^{***}$
Min–Max, interquartile range	0–45, 4–15	0–43, 2–10	
Meditation type[c]			
Zen	102 (11.5%)	110 (39.0%)	$\chi^2(4) = 369.32^{***}$
Vipassana	107 (12.0%)	136 (48.2%)	
Tibetan	54 (6.1%)	5 (1.8%)	
Yoga	348 (39.1%)	24 (8.5%)	
Other	279 (31.3%)	7 (2.5%)	

Note. [a] Based on 387 participants due to incomplete data. Based on [b] 738 and 348/[c] 890 and 282 participants, respectively, for which data were available. *** $p<.001$.

17 persons (<1%) provided incomplete data. Of the 984 persons with complete data, 891 (91%) were identified as practicing meditators and kept for further analysis. DBU, BDY, ÖBR, and participants disseminated the information on the study and the link to the survey independently and autonomously. Therefore, it is not possible to state exactly how many persons received the link to the survey and what percentage decided to participate.

The Spanish sample was recruited with help of several Spanish scientific research portals related to mindfulness and meditation. It was also sent to several mindfulness associations, Zen monasteries, and sanghas, and to a non-meditator convenience sample. A survey containing several questionnaires was developed using a commercial on-line survey system (www.surveymonkey.com; Portland, OR, USA), and a link to this website was posted on several other websites. The survey was available for response between April 2011 and December 2012. In total, 917 subjects accessed the link, while 850 (93%) voluntarily agreed to participate, of which 670 (79%) filled in the survey's scales and questionnaires fully. Of these, 384 (57%) were identified as practicing meditators and kept for further analysis.

Mindfulness. Mindfulness was assessed with the German [20] and the Spanish [21] form of the full 39-item FFMQ. Items are scored on a 5-point scale from 1 = *never or very rarely true* to 5 = *very often or always true*, assessing five facets of mindfulness, Observe, Describe, Acting with Awareness (Actaware), Nonjudging of Inner Experience (Nonjudge), and Nonreactivity to Inner Experience (Nonreact), with eight items (seven items in Nonreact) each. Cronbach alpha of the full facet scales lay between .79 (Observe) and .91 (Nonjudge) in the German sample and between .81 (Observe) and .94 (Nonjudge) in the Spanish sample, respectively; Cronbach alphas in Nonreact were satisfactory for both samples, .87 in the German and .86 in the Spanish sample.

Depression and anxiety. Symptoms of depression and anxiety were assessed with the depression and anxiety scales of the Brief Symptom Inventory (BSI; German form [39]) in the German sample, and the Depression, Anxiety and Stress scale (DAS-21 [40]; Spanish form [41]) in the Spanish sample. The BSI assesses the prevalence and distress caused by a variety of symptoms during the last seven days. Depression and anxiety are assessed with six items each, scored on a 5-point scale from 0 = *not at all* to 4 = *extremely*. The DAS-21 has three subscales that measure depression, anxiety, and stress with seven items each. Subjects assess the frequency/severity of 21 negative emotional symptoms during the previous week. Each item comprises a statement and four short response options to reflect severity and scored from 0 = *did not apply to me at all* to 3 = *applied to me very much, or most of the time*. Cronbach alpha was.81 (depression) and.80 (anxiety) in the German sample and.90 and.85, respectively, in the Spanish sample.

For multigroup analysis, scores of the two samples were equated, using methods described by [42]. Equating allows the mapping of scores of different groups or measures on a common scale, ensuring that scores relate to the same underlying dimension. For equating, we identified similar items that had been devised in both groups. Items 10, 13, 16, and 17 of the DAS-21 depression scale were similar in content to Items 5, 2, 6, and 3 of the BSI depression scale, assessing feelings of hopelessness, depressed mood, lack of interest, and feelings of worthlessness (in this order); Items 7, 15, and 20 of the DAS-21 anxiety scale were similar in content to Items 10, 11, and 9 of the BSI anxiety scale, assessing tremulousness, fits of panic and fear, and being scared without reason (in this order). These sets of similar items were used for equating, utilizing structural equation modeling (see the Statistical analysis section).

Perceived stress. Perceived stress was assessed in the German sample with the German form the revised Perceived Stress Questionnaire (PSQ [43]), an economic and well-validated 20-item measure with four scales: Stress, Worries, Tension, Joy, and Demands, assessed with five items each. Items are scored on a 4-point scale from 1 = *almost never* to 4 = *usually*, asking respondents to rate the frequency of having experienced various stress reactions (Worries, Tension, Joy) and stressors (Demands) during the last four weeks. Cronbach alpha lay between.86 and.87 in the four scales.

Mechanisms of mindfulness. A number of likely mechanisms of mindfulness [6], were assessed in the Spanish sample with the Effortful Control Scale (EC [44]; Spanish form [45]), the Scale of Body Connection (SBC [46]; Spanish form [47]), the Experience Questionnaire (EQ [48]; Spanish form [2]), the Difficulties in Emotion Regulation Scale (DERS [49]; Spanish form [50]), and the Nonattachment Scale (NAS [51]).

The 19-item EC measured executive attention with three subscales: Attentional Control (seven items; the ability to intentionally shift and focus attention), Inhibitory Control (five items; the ability to inhibit a dominant, positively toned, response that may entail approach behavior), and Activation Control (seven items; the ability to suppress a dominant, negatively toned, response that may entail avoidance behavior). Items are rated on a 7-point Likert scale (1 = *extremely untrue of you* to 7 = *extremely true of you*). Cronbach alpha was .76.

The 20-item SBC measured Body Awareness (12 items; conscious attention to sensory signals that indicate the state of the body, i.e., tension, nervousness, relaxation) and Body Dissociation (eight items; body connection and separation, including emotional connection with one's body). Items are scored on a 5-point Likert scale, ranging from 0 = *not at all* to 4 = *all the time*. Cronbach alpha was.86 (Body Awareness) and.67 (Body Dissociation). For ease of interpretation, the Body Dissociation scale was reverse scored and termed Body Association (higher scores indicating higher bodily association) for purposes of the present study.

Aspects of emotion regulation were measured with the EQ and the DERS. The 11-item EQ measures decentering, i.e., the capacity to observe one's thoughts and feelings as temporary and objective events of the mind [2,48]. Decentering is a unidimensional construct, related to metacognitive awareness [52], and comprises three facets: The ability to view one's self as not synonymous with one's thoughts, the ability not to habitually react to one's negative experiences, and the capacity for self-compassion (i.e., a positive and caring stance towards the self). Given that decentering is the ability of not being entangled with emotions and other internal events [48], it has been considered an aspect of emotional regulation in the present study. Items are rated on a 5-point Likert scale ranging from 1 = *never or very rarely true* to 5 = *very often or always true*. Cronbach alpha was .89.

The DERS measured difficulties in emotion regulation. The Spanish form [50], that was utilized in this study, comprises 28 items and five scales, instead of the 36 items and six scales of the English form (Non acceptance of Emotions, Difficulties Engaging in Goal-Directed Behavior When Distressed, Impulse Control Difficulties, Lack of Emotional Awareness, Limited Access to Emotion Regulation Strategies, Lack of Emotional Clarity; items of the Impulse Control Difficulties and Limited Access to Emotion Regulation Strategies scales form a single scale in the Spanish form). For ease of interpretation, the DERS scales were reverse scored in the present study so that higher scores reflected greater ability, not more problems with emotion regulation. We termed the scales in the present study in the following way: Acceptance of

Emotions (seven items), Goals (four items), Control & Regulation (nine items; containing items of the Impulse Control Difficulties and Limited Access to Emotion Regulation Strategies scales), Emotional Awareness (four items), and Emotional Clarity (four items). With regard to their theoretical status, see [6], Acceptance of Emotions, Emotional Awareness, and Emotional Clarity each tap into the revalorization dimension of emotion regulation, whereas Goals and Control & Regulation into the exposure and reconsolidation dimension. Items are rated on a 5-point scale from 1 = *almost never* to 5 = *almost always*. Internal consistency in the present sample was .89.

Changes in perspective on the self were measured with the 30-item NAS. The NAS measures nonattachment, i.e., a subjective quality characterized by a relative absence of fixation on ideas, images, or sensory objects, as well as an absence of internal pressure to get, hold, avoid, or change circumstances or experiences [51]. Items are scored on a 6-point scale from 1 = *disagree strongly* to 6 = *agree strongly*. Cronbach alpha was .92.

Statistical analysis

Structural analysis of the FFMQ and construction of a short form. The structure and measurement characteristics of the full FFMQ were assessed with multigroup structural equation modeling (SEM) in the two samples, testing for configural invariance (i.e., equality of the factor structure across the samples) of a correlated five-factor model [14].

A short form was then constructed, informed also by the results of a multigroup exploratory structural equation modeling (ESEM [53]) analysis that tested for item cross-loadings that may otherwise be overlooked in traditional SEM analysis. ESEM integrates exploratory (EFA) and confirmatory factor analysis (CFA) and allows the free estimation of cross-loadings as in EFA, but also provides standard errors and goodness-of-fit statistics as in CFA and SEM. ESEM was previously used to investigate the higher-order structure of the FFMQ in samples of non-meditators [20], but not the multidimensional structure of the items themselves. Items were then selected that: (1) loaded highest on their designated factor; (2) had no cross-loadings on the other factors; (3) were not redundant with other items in their scale; (4) maximized fit of a one-factor model (unidimensionality of facets) in both samples.

Structural invariance was re-assessed with the short form, testing: (a) configural invariance; (b) (full) measurement invariance (i.e., constraining all item loadings and thresholds to equality across samples); (c) partial measurement invariance, relaxing equality constraints for items where indicated by modification indices. The analyses (b) and (c) served to examine whether items in the FFMQ had the same measurement properties in the two samples and to determine a common origin and scale for estimating mindfulness in the two samples. Improvement of data fit of the partial measurement model versus the full measurement model was investigated with Mplus's DIFFTEST option.

Structural analyses were conducted with Mplus 6.11 [54], using the weighted least square mean- and variance-adjusted (WLSMV) estimator that is based on the polychoric item correlation matrix and that provides estimates of item loadings and thresholds. WLSMV estimation is suited for ordered categorical variables and provides robust parameter estimates, standard errors, and tests of model fit [55]. WLSMV estimation was previously used in FFMQ item analyses in samples of non-meditators [20]. Model fit was assessed using widely-used benchmarks [56], utilizing the comparative fit index (CFI), the Tucker-Lewis index (TLI; CFI and TLI: good fit: ≥.95, acceptable fit: ≥.90), and the root mean square error of approximation (RMSEA; good fit: <.06, acceptable fit: <.08). In models with small degrees of freedom (*df*), as in the ESEM analyses and analyses of unidimensionality of facets, model fit was primarily assessed with CFI and TLI as RMSEA may then be overinflated [57].

Higher-order structure of mindfulness. ESEM analysis currently does not allow the direct investigation of higher-order structures in item analysis; hence, facet factor scores of the final partial measurement invariance model were used to investigate the higher-order structure of the FFMQ with multigroup ESEM analysis, fitting a two-factor model to the data and using QUARTIMAX rotation and a maximum likelihood estimator that approximates the standard errors by first-order derivatives (MLF) [20].

Effects and mechanisms of mindfulness. Higher-order factor scores were then utilized in multigroup path models to investigate the effects of mindfulness on depression and anxiety, on perceived stress (German meditators only), on mechanisms of mindfulness (Spanish meditators only), and of mechanisms of mindfulness on depression and anxiety (Spanish meditators only), controlling also for meditation experience in each analysis. As meditation experience was positively skewed (skewness = 1.41 across both samples), the logarithm of meditation experience in months was used for all correlational analyses. Age and meditation experience correlated with $r = .41$ ($p < .001$) across both samples. In the presence of meditation experience, age exerted no significant ($p > .05$) or substantial effect (standardized parameter estimates <.10) on the other variables in any of the investigated models and was therefore excluded from all path analyses. Mplus 6.11 was used for path analyses, using the robust maximum likelihood (MLR) estimator that allows and corrects for non-normality in continuous scores and provides robust standard errors, based on a sandwich estimator. Mplus' full-information maximum likelihood (FIML) option was utilized, using all available data for parameter estimation, allowing the inclusion of participants with missing data regarding their meditation experience (see Table 1). Participants with missing data in meditation experience differed neither with regard to sex ($\chi^2(1) = 0.04$, $p = .849$), age ($t(1280) = 0.08$, $p = .938$), nor education ($\chi^2(2) = 1.76$, $p = .414$) from other participants, but reported a lower frequency of meditation than other participants ($\chi^2(2) = 758.45$, $p < .001$). Thus, participants with missingness regarding their meditation experience were likely less experienced meditators.

Equating depression and anxiety scores for multigroup analysis. Items with similar content in the DAS-21 and BSI were used to equate factor scores of depression and anxiety in the two samples. Multigroup 1-factor models were fit to the data, constraining in a first step the loadings of the equated items to equality across groups (full measurement invariance), but relaxing these constraints in subsequent steps (partial measurement invariance), where necessary. Mplus 6.11 was used, utilizing WLSMV estimation. The BSI is scored on a 5-point scale, the DAS-21 on a 4-point scale; thus, the two highest response options were combined in the BSI items. Factor scores on a common scale were then used in multigroup analysis to investigate the effects of mindfulness on depression and anxiety.

Results

Construction of a short form and invariance testing

Fit of the configural invariance five-factor model in the full FFMQ is displayed in Table 2. While RMSEA appeared acceptable (<.06), CFI and TLI were below a cutoff of.95 each, indicating that fit could be still improved. A five-factor multigroup ESEM model fitted the data considerably better than the confirmatory model, $\chi^2(1394) = 2904.15$, CFI = .971, TLI = .969, RMSEA = .041 [.039,.043]. Factor loadings are displayed in Table S1. Some items in Describe (Items 12 and 16) and Actaware (Items 23, 28, 34, and 38) displayed non-negligible cross-loadings on the Observe factor, while loadings of items in Observe where overall low (lowest in Items 11 and 36) and items had also cross-loadings on the Nonreact factor (Items 1 and 36). Item 13 in Actaware had a cross-loading on the Nonreact factor as well.

Final item selections and Cronbach alpha coefficients of the short scales are displayed in Table 3. Elimination of items improved unidimensionality of all five facets, strongest in Observe, Describe, and Actaware with regard to CFI and TLI (Table 4). Despite a cross-loading on the Nonreact factor, Item 13 was kept in Actaware as it had the highest loading of all items on its designated factor. Item selections were fully concordant with a previous item selection in samples of non-meditators [20] in Observe and Actaware, and partially concordant (three items) in Nonjudge. In Describe only one item (Item 32) was concordant, with Item 2 being similar in content to Item 37 that was selected in non-meditators instead. Largest differences were observed in Nonreact, where only the selection of one item (Item 21) matched across studies. Differences in item selections likely stemmed from differences in meditation experience, especially with regard to Nonreact that was found to be psychometrically weak among non-meditators [20]. Differences, however, may have also stemmed from differences in methodology, as the item selection in the present study also controlled for, and minimized, item cross-loadings via ESEM analysis.

The configural invariance five-factor model fitted considerably better to the short form than to the full FFMQ (Table 2). Descriptively, a full measurement invariance model fitted the data as well. However, a partial measurement invariance model, estimating loadings and thresholds of five items, one per scale, freely across samples, improved the model fit significantly (DIFFTEST: $\chi^2(25)$ = 249.78, $p<.001$).

Table 3 displays standardized loadings in the final partial measurement invariance model. Even though unidimensionality was not violated in the respective scales in either sample, Item 20 had only a low loading in the German sample, whereas Item 32 in the Spanish sample, indicating differences in psychometric properties across samples/languages even in this purified FFMQ item selection. Based on estimates derived from the partial measurement model, samples differed significantly in three of the five FFMQ facets: The German meditators had slightly lower values in Observe ($d = -0.15$, $p = .028$), but higher values in Actaware ($d = 0.44$, $p<.001$) and Nonjudge ($d = 0.21$, $p = .003$) than the Spanish meditators (Describe: $d = -0.06$, $p = .363$; Nonreact: $d = 0.07$, $p = .305$).

Table 5 displays factor intercorrelations in the unconstrained configural invariance five-factor model in the full FFMQ and the final partial measurement invariance model in the short form. As can be seen, the factor intercorrelation pattern was similar in the two samples and was closely reproduced in the short form; however, consistent with observed cross-loadings, correlations of Actaware with Observe and Describe, and of Nonreact with Observe, were somewhat higher in the full FFMQ than in the short form. As items in the short form were free of cross-loadings, one may therefore infer that factor intercorrelations were more accurately estimated in the short form.

Higher-order structure

Multigroup ESEM analysis of the facet factor scores indicated that the fit of a two-factor higher-order model could be still improved, $\chi^2(11)$ = 126.26, CFI = .956, TLI = .920, RMSEA = .128 [.108,.148]. Modification indices suggested a residual dependence of Observe and Describe. Allowing for this dependence, and constraining the variance of Nonreact to be positive, to ensure a positive definite correlation matrix, model fit was improved, $\chi^2(10) = 88.43$, CFI = .970, TLI = .940, RMSEA = .111 [.090,.132].

Facet factor loadings of this final model are displayed in Table 6. Residual variances of Observe and Describe correlated with $r = .36$ ($p<.001$) in the German and $r = .13$ ($p = .018$) in the Spanish sample. The loading pattern was broadly similar to the pattern in non-meditating samples [20]; however, Nonreact, not Observe, appeared to be the most important facet of Self-regulated Attention. In turn, Nonreact did not load on Orientation to Experience as among non-meditators. Nonjudge had a small positive loading on Self-regulated Attention. Similar to previous results, Actaware was the most important facet of Orientation to Experience, followed by Nonjudge. Observe had a small, but positive (negative in [20]), loading on this higher-order factor as well. The two higher-order factors correlated with $r = .69$ and .62 ($ps<.001$), respectively, considerably higher than in non-meditating samples [20].

Based on estimates derived from this model, the German meditators had, with a medium effect size, higher scores than the Spanish meditators in Orientation to Experience ($d = 0.53$, $p<.001$), but not in Self-regulated Attention ($d = -0.06$, $p = .316$).

Effects of meditation experience and mindfulness

Depression and anxiety. Clinically relevant levels of depression and anxiety in the German sample were similar to levels expected in the general population, according to the norm data of the BSI: With regard to depression 19.9% of participants, and with regard to anxiety 13.6% participants had a T value (adult

Table 2. Fit of Five-Factor Multigroup Models on All Five Facets.

	χ^2 (*df*)	CFI	TLI	RMSEA [90%-CI]
Full FFMQ				
Configural invariance	4130.30 (1384)	.947	.944	.056 [.054,.058]
20-Item Short Form				
Configural invariance	1028.76 (320)	.971	.965	.059 [.055,.063]
Measurement invariance	1400.26 (410)	.959	.962	.061 [.058,.065]
Partial measurement invariance*	1167.52 (385)	.968	.968	.056 [.053,.060]

Note. * Estimating loadings and thresholds of Items 4, 17, 18, 20, and 32 freely in both groups.

Table 3. Factor Loadings in the Partial Measurement Invariance Five-Factor Model.

Observe			Describe			Actaware			Nonjudge			Nonreact		
Item	Ger	Span	Item	Ger	Span	Item	Ger	Span	Item	Ger	Span	Item	Ger	Span
15	.82	.78	**2**	.81	.85	**5R**	.81	.84	17R*	.74	.82	4*	.63	.75
20*	.49	.74	7	.81	.85	**8R**	.74	.78	**25R**	.90	.90	**21**	.75	.71
26	.81	.76	27	.79	.83	**13R**	.87	.91	**30R**	.90	.90	29	.79	.74
31	.73	.69	**32***	.68	.48	**18R***	.76	.85	**35R**	.83	.83	33	.87	.82
α	.75	.77		.81	.80		.83	.86		.87	.89		.80	.79

Note. Ger = German sample; Span = Spanish sample. α = Cronbach Alpha. Numbers refer to standardized factor loadings in the partial measurement invariance model where unstandardized loadings and thresholds were constrained to equality across samples. Items that were similarly retained in non-meditating samples (see text) are printed boldface. * Loadings and thresholds estimated freely in both groups. All *ps*<.001.

norm of the BSI) at or greater than 63, considered reliably indicative of clinically relevant symptoms. This compares to around 16% that would have been expected with regard to normative data. In the Spanish sample 6.5% of participants reported severe or extremely severe symptoms in depression, whereas 7.1% in anxiety, according to the scoring of the DAS-21. Structural equation modeling revealed a good fit of a 1-factor model with full measurement invariance to the depression ratings of the German and Spanish meditators on the four common items of the BSI and DAS-21, $\chi^2(18)$ =91.80, p<.001, CFI=.979, TLI=.986, RMSEA=.081 [.065,.097]. Relaxing equality assumptions for Item pair 7 (DAS-21) and 10 (BSI), fit of a 1-factor model with partial measurement invariance was also good for the three common anxiety items, $\chi^2(6)$ = 24.21, p <.001, CFI = .986, TLI = .986, RMSEA = .069 [.042,.099]. A path model was fitted on the equated factor scores to explain the associations of the higher-order factors with depression and anxiety and of meditation experience on mindfulness (see Table S2 for the correlational pattern in raw scores). Equated factor scores correlated.91 and.84 (both ps<.001) with the standardized depression and anxiety raw scores across both samples.

The multigroup model, depicted in Figure 1, had a good fit to the data, $\chi^2(4)$ =2.11, p =.716, CFI = 1.000, TLI =1.000, RMSEA =.000 [.000,.044]. There was an overall tendency that Self-regulated Attention was slightly less indicative of depression and anxiety than Orientation to Experience. However, there were also substantive differences between the two samples: Effects of Orientation to Experience on anxiety were markedly higher among the Spanish than the German meditators. In turn, the contribution of Self-regulated Attention on anxiety was negligible among Spanish meditators, but of similar size to that of Orientation to Experience among the German meditators. Overall, the model explained 24% (24%) of the variance of depression scores in German and Spanish meditators, respectively, and 18% (27%) of anxiety scores. The total effect (standardized estimates) of meditation experience on depression and anxiety scores amounted to -.15/-.15 (depression), and -.13/-.14 (anxiety; all ps <.001) in German and Spanish meditators, respectively.

Perceived stress. German meditators were similar in their reported levels of perceived stress (Table S3) to healthy adults [43]. A similar path model as for depression and anxiety was fitted to the German data regarding perceived stress (Table S3). The model fitted the data well, $\chi^2(4)$ = 5.95, p =.203, CFI =.999, TLI =.997, RMSEA =.023 [.000,.060], and is depicted in Figure 2. Orientation to Experience was, again, a slightly stronger predictor of all facets of perceived stress save Joy than Self-regulated Attention, corroborating the pattern obtained before with regard to depression and anxiety. Overall, the model explained 36% to 38% of the variance of Worries, Tension, and Joy scores, respectively, and 16% of the Demands score variance. The total effect (standardized estimates) of meditation experience on the former three scores was around.18 each (ps <.001) and.12 (p <.001) on Demands scores.

Mechanisms of mindfulness

Two final path models were fitted on the Spanish data (Table S4) to explore (1) mechanisms of mindfulness and (2) to identify those mechanisms that exerted unique beneficial effects on mental health. The first path model incorporated paths from meditation experience to the higher-order factors of mindfulness that, in turn, had paths to all proposed mechanisms. Paths of the higher-order factors to mechanisms were then deleted, where insignificant (p> .05). The final model had a good fit to the data, $\chi^2(18)$ = 35.42, p<.001, CFI =.993, TLI =.960, RMSEA =.050 [.025,.074].

Table 4. Fit of One-Factor Multigroup Models in Individual Facets.

	χ^2 (*df*)	CFI	TLI	RMSEA [90%-CI]
Observe	263.48 (40)	.959	.943	.093 [.083,.104]
Observe-short	11.48 (4)	.998	.993	.054 [.019,.092]
Describe	680.16 (40)	.965	.950	.158 [.148,.168]
Describe-short	6.60 (4)	1.000	.999	.032 [.000,.073]
Actaware	867.30 (40)	.941	.918	.179 [.169,.190]
Actaware-short	39.64 (4)	.995	.986	.118 [.086,.152]
Nonjudge	225.08 (40)	.991	.988	.085 [.074,.096]
Nonjudge-short	18.79 (4)	.999	.996	.076 [.044,.112]
Nonreact	232.85 (28)	.982	.973	.107 [.094,.120]
Nonreact-short	10.50 (4)	.999	.996	.050 [.013,.089]

Standardized path coefficients, explained variance, and total effects of meditation experience on mechanisms are presented in Table 7. Mindfulness was associated with all proposed mechanisms, strongest with Decentering and Nonattachment. Mindfulness was weakest associated with Emotional Awareness and Activation Control. Notably, a number of mechanisms were differentially associated with the higher-order factors of mindfulness: Acceptance of Emotions, Control & Regulation, Emotional Clarity, Attentional Control, Goals, Bodily Association, and Activation Control were stronger or exclusively associated with Orientation to Experience, whereas Body Awareness, Inhibitory Control,and Emotional Awareness with Self-regulated Attention. For Decentering and Nonattachment associations with the higher-order factors were of similar magnitude.

In the second model, depression and anxiety were included as endogenous variables, connected with paths to the mechanisms that were now mediating variables. Paths of mechanisms to depression and anxiety that were insignificant ($p>.05$), and mechanisms themselves that had no remaining significant paths, were then deleted in a stepwise procedure. The final model had a good fit to the data, $\chi^2(16)$ = 10.87, p =.818, CFI = 1.000, TLI = 1.000, RMSEA =.000 [.000,.029], it is depicted in Figure 3. Body Awareness, Acceptance of Emotions, Control & Regulation, Emotional Clarity, and Nonattachment remained in the model. For both depression and anxiety, Acceptance of Emotions, Control & Regulation, and Emotional Clarity were important mechanisms, Acceptance of Emotions most important regarding depression, Emotional Clarity most important regarding anxiety. Otherwise, Nonattachment was a further important and specific mechanism regarding depression, whereas Body Awareness regarding anxiety. Overall, the model explained 59% of the variance of depression scores and 57% of the variance of anxiety scores. The total effect (standardized estimates) of the higher-order factors (Self-regulated Attention/Orientation to Experience) on depression and anxiety scores amounted to -.33/-.31 (depression) and -.26/-.32 (anxiety; all *ps* <.003).

Discussion

In two large and independent samples of German and Spanish meditators we investigated the psychometric and structural properties of the FFMQ, constructed a short form of the FFMQ, and confirmed a two-factor higher-order structure of mindfulness, delineating Self-regulated Attention and Orientation to Experience, previously reported in samples of non-meditators [20]. The higher-order factors contributed mostly similarly to mental health and, among the proposed mechanisms of action, fostered strongest emotion regulation and a detached, but adaptive, perspective on thoughts, emotions, and the self. Body and emotional awareness, and inhibitory control (i.e., control over responses that entail approach behavior) had unique, or stronger, paths to Self-regulated Attention, whereas bodily association, and attentional and activation control (i.e., the intentional management of attention and control over responses that entail avoidance behavior) to Orientation to Experience. Body awareness, a detachment from identifying with a static self, and, especially, the accepting and regulating aspects of emotion regulation were found to be mediators that uniquely explained the associations of meditation and mindfulness with depression and anxiety. We discuss our findings in detail in the following.

Table 5. Factor Intercorrelations in the Five-Factor Multigroup Models.

	Observe	Describe	Actaware	Nonjudge	Nonreact
Observe		.50/.48	.50/.48	.37/.33	.64/.71
Describe	.49/.47		.45/.43	.40/.44	.51/.51
Actaware	.35/.39	.33/.28		.61/.55	.54/.49
Nonjudge	.35/.32	.34/.33	.54/.54		.53/.55
Nonreact	.50/.66	.47/.56	.50/.42	.51/.53	

Note. Figures in the upper triangular matrix display factor intercorrelations in the configural invariance model in the full FFMQ (left: German sample; right: Spanish sample), whereas figures in the lower triangular matrix factor intercorrelations in the partial measurement invariance model in the short form. All *ps*<.001.

Table 6. Facet Factor Loadings in the Two-Factor Higher-Order Multigroup ESEM Analysis.

	Self-regulated Attention		Orientation to Experience	
	German	Spanish	German	Spanish
Observe	.57***	.60***	.12*	.14*
Describe	.55***	.54***	.07	.08
Actaware	-.03	-.03	.90***	.89***
Nonjudge	.27***	.25***	.50***	.51***
Nonreact	.99***	.98***	-.03	-.03

Note. * $p<.05$, *** $p<.001$.

FFMQ short form

Our item selection in meditator samples broadly reproduced the previous item selection in non-meditator samples [20]. Item selections were identical, or mostly identical, in Observe, Actaware, and Nonjudge, but differed in Describe and, even more so, in Nonreact. Shortening the FFMQ raised model fit and improved psychometric properties, as in previous research with non-meditators [20]. Differences in item selections may be explained by differences between meditators and non-meditators in comprehending the item contents of the FFMQ [7]. Van Dam et al. [7] reported that non-meditators, but not meditators, responded differently to positively and negatively worded items. Nonreact had only weak psychometric properties in non-meditating samples [14,20], but it was the most salient facet of Self-regulated Attention in the meditator samples in the present study, surpassing Observe, that proved the most salient facet in non-meditating samples [20]. Nonreact may thus measure different constructs in meditating and non-meditating samples. It has been previously suggested [58] that among meditator samples Observe and Nonreact could be especially sensitive to formal meditation practice [25,59]. Considering this, both facets, along with decentering, seem to efficiently differentiate among those who have daily practice meditation from those who never have meditated [2,59].

Given the seemingly paradoxical positive associations of Observe with symptoms of anxiety in non-meditating samples in previous research [14,20,25], it is of interest that the selection of Observe items among meditators here was fully consistent with the previous item selection among non-meditators; i.e., even though Observe differs with regard to its effects among meditators and non-meditators, items appear to measure one-and-the-same construct.

In conclusion, the previous FFMQ item selection obtained in non-meditating samples [20] was mostly replicated in the meditating samples in the present study, suggesting that the previously proposed short form is mostly also valid for meditators, and this not only in German language, but also in Spanish. With regard to Nonreact, it is recommended to use the full scale in future assessments with meditators and non-meditators, as item selections, psychometric properties, and possibly also measured trait, differed for this scale between meditators and non-meditators.

Higher-order structure of mindfulness

Replicating previous results [20], a two-factor higher-order structure of mindfulness was recovered in the meditating samples in the present study, with very similar results among German and Spanish meditators. As predicted, the higher-order factors correlated higher among meditators, r = .69 and.62 in the German and Spanish samples, than among non-meditators, r = .18 to.27 [20]. These results may be interpreted as a direct proof, and suggest a broad applicability, of the two-component model of mindfulness [3], with regard to both the conceptualization and measurement of mindfulness in the domain of self-report. In essence, these results suggest that self-reported mindfulness is, both among meditators and non-meditators, a multi-facetted, but two-factorial construct, whose homogeneity increases with meditation experience. The two-component model is also informative for, readily compatible with, and applicable to, traditional Buddhist and contemporary meditation practices, and has also received broad neuroscientific support

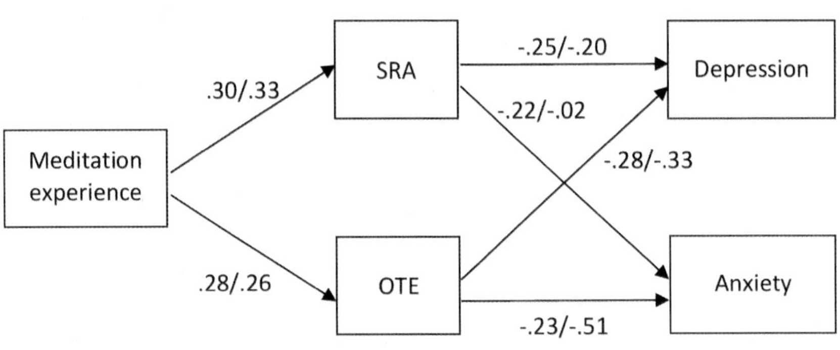

Figure 1. Multigroup path model on the effects of meditation experience on mindfulness and on depression and anxiety. Numbers are standardized path coefficients (left: German sample; right: Spanish sample). SRA = Self-regulated Attention; OTE = Orientation to Experience. Self-regulated Attention and Orientation to experience were allowed to correlate, as were depression and anxiety. All $ps < .002$, except for the path of SRA to anxiety in the Spanish sample, $p = .786$.

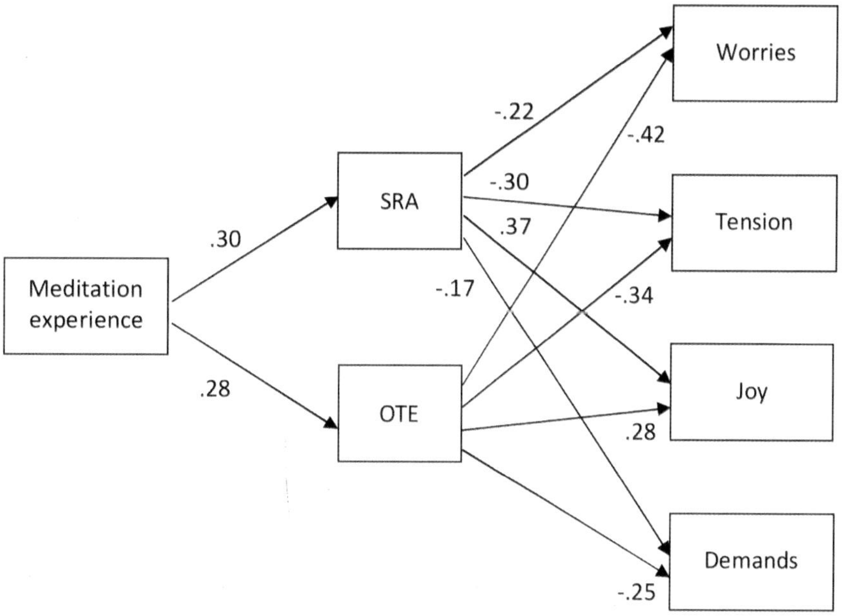

Figure 2. Path model on the effects of meditation experience on mindfulness and on facets of perceived stress in the German data. Numbers are standardized path coefficients. SRA = Self-regulated Attention; OTE = Orientation to Experience. Self-regulated Attention and Orientation to experience were allowed to correlate, as were the facets of perceived stress. All *ps*≤.001.

[7]. We thus recommend using such a two-component model as the standard model to describe and explain mindfulness.

The observed differences between Spanish and German meditators regarding mean levels in Orientation to Experience could stem from sample differences: First, the Spanish sample comprised relatively more Vipassana and Zen practitioners than the German sample. Vipassana and Zen meditation does not involve much physical motion, whereas yoga, of which the German sample included a high percentage of practitioners, has a focus on bodily movements, using postures, or *asanas*, and slow movements to center the attention, which may help training Orientation to Experience more than Vipassana or Zen.

Second, the German meditators had been practicing longer, and were thus in all likelihood more experienced, than the Spanish meditators. Previous research suggests increases of mindfulness with practice [2,22,25,59,60]. Taken at face value, our results suggest that Orientation to Experience increased at a possibly slower rate than Self-regulated Attention, or, alternatively, with a time-lag, as Self-regulated Attention did not differ between the two samples. This would fit conceptual and neuroscientific consider-

Table 7. Mechanisms of Mindfulness in Descending Order of Explained Variance.

	Standardized path coefficients			Total effect of meditation
	SRA	OTE	R^2	experience
Decentering	.45	.40	61%	.25
Nonattachment	.39	.36	47%	.22
Acceptance of Emotions[a]	.21	.46	38%	.19
Control & Regulation[a]	.25	.41	37%	.19
Emotional Clarity[a]	.23	.40	35%	.18
Attentional Control	–	.59	35%	.15
Body Awareness	.52	–	27%	.17
Inhibitory Control	.35	.21	26%	.17
Goals[a]	–	.51	26%	.14
Body Association[b]	–	.33	11%	.09
Emotional Awareness[a]	.33	–	10%	.10
Activation Control	–	.32	10%	.08

Note. Results of a path model on the effects of meditation experience on mindfulness and mechanisms of mindfulness in the Spanish data. SRA = Self-regulated Attention; OTE = Orientation to Experience. [a] DERS scales were reverse scored so that higher scores reflected greater ability, not more problems with emotion regulation. [b] The Body Dissociation scale was reverse scored so that higher scores reflected bodily association. All *ps*<.001, except the path of SRA on Control & Regulation, *p* = .002.

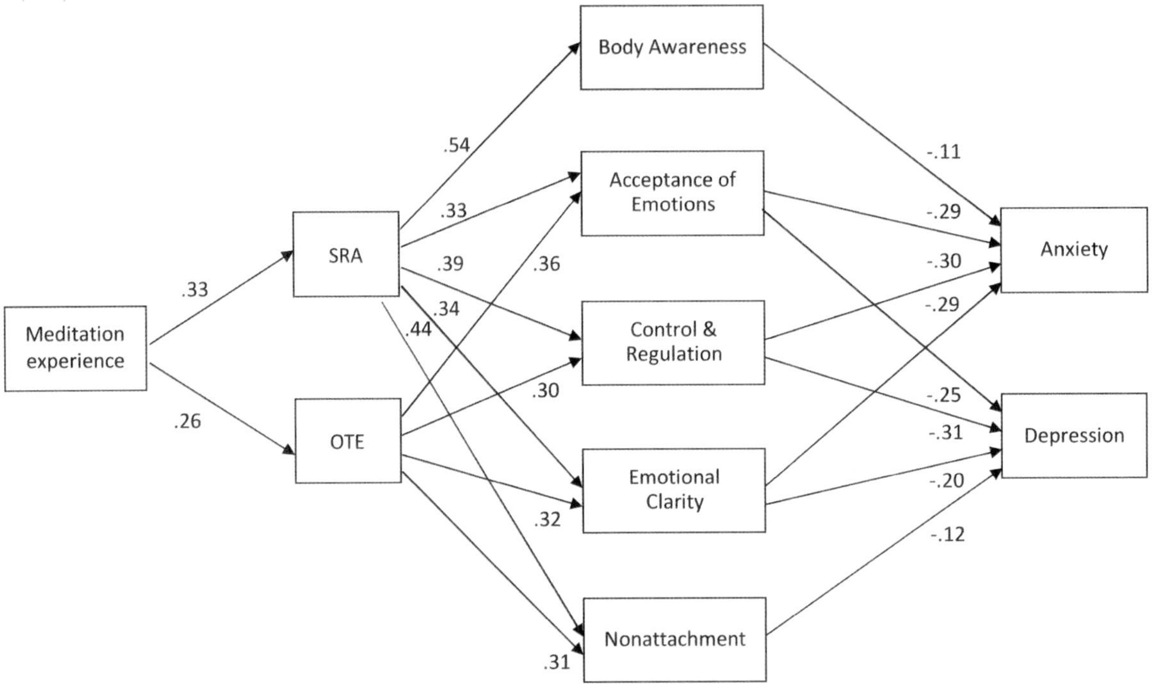

Figure 3. Path model on the effects of meditation experience on mindfulness, mechanisms of mindfulness, and depression and anxiety in the Spanish data. Numbers are standardized path coefficients. SRA = Self-regulated Attention; OTE = Orientation to Experience. Self-regulated Attention and Orientation to experience were allowed to correlate, as were mechanisms, and depression and anxiety. All *ps* <.015.

ations on meditation practice: Apparently, some training in attention regulation is needed to proceed to Orientation to Experience [6,7]. However, statistically, it may not be ruled out that age, or cohort effects, were fully or partially responsible for the observed associations of meditation practice and mindfulness [22]. Effects of meditation style and meditation experience should be investigated in more detail in future research, using longitudinal study designs.

Effects of mindfulness and meditation on mental health

Facets of mindfulness showed negative associations with anxiety and depression in both samples, similar to previous studies with meditating samples [14,25], but see [23], and also with perceived stress. Apparently (neglecting the limitations of the cross-sectional design of the present study; see above), mindfulness fully mediated the effects of meditation practice with regard to depression and anxiety [25], and with perceived stress. Orientation to Experience and Self-regulated Attention predicted anxiety, depression, and perceived stress. While the mediating effects of the two-higher factors were also similar in magnitude among the German meditators, only Orientation to Experience, but not Self-regulated Attention predicted anxiety among the Spanish meditators. This latter result compares to findings in non-meditating samples, where Orientation to Experience, but not Self-regulated Attention, showed associations with mental health [20]. This difference may be interpreted as a further indication of mindfulness being a more homogeneous construct among meditators than non-meditators, not only with regard to its latent structure (see above), but also with regard to its effects. Moreover, it suggests also differences between more and less experienced meditators and/or, alternatively, between different meditation styles.

Mechanisms of mindfulness

Decentering appeared most of all mechanisms related to meditation practice and was to the largest extent explained by the higher-order factors of mindfulness. Decentering, or metacognitive awareness, is considered a core product of mindfulness practice [2,52] and one of the main objectives of Mindfulness-Based Cognitive Therapy [61]. We obtained empirical evidence that decentering shows a substantial overlap with mindfulness and may thus be considered one of its core mechanisms in experienced meditators.

Nonattachment was found another important mechanism that, however, had not yet received broad attention [6]. Nonattachment may not only be a consequence of practice, but it is also a core concept of Buddhism. In the present study, both samples included, with high percentages, Buddhist meditators, which could have affected the obtained results. Further research is needed to investigate whether nonattachment is a general consequence of meditation practice and training, and a general correlate of mindfulness, or whether this association depends on a specific Buddhist background of meditation practice.

Even though decentering and nonattachment were mechanisms of action that were most closely associated with mindfulness, it was mostly *other* mechanisms, or in the case of decentering, more specific mechanisms, that were found to uniquely explain the beneficial effects of mindfulness and meditation on mental health. Consistent with neuroscientific evidence [7], aspects of emotion regulation, i.e., the accepting and nonjudgmental attitude towards one's emotions, emotional clarity, and the capacity to control and regulate emotional reactions, appeared in this study the most important mechanisms of action with regard to symptoms of both depression and anxiety.

Bodily awareness appeared to convey a specific anxiolytic effect, whereas nonattachment a specific antidepressant effect. Even though these effects were rather small, these findings corroborate that mindfulness affects symptoms of depression and anxiety via different pathways [37]. As predicted previously [20], it appears that the exposure to bodily sensory information in meditation gradually brings about a change in how this information is processed: Meditators in this study obviously interpreted bodily sensory information less as a sign of anxious arousal compared to non-meditators who, in contrast, show ruminative tendencies and positive associations of Observe with anxiety [14,20,25]. Besides setting a focus on emotion regulation, MBIs for anxiety disorders may thus benefit from including elements that specifically focus on bodily awareness. Vice versa, one may further expect that interventions, which already include a focus on bodily awareness, increase also mindfulness, regardless of their theoretical basis. This needs to be followed up in future research.

The potential of nonattachment for a specific antidepressant effect, as observed in the present study, appears to be a new finding (but see also [51]). Buddhist thought (for a Western perspective see, e.g., [62,63]) highlights that attachment (i.e., the mental fixation on ideas, images, or sensory objects, combined with an internal pressure to get, hold, avoid, or change circumstances or experiences) is a constant source of suffering. Nonattachment may facilitate "to 'let go' of psychological strategies that unintentionally promote or prolong suffering" [51] (p. 121). Nonattachment needs to be investigated in more detail in future studies. Its specific effects in MBIs for the treatment of depression need to be more closely examined. It should also be checked whether its effects depend on a Buddhist background of mediation (see above).

Different aspects of attention control were found to be differently associated with Self-regulated Attention and Orientation to Experience. This result appears interesting, as the two-component model of mindfulness [3] remains somewhat ambiguous with regard to attention control. Our results suggest that the voluntary allocation of attention (attentional control) and the capacity to control responses that entail avoidance behavior (activation control) are mechanisms of Orientation to Experience, whereas the capacity to control responses that entail approach behavior (inhibitory control) is more strongly governed by Self-regulated Attention, corroborating the specific assumptions of the two-component model [3] in this regard. However, more research is needed here, especially with regard to approach and avoidance behaviors that are implied by these different attentional processes.

Limitations

The Spanish meditator sample was recruited through the Internet, which could have resulted in a selection bias regarding the underrepresentation of specific groups of persons or meditation types (e.g., Tibetan or yoga meditation that were much more frequent in the German sample). Generally, it is not assured that the proportions of meditation styles as observed in the present study, or the sociodemographic characteristics of the participants, were in any way representative of meditators in German-speaking countries or Spain, as participation was wholly self-assigned.

Given the cross-sectional design of the study, causal inferences were not possible. In principle, assumed effects of meditation experience could have been caused, partially or fully, by age or cohort effects that could not be disentangled, and examined directly, in the present study.

All analyses reported in the present study relied on self-report data. Thus, results may not be generalized to other types of data and may have been affected by social desirable responding, recall bias or other forms of bias applicable to self-report data.

Conclusions

The present study broadly confirmed a previous item selection for a short form of the FFMQ and replicated a higher-order structure with two factors, Orientation to Experience and Self-regulation Attention, in samples of experienced German and Spanish meditators. The obtained results may be regarded as empirical validation of the two-component model of mindfulness [3], for which direct evidence among meditators was previously lacking. Adopting a two-component conceptualization for the FFMQ and for the study of the mindfulness as a psychological construct, is thus recommended for future research. This may specifically benefit research on mindfulness-based interventions, but also on the psychological mechanisms underlying mindfulness practice and meditation. Mechanisms of bodily awareness and nonattachment need to be further investigated in the future with regard to their specific effects on symptoms of anxiety and depression.

Supporting Information

Table S1 Factor Loadings in the Five-Factor Multigroup ESEM Analysis.

Table S2 Correlations of FFMQ Factor Scores (Short Form) with Meditation Experience, Depression, and Anxiety in Both Samples, and Means and Standard Deviations of Factor Scores and of Depression and Anxiety, Differentiated By Sample.

Table S3 Correlations of Perceived Stress (PSQ) with Meditation Experience and Higher-Order Factor Scores of Mindfulness, and Means and Standard Deviations in the German Sample.

Table S4 Correlations of Proposed Mechanisms of Mindfulness with Meditation Experience, Higher-Order Factor Scores of Mindfulness, Depression, and Anxiety, and Means and Standard Deviations in the Spanish Sample.

Acknowledgments

CIBEROBN is an initiative of ISCIII (Instituto de Salud Carlos III). Thanks are extended to the *Deutsche Buddhistische Union*, the *Berufsverband der Yogalehrenden in Deutschland*, and the *Österreichische Buddhistische Religionsgemeinschaft* for supporting the data collection of the German-speaking meditating sample.

Author Contributions

Conceived and designed the experiments: UST AC TMG. Performed the experiments: AC TvM. Analyzed the data: UST. Wrote the paper: UST AC TMG JS JG-C TvM.

References

1. Khoury B, Lecomte T, Fortin G, Masse M, Therien P, et al. (2013) Mindfulness-based therapy: A comprehensive meta-analysis. Clin Psychol Rev 33: 763-771.

2. Soler J, Franquesa A, Feliu-Soler A, Cebolla A, Garcia-Campayo J, et al. (in press) Assessing decentering: Validation of the psychometric properties and

clinical usefulness of the Experiences Questionnaire in a Spanish sample. Behav Ther.
3. Bishop SR, Lau M, Shapiro S, Carlson L, Anderson ND, et al. (2004) Mindfulness: A proposed operational definition. Clin Psychol: Sci Pract 11: 230-241.
4. Chiesa A (2012) The difficulty of defining mindfulness: Current thought and critical issues. Mindfulness 4: 255-268.
5. Bergomi C, Tschacher W, Kupper Z (2012) The assessment of mindfulness with self-report measures: Existing scales and open issues. Mindfulness 4: 191-202.
6. Hölzel BK, Lazar SW, Gard T, Schuman-Olivier Z, Vago DR, et al. (2011) How does mindfulness meditation work? Proposing mechanisms of action from a conceptual and neural perspective. Persp Psychol Sci 6: 537-559.
7. Lutz A, Slagter HA, Dunne JD, Davidson RJ (2008) Attention regulation and monitoring in meditation. Trends Cogn Sci 12:163-169.
8. Cardaciotto L, Herbert JD, Forman EM, Moitra E, Farrow V (2008) The assessment of present-moment awareness and acceptance: The Philadelphia Mindfulness Scale. Assessment 15: 204-223.
9. Tejedor R, Feliu-Soler A, Pascual JC, Cebolla A, Portella M, et al. (in press). Propiedades psicométricas de la versión española de la escala Philadelphia Mindfulness Scale (PHLMS). Revista de Salud Mental y Psiquiatría.
10. Brown KW, Ryan RM (2003) The benefits of being present: Mindfulness and its role in psychological well-being. J Pers Soc Psychol 84: 822-848.
11. Deci EL, Ryan RM (1985) Intrinsic motivation and self-determination in human behavior. New York: Plenum. 371 p.
12. Baer RA, Smith GT, Allen KB (2004) Assessment of mindfulness by self-report: The Kentucky Inventory of Mindfulness Skills. Assessment 11: 191-206.
13. Linehan MM (1993) Cognitive behavioral treatment of borderline personality disorder. New York: Guilford Press. 558 p.
14. Baer RA, Smith GT, Hopkins J, Krietemeyer J, Toney L (2006) Using self-report assessment methods to explore facets of mindfulness. Assessment 13: 27-45.
15. Buchheld N, Grossman P, Walach H (2001) Measuring mindfulness in insight meditation (Vipassana) and meditation-based psychotherapy: The development of the Freiburg Mindfulness Inventory (FMI). J Meditation Res 1:11-34.
16. Chadwick P, Hember M, Mead S, Lilley B, Dagnan D (2005) Responding mindfully to unpleasant thoughts and images: Reliability and validity of the Mindfulness Questionnaire. Unpublished manuscript.
17. Feldman GC, Hayes AM, Kumar SM, Greeson JM (2004) Development, factor structure, and initial validation of the Cognitive and Affective Mindfulness Scale. Unpublished manuscript.
18. Hou J, Wong SY, Lo HH, Mak WW, Ha HS (2013) Validation of a Chinese Version of the Five Facet Mindfulness Questionnaire in Hong Kong and development of a short form. Assessment 16: 363-371.
19. Veehof MM, ten Klooster PM, Taal E, Westerhof GJ, Bohlmeijer ET (2011) Psychometric properties of the Dutch Five Facet Mindfulness Questionnaire (FFMQ) in patients with fibromyalgia. Clin Rheumatol 30: 1045-1054.
20. Tran US, Glück TM, Nader IW (2013) Investigating the Five Facet Mindfulness Questionnaire (FFMQ): Construction of a short form and evidence of a two-factor higher order structure of mindfulness. J Clin Psychol 69: 951-965.
21. Cebolla A, García-Palacios A, Soler J, Guillen V, Baños R, et al. (2012) Psychometric properties of the Spanish validation of the Five Facets of Mindfulness Questionnaire (FFMQ). Europ J Psychiat 26: 118-126.
22. Lilja JL, Frodi-Lundgren A, Hanse JJ, Josefsson T, Lundh LG, et al. (2011) Five Facets Mindfulness Questionnaire – reliability and factor structure: A Swedish version. Cogn Behav Ther 40: 291-303.
23. de Bruin EI, Topper M, Muskens JGAM, Bögels SM, Kamphuis JH (2012)Psychometric properties of the Five Facets Mindfulness Questionnaire (FFMQ) in a meditating and non-meditating sample. Assessment 19: 187-197.
24. Williams MJ, Dalgleish T, Karl A, Kuyken W (2014) Examining the factor structures of the Five Facet Mindfulness Questionnaire and the Self-Compassion Scale. Psychol Assess 3.
25. Baer RA, Smith GT, Lykins E, Button D, Krietemeyer J, et al. (2008) Construct validity of the five facet mindfulness questionnaire in meditating and non meditating samples. Assessment 15: 329-342.
26. Bohlmeijer E, ten Klooster PM, Fledderus M, Veehof M, Baer R (2011) Psychometric properties of the Five Facet Mindfulness Questionnaire in depressed adults and development of a short form. Assessment 18: 308-320.
27. Van Dam NT, Earlywine M, Danoff-Burg S (2009) Differential item function across meditators and non-meditators on the Five Facet Mindfulness Questionnaire. Pers Indiv Diff 47: 516-521.
28. Thompson BL, Waltz J (2010) Mindfulness and experiential avoidance as predictors of posttraumatic stress disorder avoidance symptom severity. J Anxiety Disord 24: 409-415.
29. Cash M, Wittingham K (2012) What facets of mindfulness contribute to psychological well-being and depressive, anxious, and stress-related symptomatology? Mindfulness 1: 177-182.
30. Baer RA, Carmody J, Hunsinger M (2012) Weekly changes in mindfulness and perceived stress in a mindfulness-based stress reduction program. J Clin Psychol 68: 755-765.
31. Keng SL, Smoski MJ, Robins CJ (2011) Effects of mindfulness on psychological health: A review of empirical studies. Clin Psychol Rev 31: 1041-1056.
32. Hill CL, Updegraff JA (2012) Mindfulness and its relationship to emotional regulation. Emotion 12: 81-90.
33. Burg JM, Michalak J (2010) The healthy quality of mindful breathing: Associations with rumination and depression. Cogn Ther Res 35: 179-185.
34. Keune PM, Bostanov V, Kotchoubey B, Hautzinger M (2012) Mindfulness versus rumination and behavioral inhibition: A perspective from research on frontal brain asymmetry. Pers Indiv Diff 53: 323-328.
35. Ehring T, Watkins ER (2008) Repetitive negative thinking as a transdiagnostic Process. Int J Cogn Ther 1: 192-205.
36. Aldao A, Nolen-Hoeksema S, Schweizer S (2010) Emotion-regulation strategies across psychopathology: A meta-analytical review. Clin Psychol Rev 30: 217-237.
37. Desrosiers A, Vine V, Klemanski DH, Nolen-Hoeksema S (2013) Mindfulness and emotion regulation in depression and anxiety: Common and distinct mechanisms of action. Depress Anxiety 30: 654-661.
38. Kerr CE, Sacchet MD, Lazar SW, Moore CI, Jones SR (2013) Mindfulness starts with the body: Somatosensory attention and top-down modulation of cortical alpha rhythms in mindfulness meditation. Front Hum Neurosci 7: e12.
39. Franke GH (2000) Brief Symptom Inventory von L. R. Derogatis. Göttingen: Beltz. 120 p.
40. Antony MM, Bieling PJ, Cox BJ, Enns MW, Swinson RP (1998) Psychometric properties of the 42-item and 21-item versions of the Depression Anxiety Stress Scales in clinical groups and a community sample. Psychol Assess 10: 176-181.
41. Bados A, Solanas A, Andrés R (2005) Psychometric properties of the Spanish version of Depression, Anxiety and Stress Scales (DASS). Psicothema 17: 679-683.
42. Curran PJ, Hussong AM (2009) Integrative data analysis: The simultaneous analysis of multiple data sets. Psychol Meth 14: 81-100.
43. Fliege H, Rose M, Arck P, Walter OB, Kocalevent RD, et al. (2005) The Perceived Stress Questionnaire (PSQ) reconsidered: Validation and reference values from different clinical and healthy adult samples. Psychosom Med 67: 78-88.
44. Evans DE, Rothbart MK (2007) Developing a model for adult temperament. J Res Pers 41: 868-888.
45. Tortella-Feliu M, Ibáñez I, de la Banda GG, Balle M, Aguayo-Siquier B, et al. (2013) The Effortful Control Scale for adults: Psychometric properties of the Catalan version and its relationship to cognitive emotion regulation. Anales de Psicología 29: 953-964.
46. Price CJ, Thompson EA (2007) Measuring dimensions of body connection: Body awareness and bodily dissociation. J Altern Complement Med 13: 945-953.
47. Quezada LC, Gonzalez-Ramirez MT, Cebolla A, Soler J, Garcia-Campayo J (2014) Body awareness and mindfulness: Validation of the Spanish version of the Scale of Body Connection. Actas Esp Psiquiatr 42: 57-67.
48. Fresco DM, Moore MT, van Dulmen MHM, Segal ZV, Ma SH, et al. (2007) Initial psychometric properties of the experiences questionnaire: Validation of a self-report measure of decentering. Behav Ther 38: 234-246.
49. Gratz KL, Roemer L (2004) Multidimensional assessment of emotion regulation and dysregulation: Development, factor structure, and initial validation of the Difficulties in Emotion Regulation Scale. J Psychopathol Behav Assess 26: 41-54.
50. Hervás G, Jódar R (2008) Adaptación al castellano de la Escala de Dificultades en la Regulación Emocional. Clínica y Salud 19: 139-156.
51. Sahdra BK, Shaver PR, Brown KW (2010) A scale to measure nonattachment: A Buddhist complement to Western research on attachment and adaptive functioning. J Pers Assess 92: 116-127.
52. Teasdale JD, Moore RG, Hayhurst H, Pope M, Williams S, et al. (2002) Metacognitive awareness and prevention of relapse in depression: Empirical evidence. J Consult Clin Psychol 70: 275-287.
53. Asparouhov T, Muthén B (2009) Exploratory structural equation modeling. Struct Equ Modeling 16: 397-438.
54. Muthén LK, Muthén BO (2008) Mplus user's guide. Los Angeles, CA: Muthén & Muthén. 676 p.
55. Beauducel A, Herzberg PY (2006) On the performance of maximum likelihood versus means and variance adjusted weighted least squares estimation in CFA. Struct Equ Modeling 13: 186-203.
56. Hu LT, Bentler PM (1999) Cutoff criteria for fit indexes in covariance structure analysis: Conventional criteria versus new alternatives. Struct Equ Modeling 6: 1-55.
57. Kenny DA, Kaniskan B, McCoach DB (2014) The performance of RMSEA in models with small degrees of freedom. Sociol Meth Res. doi: 10.1177/0049124114543236
58. Lilja JL, Lundh LG, Josefsson T, Falkenström F (2012) Observing as an essential facet of mindfulness: A comparison of FFMQ patterns in meditating and non-meditating individuals. Mindfulness 4: 1-10.
59. Soler J, Cebolla A, Feliu-Soler A, Demarzo M, Pascual JC, et al. (2014) Relationship between meditative practice and self-reported mindfulness: The MINDSENS composite index. PLOS ONE 9: e86622.
60. Baer RA (2009) Self-focused attention and mechanisms of change in mindfulness-based treatment. Cogn Behav Ther 38: 15-20.
61. Segal ZV, Williams JMG, Teasdale JD (2001) Mindfulness-based cognitive therapy for depression: A new approach to preventing relapse. New York: Guilford Press. 351 p.
62. Ekman P, Davidson RJ, Ricard M, Wallace BA (2005) Buddhist and psychological perspectives on emotions and well-being. Curr Dir Psychol Sci 14: 59-63.
63. Wallace BA, Shapiro SL (2006) Mental balance and well-being: Building bridges between Buddhism and Western psychology. Am Psychol 61: 690-701.

Genetic Prediction of Antidepressant Drug Response and Nonresponse in Korean Patients

Shinn-Won Lim[1¶], Hong-Hee Won[1¶], Hyeran Kim[2¶], Woojae Myung[2], Seonwoo Kim[3], Ka-Kyung Kim[4], Bernard J. Carroll[5], Jong-Won Kim[4]*, Doh Kwan Kim[2]*

1 Center for Clinical Research, Samsung Biomedical Research Institute, Seoul, Korea, **2** Department of Psychiatry, Samsung Medical Center, Sungkyunkwan University School of Medicine, Seoul, Korea, **3** Biostatistics Unit, Samsung Biomedical Research Institute, Seoul, Korea, **4** Department of Laboratory Medicine and Genetics, Samsung Medical Center, Sungkyunkwan University School of Medicine, Seoul, Korea, **5** Pacific Behavioral Research Foundation, Carmel, California, United States of America

Abstract

Genetic polymorphism contributes to variation in response to drug treatment of depression. We conducted three independent 6-week treatment studies in outpatients with major depressive disorder (MDD) to develop a pharmacogenomic model predicting response and nonresponse. We screened candidate genomic markers for association with response to selective serotonin reuptake inhibitors (SSRIs). No patients had received any antidepressant drug treatment in the current episode of depression. Outcome evaluation was blinded to drug and genotype data. The prediction model derived from a development sample of 239 completer cases treated with SSRIs comprised haplotypes and polymorphisms related to serotonin synthesis, serotonin transport, glutamate receptors, and GABA synthesis. The model was evaluated prospectively for prediction of outcome in a validation sample of 176 new SSRI-treated completer cases. The model gave a prediction in 60% of these cases. Predictive values were 85% for predicted responders and 86% for predicted nonresponders, compared to prior probabilities of 66% for observed response and 34% for observed nonresponse in those cases (both $P<0.001$). Convergent cross-validation was obtained through failure of the model to predict outcomes in a third independent sample of 189 completer cases who received non-SSRI antidepressants. We suggest proof of principle for genetic guidance to use or avoid SSRIs in a majority of Korean depressed patients.

Editor: Judith Homberg, Radboud University, Netherlands

Funding: This study was supported by grants from National Research Foundation of Korea funded by the Korea government (MEST, R0A 2007-000-20129-0, to D.K.K.), the Korean Health Technology R&D Project, Ministry of Health & Welfare, Republic of Korea (A110339, to D.K.K.), and the Brain Research Program through the National Research Foundation of Korea, funded by the Ministry of Science, ICT, and Future Planning (NRF-2013M3C7A1073000, to J.W.K.). The funders had no role in study design, data collection and analysis, decision to publish, or preparation of the manuscript.

Competing Interests: Hyeran Kim and Woojae Myung are affiliated to Samsung Medical Center. Samsung Medical Center is a public utility foundation which is administratively separate from the Samsung Corporation

* Email: paulkim@skku.edu (DKK); kimjw@skku.edu (J-WK)

¶ These authors contributed equally to this work.

Introduction

Response rates in drug treatment of major depression are variable and often less than 50% in "real world" studies [1], and there are no biomarkers to direct choice of antidepressant drug class. Genetic markers hold promise for improving this record [2–4].

Many studies have focused on a few genes related to the primary actions of the drugs. Genetic polymorphism in the serotonin transporter (5-hydroxytryptamine transporter, 5-HTT), has been linked to antidepressant response to selective serotonin reuptake inhibitors (SSRIs) [5–7], although not in all studies [8]. Among the factors affecting functional response to antidepressant drugs are multiple secondary neurobiological mechanisms, environmental factors, ethnicity, and drug class. Based on our earlier reports [5,9], we adopted an expanded survey of candidate genes using single nucleotide polymorphism (SNP) microarray methods. Candidate genes were selected for the primary targets and secondary mechanisms affected by antidepressant drugs. We used a candidate gene strategy rather than an exploratory genome wide association study (GWAS) which requires much larger sample sizes [10].

Here we report on a 3-stage study (Figure 1) of multiple candidate genes for predicting response and nonresponse to SSRIs in depressed patients. After identifying a predictive model for SSRI response in the derivation sample, we subjected the model to validation testing in the second, independent, sample of patients, who also received SSRI treatment. The cross-validation sample, also independent, was treated with non-SSRI drugs. This third sample served 3 purposes – as a partial solution to the absence of a placebo-treated group; to evaluate whether the predictive SSRI model generalized to another class of antidepressant drug; and for exploration of gene markers of response to non-SSRI agents. We hypothesized that the predictive model for SSRI response would predict response to SSRI treatment in the validation sample, whilst it would not predict response to non-SSRI drugs in the cross-validation sample. These predictions are consistent with other reports of drug class differences [9,11].

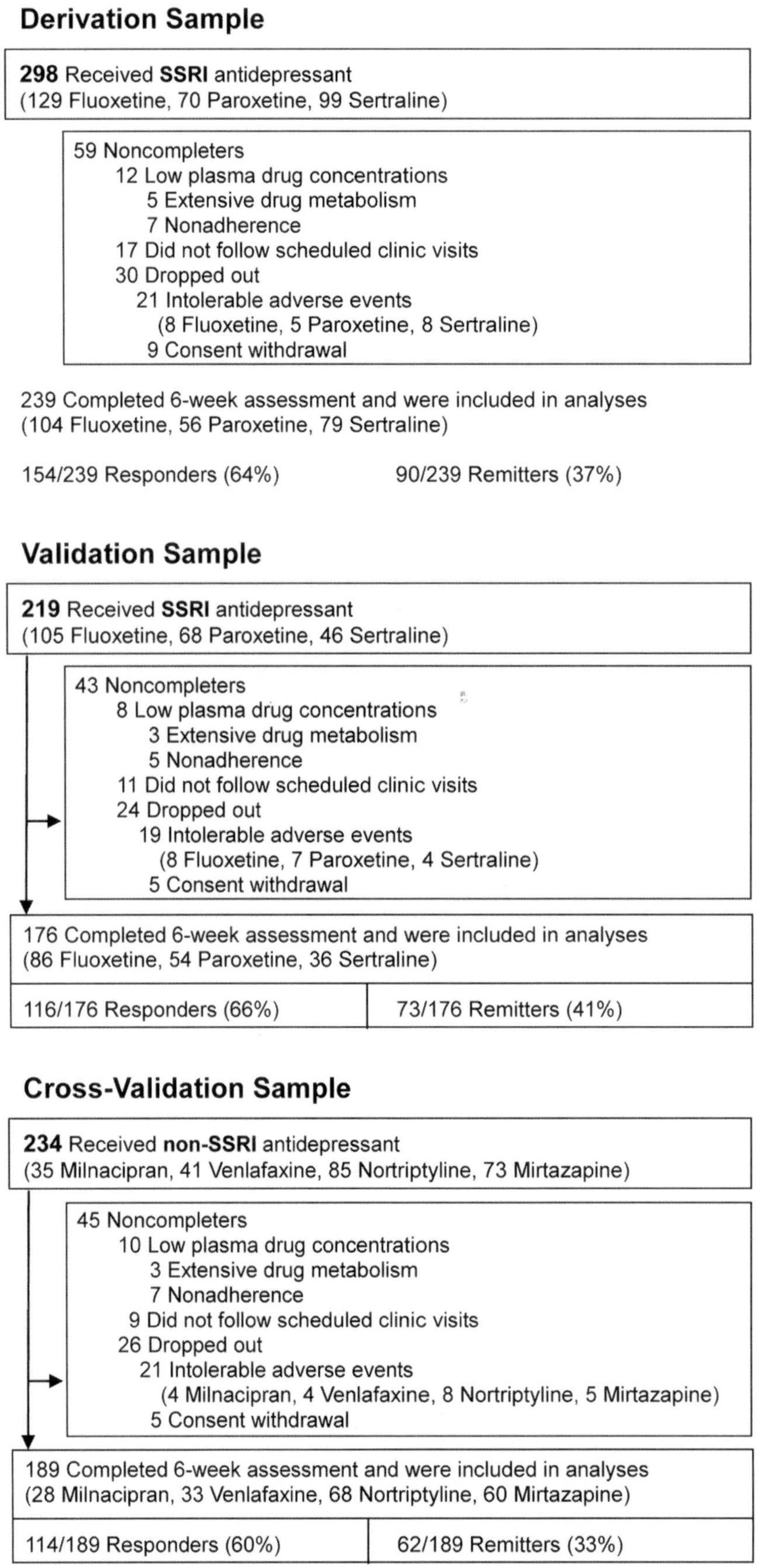

Figure 1. Enrollment, attrition, drug treatments, and outcomes of patients in all samples.

Methods

Participants

We studied 3 independent cohorts totaling 751 Korean adult outpatients with major depression. These samples were completely separate from our previous reports [5,9]. The first (derivation) sample (N = 298) received SSRI drugs. The second (validation) sample (N = 219) also received SSRI drugs. The third (cross-validation) sample (N = 234) received non-SSRI drugs. No patients had received any antidepressant drug treatment during the current episode of depression. The study was conducted in a naturalistic clinical setting rather than in a placebo-controlled clinical trial [12,13]. The protocol was approved by the ethics review board of Samsung Medical Center, Seoul, Korea. Signed informed consent was obtained from all participants. The study is registered (NCT00817375) in ClinicalTrials.gov.

The assessment and quality control procedures have been fully described previously [5,9]. A total 782 participants were recruited from patients seeking care for depression at a university hospital from October 1997 through July 2007. Thirty-one cases were excluded: 6 patients did not have a significant other to obtain collateral diagnostic information, 4 patients had significant medical conditions, 7 patients had a concomitant Axis I psychiatric disorder, and 16 patients did not have a minimum 17-item HAM-D score of 15. Two cases met 2 of these exclusion criteria. Thus, a total of 751 Korean outpatients with MDD were enrolled. All were clinically referred and all were of unrelated Korean ancestry. Figure 1 displays retention and attrition data for the 3 independent clinical samples. As this is a discovery project, outcome analyses included only subjects who completed 6 weeks of treatment with adequate blood levels (Figure 1). Extensive drug metabolizers were distinguished from nonadherent cases by clinical review after a low blood level was detected. Overall, 604 patients (80.4%) completed the protocol.

Enrolled patients met the *Diagnostic and Statistical Manual of Mental Disorders, Fourth Edition* (DSM-IV) criteria for MDD without psychotic features. The diagnosis was based on an initial clinical interview, followed by a structured research interview, the Samsung Psychiatric Evaluation Schedule (SPES). The affective disorder section of the SPES uses the Korean version of the *Structured Clinical Interview for the Diagnostic and Statistical Manual of Mental Disorders, Fourth Edition*. The SPES provides additional information including cognitive screening, comorbid psychiatric diagnoses, psychosocial variables (age, sex, age of onset, duration of current episode, episode number), family history and initial Hamilton Depression Rating Scale (HAM-D) [14] severity score. These diagnostic interviews involved the patient and at least one family member. The final diagnosis was made after review of ongoing clinical observations, medical records, past histories, and the DSM-IV criteria, by a board-certified psychiatrist. Inclusion criteria were 18 years of age or older, the existence of a current nonpsychotic unipolar major depressive episode as verified by DSM-IV criteria, a minimum 17-item HAM-D score of 15, and ability to provide informed consent. To be included in these discovery analyses, patients also were required to adhere to prescribed medication and to have an adequate plasma antidepressant drug level measured at 6 weeks. Exclusion criteria were pregnancy, significant medical conditions, abnormal baseline laboratory values, unstable psychiatric features (e.g., suicide attempt), histories of alcohol or drug dependence, seizure disorder, neurological illness including significant cognitive impairment, or concomitant Axis I psychiatric disorder. Patients with MDD who met DSM-IV criteria for the specifier '*Severe With Psychotic Features*' were excluded because they would normally receive concurrent antipsychotic medication. As stated above, no patients had received antidepressant drug treatment in the current episode before enrolment in this study. In addition, no patient had received non-antidepressant psychotropic medication within 2 weeks of the study. We also verified that no patients had received fluoxetine, which has a long half-life, for any reason within the preceding 4 weeks.

Procedures

Patients received monotherapy for 6 weeks with one of three commonly used SSRI drugs or one of four non-SSRI antidepressants, by clinician's choice (Figure 1). In this naturalistic study, choice of drug was driven by the preference of the physician, with consideration of anticipated side effects in at-risk individuals [15]. Dose titration was completed within two weeks. Trough plasma samples were drawn at the end of week 6 for plasma drug concentrations. Lorazepam 0.5–1 mg was allowed at bedtime for insomnia. Patients were seen by a psychiatrist, who monitored their adverse events by the Udvalg for Kliniske Undersogelser (UKU) scale [16] at weeks 0, 1, 2, 4, and 6. The 17-item Hamilton scale for depression (HAM-D) [14] was administered by a single trained rater every two weeks. The rater and genotyper were blinded to the hypotheses and to drug assignment. HAM-D and genotype data were not disclosed to the psychiatrist, and the rater was blinded to the genotype data. To maintain the blindness, a trained research coordinator managed the data and schedules. At six weeks, response was defined according to standard conventions [4] as ≥50% decrease in the HAM-D score, and remission as a HAM-D score ≤7.

The protocol completion rates were 80% (derivation sample), 80% (validation sample), and 81% (cross-validation sample) (Figure 1). For comparison, protocol completion rates in controlled clinical trials of antidepressant drugs typically are 70–75% [17]. As shown in Figure 1, dropouts occurred for the usual clinical and administrative reasons, and we excluded cases with evidence of nonadherence or extensive drug metabolism inferred from the finding of low plasma drug concentrations at week 6. The clinical characteristics of non-completers did not differ significantly from completers in any cohort (data not shown). The data reported in the Results apply to the 604 completer cases: 239 in the derivation cohort; 176 in the validation SSRI cohort; and 189 in the cross-validation non-SSRI cohort (Figure 1).

Candidate genes and selection of SNP markers

We focused on candidate genes of neurotransmitter metabolic enzymes, transporters and receptors (Table S1). We selected 79 candidate genes, based on their likely importance for immediate or delayed mechanisms of antidepressant action. We combined knowledge-based and function-based tagging selection approaches (Figure S1). We selected 155 SNPs through a literature survey on the significant SNPs related to antidepressant response, and 1657 SNPs by tagging based on potential functional importance (Table S2).

After screening for availability of Golden Gate Bead Array analysis (Illumina, Inc. San Diego, CA), 1502 SNPs were genotyped. 67 SNPs with a call rate of less than 95% and 35 SNPs with a minor allele frequency less than 5% were excluded. Finally, 1400 SNPs were prepared.

To enable comparison with SNP data using different SNP genotyping platforms, we imputed genotypes for untyped SNPs using the IMPUTE software [18].

Table 1. Characteristics of patients in derivation sample, validation sample, and cross-validation sample.

Characteristics	Derivation Sample			Validation Sample				Cross-Validation Sample			
	SSRI Treated Group			SSRI Treated Group			P^{+}	Non-SSRI Treated Group			P^{++}
	Responder	Nonresponder	P	Responder	Nonresponder	P		Responder	Nonresponder	P	
Response Rate (%)[a]	154/239 (64.4%)			116/176 (65.9%)			1.00	114/189 (60.3%)			0.84
Remission Rate (%)[a]	90/239 (37.7%)			73/176 (41.5%)			0.96	62/189 (32.8%)			0.62
Gender, Female (%)[a]	180/239 (75.3%)			136/176 (77.3%)			1.00	137/189 (72.5%)			1.00
	119/154 (66.1%)	61/85 (71.8%)	0.35	91/116 (78.5%)	45/60 (75.0%)	0.70		83/114 (72.8%)	54/75 (72.0%)	1.00	
Age, Mean±SD (Range), Year[b]	59.8±13.7 (19–86)			62.3±12.7 (24–87)			0.11	58.7±13.3 (22–82)			0.82
	59.1±14.0 (19–86)	61.1±13.2 (24–85)	0.35	62.0±12.3 (27–87)	62.7±13.4 (24–83)	0.47		58.7±13.0 (22–82)	59.4±13.9 (25–82)	0.21	
Family History of Depression (%)[a]	46/239 (19.3%)			34/176 (19.3%)			1.00	39/189 (20.6%)			1.00
	33/154 (21.4%)	13/85 (15.3%)	0.30	23/116 (19.8%)	11/60 (18.3%)	1.00		23/114 (20.2%)	16/75 (21.3%)	0.86	
Duration of Index Episode, Mean±SD (Range), Month[b]	9.6±14.1 (1–92)			8.8±13.2 (1–92)			1.00	10.8±15.9 (1–120)			0.82
	9.1±15.3 (1–92)	10.5±11.4 (1–71)	0.04	8.2±12.1 (1–63)	10.0±15.2 (1–92)	0.36		11.1±18.7 (1–120)	10.4±10.5 (1–37)	0.13	
No. of Episodes, Mean±SD (Range)[b]	2.2±1.8 (1–16)			2.3±2.0 (1–16)			1.00	2.2±2.1 (1–19)			1.00
	2.2±2.0 (1–16)	2.1±1.2 (1–6)	0.31	2.3±2.2 (1–16)	2.2±1.8 (1–12)	0.86		2.1±1.8 (1–11)	2.4±2.4 (1–19)	0.20	
Age at First Episode, Mean±SD (Range), Year[b]	53.0±15.1 (16–82)			55.6±14.5 (15–82)			0.18	51.2±15.0 (15–77)			0.56
	52.4±15.7 (16–81)	54.3±13.9 (19–82)	0.47	55.4±14.4 (20–81)	56.0±15.0 (15–82)	0.66		51.5±14.4 (15–77)	50.9±15.9 (15–75)	0.90	
HAM-D Baseline, Mean±SD (Range)[b]	20.9±4.8 (15–40)			19.2±3.4 (15–32)				21.5±5.1 (15–40)			
	20.8±5.3 (15–40)	21.0±4.0 (15–31)	0.45[c]	19.1±3.2 (15–29)	19.4±3.7 (15–32)	1.00		21.4±5.1 (15–40)	21.6±5.2 (15–36)	1.00[c]	
HAM-D After, Mean±SD (Range)[b]	10.2±5.6 (0–26)			9.5±5.3 (0–30)				11.7±6.5 (1–35)			
	7.0±3.1 (0–15)	16.0±4.3 (9–26)	<0.01[c]	6.5±2.8 (0–14)	15.3±4.0 (9–30)	<0.01		7.4±3.1 (1–17)	18.1±4.6 (10–35)	<0.01[c]	

Abbreviations: SSRI, selective serotonin reuptake inhibitor; HAM-D, Hamilton depression rating score.
[a]Fisher's exact test.
[b]Mann-Whitney test.
[c]Corrected by Bonferroni's correction for multiple testing.
[+]Comparison between derivation sample and validation sample.
[++]Comparison between derivation sample and cross-validation sample.

Statistical analysis

We performed tests of five genetic modes (dominant, recessive, genotype, allele, and additive) for each SNP with the use of Fisher's exact test and the Cochran-Armitage test [19]. The mode most strongly associated with response was considered the best-fitting genetic mode for each SNP. These significance levels were calculated and corrected with the false discovery rate (FDR) control [20].

Haplotype blocks were defined in the derivation sample by confidence intervals using Haploview [21,22]. Associations between haplotype blocks and response were tested using Fisher's exact test with the FDR control. Multivariable analyses for SNPs and for haplotype blocks found to be significant in univariable analyses were performed using multiple logistic regression and the Generalized Estimating Equations method [23], respectively.

Prediction models for response and nonresponse were constructed using multiple logistic regression. We constructed two types of prediction model. First, only polymorphic markers were considered (polymorphism model, section 4 of Text S2). Second, in addition to SNPs and VNTR markers, haplotypes were included and considered in the model (HAP-SNP model). Before constructing a combined haplotype-SNP (HAP-SNP) model, haplotypes were re-defined as a pair of two haplotypes (for example, *TPH2* H3-A is defined as a pair of two haplotypes (GCATGG and GCATGG) because the haplotypes are clustered data. We used the operational criteria of probability>0.8 for predicting response (better than the optimal response rate expected with combined drug and cognitive behavioral therapy in common psychiatric disorders such as depression and anxiety) [24,25], and response probability <0.3 for predicting nonresponse (lower than conservative estimates of the expected response rate with placebo in controlled clinical trials for depression [26]). This approach stratified each sample as predicted responders, predicted nonresponders, and indeterminate cases (no prediction). Excluding the indeterminate cases, we calculated overall accuracy, positive predictive value (PPV), negative predictive value (NPV), sensitivity and specificity, and areas under the receiver operating curve (AUC). The significance of the change from prior probabilities in the absence of genotyping to posterior probabilities from the prediction model was tested by the Chi square Goodness of Fit method. The PPVs and NPVs between the derivation set and the validation set were compared by Fisher's exact test.

The study was powered for the outcomes of observed response and nonresponse (see Text S1, section 4). All p values were reported as two-sided, and *P* values <0.05 were considered statistically significant. Analyses were performed with the use of the SAS software, version 9.13.

Detailed methods of function-based tagging selection of SNP markers, genotyping, power analysis and quantification of plasma drug levels are described in Text S1 (Supplementary Method).

Results

Clinical characteristics

Demographic variables, response and remission rates, severity ratings, and salient clinical variables of the three samples are shown in Table 1. HAM-D scores indicated moderate to severe depression. Observed response rates exceeded 60% in all groups. Responders and nonresponders did not differ at baseline on any variable, except for duration of episode in the derivation sample. Choice of SSRI drug did not influence outcomes overall (response rate to fluoxetine, paroxetine and sertraline: 65.4%, 64.3% and 63.3%, see Table S3) or in relation to any genotype (Table S3). Plasma drug levels in responders and nonresponders were not significantly different (Table S4).

Significant polymorphic markers for SSRI response

In the derivation sample, ten of 1400 candidate SNPs showed significant associations ($P<0.05$) with response after FDR correction (Table 2). These resided in four genes: four in *TPH2*, two in *GRIK2*, two in *GAD1*, and two in *SLC6A4*. The *TPH2* gene was most strongly associated with SSRI response. The rs4760815 in intron 6 of *TPH2* showed the strongest association ($P=1.26\times10^{-5}$), and rs11179027, rs17110532 and rs17110747 in *TPH2* were also significantly associated ($P=1.57\times10^{-5}$, 8.86×10^{-5} and 1.94×10^{-4}).

The second strongest associations with response to SSRIs were found in rs543196 and rs572487 in intron 2 of *GRIK2* ($P=4.84\times10^{-5}$ and 1.36×10^{-4}). Another strong association was found in *GAD1*, where rs3828275 in intron 3 and rs12185692 located ~2.5 kb upstream of this gene showed strong association ($P=6.89\times10^{-5}$ and 2.33×10^{-4}).

Two SNPs, rs2066713 and rs2020942, in the serotonin transporter gene (*SLC6A4*) also showed strong association with SSRI response ($P=1.26\times10^{-4}$ and 2.96×10^{-4}). Previously, we reported that 44 bp insertion/deletion polymorphisms in the promoter region (*5-HTTLPR*) and variable number of tandem repeat (VNTR) *s/l* polymorphisms in intron 2 (*STin2*) of *SLC6A4* were associated with response to SSRIs [5,9]. We also genotyped these two VNTRs, and they once again showed significant associations with response to SSRIs ($P<0.01$) (Table 2).

Haplotype analysis for SSRI response

We further analyzed the four major genes (*TPH2*, *GRIK2*, *GAD1* and *SLC6A4*) which have multiple significant SNPs by examining linkage disequilibrium (LD) structures and haplotypes. Six haplotype blocks in those genes except *GAD1* were significantly associated with SSRI response (FDR corrected $P<0.05$). Among five haplotype blocks observed in *TPH2*, the third (H3), fourth (H4) and fifth (H5) blocks were significantly associated with response ($P<0.01$) (Figure 2A). When we examined haplotypes and LD structure separately for the responders and nonresponders to SSRI drugs, LD was stronger and haplotype blocks were longer in the responders than the nonresponders (Figure S2).

Among 16 haplotype blocks constructed from 78 SNPs of *GRIK2*, the eighth ($P=9.6\times10^{-4}$) and ninth ($P=9.6\times10^{-4}$) haplotype blocks were significantly associated with SSRI response (Figure 2B). Only one haplotype block from 12 SNPs of *SLC6A4* was significantly associated ($P=1.3\times10^{-2}$) (Figure 2C). However, two haplotype blocks from ten SNPs of *GAD1* were not significantly associated with response to SSRI drugs (Figure 2D).

Prediction model for SSRI response

Using the stated operational criteria for predicting observed response and nonresponse to SSRIs (see Method; statistical analysis), the two prediction models demonstrated similar predictive performance. The HAP-SNP model made predictions for 54% of cases (129/239), compared with 46% (110/239) of patients using the polymorphism model. For this reason, we report on the HAP-SNP model as the optimal prediction model for response to SSRI treatment in this study. Genotypic combinations of the HAP-SNP model are presented in Table 3.

Moreover, we examined the effect of duration of episode, which differed between responders and nonresponders (Table 1), in the modeling but found that this clinical feature did not contribute significantly.

Table 2. The SNPs most strongly associated with SSRI response ($P < 0.05$ after FDR correction) and the strongly associated polymorphisms in *SLC6A4* from our previous study [9].

Gene	Chromosome	Position[a]	SNP	Responsive Allele	RAF in Responders	RAF in Nonresponders	MAF	*P* Value[b]	*P* Value by Bonferroni's Correction	*P* Value by Controlling FDR	Genetic Mode	Heterozygote Odds Ratio (95% CI)	Homozygote Odds Ratio (95% CI)
TPH2	12	70658496	rs4760815	T	0.60	0.41	0.50	1.26×10^{-5}	0.02	0.02	Dominant	3.77 (3.55–4.00)	4.39 (2.08–9.29)
TPH2	12	70663579	rs11179027	C	0.55	0.34	0.44	1.57×10^{-5}	0.02	0.02	Allele	2.69 (1.45–4.99)	4.77 (2.17–10.49)
GRIK2	6	102158042	rs543196	C	0.65	0.46	0.44	4.84×10^{-5}	0.07	0.02	Additive	1.69 (0.83–3.45)	5.02 (2.18–11.53)
GAD1	2	171390986	rs3828275	G	0.72	0.64	0.31	6.89×10^{-5}	0.10	0.02	Genotype	0.31 (0.17–0.55)	1.24 (0.43–3.62)
TPH2	12	70650935	rs17110532	C	0.42	0.24	0.33	8.86×10^{-5}	0.12	0.02	Allele	2.02 (1.14–3.59)	5.36 (1.93–14.87)
SLC6A4	17	25575791	rs2066713	C	0.96	0.86	0.07	1.26×10^{-4}	0.18	0.03	Recessive	0.48 (0.03–8.42)	2.27 (0.14–36.87)
GRIK2	6	102157181	rs572487	G	0.59	0.41	0.48	1.36×10^{-4}	0.19	0.03	Additive	1.65 (1.54–1.77)	4.76 (2.09–10.86)
TPH2	12	70712221	rs17110747	A	0.31	0.16	0.25	1.94×10^{-4}	0.27	0.03	Allele	2.53 (1.37–4.69)	3.88 (1.25–11.99)
GAD1	2	171379072	rs12185692	C	0.71	0.65	0.31	2.33×10^{-4}	0.33	0.04	Genotype	0.35 (0.20–0.62)	1.57 (0.49–5.03)
SLC6A4	17	25571040	rs2020942	G	0.95	0.85	0.09	2.96×10^{-4}	0.42	0.04	Additive	1.27 (1.21–1.34)	4.56 (0.41–51.22)

Gene	Chromosome	VNTR	*P* Value[b]	*P* Value by Bonferroni's Correction	*P* Value by Controlling FDR	Genetic Mode	Odds Ratio (95% CI)
SLC6A4	17	*5-HTT* VNTR in promoter (*5-HTTLPR*)	6.00×10^{-3}	NA	NA	*ss* vs. *sl+ll*	2.18 (1.27–3.75)
SLC6A4	17	*5-HTT* VNTR in intron 2 (*STin2*)	2.00×10^{-4}	NA	NA	*ll* vs. *sl+ss*	3.86 (1.90–7.84)

Abbreviations: SNP, single-nucleotide polymorphism; SSRI, selective serotonin reuptake inhibitor; RAF, responsive allele frequency; FDR, false discovery rate; VNTR, variable number of tandem repeat; MAF, minor allele frequency; NA, not applicable.

[a]Genomic position (NCBI Build 36).

[b]Fisher's exact test.

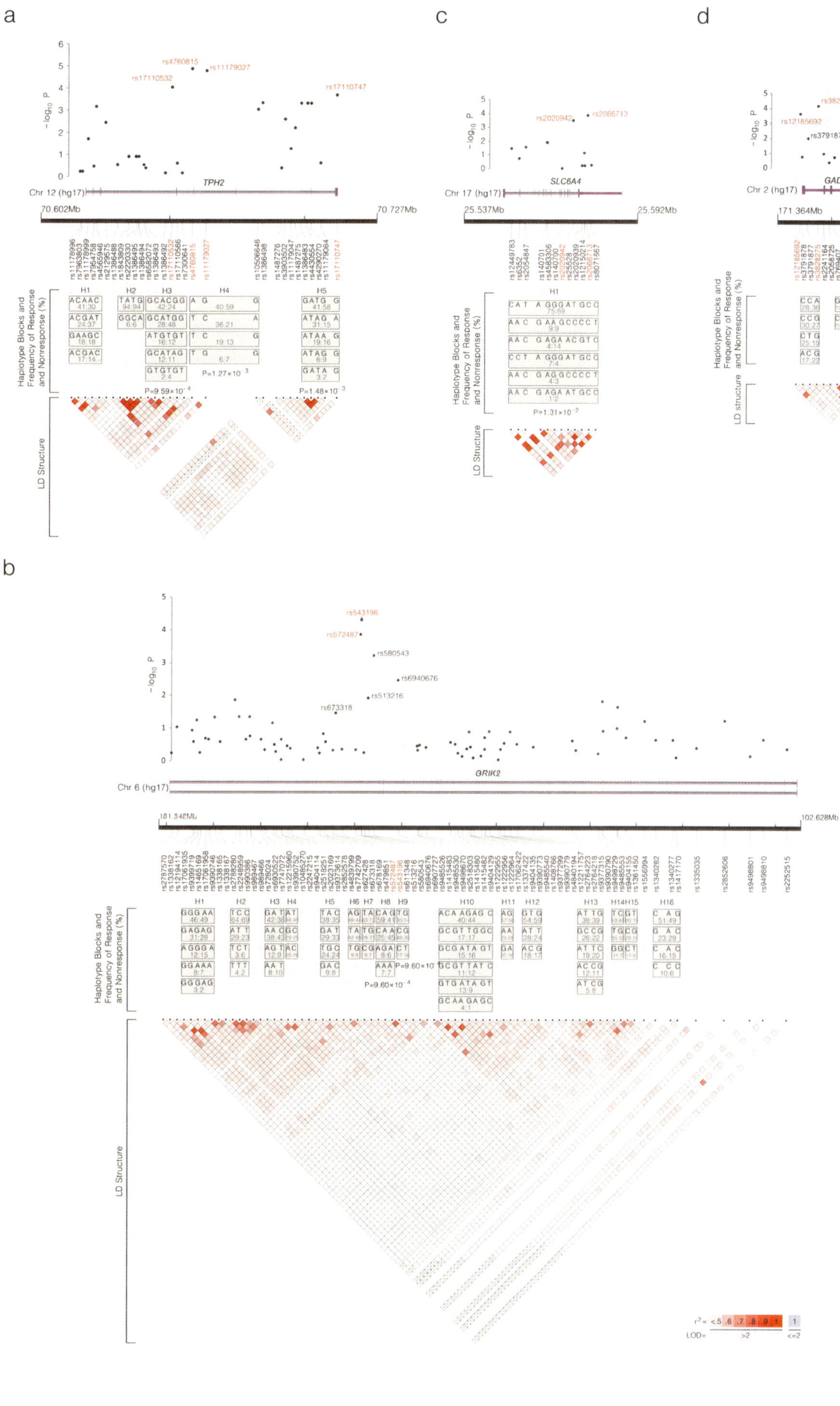
a
b
c
d
TPH2
Chr 12 (hg17)
70.602Mb
70.727Mb
rs4760815
rs11179027
rs17110532
rs17110747
SLC6A4
Chr 17 (hg17)
25.537Mb
25.592Mb
rs2020942
rs2066713
GAD1
Chr 2 (hg17)
171.364Mb
171.438Mb
rs3828275
rs12185692
rs3791877
GRIK2
Chr 6 (hg17)
102.628Mb
rs543196
rs572487
rs580543
rs6940676
rs513216
rs673318
−log10 P
Haplotype Blocks and Frequency of Response and Nonresponse (%)
LD Structure
LD structure
P=9.59×10⁻⁴
P=1.27×10⁻³
P=1.48×10⁻³
P=1.31×10⁻²
P=9.60×10⁻⁴
r² = <.5 .6 .7 .8 .9 1
LOD=
>2
<=2

Figure 2. Linkage disequilibrium (LD) and haplotype structure of (a) *TPH2,* (b) *GRIK2,* (c) *SLC6A4,* and (d) *GAD1.* The LD structure in the lower panel is based on the measure of r^2. Dark red indicates strong LD between two markers with high r^2 and a logarithm of odds (LOD) score of greater than 2.0. Haplotype frequencies of responders and nonresponders are also shown in each box in order (responders: nonresponders). The figure was prepared with LocusView2.0 (http://www.broad.mit.edu/mpg/locusview). Significant SNPs inscribed in red are plotted with their association analysis p values (as $-\log_{10}$ values) in the upper panel. Haplotype blocks and estimated haplotypes for each block are presented in the middle panel. (a) Among 30 SNPs screened in *TPH2,* four SNPs (colored red), rs17110532, rs4760815, rs11179027 and rs17110747, were significantly associated (see Table 2). The third (H3), fourth (H4) and fifth haplotype (H5) blocks were significantly associated with drug response ($P<0.05$ after FDR correction). (b) Among 78 SNPs in *GRIK2,* two SNPs (colored red), rs543196 and rs572487, were significantly associated. Four SNPs, rs580543, rs6940676, rs513216, and rs673318, adjacent to the peak SNPs also showed high associations. The eighth (H8) and ninth (H9) blocks were significantly associated with response ($P<0.05$ after FDR correction). (c) Among 12 SNPs in *SLC6A4,* two SNPs (colored red), rs2066713 and rs2020942, were significantly associated with response. The first haplotype (H1) block was significantly associated with response ($P<0.05$ after FDR correction). (d) Among ten SNPs in *GAD1,* two SNPs (colored red), rs3828275 and rs12185691, were significantly associated (see Table 2). No haplotype blocks were significantly associated with response.

The HAP-SNP model contained polymorphic markers and haplotype blocks: *TPH2* (H3) ($P<0.001$), *SLC6A4* (H1) ($P<0.001$), rs543196 of *GRIK2* ($P<0.001$), rs3828275 of *GAD1* ($P=0.01$), and *5-HTTLPR* of *SLC6A4* ($P=0.04$), and showed an AUC of 0.82, which is considered an overall good performance [27]. The model predicted outcome for 54% of completer cases (129/239) in the derivation sample, with 90 predicted responders (>80% predicted probability of response) and 39 predicted nonresponders (<30% predicted probability of response) (Figure 3A). The observed outcomes in these 129 cases were 85 responders and 44 nonresponders (observed response rate 66%). For these 129 cases, 79 of 85 observed responders were correctly predicted (sensitivity 93%; 95% confidence interval [CI] 88%–98%), as were 33 of 44 observed nonresponders (specificity 75%; [62%–88%]). The positive predictive value (PPV) was 88% (79/90; [81%–95%]) and the negative predictive value (NPV) was 85% (33/39; [74%–96%]). The overall accuracy of prediction was 112 of 129 predicted cases (87%; [81%–93%]). The prior probabilities of observed response (66%) and nonresponse (34%) in the absence of genotyping increased to posterior probabilities of 88% and 85%, respectively ($P<0.001$ in each case). For the remaining 110 cases with predicted probability of response between 30% and 80%, posterior probabilities did not differ significantly from prior probabilities of response or nonresponse.

Validation of prediction model

In the validation sample of 176 new completer cases treated with SSRI drugs, the distributions of clinical characteristics and genetic markers did not differ from the derivation sample (Table 1, Table S5). Seven of the top 10 SNPs that showed the strongest association with SSRI treatment response in the derivation sample were significantly associated in the validation sample (Table S6). In this validation cohort, the prior probabilities were 66% for response (116 of 176) and 34% for nonresponse (60 of 176) (Table 1). The HAP-SNP model made predictions for 60% (106/176) of these patients, with 84 predicted responders and 22 predicted nonresponders (Figure 3B). The observed outcomes in these 106 predicted cases were 74 responders and 32 nonresponders (Figure 3B). The overall accuracy of prediction was 85% (90/106; [78%–92%]). Sensitivity and specificity were 96% (71/74; [91%–100%]) and 59% (19/32; [42%–76%]), respectively. This specificity result was not significantly lower than in the derivation sample ($P=0.21$). Among these 106 cases, the prior probabilities of observed response (70%) and nonresponse (30%) in the absence of genotyping increased to posterior probabilities of 85% (PPV; 71/84; [77%–92%]) and 86% (NPV; 19/22; [72%–100%]), respectively ($P<0.001$ in each case). These PPV and NPV results did not significantly differ from the corresponding values (PPV = 88%, NPV = 85%) in the derivation sample (Fisher's exact test, $P=0.66$, $P=1.00$, respectively). Of note, the model predicted 59% (19 of 32) of observed nonresponders in the validation sample with 86% accuracy (Figure 3B).

Cross-validation of prediction model

In the third phase of this study we tested whether the HAP-SNP model that predicted response to SSRIs also predicted outcomes in patients treated with non-SSRI antidepressants. In an independent sample of 189 protocol completers (Figure 1), we compared response and nonresponse predicted for SSRIs by the HAP-SNP model with observed response and observed nonresponse to non-SSRI antidepressants. The distributions of clinical characteristics and genetic markers did not differ from the derivation sample in this cross-validation sample (Table 1, Table S5). The observed response rate was 60% (114/189). The genetic associations with observed response to SSRI drugs were not replicated for observed response to non-SSRI agents (Table S7). Figure S3 shows a lack of correlation between the association analysis P values of groups receiving SSRIs and non-SSRIs (Pearson $r=0.02$). No SNP markers in the non-SSRI group reached a significant level of association with response after FDR correction.

Consistent with these gene association differences, the observed responses to non-SSRI drugs differed significantly from the predictions made by the HAP-SNP model that predicted response to SSRIs. The model made predictions for 84 (44%) of the 189 cases in the cross validation sample (61 predicted responders (73%) and 23 predicted nonresponders (27%)). There were 43 observed responders (70.5%) among the 61 predicted responders (PPV), and 11 observed nonresponders (47.8%) among the 23 predicted nonresponders (NPV). These values were significantly different from the corresponding PPV and NPV values in the derivation sample. (Fisher's exact test, $P=0.01$, $P<0.01$, respectively). Within this group of 84 cases, the observed outcomes were 55 responders (65%) and 29 nonresponders (35%). These are the prior probabilities of response and nonresponse among predicted cases, not significantly different from the full cohort of 189 cases (60% and 40%, respectively).

Text S2 provides additional descriptions of secondary analyses (Supplementary Results), which describes (1) comparisons of the three cohorts in respect of genotypes, clinical characteristics, and plasma drug levels in relation to response status; (2) SNP associations with the secondary outcome of remission; (3) a test of the top 10 SNPs in the response prediction model for possible associations with the diagnosis of major depression – with no significant association being found; (4) details of the polymorphism prediction model that was replaced by the HAP-SNP model; (5) secondary conditional probability analyses in the cross-validation cohort, demonstrating a double dissociation of observed versus expected outcomes: cases predicted by the HAP-SNP model to do poorly with SSRI treatment actually had significantly better observed outcomes with non-SSRI treatment, while cases

Table 3. Genotypic combinations of haplotype-SNP (HAP-SNP) prediction model.

	TPH2 (H3)*	SLC6A4 (H1)[†]	rs543196	rs3828275	5-HTTLPR	
Predicted responder	H3-B	H1-A	CC	AA	ss	>80% (n = 90)
	H3-B	H1-A	CC	GG	ss	
	H3-B	H1-A	CC	AA	sl+ll	
	H3-B	H1-A	TC	AA	ss	
	H3-B	H1-A	CC	GG	sl+ll	
	H3-B	H1-A	TC	GG	ss	
	H3-B	H1-A	CC	AG	ss	
	H3-B	H1-A	TC	AA	sl+ll	
Predicted Nonresponder	H3-B	H1-B	TT	GG	ss	<30% (n = 39)
	H3-B	H1-B	TC	AG	ss	
	H3-A	H1-A	TT	AA	ss	
	H3-A	H1-B	CC	AA	ss	
	H3-A	H1-A	TC	GG	sl+ll	
	H3-A	H1-A	CC	AG	sl+ll	
	H3-B	H1-B	TT	AA	sl+ll	
	H3-A	H1-A	TT	GG	ss	
	H3-A	H1-A	TC	AG	ss	
	H3-A	H1-B	CC	GG	ss	
	H3-B	H1-B	TT	GG	sl+ll	
	H3-B	H1-B	TC	AG	sl+ll	
	H3-A	H1-A	TT	AA	sl+ll	
	H3-B	H1-B	TT	AG	ss	
	H3-A	H1-B	CC	AA	sl+ll	
	H3-A	H1-B	TC	AA	ss	
	H3-A	H1-A	TT	GG	sl+ll	
	H3-A	H1-A	TC	AG	sl+ll	
	H3-A	H1-B	CC	GG	sl+ll	
	H3-A	H1-A	TT	AG	ss	
	H3-A	H1-B	TC	GG	ss	
	H3-A	H1-B	CC	AG	ss	
	H3-B	H1-B	TT	AG	sl+ll	
	H3-A	H1-B	TC	AA	sl+ll	
	H3-A	H1-B	TT	AA	ss	
	H3-A	H1-A	TT	AG	sl+ll	
	H3-A	H1-B	TC	AA	sl+ll	
	H3-A	H1-B	CC	AG	sl+ll	
	H3-A	H1-B	TT	GG	ss	
	H3-A	H1-B	TC	AG	ss	
	H3-A	H1-B	TT	AA	sl+ll	
	H3-A	H1-B	TT	GG	sl+ll	
	H3-A	H1-B	TC	AG	sl+ll	
	H3-A	H1-B	TT	AG	ss	
	H3-A	H1-B	TT	AG	sl+ll	

Abbreviations: SNP, single-nucleotide polymorphism; *5-HTTLPR*, serotonin-transporter-linked polymorphic region.
*H3-A is defined as a pair of two haplotypes (GCATGG and GCATGG), and H3-B as the other cases.
[†]H1-A is defined as any pairs constituting of the CATAGGGATGCC, CATAGGGACGCC, CATAGGAACGTC, CCTAGGGATGCC, AATAGGGATGCC, AACGAGGCCCCT, AACGAGAATGCC and AACGAAGCCCCT haplotypes, and H1-B as any pairs including at least one haplotype among the AACGAGAACGTC, CATAGGGCCCCC and CATGAGGATGCC haplotypes.

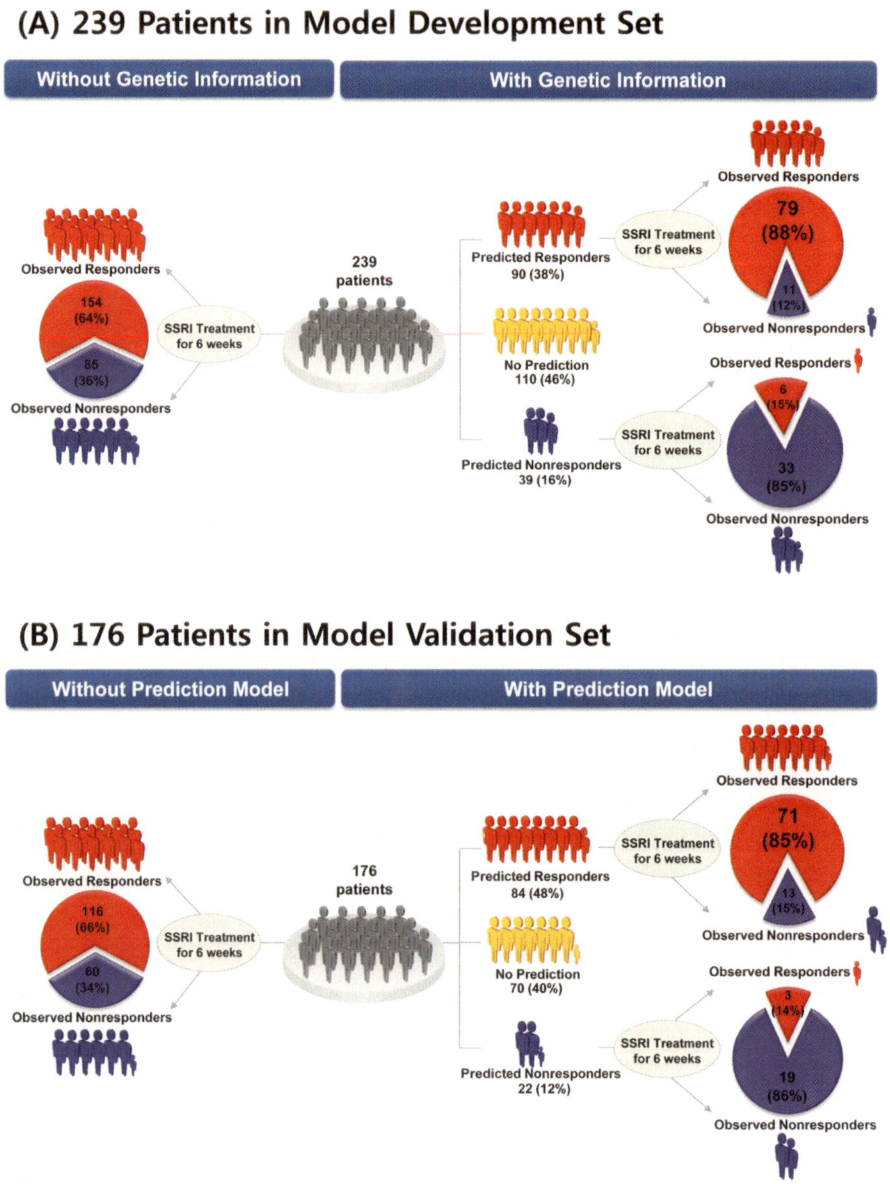

Figure 3. Clinical performance of selective serotonin reuptake inhibitor (SSRI) response prediction model using genetic information. Results of genetic prediction of response or nonresponse to SSRIs (a) in initial derivation sample (n = 239) and (b) validation sample (n = 176) of completer patients with major depression.

predicted by the HAP-SNP model to do well with SSRI treatment actually had significantly worse observed outcomes with non-SSRI drugs.

Discussion

The markers associated with response to SSRI drugs comprised ten SNPs from the *TPH2, SLC6A4, GRIK2,* and *GAD1* genes and six haplotypes from the *TPH2, SLC6A4,* and *GRIK2* genes (Table 2 and Figure 2). Thus, SSRI response was associated with polymorphisms in serotonin, glutamate, and GABA related genes. *TPH2* showed the most significant association with SSRI response. *TPH2* encodes the rate-limiting enzyme of brain serotonin production [28].

Comparison with previous studies

Our finding of association between *TPH2* and SSRI response is consistent with prior evidence from studies in an animal model and human post mortem neurochemistry [29,30]. We found associations of SSRI response with 4 SNPs in *TPH2* (rs4760815, rs11179027, rs17110532, and rs17110747). A previous small study found that three SNPs in *TPH2*, rs1843809 and rs1386492 of intron 5, and rs1487276 of intron 8, were associated with drug response after 12 weeks of SSRI treatment (Figure S4) [31]. However, there was no significant association between those three SNPs and SSRI response in the present study.

Another study performed in a European population investigated nine SNPs in the *TPH2* gene, and found two SNPs, rs10879346 and rs1487278, were significantly related to antidepressant response [32]. Additionally, rs2171363 was significant in a

Chinese population [33]. We imputed these three SNPs using genotype data, because they were not genotyped in our study. The imputed SNPs showed significant associations with SSRI response (Figure S4). These results from imputed data increase the possibility that the predictive markers suggested in our data will be replicable in other populations.

Our previous studies indicated that two VNTRs in the 2nd intron (*STin2*) and promoter (*5-HTTLPR*) of *SLC6A4* are associated with SSRI response [5,9]. In this study, we examined the two VNTRs and 12 SNPs in the *SLC6A4* gene, and found both VNTRs and two SNPs were significantly associated with SSRI response (Table 2). The two SNPs, rs2066713 and rs2020942, were located in intron 1 and intron 3, respectively. A previous study reported that these two SNPs have no association with SSRI response at 12 weeks in an ethnically mixed population [31], but another U.S. study reported that rs2066713 showed a trend towards association with SSRI response [34]. Three polymorphisms significantly associated with SSRI response, rs2066713 of intron 1, VNTR of intron 2, and rs2020942 of intron 3, were tightly linked (Table S8). When we constructed a haplotype from 12 SNPs of the *SLC6A4* gene, the haplotype was significantly associated with SSRI response (Figure 2C). It was also reported in a Caucasian population that a haplotype constructed from 21 SNPs of the *SLC6A4* gene was significant [31]. Thus, our results here and previously [5,9] are consistent with much previous work and with a previous meta-analysis [35] which concluded that the *SLC6A4* gene is an informative genetic marker for SSRI response. Moreover, a recent meta-analysis study [36] that examined Caucasian and Asian populations separately confirmed the importance of ethnicity for interpreting pharmacogenetic studies [37]. This is in contrast to an earlier meta-analysis [38] that disregarded ethnicity and found no overall association of *5-HTTLPR* genotype and responsiveness. Porcelli and colleagues reported in Caucasians that *5-HTTLPR* may be a predictor of antidepressant response, while in Asians it is not. These inconsistencies in the evidence for an association between *5-HTTLPR* and antidepressant response in Asian populations may result also from the established genetic variability within broad Asian ethnic groups. For instance, the genotype distribution of *5-HTTLPR* in Han Chinese is closer to the Caucasian profile than to the Japanese or Korean profile [37].

We did not confirm the claim that the serotonin receptor gene *HTR2A* is associated with SSRI response [8]. We found no association for any of the 28 markers in the *HTR2A* gene in our population (rs7997012, FDR corrected $P = 0.47$). In addition, the original report [8] has not been consistently replicated [12,39].

We found that both glutamate (*GRIK2*) and GABA (*GAD1*) related genes are associated with SSRI response. Both these abundant neurotransmitters are implicated in mood circuitry. Our result with *GRIK2* might be related to a report claiming *GRIK4* is associated with response to the SSRI citalopram [40]. We found that two SNPs in intron 1 of the *GRIK2* gene (rs543196 and rs572487) and two haplotypes including each SNP were significantly associated with SSRI response, and several neighboring SNPs showed a trend towards association (Table 2 and Figure 2B). The *GRIK2* gene encodes glutamate receptors, which respond to glutamate for excitatory transmission in mood circuits. There are abnormalities in glutamatergic neurotransmission in depressed patients [41], and the glutamate system is influenced by SSRIs [42,43].

We know of no previous reports that GABA (*GAD1*) related genes are associated with SSRI response. *GAD1* is the key enzyme of the GABA neurotransmitter system. We found that two SNPs in the *GAD1* gene (rs3828275 of intron3 and rs12185692 of 5′-untranslated region) were significantly associated with SSRI response (Table 2). Abnormalities in GABA neurotransmission have been noted in depression [44]. Overall, the genetic profile of our HAP-SNP model for prediction of response to SSRIs is consistent with drug actions involving the neuromodulator serotonin, followed by effects on the mood circuits that employ glutamate and GABA [45].

Study limitation and strength

A recent meta-analysis identified no individual SNP associations with a genome-wide significance for response to SSRI drugs in depression. That null result includes our own findings [46]. One candidate reason for this apparent non-confirmation may be the ethnic distinctiveness of our population. It is previously reported that response to the SSRI citalopram in African American depressed patients was poorer than in Caucasian Americans and it was suggested that this variance in response may be explained by an allelic frequency difference in rs7997012 of *HTR2A* between the two population samples [8]. Three recent genome-wide association studies [12,13,47] failed to identify gene associations with response to antidepressant drugs in depression. These failures underscore the heterogeneity of the clinical depression phenotype, and the complex gene-environment nature of the disorder. In addition, these large, multi-site studies risk incurring methodological problems such as heterogeneity of case material, ethnic heterogeneity, measurement error, and variable recruitment practices [48,49]. By comparison, strengths of our study design include single site performance by an experienced research team, strictly blinded quality control, ethnic homogeneity, inclusion of only clinically referred cases, clinical diagnoses by experienced psychiatrists in advance of confirmatory research diagnostic interviews [50], outcome assessments in person rather than by telephone, and verification of adequate antidepressant blood levels. We also required that all cases were unexposed to antidepressant drugs in the current episode of depression before enrolment in this study. By these means, heterogeneity and confounding of the case material were controlled, and we succeeded in identifying and validating significant genetic predictors of response with manageable sample sizes.

The prediction model examined *observed* response and nonresponse: without a placebo control group we have no basis to predict specific drug response. The gain of information from the predictive model is substantial, especially in the prediction of nonresponse. For the 16% of completer cases (39/239) that our HAP-SNP model predicts will be nonresponders in the derivation sample (Figure 3A), the relative risk of observed nonresponse is 3.3 in comparison to all other cases, and 6.9 in comparison to the cases whom the model predicts will be responders. In the validation sample, these relative risks are 3.2 and 5.6, respectively (Figure 3B). For comparison, the relative risk of a poor outcome is 1.5 in the 27% of patients receiving clopidogrel who have loss of function polymorphisms in *CYP2C19* [51].

The genetic determinants of observed response to SSRI drugs (Table 2) were not associated with response to non-SSRI antidepressant drugs (Table S7). Thus, these results are consistent with the previous reports [9,11] that pharmacologically different antidepressants are associated with different genetic determinants of response. A further, indirect, inference is that the significant markers for observed response to SSRI drugs may be unrelated to nonspecific response factors ("placebo effect") in our patients. However, we should mention that previous antidepressant treatment history in prior episodes of depression might have influenced the clinicians' choice of non-SSRI treatment in the cross-validation sample. We cannot positively rule out this possible confound in this naturalistic study, even though the cross-validation sample closely resembled the SSRI-treated samples on relevant clinical variables (Table 1).

The convergent data from the validation and cross-validation samples suggest that for approximately half the total cases who adhere to treatment, a gene-based recommendation of SSRI or non-SSRI agent as first-line treatment may be possible with 85% confidence, and that this represents a significant improvement over base rates of response and nonresponse in the absence of genotype information for those cases.

The ethnic homogeneity of our sample may be viewed as either a strength or a limitation, and our prediction model needs to be evaluated in other populations. However, the predictive markers suggested in the European [32] and Chinese studies [33] were replicable in our population from imputed data of *TPH2* (Figure S4). Moreover, the ethnic homogeneity of our sample with the appropriate power may overcome the problems of population stratification which can occur in ethnically mixed populations [8]. Additionally, we could not detect any evidence of population stratification between responders and nonresponders in the 1400 genetic markers of our subjects by the Structure 2.2 software [52] and by quantile-quantile plots of the association results (Figure S5 and Figure S6).

Our prediction model does not include clinical variables. Duration of depressive episode was the only clinical or demographic variable that differed between responders and nonresponders, and only in the derivation sample (Table 1). This clinical variable was eliminated when it was found to be nonsignificant in the logistic regression analyses. Thus, while clinical features are somewhat related to antidepressant response, they may not be independently predictive after correction for genomic factors [32].

Implications

Our HAP-SNP model appears to achieve the goal of gene-based selection of drug class in just over 50% of adherent cases. Though it remains an objective, we do not yet know whether it is realistic to expect significantly better predictive power than 50% in such a complex and heterogeneous disorder as DSM-IV defined major depression. Nevertheless, this extent of genetic prediction is potentially cost-effective [53]. In particular, 59% of the anticipated nonresponders could be identified without the expense and delay associated with a failed trial of SSRIs. In order to evaluate the applicability of genetic predictors in clinical practice, Intent-to-Treat (ITT) analyses and cost analyses will be required. However, ITT is not the appropriate framework for discovery purposes such as this study. Moreover, all potential biomarkers for prediction of antidepressant response in practice settings are destined to be subject to the attrition that we observed (at least 20%), if not much more [54]. While our results need to be confirmed in other populations, and will doubtless be refined with further experience, to the best of our knowledge, no genetic models possessing comparable power have been proposed and validated for the prediction of antidepressant drug class response.

Web Resources

dbSNP: http://www.ncbi.nlm.nih.gov/projects/SNP

FESD: http://sysbio.kribb.re.kr:8080/fesd

HapMap: http://hapmap.org

Tagger: http://www.broad.mit.edu/mpg/tagger

Supporting Information

Figure S1 Selection of 1502 candidate SNPs from 79 candidate genes.

Figure S2 Difference in linkage disequilibrium (LD) structure of TPH2 between responders and nonresponders. The LD structure is based on the measure of r^2. LD was stronger among responders than among nonresponders. The region including three different haplotype blocks, H2, H3, and a part of H4 in the nonresponder group was observed as a single long haplotype, H2 (12 SNPs) in the responder group.

Figure S3 Association analysis of SSRI and non-SSRI treated groups. Association analysis p values (as $-\log_{10}$ values) of 1400 polymorphic markers were plotted. No correlation of p values between SSRI treated and non-SSRI treated groups was observed. (A) Association analysis p values between antidepressant response and single-nucleotide polymorphisms (SNPs) in the SSRI treated group are sorted in descending order. The plot of the p values of the SSRI treated group is distributed by continuous curve form and that of the non-SSRI treated group by scattered form. (B) The distribution of high $-\log_{10}$ p values on each axis demonstrates that distinct SNPs were associated with response to each class of antidepressant drug.

Figure S4 Comparison of association analysis results for *TPH2* with previous studies. Red filled diamonds indicate genotyped SNPs in this study and red blank diamonds imputed SNPs. Blue filled triangles, blue blank triangles, and dark green crosses indicate association results studied in Tzvetkov et al. 2008, Peters et al. 2004, and Tsai et al. 2009, respectively. The same SNPs between studies are linked by dotted lines. The significant SNPs, rs10879346 and rs1487278, in Tzvetkov et al. 2008 study and rs2171363 in Tsai et al. 2009 study were replicated in our imputation study, suggesting that associations in the current study might be replicable in other populations (See Discussion of Manuscript).

Figure S5 Population structure in the derivation sample of SSRI treated patients. Population structure was estimated from 10 000 iterated simulations using the Structure 2.2 software. Red and green circles indicate responders and nonresponders, respectively. We set the number (K) of possible sub-populations as three (cluster 1, cluster 2 and others). If there was population stratification, individual circles would be grouped near one of the clusters according to their overall genetic similarity. We did not observe any clear pattern of clustering between responders and nonresponders. No evidence of population stratification between two groups was observed in our sample.

Figure S6 Quantile-quantile (QQ) plots for association tests of 1400 SNPs. For each of five genetic modes of (A) genotype, (B) additive, (C) allele, (D) dominant, and (E) recessive, QQ plots of the results of association with selective serotonin reuptake inhibitor (SSRI) response are shown in blue. No overall departures of the observed p values from the expected p values were observed in the QQ plots. Median value of $-\log_{10} P$ values ranged from 0.24 to 0.34 according to the genetic mode.

Table S1 Candidate genes and 1502 selected SNPs.

Table S2 Summary of selected SNPs according to SNP selection method.

Table S3 Associations of significant SNP markers with response for individual SSRI drugs in derivation sample.

Table S4 Plasma levels of antidepressants for responders and nonresponders.

Table S5 Distribution of genotypes of the SNPs most strongly associated with response to SSRIs in derivation sample, in validation sample, and in cross-validation sample.

Table S6 Association analysis results in validation samples of top 10 SNPs significantly associated with SSRI response in derivation samples.

Table S7 SNPs most strongly associated with response to non-SSRI drugs.

Table S8 Linkage disequilibrium (LD) between predictive markers.

Text S1 Supplementary Methods: 1. Function-based tagging selection of single-nucleotide polymorphism markers; 2. Genotyping, 3. Plasma drug levels; 4. Power analysis.

Text S2 Supplementary Results: 1. Characteristics of study subjects; 2. SNPs most strongly associated with remission in SSRI treated group; 3. Association with depression diagnosis for top 10 SNPs significantly associated with SSRI response; 4. Polymorphism prediction model for SSRI treatment; 5. Cross validation results with HAP-SNP prediction model.

Acknowledgments

We thank Sang-En Lee and Heejin Bae from Medical Information and Medical Service of Samsung Medical Center for their assistance in drawing Figure 3 and text editing. And we thank Jong Min Woo from Inje University for his advice on the likely cost-effectiveness of genetic screening in depression. We also thank William H. Wilson from Duke University Medical Center for advice on statistical analyses.

Author Contributions

Conceived and designed the experiments: DKK SL HW WM HK SK JK BJC. Performed the experiments: SL HW JK. Analyzed the data: HW SK BJC. Contributed reagents/materials/analysis tools: SL KK. Wrote the paper: DKK JK SL HW WM SK BJC.

References

1. Trivedi MH, Rush AJ, Wisniewski SR, Nierenberg AA, Warden D, et al. (2006) Evaluation of outcomes with citalopram for depression using measurement-based care in STAR*D: implications for clinical practice. Am J Psychiatry 163: 28–40.
2. Laje G, Perlis RH, Rush AJ, McMahon FJ (2009) Pharmacogenetics studies in STAR*D: strengths, limitations, and results. Psychiatr Serv 60: 1446–1457.
3. Licinio J, Wong ML (2010) Pharmacogenomics of antidepressants: what is next? Mol Psychiatry 15: 445.
4. Kato M, Serretti A (2010) Review and meta-analysis of antidepressant pharmacogenetic findings in major depressive disorder. Mol Psychiatry 15: 473–500.
5. Kim DK, Lim SW, Lee S, Sohn SE, Kim S, et al. (2000) Serotonin transporter gene polymorphism and antidepressant response. Neuroreport 11: 215–219.
6. Pollock BG, Ferrell RE, Mulsant BH, Mazumdar S, Miller M, et al. (2000) Allelic variation in the serotonin transporter promoter affects onset of paroxetine treatment response in late-life depression. Neuropsychopharmacology 23: 587–590.
7. Smeraldi E, Zanardi R, Benedetti F, Di Bella D, Perez J, et al. (1998) Polymorphism within the promoter of the serotonin transporter gene and antidepressant efficacy of fluvoxamine. Mol Psychiatry 3: 508–511.
8. McMahon FJ, Buervenich S, Charney D, Lipsky R, Rush AJ, et al. (2006) Variation in the gene encoding the serotonin 2A receptor is associated with outcome of antidepressant treatment. Am J Hum Genet 78: 804–814.
9. Kim H, Lim SW, Kim S, Kim JW, Chang YH, et al. (2006) Monoamine transporter gene polymorphisms and antidepressant response in Koreans with late-life depression. JAMA 296: 1609–1618.
10. McMahon FJ (2010) Pioneering first steps and cautious conclusions. Biol Psychiatry 67: 99–100.
11. Perlis RH, Fijal B, Dharia S, Heinloth AN, Houston JP (2010) Failure to replicate genetic associations with antidepressant treatment response in duloxetine-treated patients. Biol Psychiatry 67: 1110–1113.
12. Ising M, Lucae S, Binder EB, Bettecken T, Uhr M, et al. (2009) A genomewide association study points to multiple loci that predict antidepressant drug treatment outcome in depression. Arch Gen Psychiatry 66: 966–975.
13. Garriock HA, Kraft JB, Shyn SI, Peters EJ, Yokoyama JS, et al. (2010) A genomewide association study of citalopram response in major depressive disorder. Biol Psychiatry 67: 133–138.
14. Hamilton M (1967) Development of a rating scale for primary depressive illness. Br J Soc Clin Psychol 6: 278–296.
15. Karasu TB, Gelenberg A, Merriam A, Wang P (2000) Treatment of patients with major depressive disorder. In: McIntyre JS, Charles SC, editors.American Psychiatric Association Practice Guidelines for the Treatment of Psychiatric Disorders Compendium 2000. 2nd ed.Arlington, Virginia: American Psychiatric Association. pp. 413–495.
16. Lingjaerde O, Ahlfors UG, Bech P, Dencker SJ, Elgen K (1987) The UKU side effect rating scale. A new comprehensive rating scale for psychotropic drugs and a cross-sectional study of side effects in neuroleptic-treated patients. Acta Psychiatr Scand Suppl 334: 1–100.
17. Cipriani A, Furukawa TA, Salanti G, Geddes JR, Higgins JP, et al. (2009) Comparative efficacy and acceptability of 12 new-generation antidepressants: a multiple-treatments meta-analysis. Lancet 373: 746–758.
18. Marchini J, Howie B, Myers S, McVean G, Donnelly P (2007) A new multipoint method for genome-wide association studies by imputation of genotypes. Nat Genet 39: 906–913.
19. Armitage P (1955) Tests for linear trends in proportions and frequencies. Biometrics 11: 375–386.
20. Storey JD, Tibshirani R (2003) Statistical significance for genomewide studies. Proc Natl Acad Sci U S A 100: 9440–9445.
21. Barrett JC, Fry B, Maller J, Daly MJ (2005) Haploview: analysis and visualization of LD and haplotype maps. Bioinformatics 21: 263–265.
22. Gabriel SB, Schaffner SF, Nguyen H, Moore JM, Roy J, et al. (2002) The structure of haplotype blocks in the human genome. Science 296: 2225–2229.
23. Liang KY, Zeger SL (1986) Longitudinal data analysis using generalized linear models. Biometrika 73: 13–22.
24. Keller MB, McCullough JP, Klein DN, Arnow B, Dunner DL, et al. (2000) A comparison of nefazodone, the cognitive behavioral-analysis system of psychotherapy, and their combination for the treatment of chronic depression. N Engl J Med 342: 1462–1470.
25. Walkup JT, Albano AM, Piacentini J, Birmaher B, Compton SN, et al. (2008) Cognitive behavioral therapy, sertraline, or a combination in childhood anxiety. N Engl J Med 359: 2753–2766.
26. Walsh BT, Seidman SN, Sysko R, Gould M (2002) Placebo response in studies of major depression: variable, substantial, and growing. JAMA 287: 1840–1847.
27. Wigton RS, Connor JL, Centor RM (1986) Transportability of a decision rule for the diagnosis of streptococcal pharyngitis. Arch Intern Med 146: 81–83.
28. Zhang X, Beaulieu JM, Sotnikova TD, Gainetdinov RR, Caron MG (2004) Tryptophan hydroxylase-2 controls brain serotonin synthesis. Science 305: 217.
29. Shishkina GT, Kalinina TS, Dygalo NN (2007) Up-regulation of tryptophan hydroxylase-2 mRNA in the rat brain by chronic fluoxetine treatment correlates with its antidepressant effect. Neuroscience 150: 404–412.
30. Lim JE, Pinsonneault J, Sadee W, Saffen D (2007) Tryptophan hydroxylase 2 (TPH2) haplotypes predict levels of TPH2 mRNA expression in human pons. Mol Psychiatry 12: 491–501.
31. Peters EJ, Slager SL, McGrath PJ, Knowles JA, Hamilton SP (2004) Investigation of serotonin-related genes in antidepressant response. Mol Psychiatry 9: 879–889.
32. Tzvetkov MV, Brockmoller J, Roots I, Kirchheiner J (2008) Common genetic variations in human brain-specific tryptophan hydroxylase-2 and response to antidepressant treatment. Pharmacogenet Genomics 18: 495–506.
33. Tsai SJ, Hong CJ, Liou YJ, Yu YW, Chen TJ, et al. (2009) Tryptophan hydroxylase 2 gene is associated with major depression and antidepressant treatment response. Prog Neuropsychopharmacol Biol Psychiatry 33: 637–641.
34. Kraft JB, Peters EJ, Slager SL, Jenkins GD, Reinalda MS, et al. (2007) Analysis of association between the serotonin transporter and antidepressant response in a large clinical sample. Biol Psychiatry 61: 734–742.
35. Serretti A, Kato M, De Ronchi D, Kinoshita T (2007) Meta-analysis of serotonin transporter gene promoter polymorphism (5-HTTLPR) association with

selective serotonin reuptake inhibitor efficacy in depressed patients. Mol Psychiatry 12: 247–257.
36. Porcelli S, Fabbri C, Serretti A (2012) Meta-analysis of serotonin transporter gene promoter polymorphism (5-HTTLPR) association with antidepressant efficacy. Eur Neuropsychopharmacol 22: 239–258.
37. Myung W, Lim SW, Kim S, Kim H, Chung JW, et al. (2013) Serotonin transporter genotype and function in relation to antidepressant response in Koreans. Psychopharmacology (Berl) 225: 283–290.
38. Taylor MJ, Sen S, Bhagwagar Z (2010) Antidepressant response and the serotonin transporter gene-linked polymorphic region. Biol Psychiatry 68: 536–543.
39. Peters EJ, Slager SL, Jenkins GD, Reinalda MS, Garriock HA, et al. (2009) Resequencing of serotonin-related genes and association of tagging SNPs to citalopram response. Pharmacogenet Genomics 19: 1–10.
40. Paddock S, Laje G, Charney D, Rush AJ, Wilson AF, et al. (2007) Association of GRIK4 with outcome of antidepressant treatment in the STAR*D cohort. Am J Psychiatry 164: 1181–1188.
41. Rosenberg DR, Mirza Y, Russell A, Tang J, Smith JM, et al. (2004) Reduced anterior cingulate glutamatergic concentrations in childhood OCD and major depression versus healthy controls. J Am Acad Child Adolesc Psychiatry 43: 1146–1153.
42. Barbon A, Popoli M, La Via L, Moraschi S, Vallini I, et al. (2006) Regulation of editing and expression of glutamate alpha-amino-propionic-acid (AMPA)/kainate receptors by antidepressant drugs. Biol Psychiatry 59: 713–720.
43. Martinez-Turrillas R, Frechilla D, Del Rio J (2002) Chronic antidepressant treatment increases the membrane expression of AMPA receptors in rat hippocampus. Neuropharmacology 43: 1230–1237.
44. Kalueff AV, Nutt DJ (2007) Role of GABA in anxiety and depression. Depress Anxiety 24: 495–517.
45. Price JL, Drevets WC (2010) Neurocircuitry of mood disorders. Neuropsychopharmacology 35: 192–216.
46. GENDEP Investigators, MARS Investigators, STAR*D Investigators (2013) Common genetic variation and antidepressant efficacy in major depressive disorder: a meta-analysis of three genome-wide pharmacogenetic studies. Am J Psychiatry 170: 207–217.
47. Tansey KE, Guipponi M, Perroud N, Bondolfi G, Domenici E, et al. (2012) Genetic predictors of response to serotonergic and noradrenergic antidepressants in major depressive disorder: a genome-wide analysis of individual-level data and a meta-analysis. PLoS Med 9: e1001326.
48. Demitrack MA, Faries D, Herrera JM, DeBrota D, Potter WZ (1998) The problem of measurement error in multisite clinical trials. Psychopharmacol Bull 34: 19–24.
49. Kraemer HC, Glick ID, Klein DF (2009) Clinical trials design lessons from the CATIE study. Am J Psychiatry 166: 1222–1228.
50. Carroll BJ (1984) Problems with diagnostic criteria for depression. J Clin Psychiatry 45: 14–18.
51. Mega JL, Close SL, Wiviott SD, Shen L, Hockett RD, et al. (2009) Cytochrome p-450 polymorphisms and response to clopidogrel. N Engl J Med 360: 354–362.
52. Pritchard JK, Stephens M, Donnelly P (2000) Inference of population structure using multilocus genotype data. Genetics 155: 945–959.
53. Braithwaite RS, Meltzer DO, King JT, Jr., Leslie D, Roberts MS (2008) What does the value of modern medicine say about the $50,000 per quality-adjusted life-year decision rule? Med Care 46: 349–356.
54. Lawrenson RA, Tyrer F, Newson RB, Farmer RD (2000) The treatment of depression in UK general practice: selective serotonin reuptake inhibitors and tricyclic antidepressants compared. J Affect Disord 59: 149–157.

Characteristics of Effective Collaborative Care for Treatment of Depression: A Systematic Review and Meta-Regression of 74 Randomised Controlled Trials

Peter A. Coventry[1]*, Joanna L. Hudson[2], Evangelos Kontopantelis[3], Janine Archer[4], David A. Richards[5], Simon Gilbody[6], Karina Lovell[4], Chris Dickens[5], Linda Gask[1], Waquas Waheed[7], Peter Bower[3]

1 Collaboration for Leadership in Applied Health Research and Care, Centre for Primary Care and Manchester Academic Health Science Centre, University of Manchester, Manchester, United Kingdom, **2** Health Psychology Section, Psychology Department, Institute of Psychiatry, King's College London, London, United Kingdom, **3** NIHR School for Primary Care Research, Centre for Primary Care and Manchester Academic Health Science Centre, University of Manchester, Manchester, United Kingdom, **4** School of Nursing, Midwifery & Social Work, University of Manchester, Manchester, United Kingdom, **5** Institute of Health Service Research, University of Exeter Medical School, University of Exeter, Exeter, United Kingdom, **6** Mental Health Research Group, Department of Health Sciences and Hull York Medical School, University of York, York, United Kingdom, **7** Lancashire Care NHS Foundation Trust, Preston, United Kingdom

Abstract

Background: Collaborative care is a complex intervention based on chronic disease management models and is effective in the management of depression. However, there is still uncertainty about which components of collaborative care are effective. We used meta-regression to identify factors in collaborative care associated with improvement in patient outcomes (depressive symptoms) and the process of care (use of anti-depressant medication).

Methods and Findings: Systematic review with meta-regression. The Cochrane Collaboration Depression, Anxiety and Neurosis Group trials registers were searched from inception to 9th February 2012. An update was run in the CENTRAL trials database on 29th December 2013. Inclusion criteria were: randomised controlled trials of collaborative care for adults ≥18 years with a primary diagnosis of depression or mixed anxiety and depressive disorder. Random effects meta-regression was used to estimate regression coefficients with 95% confidence intervals (CIs) between study level covariates and depressive symptoms and relative risk (95% CI) and anti-depressant use. The association between anti-depressant use and improvement in depression was also explored. Seventy four trials were identified (85 comparisons, across 21,345 participants). Collaborative care that included psychological interventions predicted improvement in depression (β coefficient −0.11, 95% CI −0.20 to −0.01, p = 0.03). Systematic identification of patients (relative risk 1.43, 95% CI 1.12 to 1.81, p = 0.004) and the presence of a chronic physical condition (relative risk 1.32, 95% CI 1.05 to 1.65, p = 0.02) predicted use of anti-depressant medication.

Conclusion: Trials of collaborative care that included psychological treatment, with or without anti-depressant medication, appeared to improve depression more than those without psychological treatment. Trials that used systematic methods to identify patients with depression and also trials that included patients with a chronic physical condition reported improved use of anti-depressant medication. However, these findings are limited by the observational nature of meta-regression, incomplete data reporting, and the use of study aggregates.

Editor: Phillipa J. Hay, University of Western Sydney, Australia

Funding: This study was funded by a Research and Capability Funding grant awarded by the NIHR Collaboration for Leadership in Applied Health Research and Care for Greater Manchester (ref:RCF_R10_PC). The funders had no role in study design, data collection and analysis, decision to publish, or preparation of the manuscript.

Competing Interests: The authors have been/are involved in the conduct of trials of collaborative care in the United Kingdom funded by the Medical Research Council and the National Institute for Health Research.

* Email: peter.a.coventry@manchester.ac.uk

Introduction

Major depressive disorder accounted for 8.2% of years living with disability in 2010, making it the second leading direct cause of global disease burden [1]. People with depression and a chronic physical disease have worse health status than people with depression alone or people with any combination of chronic physical disease without depression [2].

Significant advances have occurred in primary care in recent years to improve the management of chronic disease, principally by introducing structured disease management programmes that draw on the Chronic Care Model [3]. The chronic care model promotes a more proactive, planned and population-based approach to disease management and has been instrumental in transforming ambulatory care in primary care [4]. The concept and components of the chronic care model are fully specified here: http://www.improvingchroniccare.org/. Depression shares with other chronic diseases many features that can be addressed by the chronic care model, such as multiple recurrent episodes [5], where successful management hinges on regular monitoring, care coordination, enhancing providers' expertise, and supporting patients to self-manage. Interventions that include at least one component of the chronic care model have been shown to improve clinical outcomes and the process of care for people with chronic disease, including depression [6].

'Collaborative care' is the most promising chronic care model-based strategy for improving care of depression. While the make-up of collaborative care interventions for treatment of depression vary, they typically include a multi-professional approach to patient care, structured management, scheduled patient follow-ups, and enhanced inter-professional communication [7]. A recent Cochrane review that included 79 randomised controlled trials (RCTs) and 24,308 participants conclusively showed that collaborative care is more effective than usual care for both depression and anxiety after treatment, and up to two years later [8]. There is also ample evidence that these benefits are cost effective [9].

However, while some authors suggest that there is now sufficient evidence about effectiveness and that research should now shift to implementation [10], collaborative care is a complex intervention and there is significant variation in the exact nature of the intervention between trials, as well as differences in patient populations, contexts, comparators, and design. A number of these factors have already been shown to be related to estimates of effect: setting (i.e. country), recruitment of patients using systematic or population health approaches (e.g. disease registers), using case managers with a mental health background, and regular clinical supervision of case managers [11]. There has since been considerable international expansion of collaborative care outside of the United States and extension of this care model to populations with depression and chronic physical disease. We have therefore used meta-regression with a comprehensive and updated data set of randomised controlled trials of collaborative care to identify factors associated with improvement in patient outcome (i.e. depressive symptoms) and/or the process of care (i.e. anti-depressant use). The results will be used to distinguish which features of collaborative care effectively improve patient outcomes and/or the process of care and which do not.

Methods

This systematic review and meta-regression is reported in accordance with the Preferred Reporting Items for Systematic Reviews and Meta-Analyses Statement (see Figure 1 and Checklist S1) [12].

Information sources

The Cochrane Collaboration Depression, Anxiety and Neurosis Group (CC-DAN) trials registers (including both the references register and the studies register) were searched from inception to 9th February 2012. The CC-DAN registers include Randomised Controlled Trials indexed in MEDLINE, EMBASE, PsycINFO, CENTRAL, World Health Organisation's trials portal (ICTRP), Clinicaltrials.gov, and CINAHL. Details of the search strategy used can be found in Archer et al [8]. The CENTRAL search used in the Cochrane review by Archer et al [8] was updated on 29th December 2013 (see Methods S1 for search strategy). For the purposes of an update the comprehensive coverage of the CENTRAL database makes exhaustive searching of individual bibliographic databases unnecessary [13]. All reference lists of included studies and previously published reviews were checked.

Characteristics of collaborative care and conceptual model to be tested

For the purposes of this review we used a definition of collaborative care derived from a systematic review of complex interventions for managing depression in primary care [7]. Collaborative care consists of four key criteria: multi-professional approach to patient care, structured management, scheduled patient follow-ups, and enhanced inter-professional communication (Table 1).

A key innovation arising from collaborative care is the introduction of a non-medical case or care manager who works with a medical practitioner and under the supervision of a mental health specialist to deliver and coordinate psychological treatment, and to monitor progress with psychological and/or pharmacological treatment [14]. While chronic disease management interventions that include one or more features of patient or provider education, feedback, and reminders can lead to improved disease control and adherence to guidelines [15] enhanced roles in primary care for case managers are seen as central to the provision of effective and integrated interventions for depression [16]. Based on current understanding about how the intervention might work and based on previous knowledge about mechanisms of change and active ingredients of collaborative care we tested 10 factors (study covariates) that could potentially moderate patient and process outcomes (Table 2).

Eligibility criteria

Studies were included in this meta-analysis and meta-regression if they:

1) Were RCTs or clustered RCTs of collaborative care delivered in primary care settings or community settings. Primary care was defined as a person's first and ongoing contact point for health care [17].
2) Included adults over the age of 18 with a primary diagnosis of depression or mixed anxiety and depressive disorder according to clinical diagnosis or research assessment (observer interview or validated self-report measure). No restrictions on severity or chronicity of depression were made.
3) Compared the effectiveness of collaborative care with standard or enhanced usual care.

Standard usual care was defined as care routinely provided by primary care providers to patients with depression or mixed anxiety and depressive disorder. This could include onward referral to mental health teams or feedback on participants' depressive status if specified in the protocol.

Enhanced usual care was defined as care where any one or more of the following were present:

i. The patient received additional resources (i.e. educational leaflets, lists of locally available resources, letter from research team with self-help advice) OR the patient had access to enhanced care systems (i.e. consultation-liaison, enhanced referral systems to psychology services, case reviews between health professionals, equal contact time with a health professional, medication management, patient-primary care provider electronic messaging system, person-

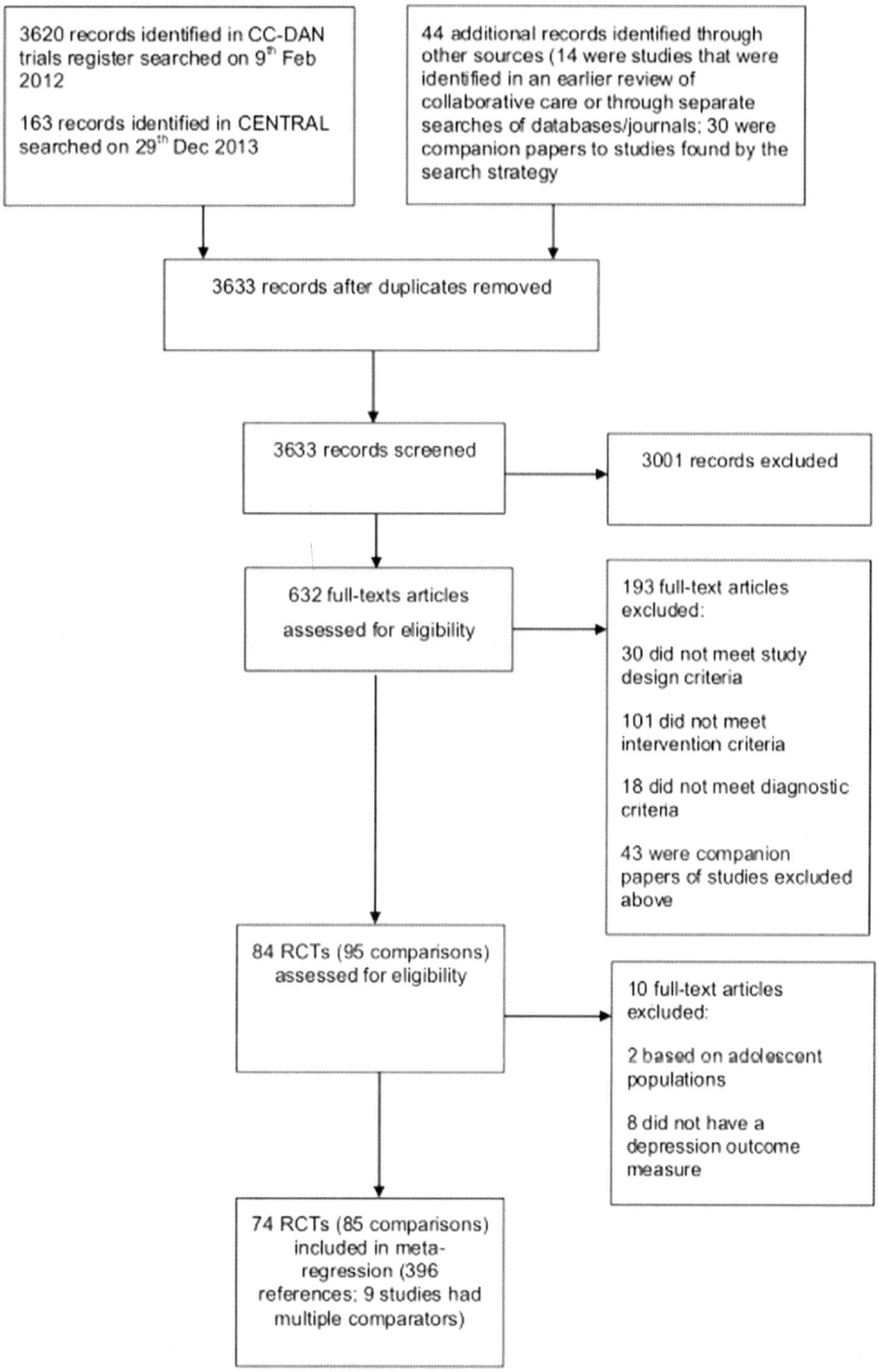

Figure 1. PRISMA Flow Diagram.

alised patient treatment plans from the principal investigator).

ii. Didactic training for the primary care provider.

iii. Primary care providers were supplied with manualised treatment algorithms or evidence based guidelines.

iv. Primary care providers received educational materials other than evidence based guidelines (e.g. educational DVD).

4) Measured change in self-reported or observer rated depression scores as a continuous or dichotomous measure (e.g. ≥ 50% decrease in symptom scores from baseline or remission)

AND/OR

Measured change in use of anti-depressant medication (e.g. proportion of patients taking medication or proportion of patients adhering appropriately to predefined criteria/guidelines), based on self-report or administrative records data.

Table 1. Key characteristics of collaborative care.

A multi-professional approach to patient care
A general practitioner (GP) or family physician and at least one other health professional (e.g. nurse, psychologist, psychiatrist, pharmacist) were involved with patient care, usually acting as a case or care manager to coordinate and/or deliver care for the depressed person
A structured management plan
Evidence based guidelines or treatment protocols. Interventions could include both pharmacological (e.g. antidepressant medication) and non-pharmacological interventions (e.g. patient screening, patient and provider education, counselling, cognitive behaviour therapy)
Scheduled patient follow-ups
An organised approach to patient follow-up that could include one or more scheduled telephone or in-person follow-up appointments to provide specific interventions, facilitate treatment adherence, or monitor symptoms or adverse effects
Enhanced inter-professional communication
Mechanisms to facilitate communication between professionals caring for the depressed person: team meetings, case-conferences, individual consultation/supervision, shared medical records, patient-specific written or verbal feedback between care-givers

Study selection

We identified eligible studies included in the Cochrane review of collaborative care for depression and anxiety [8] and also from eligible studies identified by the updated search of the CENTRAL trials database. Three authors (JH, PB, PC) independently screened non-overlapping subsets of studies against the inclusion criteria for this meta-regression.

Data extraction

Intervention content. Characteristics of collaborative and usual care intervention groups were independently extracted verbatim and coded using a standardised data extraction form and coding manual, specifically tailored to the content of collaborative care interventions (Methods S2).

Patient and process outcomes. The primary patient outcome was reduction in depressive symptoms as measured by observer or patient self-report. Outcomes were extracted for all reported follow-up time points (e.g. six months, twelve months). Most studies reported outcomes at six months follow-up and our analysis was therefore restricted to this time point to maximise both consistency and the number of studies included in the meta-regression. If eligible studies (n = 9) reported outcomes at follow-ups beyond six months we used short term follow-up data closest in time to six months. Where the studies reported two comparisons versus a control group, sample sizes were halved to avoid double counting.

To allow both continuous and dichotomous outcomes to be included in the same meta-regression, we translated dichotomous outcomes into standardised mean differences and standard errors using the *metaeff* Stata command [18].

Collaborative care improves the process of depression care, and use of anti-depressant medications may be a key driver for depressive outcomes. Anti-depressant use as a dichotomous process outcome was extracted; we used risk ratios with log-transformations applied [19].

When studies applied cluster randomisation procedures we accounted for increased Type I error rates by applying the "effective sample sizes" procedure outlined in the Cochrane Handbook [20]. An intraclass correlation coefficient (ICC) of 0.02 [21] was used and sensitivity analyses were performed to explore the impact of adjustments for clustering using an ICC of 0.00 and 0.05 [22]. We also used study sample sizes as a proxy for publication bias [23]. We explored using meta-regression whether there was an inverse relationship between study sample sizes and reported effect sizes. Allocation concealment, an important feature of trials known to reduce risk of bias, was assessed using a binary measure [24].

Analysis

Stata's (Version 12 for Windows) *metan* [25] and *metareg* [26] commands were used to calculate an overall effect size estimate of collaborative care on depressive symptoms and anti-depressant medication use. Consistent with the recommendations of Thompson and Higgins [27], ten covariates were hypothesised to have an effect on these outcomes *a priori* (See Table 2) [11]. In contrast to Bower et al [11] we revised the conceptualisation of enhanced usual care to include an ordinal measure of enhanced usual care in place of primary care provider training (See Methods S2 for the coding and scoring of enhanced usual care).

We used a DerSimonian-Laird [28] random-effects model to calculate the overall effect of collaborative care, accounting for estimated heterogeneity. To quantify the estimated heterogeneity we used the I^2 index, which represents the percentage of estimated between-study variability in the total variability [29]. By convention I^2 values of 25% are considered low, 50% moderate, and 75% high [20]. The main analysis used random-effects meta-regression to estimate a regression coefficient with 95% CIs between study level covariates and outcomes for:

i) Meta-regression model one (multivariable): study level covariates as predictors of depressive symptoms.
ii) Meta-regression model two (multivariable): study level covariates as predictors of anti-depressant use.
iii) Meta-regression model three (univariable; mechanisms of change): anti-depressant use as a predictor of depressive symptoms. This model tested whether use of anti-depressant medication predicted the treatment effect on depressive symptoms.

We explored the potential for confounding or collinearity across the 10 covariates using logistic regression analyses to perform pairwise comparisons. Shared variance between each pair was low (≤ 0.14), indicating that there is a very small risk of measured confounding or collinearity in our measured variables. To retain statistical power we identified covariates for testing in the multivariable meta-regression models by initially performing a series of separate univariable meta-regression analyses, using a significance criterion of $p \leq 0.10$. The $p \leq 0.10$ threshold was chosen to avoid prematurely discounting potentially important

Table 2. Study level covariates (N = 85 comparisons).

Characteristic	Description	N
Country		
US	Study setting	60
Non-US	Study setting	25
Recruitment method		
Systematic identification	Patients were referred into the study if they were: i) identified from a clinical database as having depression or ii) screened positive for depression on an outcome measure and/or diagnostic clinical interview	69
Referral by clinicians	Patients were referred into the study by their clinician	16
Patient sample		
Anti-depressant medication NOT inclusion criteria	Participants did not have to be on or willing to take anti-depressant medication as part of the study's inclusion criteria	62
Anti-depressant medication part of inclusion criteria	Participants had to be currently taking or willing to take anti-depressant medication as part of the study's inclusion criteria	23
Chronic physical health condition		
Present	Participants with a chronic physical health condition were actively recruited as part of the study's inclusion criteria	19
Absent	Participants with a chronic physical health condition were NOT actively recruited as part of the study's inclusion criteria	66
Case manager professional background		
Mental health professional	Trained in mental health disciplines outside of the context of the trial (i.e. psychologist, psychiatric nurse, social worker)	47
Non-mental health professional	No extensive training in mental health other than that provided by the trial	38
Intervention content		
Medication management	Intervention included a medication management plan to ensure optimal levels of adherence to pharmacotherapy. This does not represent degree of adherence (i.e. anti-depressant use).	38
Psychological or both	Intervention included a recognised psychological treatment model (i.e. behavioural activation, problem solving) either on its own or combined with medication.	47
Number of sessions		
Continuous variable	Based on number of planned sessions in the first six months. If the number of sessions differed based on the treatment modality offered (i.e. participants could choose between medication management or psychological therapy) then a mean score was calculated.	
Supervision frequency		
Ad hoc	No regular patterns of supervision.	29
Scheduled	Supervision occurred on a regular basis (i.e. weekly).	52
Not applicable	Applies to studies whose collaborative care intervention included only the primary care provider but the case manager was a certified mental health practitioner (e.g. psychiatrist, psychologist, psychotherapist).	4
Enhanced usual care		
Ordinal variable (based on summed score, 0 4)	See description provided in Methods S2	
Allocation concealment		
Low risk of bias	Coded according to Cochrane risk of bias tool	39
High risk of bias	Coded according to Cochrane risk of bias tool	4

explanatory variables. Table 2 summarises all ten study level covariates included in both meta-regression models one and two.

Results

Characteristics of included studies

Seventy four trials met our inclusion criteria for the meta-regression (including 85 relevant comparisons, across 21,345 participants); 84 comparisons had data on depressive symptoms (across 21,284 participants), and 59 comparisons had data on anti-depressant use (across, 14, 465 participants). See Figure 1.

Of the 85 comparisons included in the meta-regression 25 (29%) were conducted outside the United States; only 4% were conducted in low to middle income countries (Table S1). Nineteen (22%) comparisons specifically recruited patients with chronic physical disease. As stated in the methods section trials had to meet the four criteria for collaborative care to be included in the review. Key factors that differentiated the type of interventions tested in the meta-regression were case manager background and content of the structured management plan. In 47 (55%) comparisons the case manager was a mental health practitioner, and in 38 (45%) comparisons case managers were drawn from a variety of non-mental health backgrounds. In 39 (46%) comparisons the

Table 3. Characteristics of collaborative care.

Author	Multi-professional approach to patient care		Structured management plan	Number of scheduled follow-ups	Enhanced inter professional communication	
	Medical professional	**Case manager background**			**CM liaison with PCP**	**Supervision frequency**
Adler 2004	Doctor	Non-mental health practitioner	Medication management	6	Shared note system	Scheduled
Araya 2003	Doctor	Mental health practitioner	Both	9	Shared note system	Ad hoc
Bartels 2004	Doctor	Mental health practitioner	Medication management	Not reported	Multiple methods	Not reported
Blanchard 1995	Doctor	Mental health practitioner	Both	12	Verbal	Ad hoc
Bogner 2008	Mixed	Mental health practitioner	Medication management	5	Liaison method	Scheduled
Bogner 2010	Mixed	Non-mental health practitioner	Medication management	5	Liaison method	Scheduled
Bogner 2012	Doctor	Non-mental health practitioner	Medication management	5	Verbal	Ad hoc
Bruce 2004	Doctor	Mental health practitioner	Both	15	Liaison method	Scheduled
Buszewicz 2011	Doctor	Non-mental health practitioner	Both	4	Verbal	Ad hoc
Capoccia 2004	Doctor	non-mental health practitioner	Medication management	10	Shared note system	Scheduled
Chaney 2011	Doctor	Non-mental health practitioner	Medication management	5	Multiple methods	Scheduled
Chew-Graham 2007	Doctor	Mental health practitioner	Both	11	Multiple methods	Scheduled
Ciechanowski 2004	Doctor	Mental health practitioner	Psychological therapy	9	Other	Scheduled
Ciechanowski 2010	Specialist	Mental health practitioner	Psychological therapy	9	Other	Scheduled
Cole 2006	Doctor	Non-mental health practitioner	Both	24	Liaison method	Ad hoc
Datto 2003	Doctor	Mental health practitioner	Medication management	6	Written communication	Scheduled
Davidson 2013	Doctor	Mental health practitioner	Both	11	Verbal	Scheduled
Dietrich 2004	Doctor	Mental health practitioner	Medication management	6	Written communication	Scheduled
Dwight-Johnson 2005	Doctor	Mental health practitioner	Both	7	Multiple methods	Scheduled
Dwight-Johnson 2010	Doctor	Mental health practitioner	Both	12	Liaison method	Scheduled
Dwight-Johnson 2011	Specialist	Mental health practitioner	Psychological therapy	8	Liaison method	Scheduled
Ell 2007	Doctor	Mental health practitioner	Both	12	Liaison method	Ad hoc
Ell 2008	Specialist	Mental health practitioner	Both	21	Multiple methods	Scheduled
Ell 2010	Doctor	Mental health practitioner	Both	18	Liaison method	Scheduled
Finley 2003	Doctor	Non-mental health practitioner	Medication management	8	Multiple methods	Scheduled
Fortney 2007	Doctor	Non-mental health practitioner	Medication management	26	Shared note system	Scheduled
Fritsch 2007	Doctor	Non-mental health practitioner	Medication management	6	Other	Ad hoc
Gensichen 2009	Doctor	Non-mental health practitioner	Both	13	Written communication	Ad hoc

Table 3. Cont.

Author	Multi-professional approach to patient care		Structured management plan	Number of scheduled follow-ups	Enhanced inter professional communication	
	Medical professional	Case manager background			CM liaison with PCP	Supervision frequency
Gjerdingen 2008	Doctor	Mental health practitioner	Medication management	12	Written communication	Ad hoc
Hedrick 2003	Doctor	Mental health practitioner	Both	Not reported	Shared note system	Scheduled
Huffman 2011	Doctor	Mental health practitioner	Medication management	4	Liaison method	Scheduled
Huijbregts 2013	Doctor	Non-mental health practitioner	Both	12	Share note system	Scheduled
Hunkeler 2000	Doctor	Non-mental health practitioner	Both	14	Liaison method	Scheduled
Katon 1995a	Doctor	Mental health practitioner	Both	2	Multiple methods	Not reported
Katon 1995b	Doctor	Mental health practitioner	Both	2	Multiple methods	Not reported
Katon 1996a	Doctor	Mental health practitioner	Both	10	Multiple methods	Scheduled
Katon 1996b	Doctor	Mental health practitioner	Both	10	Multiple methods	Scheduled
Katon 1999	Doctor	Mental health practitioner	Medication management	3	Multiple methods	Not reported
Katon 2001	Doctor	Mental health practitioner	Both	4	Multiple methods	Scheduled
Katon 2004	Doctor	Non-mental health practitioner	Both	7	Multiple methods	Scheduled
Katon 2010	Doctor	Non-mental health practitioner	Both	Not reported	Liaison method	Scheduled
Katzelnick 2000	Doctor	Non-mental health practitioner	Medication management	3	Multiple methods	Ad hoc
Kroenke 2010	Doctor	Non-mental health practitioner	Medication management	4	Other	Scheduled
Landis 2007	Doctor	Mental health practitioner	Medication management	9	Liaison method	Scheduled
Lobello 2010	Doctor	Non-mental health practitioner	Medication management	3	Written communication	Ad hoc
Ludman 2007a	Doctor	Non-mental health practitioner	Medication management	3	Multiple methods	Scheduled
Ludman 2007b	Doctor	Non-mental health practitioner	Both	15	Multiple methods	Scheduled
Ludman 2007c	Doctor	Non-mental health practitioner	Both	25	Multiple methods	Scheduled
Mann 1998	Doctor	Non-mental health practitioner	Medication management	Not reported	Multiple methods	Ad hoc
McCusker 2008	Doctor	Mental health practitioner	Psychological therapy	5	Written communication	Ad hoc
McMahon 2007	Doctor	Mental health practitioner	Medication management	6	Liaison method	Scheduled
Menchetti 2013	Doctor	Non-mental health practitioner	Both	Not reported	Verbal	Scheduled
Morgan 2013	Doctor	Non-mental health practitioner	Both	2	Written communication	Ad hoc
Oslin 2003	Doctor	Mental health practitioner	Medication management	8	Liaison method	Scheduled
Patel 2010	Doctor	Non-mental health practitioner	Both	Not reported	Liaison method	Ad hoc
Piette 2011	Doctor	Mental health practitioner	Psychological therapy	15	Multiple methods	Scheduled

Table 3. Cont.

Author	Multi-professional approach to patient care		Structured management plan	Number of scheduled follow-ups	Enhanced inter professional communication	
	Medical professional	**Case manager background**			**CM liaison with PCP**	**Supervision frequency**
Pyne 2011	Specialist	Non-mental health practitioner	Medication management	Not reported	Shared note system	Scheduled
Richards 2008a	Doctor	Mental health practitioner	Both	10	Multiple methods	Scheduled
Richards 2008b	Doctor	Mental health practitioner	Both	10	Multiple methods	Scheduled
Richards 2012	Specialist	Mental health practitioner	Both	12	Liaison method	Scheduled
Rojas 2007	Doctor	Non-mental health practitioner	Both	8	Not reported	Ad hoc
Rollman 2009	Doctor	Non-mental health practitioner	Both	10	Multiple methods	Scheduled
Ross 2008	Doctor	Mental health practitioner	Medication management	5	Liaison method	Ad hoc
Rost 2002a	Doctor	Non-mental health practitioner	Medication management	6	Written communication	Ad hoc
Rost 2002b	Doctor	Non-mental health practitioner	Medication management	6	Written communication	Ad hoc
Rubenstein 2006	Doctor	Non-mental health practitioner	Medication management		Other	Ad hoc
Simon 2000a	Doctor	Mental health practitioner	Medication management	3	Multiple methods	Scheduled
Simon 2000b	Doctor	Mental health practitioner	Medication management	3	Multiple methods	Scheduled
Simon 2004a	Doctor	Mental health practitioner	Both	3	Multiple methods	Scheduled
Simon 2004b	Doctor	Mental health practitioner	Both	11	Multiple methods	Scheduled
Simon 2011	Doctor	Mental health practitioner	Medication management	4	Shared note system	Scheduled
Smit 2005a	Doctor	Mental health practitioner	Both	4	Written communication	Ad hoc
Smit 2005b	Doctor	Mental health practitioner	Both	4	Written communication	Ad hoc
Smit 2005c	Doctor	Mental health practitioner	Both	8	Written communication	Ad hoc
Strong 2008	Doctor	Non-mental health practitioner	Both	13	Multiple methods	Scheduled
Swindle 2003	Doctor	Mental health practitioner	Medication management	4	Liaison method	Ad hoc
Uebelacker 2011	Doctor	Non-mental health practitioner	Both	8	Written communication	Scheduled
Unutzer 2002	Doctor	Mental health practitioner	Both	15	Shared note system	Scheduled
Vera 2010	Doctor	Mental health practitioner	Medication management	Not reported	Liaison method	Scheduled
Vlasveld 2011	Specialist	Non-mental health practitioner	Both	9	Liaison method	Ad hoc
Wells 2000a	Doctor	Non-mental health practitioner	Medication management	8	Written communication	Ad hoc
Wells 2000b	Doctor	Mental health practitioner	Psychological therapy	Not reported	Written communication	Ad hoc
Wilkinson 2003	Doctor	Non-mental health practitioner	Medication management	5	Not reported	Ad hoc
Williams 2007	Mixed	Non-mental health practitioner	Medication management	7	Liaison method	Scheduled

Table 3. Cont.

Author	Multi-professional approach to patient care		Structured management plan	Number of scheduled follow-ups	Enhanced inter professional communication	
	Medical professional	Case manager background			CM liaison with PCP	Supervision frequency
Yeung 2010	Doctor	Non-mental health practitioner	Medication management	8	Other	Scheduled

CM = case manager; PCP = primary care provider.

intervention included both psychological therapy and antidepressant medication management; 40 (47%) included medication management alone; and 6 (7%) included psychological therapy alone. Table 3 describes characteristics of collaborative care used in the included trials. A reference list of included trials is presented in Results S1.

Meta-analysis of the effect of collaborative care on depressive symptoms and anti-depressant use

Compared with usual care, collaborative care was associated with improvements in depressive symptoms (standardised mean difference, SMD −0.28, 95% CI −0.33 to −0.23; $I^2 = 62.2\%$, 95% CI 52.2% to 70.1%; Figure S1) and increased anti-depressant use (relative risk, RR 1.53, 95% CI 1.40 to1.68; $I^2 = 80.8\%$, 95% CI 75.8% to 84.8%; Figure S2).

Meta-regression model one: predictors of depressive symptoms

The results of the univariable analyses of study-level and patient-aggregate covariates on depressive symptoms are shown in Table 4 and the multivariable analyses are shown in Table 5. Four covariates were identified for inclusion in the multivariable meta-regression model: recruitment by systematic identification using either interviews, outcome measures or electronic medical records (study-level; ß −0.16, 95% CI −0.30 to −0.02), people with a chronic physical condition as an inclusion criterion (study-level; ß −0.17, 95% CI −0.28 to −0.05), psychological interventions, alone or with medication (study-level; ß −0.13, 95% CI −0.23 to −0.03), and scheduled supervision (study-level; ß −0.12, 95% CI −0.23 to −0.02). In the multivariable model only psychological intervention remained as a statistically significant predictor of depressive symptoms (study-level; ß −0.11, 95% CI −0.20 to −0.01). Studies that included psychological interventions (alone or with medication) reported greater improvements in depressive outcomes, compared with those studies that included medication management alone.

The beta coefficient reported for the multivariable predictors of depressive symptoms can be back-transformed from an SMD to a mean difference under certain assumptions for the variance of the effect [30]. We only proceeded to back-transform to the patient health questionnaire-9, for which we observed similar within variability across studies reporting on the same scale, and the beta was equivalent to a decrease of 0.67 (95% CI −1.23 to 0.06). The multivariable model reduced the I^2 statistic from 62.2% (95% CI 52.2% to 70.1%) to 47.8% (95% CI 32.6 to 59.6).

Meta-regression model two: predictors of anti-depressant use

The results of the univariable analyses of study level covariates on antidepressant medication use are shown in Table 6 and multivariable analyses are shown in Table 7. Two study level covariates were identified for inclusion in the multivariable meta-

Table 4. Univariable predictors on depressive symptoms (N = 84).

Variable		Regression Coefficient (95% CI)	SE	P	I^2 (95% CI)
Dichotomous or categorical					
Country	Non-US (vs US)	−0.04 (−0.16 to 0.07)	.06	.47	62.4 (52.5 to 70.3)
Recruitment method	Systematic (vs GP referral)	−0.16 (−0.30 to −0.02)	.07	.03	60.8 (50.3 to 69.1)
Patient sample	Medication inclusion criteria (vs not inclusion criteria)	0.08 (−0.04 to 0.20)	.06	.21	62.3 (52.3 to 70.2)
Chronic physical health condition	Present (vs absent)	−0.17 (−0.28 to −0.05)	.06	.01	58.9 (47.7 to 67.7)
Case manager background	Mental health (vs non-mental health)	0.03 (−0.07 to 0.14)	.05	.53	62.5 (52.6 to 70.3)
Intervention content	Psychological intervention or both (vs medication only)	−0.13 (−0.23 to −0.03)	.05	.01	56.8 (44.9 to 66.1)
Supervision frequency	Scheduled (vs ad hoc)	−0.12 (−0.23 to −0.02)	.05	.02	53.7 (40.7 to 63.9)
	Not applicable (vs ad hoc)	0.10 (−0.13 to 0.33)	.12	.38	
Allocation concealment	High risk (vs low risk)	0.06 (−0.03 to 0.16)	.05	.20	62.0 (51.9 to 70.0)
Continuous					
Enhanced usual care*¶		0.02 (−0.03 to 0.08)	.03	.37	62.0 (51.9 to 70.0)
Number of sessions*¶		−0.01 (−0.02 to 0.00)	.01	.26	50.7 (35.5 to 62.3)

*N of 74 comparisons.
¶model intercepts (constants) not reported.

Table 5. Multivariable predictors of depressive symptoms (N = 84).

Variable	Regression Coefficient (95% CI)	SE	P
Recruitment method (Systematic)	−0.12 (−0.26 to 0.02)	.07	.10
Chronic physical health condition (Present)	−0.10 (−0.22 to 0.02)	.06	.11
Intervention content (Psychological intervention or both)	−0.11 (−0.20 to −0.01)	.05	.03
Supervision frequency (Scheduled)*	−0.08 (−0.19 to 0.02)	.05	.13
Supervision frequency (Not applicable)*	0.06 (−0.15 to 0.28)	.11	.57
Intercept (constant)	−0.05 (−0.20 to 0.10)	.08	.53

I^2 = 47.8% (95% CI 32.6 to 59.6).
*Compared with the reference category, ad hoc supervision.

regression model: studies that recruited participants using systematic identification (RR 1.55, 95% CI 1.22 to 1.97) and studies that included participants with a chronic physical condition (RR 1.45, 95% CI 1.16 to 1.83). In the multivariable meta-regression model studies that recruited participants systematically (RR 1.43, 95% CI 1.12 to 1.81) and included participants with a chronic physical condition (RR 1.32, 95% CI 1.05 to 1.65) remained statistically significant predictors of anti-depressant use. Studies including participants who were systematically identified and those with a chronic physical condition adhered more to their anti-depressant medications. The multivariable model reduced the I^2 statistic from 80.8% (95% CI 75.8% to 84.8%) to 75.2% (95% CI 68.1% to 80.7%).

Sensitivity analyses using intraclass correlation coefficients of 0.00 and 0.05 for cluster trials did not impact greatly on the multivariable meta-regression findings (see Results S2 and Results S3). The subgroup analysis exploring the relationship between sample size and effect size for both depressive symptoms and medication use was statistically non-significant, thus decreasing the likelihood that our findings are susceptible to publication bias (Results S4).

Meta-regression model three: the effect of change in anti-depressant use on depressive symptoms

Increased anti-depressant use was not associated with improvement in depressive symptoms (ß −0.13, 95% CI −0.27 to 0.004, p = 0.06).

Discussion

Overall, collaborative care successfully improves both patient outcomes and the process of care for depression. Studies that included psychological interventions, (alone or with medication management), as part of collaborative care were associated with greater improvements in depressive symptoms compared with studies that only included medication management alone. Use of antidepressants was increased in studies that included participants with a chronic physical health condition and in studies that recruited participants through a process of systematic identification.

Strengths and limitations

Our analyses were based on a priori decisions about covariates likely to moderate the treatment effect of collaborative care [11] and included the largest and most comprehensive dataset about

Table 6. Univariable predictors of antidepressant use (N = 59).

Variable		Relative risk (95% CI)	SE	P	I^2 (95% CI)
Dichotomous or categorical					
Country	Non-US (vs US)	0.89 (0.71 to 1.13)	.11	.34	80.1 (74.8 to 84.3)
Recruitment method	Systematic (vs GP referral)	1.55 (1.22 to 1.97)	.19	<.001	77.3 (71.0 to 82.2)
Patient sample	Medication inclusion criteria (vs not inclusion criteria)	0.85 (0.68 to 1.07)	.10	.16	80.6 (75.5 to 84.6)
Chronic physical health condition	Present (vs absent|)	1.45 (1.16 to 1.83)	.17	.001	78.2 (72.2 to 82.9)
Case manager background	Mental health (vs non-mental health)	1.06 (0.85 to 1.31)	.12	.61	80.9 (75.9 to 84.9)
Intervention content	Psychological intervention or both (vs medication only)	0.92 (0.74 to 1.14)	.10	.44	81.1 (76.2 to 85.0)
Supervision frequency	Scheduled (vs ad hoc)	1.03 (0.82 to 1.29)	.12	.83	81.3 (76.4 to 85.2)
	Not applicable (vs ad hoc)	0.94 (0.44 to 2.02)	.37	.87	
Allocation concealment	High risk (vs low risk)	0.89 (0.72 to 1.09)	.09	.25	80.9 (75.9 to 84.9)
Continuous					
Enhanced usual care		0.93 (0.85 to 1.03)	.05	.17	81.0 (76.0 to 84.9)
Number of sessions*¶		0.99 (0.97 to 1.01)	.01	.54	78.2 (71.9 to 83.1)

*N of 53 comparisons.
¶model intercepts (constants) not reported.

Table 7. Multivariable predictors of antidepressant use (N = 59).

Variable	Relative risk (95% CI)	SE	P
Recruitment method (systematic)	1.42 (1.12 to 1.81)	.17	.004
Chronic physical health condition (Present)*	1.32 (1.05 to 1.65)	.15	.02
Intercept (constant)	1.08 (0.88 to 1.32)	.11	.46

$I^2 = 75.2\%$ (95% CI 68.1% to 80.7%).
*Compared with the reference category, physical health condition absent.

collaborative care. By searching extensively, we were able to include almost twice as many trials as previous reviews, and this substantially enhanced our ability to quantify and explore heterogeneity with a greater level of statistical power, thus reducing the chance of spurious findings [31]. In addition, the large number of studies gives us more confidence in the asymptotic meta-analysis methods employed [32], even if the study effects are not normally distributed [33]. The high levels of estimated heterogeneity are a positive finding since it appears heterogeneity levels are being consistently underestimated in meta-analyses [34]. Although there is a link between meta-analysis size and heterogeneity levels and we would expect to detect high levels given the size of our review [34], as we do, the large between-study variability implies that there might be other study or patient-level variables that could explain some of it (e.g. depression severity, ethnicity of patients, fidelity to intervention, quality of case manager training, and level of engagement in psychological treatment).

Additionally, meta-regression can be weakened by other statistical considerations and poor reporting. For example, we were not able to include demographic variables in the regression models due to a lack of variability, and we were unable to model a dose response relationship between treatment effects and case management sessions because most trials did not report data about the frequency, intensity, and duration of psychological treatments. We contacted authors for this information but this process did not overcome this limitation pointing to the need for more comprehensive reporting about the delivery of treatments in psychological therapy trials. More severely depressed patients are more responsive to psychological [35] and pharmacological interventions [36] but we were unable to replicate these analyses in trials of collaborative care because depression severity was inconsistently reported; contacting authors did not overcome this issue. Failure to include these covariates may have biased our results [37]. This limitation also highlights the need for more consistent and comprehensive reporting about the content of complex mental health interventions and efforts to strengthen reporting and specification of complex behaviour change are a step forward to overcoming this limitation [38].

In the absence of individual patient data we had to rely on analyses of mean study effects which are prone to bias ('ecological fallacy': deducing for an individual from a group mean), which are difficult to interpret since the relationships within- and between-studies might differ, making evidence from such analyses inconclusive [27]. In addition, we could not use a single structural equation model to properly account for mediating and moderating effects and the relationships between antidepressant use and depressive symptoms.

Most trials included in this review only reported short-term follow-up limiting opportunities to conduct sensitivity analyses of moderators of long term effectiveness of collaborative care. The absence of long term follow-up data among the group of trials included in this review resembles the findings of Deshauer et al., who screened more than 2000 records for classic placebo-controlled RCTs of selective serotonin reuptake inhibitors and identified only six studies with follow-up of 6 months or greater [39]. There is a clear need to build longer term follow-up into trials of treatment of depression given that depression is episodic and the ultimate goal of treatment is to bring about sustained recovery. Additionally, most trials did not report if the trial population included patients with comorbid chronic physical health conditions, further reducing the number of comparisons entered into the regression models. Furthermore, it is reasonable to assume that all studies that included older adults will have included patients with unreported comorbidity, potentially rendering comparisons of collaborative care in chronic physical health conditions redundant. However, our analysis suggests that presence of a chronic physical health condition as a study inclusion criteria remained a key moderator of medication adherence irrespective of the presence of unreported comorbidities, suggesting that this issue has substantive significance, and does not represent confounding.

We analysed ten theoretically plausible covariates that might determine the effectiveness of collaborative care on both depressive symptoms and medication use using an initial p value of 0.10. Assuming statistical independence then approximately one in ten of our tests was susceptible to type I error but we did not adjust for multiple testing. However, we felt justified in this approach. Although adopting a more conservative approach to hypothesis testing using multiplicity adjustments would have decreased our chances of making a Type I error, we would have also increased our chances of Type II errors (i.e. false negatives), and thus rejected important predictors of the effectiveness of collaborative care outcomes [40].

Comparisons with the previous meta-regression analysis

A novel finding of our meta-regression is that including psychological therapy, either alone or with antidepressant medication, conferred additional benefit, at least for depressive symptoms. Compared with previous analyses [11] we included a greater number of trials (+50) in our analysis which means that our analysis is the first to be powered to detect this finding. In addition, we showed that studies that systematically identified patients were important moderators of anti-depressant medication use. This finding may also be due to increased statistical power generated by our meta-regression. Additionally, we also showed that the presence of a chronic physical condition moderated use of anti-depressant medications – trials that included patients with chronic physical conditions reported increased use of anti-depressant medication. This patient characteristic was not explored in the previous meta-regression.

Contrary to the findings of a previous meta-regression [11], case-manager background did not predict reduction in depressive symptoms. Despite improvements there are still shortages of psychologists and psychotherapists, especially in low and middle-income countries [41], but case management of depression in the context of collaborative care might not need be delivered by a mental health professional. Indeed there is emerging evidence, mainly from the United States, that nurse-led collaborative care is more effective than usual care for treating depression in people with chronic physical disease [42], suggesting that non-mental health trained primary care nurses are as well placed as mental health professionals to work as case managers for certain types of patients. However, where case managers are drawn from non-mental health professions there may need to be more emphasis on ensuring that there are satisfactory arrangements in place for regular specialist supervision.

Clinical supervision of psychological therapists can positively affect the process of treatment, leading to greater confidence, self-awareness, and competence among therapists [43], and, in the context of brief psychological treatment, possibly improved patient outcomes [44]. Our initial univariable analysis adds weight to previous findings [11] that compared with ad hoc supervision the availability of scheduled case manager supervision from a mental health specialist predicted improved depressive symptom outcomes. This finding has important implications for patient benefit given that large scale epidemiological studies have shown that depression is under-treated because of inadequate anti-depressant medication management by health care providers, along with poor clinical supervision and patient follow-up [45]. Inadequate anti-depressant treatment of depression is more pronounced in people with chronic physical conditions [46]. Recurrence of symptoms is also common, but patients who continue treatment with anti-depressants reduce the risk of recurrence by 70% compared with those who discontinue treatment [47], although it is not clear whether reduction in relapse represents true long term efficacy or avoidance of relapse precipitated by antidepressant withdrawal [48]. Additionally, few patients respond to an initial 20 mg dose of citalopram and only about 40% of patients achieve remission after receiving the full therapeutic dosage of an anti-depressant medication [49]. Furthermore, up to 20% of patients remain depressed after completing an initial phase of treatment [50]. Regular supervision within collaborative care could thus help to overcome therapeutic impasse by supporting case managers to identify and manage patients who do not initially respond to or discontinue treatment by facilitating changes to anti-depressant dosage, augmentation of medication with another therapy, or recommending switching to another treatment.

Implications for policy and practice

Our findings show that structured management plans that included psychological interventions either as a standalone therapy or in combination with antidepressant medication predicted reductions in depressive symptoms more so than collaborative care that only offered patients anti-depressant medication. While the additional effects associated with psychological treatment were small this result does highlight the importance of patient choice in the delivery of health care for depression. Across a diverse range of psychiatric conditions and health care settings patients have reported a 3-fold preference for psychological treatment over pharmacological treatment, underscoring the need to link treatment strategies to patient preference [51].

We showed that certain types of patients appear to be better at taking anti-depressant medications than others. In the absence of collaborative care depression is under-treated with anti-depressant medication in older adults with chronic physical conditions [46]. However, our findings show that this patient group showed improved levels of anti-depressant use compared with those without chronic physical conditions. It may be that patients with depression and chronic physical conditions are primed to respond well to structured management programmes that include anti-depressant medication because they are well versed in using medications to self-manage their chronic illness. However the burden of treatment for patients with complex, chronic physical and mental comorbidities may reduce their capacity to collaborate in their care [52].

Novel to this review was our finding that compared with recruitment by clinicians, trials that systematically identified patients were associated with increased use of anti-depressant medication. This finding goes beyond methodological considerations about how to effectively recruit patients into mental health trials. Patients referred to mental health services by clinicians tend to be patients with most to gain as they may be more severely depressed. However, the fact that we found that systems based approaches to patient identification predicted increased use of anti-depressant medication highlights the fact that population approaches to disease management can identify different types of patients who may have additional capacity to benefit, further underlining the importance of structured approaches to depression care.

Future work and conclusion

Given the premise that collaborative care is an organisational framework within which different combinations of psychological and pharmacological interventions can be used a key unanswered question relates to how interventions can be tailored, adjusted, or changed to meet the needs of patients. Most collaborative care trials have only measured adherence to anti-depressants but not frequency of changes to medication dosage or augmentation of medication with another therapy. Given that use of anti-depressant medication might be a proxy for why collaborative care is effective it is critical that future trials include process measures that can evaluate adjustment and augmentation of medication similar to those used in the Teamcare trial [53]. Additionally, meta-analysis using individual rather than study-level data would increase opportunities to detect differential treatment effects across individuals in randomised trials, and allows for more complex modelling of the association of treatment effects and patient characteristics [54].

In conclusion, these results update and expand on a previous analysis of factors that differentiate collaborative care trials that improve patient outcomes and/or the process of care from those that do not. Psychological therapy is an active ingredient in collaborative care with or without anti-depressant medication, emphasising the importance of building flexible collaborative care models that include different combinations of pharmacological and non-pharmacological therapies that meet patients' treatment preferences. Furthermore, patients systematically identified and those with chronic physical conditions are likely to adhere more to pharmacological treatments. Using systems based approaches to identify patients with depression highlights the importance of borrowing elements from chronic disease management models to improve the process of depression care.

Supporting Information

Figure S1 Forest plot of effect of collaborative care on depressive symptoms. *Meta-analysis of individual trial and* *pooled effects. Random effects model used. 95% CI = 95% confidence intervals.*

Figure S2 Forest plot of effect of collaborative care on antidepressant use. *Meta-analysis of individual trial and pooled effects. Random effects model used. 95% CI = 95% confidence intervals.*

Table S1 Characteristics of included studies.

Methods S1 Central Search Strategy.

Methods S2 Meta-regression coding manual.

Checklist S1 PRISMA Checklist.

Results S1 Reference list of included studies.

Results S2 Sensitivity analysis: Cluster Intraclass correlation coefficient of 0.00.

Results S3 Sensitivity analysis: Cluster Intraclass correlation coefficient of 0.05.

Results S4 Sensitivity analysis: Relationship between sample size and effect size.

Acknowledgments

PC is the guarantor of this work and, as such, had full access to all the data in the study and takes responsibility for the integrity of the data and the accuracy of the data analysis.

Author Contributions

Conceived and designed the experiments: PC JH EK PB. Analyzed the data: JH EK PC PB JA. Wrote the paper: PC JH EK PB. Edited the manuscript: WW LG SG DR CD KL JA.

References

1. Ferrari AJ, Charlson FJ, Norman RE, Patten SB, Freedman G, et al. (2013) Burden of Depressive Disorders by Country, Sex, Age, and Year: Findings from the Global Burden of Disease Study 2010. PLoS Med 10: e1001547.
2. Moussavi S, Chatterji S, Verdes E, Tandon A, Patel V, et al. (2007) Depression, chronic diseases, and decrements in health: results from the World Health Surveys. Lancet 370: 851–858.
3. Wagner EH, Austin BT, Michael Von K (1996) Organizing Care for Patients with Chronic Illness. The Milbank Quarterly 74: 511–544.
4. Bodenheimer T, Wagner EH, Grumbach K (2002) Improving primary care for patients with chronic illness. JAMA 288: 1775–1779.
5. Furukawa TA, Yoshimura R, Harai H, Imaizumi T, Takeuchi H, et al. (2009) How many well vs. unwell days can you expect over 10 years, once you become depressed? Acta Psychiatrica Scandinavica 119: 290–297.
6. Tsai AC, Morton SC, Mangione CM, Keeler EB (2005) A meta-analysis of interventions to improve care for chronic illnesses. American Journal of Managed Care 11: 478–488.
7. Gunn J, Diggens J, Hegarty K, Blashki G (2006) A systematic review of complex system interventions designed to increase recovery from depression in primary care. BMC Health Serv Res 6: 88.
8. Archer J, Bower P, Gilbody S, Lovell K, Richards D, et al. (2012) Collaborative care for depression and anxiety problems. Cochrane Database Syst Rev 10: CD006525.
9. Gilbody S, Bower P, Whitty P (2006) Costs and consequences of enhanced primary care for depression: systematic review of randomised economic evaluations. Br J Psychiatry 189: 297–308.
10. Katon W, Unutzer J (2006) Collaborative care models for depression: time to move from evidence to practice. Arch Intern Med 166: 2304–2306.
11. Bower P, Gilbody S, Richards D, Fletcher J, Sutton A (2006) Collaborative care for depression in primary care. Making sense of a complex intervention: systematic review and meta-regression. Br J Psychiatry 189: 484–493.
12. Liberati A, Altman DG, Tetzlaff J, Mulrow C, Gotzsche PC, et al. (2009) The PRISMA Statement for Reporting Systematic Reviews and Meta-Analyses of Studies That Evaluate Health Care Interventions: Explanation and Elaboration. Annals of Internal Medicine 151: W-65.
13. Royle P, Waugh N (2005) A simplified search strategy for identifying randomised controlled trials for systematic reviews of health care interventions: a comparison with more exhaustive strategies. BMC Medical Research Methodology 5: 23.
14. Korff MV, Goldberg D (2001) Improving outcomes in depression. BMJ 323: 948–949.
15. Weingarten SR, Henning JM, Badamgarav E, Knight K, Hasselblad V, et al. (2002) Interventions used in disease management programmes for patients with chronic illnesswhich ones work? Meta-analysis of published reports. BMJ 325: 925.
16. Gilbody S, Whitty P, Grimshaw J, Thomas R (2003) Educational and organizational interventions to improve the management of depression in primary care: a systematic review. JAMA 289: 3145–3151.
17. Boerma WG, Verhaak PF (1999) The general practitioner as the first contacted health professional by patients with psychosocial problems: a European study. Psychol Med 29: 689–696.
18. Kontopantelis E, Reeves D (2009) METAEFF: Stata module to perform effect sizes calculations for meta-analyses. Statistical Software Components.
19. Lipsey MW, Wilson D (2001) Practical Meta-Analysis. Thousand Oaks: Sage Publictions Inc.
20. Higgins JPT, Green S (2011) Cochrane Handbook for Systematic Reviews of Interventions Version 5.1.0: Cochrane Collaboration.
21. Adams G, Gulliford MC, Ukoumunne OC, Eldridge S, Chinn S, et al. (2004) Patterns of intra-cluster correlation from primary care research to inform study design and analysis. Journal of clinical epidemiology 57: 785–793.
22. Donner A, Klar N (2002) Issues in the meta-analysis of cluster randomized trials. Statistics in medicine 21: 2971–2980.
23. Pereira TV, Horwitz RI, Ioannidis JA (2012) Empirical evaluation of very large treatment effects of medical interventions. JAMA 308: 1676–1684.
24. Hewitt C, Hahn S, Torgerson DJ, Watson J, Bland JM (2005) Adequacy and reporting of allocation concealment: review of recent trials published in four general medical journals. BMJ 330: 1057–1058.
25. Harris R, Bradburn M, Deeks J, Harbord R, Altman D, et al. (2008) metan: fixed- and random-effects meta-analysis. Stata Journal 8: 3–28.
26. Harbord RM, Higgins JPT (2008) Meta-regression in Stata. Stata Journal 8: 493–519.
27. Thompson SG, Higgins JP (2002) How should meta-regression analyses be undertaken and interpreted? Stat Med 21: 1559–1573.
28. DerSimonian R, Laird N (1986) Meta-analysis in clinical trials. Controlled clinical trials 7: 177–188.
29. Higgins JP, Thompson SG (2002) Quantifying heterogeneity in a meta-analysis. Stat Med 21: 1539–1558.
30. Kontopantelis E, Reeves D (2009) MetaEasy: A Meta-Analysis Add-In for Microsoft Excel. Journal of Statistical Software 30.
31. Peduzzi P, Concato J, Kemper E, Holford TR, Feinstein AR (1996) A simulation study of the number of events per variable in logistic regression analysis. J Clin Epidemiol 49: 1373–1379.
32. Brockwell SE, Gordon IR (2001) A comparison of statistical methods for meta-analysis. Statistics in medicine 20: 825–840.
33. Kontopantelis E, Reeves D (2012) Performance of statistical methods for meta-analysis when true study effects are non-normally distributed: A simulation study. Statistical methods in medical research 21: 409–426.
34. Kontopantelis E, Springate DA, Reeves D (2013) A Re-Analysis of the Cochrane Library Data: The Dangers of Unobserved Heterogeneity in Meta-Analyses. PLoS One 8: e69930.
35. Driessen E, Cuijpers P, Hollon SD, Dekker JJ (2010) Does pretreatment severity moderate the efficacy of psychological treatment of adult outpatient depression? A meta-analysis. J Consult Clin Psychol 78: 668–680.
36. Kirsch I, Deacon BJ, Huedo-Medina TB, Scoboria A, Moore TJ, et al. (2008) Initial severity and antidepressant benefits: a meta-analysis of data submitted to the Food and Drug Administration. PLoS Med 5: e45.
37. Negassa A, Hanley JA (2007) The effect of omitted covariates on confidence interval and study power in binary outcome analysis: a simulation study. Contemp Clin Trials 28: 242–248.
38. Michie S, Richardson M, Johnston M, Abraham C, Francis J, et al. (2013) The Behavior Change Technique Taxonomy (v1) of 93 Hierarchically Clustered Techniques: Building an International Consensus for the Reporting of Behavior Change Interventions. Annals of Behavioral Medicine 46: 81–95.
39. Deshauer D, Moher D, Fergusson D, Moher E, Sampson M, et al. (2008) Selective serotonin reuptake inhibitors for unipolar depression: a systematic review of classic long-term randomized controlled trials. Canadian Medical Association Journal 178: 1293–1301.

40. Rothman KJ (1990) No adjustments are needed for multiple comparisons. Epidemiology 1: 43–46.
41. Saraceno B, van Ommeren M, Batniji R, Cohen A, Gureje O, et al. (2007) Barriers to improvement of mental health services in low-income and middle-income countries. The Lancet 370: 1164–1174.
42. Ekers D, Murphy R, Archer J, Ebenezer C, Kemp D, et al. (2013) Nurse-delivered collaborative care for depression and long-term physical conditions: A systematic review and meta-analysis. J Affect Disord 149: 14–22.
43. Milne D, James I (2000) A systematic review of effective cognitive-behavioural supervision. British Journal of Clinical Psychology 39: 111–127.
44. Bambling M, King R, Raue P, Schweitzer R, Lambert W (2006) Clinical supervision: Its influence on client-rated working alliance and client symptom reduction in the brief treatment of major depression. Psychotherapy Research 16: 317–331.
45. Salisbury C, Johnson L, Purdy S, Valderas JM, Montgomery AA (2011) Epidemiology and impact of multimorbidity in primary care: a retrospective cohort study. British Journal of General Practice 61: e12–e21.
46. Kendrick T, Dowrick C, McBride A, Howe A, Clarke P, et al. (2009) Management of depression in UK general practice in relation to scores on depression severity questionnaires: analysis of medical record data. BMJ 338: b750.
47. Dickens C, Katon W, Blakemore A, Khara A, McGowan L, et al. (2012) Does depression predict the use of urgent and unscheduled care by people with long term conditions? A systematic review with meta-analysis. Journal of Psychosomatic Research 73: 334–342.
48. El-Mallakh R, Briscoe B (2012) Studies of Long-Term Use of Antidepressants. CNS Drugs 26: 97–109.
49. Mathur R, Hull SA, Badrick E, Robson J (2011) Cardiovascular multimorbidity: the effect of ethnicity on prevalence and risk factor management. British Journal of General Practice 61: e262–e270.
50. Bower P, Macdonald W, Harkness E, Gask L, Kendrick T, et al. (2011) Multimorbidity, service organization and clinical decision making in primary care: a qualitative study. Family Practice 28: 579–587.
51. RK M, SW W, AD P, JA W, MW O (2013) Patient preference for psychological vs pharmacologic treatment of psychiatric disorders: a meta-analytic review. Journal of Clinical Psychiatry 74: 595–602.
52. May C, Montori VM, Mair FS (2009) We need minimally disruptive medicine. BMJ 339: b2803.
53. Katon WJ, Lin EH, Von Korff M, Ciechanowski P, Ludman EJ, et al. (2010) Collaborative care for patients with depression and chronic illnesses. N Engl J Med 363: 2611–2620.
54. Riley RD, Lambert PC, Abo-Zaid G (2010) Meta-analysis of individual participant data: rationale, conduct, and reporting. BMJ 340: c221.

The Impact of Social Deprivation on Paranoia, Hallucinations, Mania and Depression: The Role of Discrimination Social Support, Stress and Trust

Sophie Wickham[1]*, Peter Taylor[1], Mark Shevlin[2], Richard P. Bentall[1]

1 Institute of Psychology, Health and Society, University of Liverpool, Liverpool, Merseyside, United Kingdom, **2** School of Psychology, University of Ulster, Magee Campus, Londonderry, Northern Ireland, United Kingdom

Abstract

The negative implications of living in a socially unequal society are now well documented. However, there is poor understanding of the pathways from specific environmental risk to symptoms. Here we examine the associations between social deprivation, depression, and psychotic symptoms using the 2007 Adult Psychiatric Morbidity Survey, a cross-sectional dataset including 7,353 individuals. In addition we looked at the mediating role of stress, discrimination, trust and lack of social support. We found that the participants' neighbourhood index of multiple deprivation (IMD) significantly predicted psychosis and depression. On inspection of specific psychotic symptoms, IMD predicted paranoia, but not hallucinations or hypomania. Stress and trust partially mediated the relationship between IMD and paranoid ideation. Stress, trust and a lack of social support fully mediated the relationship between IMD and depression. Future research should focus on the role deprivation and social inequalities plays in specific manifestations of psychopathology and investigate mechanisms to explain those associations that occur. Targeting the mediating mechanisms through appropriate psychological intervention may go some way to dampen the negative consequences of living in an unjust society; ameliorating economic injustice may improve population mental health.

Editor: James G. Scott, The University of Queensland, Australia

Funding: The first author has carried out this work with funding received from the University of Liverpool to carry out her PhD. The funders had no role in study design, data collection and analysis, decision to publish, or preparation of the manuscript.

Competing Interests: The authors have declared that no competing interests exist.

* Email: slw@liverpool.ac.uk

Introduction

Social deprivation, inequality and psychosis

Since the 1970s, in much of the developed world, the wealthiest have become increasingly wealthy but the wealth of the collective poor has remained unchanged [1]. The negative implications for health and wellbeing of this increasing inequality are now well documented [2–5]. Research has identified a wide range of poor physical and psychological outcomes associated with inequality and social deprivation, including obesity [6], cardiovascular disease [7], anxiety [8], depression [9], suicide [10] and also severe mental health diagnoses, including psychosis [11]. The economic consequences of these inequalities are vast. Marmot [2] has estimated that, in the United Kingdom (UK) alone, the healthcare costs associated with social and economic deprivation exceed £5.5 billion per year. However, the mechanisms responsible for these associations are poorly understood. It seems likely that social stressors impacting on emotional regulation play an important role [12–15]. Here we examine associations between indices of deprivation, and serious mental illness, investigating associations with specific symptoms in the non-affective psychosis spectrum, and also with depression and mania. In addition we consider the mediating role of stress, discrimination, trust and lack of social support.

Links between economic deprivation and poor psychological functioning are now well established, with associations found for multiple psychopathologies [8,10,16,17]. Economically deprived areas have excessive numbers of diagnosed individuals with depression [18] and also psychosis [19–21]. In the case of depression it is estimated that living in deprivation, poverty and feeling financial strain are all significant risk factors [9]. In the case of psychosis, a significant proportion of the variance (8%) in incidence rates is attributed to characteristics associated with neighbourhood level and environmental characteristics [5]. A recent analysis has suggested that a one standard deviation increase in deprivation in England may confer an increased relative risk of psychosis of 1.28 [17].

These associations have often been explained in terms of reverse causality on the grounds that individuals with a deteriorating mental state seek out environments that are typically urban and deprived due to downward social drift (e.g. [22]). However this explanation seems unlikely as research indicates an association before the onset of the illness and especially with deprivation during childhood [23] with one research finding associations at birth [24]. There is the possibility that drift may originate in earlier generations, accounting for these findings. However, a dose-response relationship has been detected between deprivation and psychosis, with those who spend most time in urban and deprived environments being at highest risk [25,26]. Moreover, research that has controlled for possible genetic confounding suggests that growing up in deprivation puts individuals at a higher risk of a schizophrenia diagnosis, regardless of genetic risk, and perhaps more importantly for intervention strategies, that growing up with high socioeconomic status (SES) is a protective factor for those who are at genetic risk [27].

Recent studies have suggested that inequality (living in circumstances in which there are large variations in economic wellbeing) may confer risk that is additional to the risk of deprivation alone [28,29]. Kirkbride et al. [17] investigated the association of social inequality with incidence rates of affective and non-affective psychosis. They used the index of multiple deprivation (IMD; a small area statistic made available by the UK Office of National Statistics) and local Gini coefficients calculated by comparing variation in deprivation within each neighbourhood at a lower, nested level of geography, and found that both were associated with non-affective psychosis but not with affective psychosis. More recently, Tsai et al. [30], in a 10-year longitudinal study found that a combination of individual and neighbourhood economic status predicted extremely poor outcomes for psychosis, so that schizophrenia patients with low SES living in deprived neighbourhoods were at 18–22% higher risk of death than those with high SES living in advantaged neighbourhoods. Schizophrenia patients with low SES living in advantaged neighbourhoods also had better outcomes than their counterparts in disadvantaged neighbourhoods.

One limitation of the above research is that it has generally employed broad diagnostic categories as outcome variables. In the case of psychosis, especially, such categories are problematic because they encompass heterogeneous phenomena, leading some to argue that psychopathology is better understood in terms of a small number of dimensions [31] or at the symptom level [32]. Indeed, existing evidence suggests that some environmental factors may confer risk of specific symptoms, for example that childhood sexual abuse confers a specific risk of auditory verbal hallucinations (AVHs) whereas attachment-disrupting events confer a specific risk of paranoia [33,34]. However, other risk factors, for example, urbanicity [35], appear to confer risk across the broad positive symptom dimension. For example, Oher et al. [35] considered the association between deprivation and psychotic symptoms in people with first episode psychosis. They found that there were higher levels of reality distortion and depressive symptoms in the most densely populated areas, however no clear association was observed for paranoia. In addition, it was associated with hallucinations. In some cases, for example perceived discrimination, the data is inconsistent, with some studies suggesting an association with all positive symptoms [36] and some suggesting a specific association with non-clinical but not clinical paranoia [37,38]. These kinds of specificities are important because they provide clues about the mechanisms that may give rise to symptoms. In this paper, we consider whether deprivation might be linked to specific psychotic symptoms.

It seems reasonable to hypothesize that paranoid beliefs may be particularly linked to deprivation because psychological research implicates negative social comparison and experiences of victimisation (arguably more likely in deprived and unequal neighbourhoods) in these beliefs [39,40]. Consistent with this hypothesis, Mirowsky and Ross [41], in a population survey of residents of El Paso (USA) and Juarez (Mexico) found that paranoid beliefs were associated with urban areas in which individuals felt powerless and victimized, and that external locus of control and lack of trust mediated this association. More recently, in a study of a large student sample, Wickham et al. [42] found that recalled relative deprivation in childhood was associated with paranoid beliefs and hallucination-proneness in early adulthood. However, on investigating possible mechanisms to explain this association (beliefs about injustice, trust and social rank) this study found that these variables were significant mediators for paranoid beliefs but not for hallucination-proneness. Finally, experimental studies have demonstrated that walking through a deprived urban neighbourhood can provoke paranoid thoughts in both psychiatric patients [43] and ordinary people [44].

Underlying mechanisms between inequality and psychosis

Several underlying mechanism have been hypothesised to explain the pathways from environment risks to psychosis. Impaired nutrition [45] and infections [46] have been suggested to play a role, but with varying and unreliable findings [47–49]. Given that that stress is implicated in a range of mental illnesses and, in particular, psychosis [15,50,51] an alternative possibility is that experiences of deprivation, especially in highly unequal societies such as the UK or the US, are stress-inducing. Concepts such as status anxiety (SA; [52,53]), social defeat (SD; [54]) and social exclusion (SE; [55]) have all been proposed as potential mechanisms. Although these are conceptually different, a common theme is the perception of being disadvantaged compared to others and hence excluded. The SD hypothesis, in particular, has gone to some lengths to explain the role of not only deprivation but of other risk factors for psychosis such as childhood trauma, urban upbringing, low IQ, migration and illicit drug use [54,56]. A recent review suggests that the impact of population density, social fragmentation and deprivation on risk of psychosis may not be directly causal, but explained or modified by individual level social stressors (i.e. cannabis use, social adversity, exclusion and discrimination). However the authors of the review note that good research is lacking in this area [26].

In this study, we aimed to assess the association between deprivation as measured by the index of multiple deprivation (IMD) and specific mental health outcomes, using data from the 2007 Adult Psychiatric Morbidity Survey (APMS2007; [57]). For reasons reviewed above, we hypothesised deprivation to be associated with paranoia. In the light of previous research (e.g. [58]), we also predicted deprivation to be associated with depression. Predictions about hallucinations had to be more tentative. On the one hand, in our previous research [42] with student participants we did find a modest association between IMD of neighbourhood during childhood and hallucination-proneness. However, research on the cognitive processes involved in AVHs has implicated impaired source monitoring as a crucial mechanism [59] and there was no reason to predict that this mechanism would be affected by current exposure to deprived urban environments. Hence we anticipated that any association between deprivation and AVHs would be small or non-existent. Given the lack of association between manic symptoms and urbanicity [60,61], we also did not predict an association between these symptoms and deprivation.

We also tested four potential mediators of the predicted relationships which were available in APMS2007 and which we selected on the basis of previous research. Because discrimination has been implicated in psychosis in some studies [36] and paranoia in others [37,38] this was included. Trust was included in the light of evidence that it might be specifically implicated in paranoia

[41,43]. Finally, lack of social support and isolation has been implicated in paranoia [62,63].

Although our main research focus is the positive symptoms of psychosis, because depression has also been linked to poverty [9,64] and social deprivation [65,66] we included it in our models. Finally, because mania was also assessed in APMS2007, and because the research linking urbanicity to affective psychosis and bipolar disorder has been inconsistent [17,67], we also considered it in our analyses.

Methods

Ethics statement

The current study used secondary data therefore direct ethical approval was not required. However the original data collection (APMS2007) received ethical approval from the Royal Free Hospital and Medical School Research Ethics Committee (reference number 06/Q0501/71). Written consent was obtained from all participants.

Sample

The APMS2007 was carried out between October 2006 and December 2007 by the National Centre for Social Research and the University of Leicester. The survey was commissioned by the NHS Information Centre for Health and Social Care and employed a multistage stratified probability sampling design. Individuals aged 16 years and above living in private households were identified for interview in England using postcodes. From 13,171 eligible households, 7,353 individuals completed the first phase (although a second phase involved clinical interviews with a subsample, these data are not used in this study, with the exception that they contributed to the definition of probable psychosis; see below). Researchers administered computer-assisted interviews and self-completion questionnaires using laptops to obtain data on topics including physical health, mental health, service use, religion, social capital, discrimination and sexual abuse. For more information, see McManus et al [57].

Dependent variables

Psychosis. The APMS2007 screened for psychosis experiences during phase one using the Psychosis Screening Questionnaire (PSQ; [68]), and then interviewed a subsample of participants with the Schedule for Clinical Assessment in Neuropsychiatry (SCAN; [69]) in phase two. Probable psychosis and definite psychosis were binary variables derived from phase one and two data.

Probable psychosis was derived by all those who screened positive for psychosis at phase one from the PSQ and during the SCAN assessment at phase two. These were scored as probable psychosis (given a score of 1). In addition, those who did not have a SCAN assessment but met two or more positive psychosis screening criteria on the basis of their questionnaire responses were also assigned a probable psychosis outcome. A score of 0 was given to individuals who only met one positive screening criteria at phase one and who did not have a SCAN assessment, and also to all those who screened as having no psychosis experiences at phase one. The scoring of definite psychosis employed the same strategy as probable psychosis but a different restrained weighting strategy was applied to take account of non-response in phase two (see [57]). This is considered a more conservative estimate of psychotic experiences.

Paranoia, AVHs and Mania. The PSQ [68] has 5 sections to identify psychotic-like experiences that may have occurred within the past year: mania/hypomania, thought control, paranoia, strange experiences, and AVHs. Each section has an initial question followed by 1 or 2 follow-up questions to determine severity. For present purposes, paranoia, AVHs and mania/hypomania sections were of interest, and were scored as binary variables, scoring the highest level of severity as 1, and all others as 0. Here, we are using a narrow definition of paranoia, encompassing thoughts of deliberate acts of harm and plotting against an individual as has been used in a previous publication using this dataset [33].

The highest severity of paranoia was assessed using the question, "Have there been times that you felt that a group of people was plotting to cause you serious harm or injury?" The highest severity of auditory-verbal hallucination (AVH) was identified by respondents answering yes to the question: "Did you at any time hear voices saying quite a few words or sentences when there was no one around that might account for it?" The highest severity of mania/hypomania was assessed using the question, "Did people around you think it [being happy, for no reason, for days without a break] was strange or complain about it?"

Depression. A binary score for depression (1 = depression, 0 = absent) was derived from the phase one Clinical Interview Scale – Revised (CIS-R, see [70]). This score was derived from the APMS2007 coding script which included many variables from the CIS-R, including depressive ideas and depressive moods, but also fatigue and appetite. The final depression score encompasses mild, moderate and severe depression.

Mediating Variables

Stress. One item from the social functioning section of the APMS2007 asked individuals whether they saw their tasks at home and at work as very stressful. Individuals answered on a 4-point Likert scale from 0 "not at all" to 3 "most of the time".

Social Support. Seven items were used to identify the level of social support each respondent felt that they had from family and friends. Participants were asked to respond "not true" "partly true" or "certainly true" to a series of statements, including whether family and friends did things to make them happy, made them feel loved, could be relied on no matter what, would see that they were taken care of no matter what, accepted them just the way they are, made them feel an important part of their lives, and gave them support and encouragement. Each respondent could have a score between 0 and 14, creating a 15-point scale. In the current analysis, internal consistence is good (Cronbach's $\alpha = .88$).

Discrimination. An eight point scale was derived based on cumulative experiences of discrimination in the last 12 months. This was assessed using eight items from the discrimination section of the APMS2007. Respondents were asked to answer yes (1) or no (0) to identify if they had been unfairly treated in the last 12 months due to skin colour/ethnicity, sex, religious beliefs, age, mental health, other health problems or disability or sexual orientation.

Independent Variable

The Index of Multiple Deprivation. The index of multiple deprivation (IMD) 2004 data were collected for the APMS 2007. This is a derived measure of social and economic deprivation based on seven domains or neighbourhood variables: income; employment; health and disability; education, skills and training; barriers to housing and services; living environment; and crime. Data for the IMD 2004 was collected between 1997 and 2003 and the APMS2007 reported a 5 point scale, where 1 (0.59–8.35) represents the least deprived and 5 (34.21–86.36) represents most deprived.

Covariates. Covariates included in the analyses encompassed age (range = 16 to 95 with a mean of 46.35, SD = 18.60). Sex was added as a categorical variable covariate where 48.6% of respondents were male (1 = male, 0 = female). Ethnicity was also added as a categorical variable where 0 equated to white British and 1 equalled other ethnicity. In this dataset 84.6% of respondents were white British. Drug use with the last year was added as a covariate, this was added as a binary variable (1 = yes and 0 = no). In this sample 92% of the total sample reported using any drug in the year leading up to the interview. Highest education level achieved was also entered into the analysis, this included 6 categorical variables from degree (18.6%), teaching, HND and nursing (7.3%), A levels (12.7%), GCSE or equivalent (24.5%), foreign or other (3.9%) and no qualification (30.8%), with 2.3% missing data. Finally AVHs were entered as a covariate in the mediation analysis, this was to address the issue of co-occurrence of symptoms, particularly between paranoia and AVHs) as has been previously identified and used in these large epidemiological datasets (see [33,34]).

Statistical Analyses

Descriptive statistics were produced using SPSS 21 and regression and multivariate mediation models were specified and estimated using Mplus6.1. Logistic regressions were carried out to assess the association between the independent variable (IV) IMD and the dependent variables (DV) mental health outcomes (probable psychosis, definite psychosis, depression, paranoia, AVHs and mania/hypomania). This was completed three times. In the first regression IMD was regressed to definitive psychosis, as this required different weighting than for other DVs. The second regression allowed IMD to predict probable psychosis, and the final regression allowed IMD to predict to all other DVs (depression, paranoia, AVHs and mania/hypomania). All regressions used the appropriate weighting for survey design and non-response in order to be representative of English population (see [57]).

Mediation was investigated using multivariate binary logistic regression models estimated in Mplus 6.1 [71] using robust maximum likelihood estimation. In in an initial model, direct paths between the IMD and the symptoms associated with IMD were computed. Model 2 added the direct paths from covariates to symptoms including age, sex, ethnicity and AVHs. AVHs were added as a covariate due to its shared variance with both paranoia and depression [33,34]. All parameters were estimated simultaneously so that the differences in the estimates for the IMD variable between model 1 and model 2 showed the effects of controlling for comorbidity between symptoms and other potential confounders. In model 3, discrimination, stress, lack of support and trust variables were introduced in the model as mediators between IMD and symptom outcome variables, and the mediating variables were allowed to covary. The effects from IMD to the mediating variables were linear regression estimates and the effects from the mediators to the symptoms were logistic estimates reported as odds ratios (see Figure 1).

The adequacy of each model was assessed by examining three information theory based fit statistics: the Akaike Information Criterion (AIC; [72]), the Bayesian Information Criterion (BIC; [73]), and the sample size adjusted Bayesian Information Criterion (ssaBIC; [74]) with lower values indicating better model fit. These fit statistics balance model fit with parsimony in order to determine the optimum model. In addition, chi-square difference tests were used to determine the best fitting model.

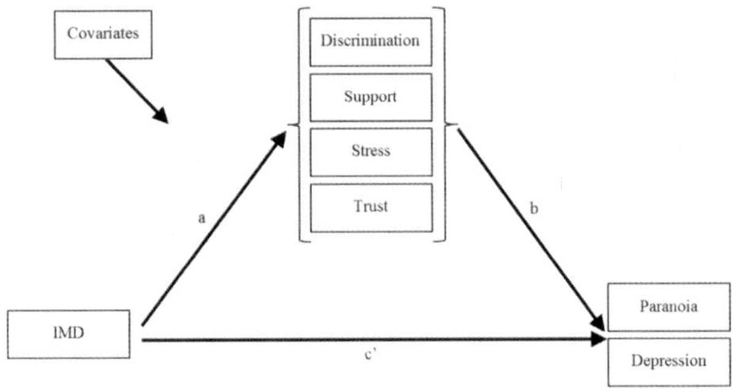

Figure 1. Illustration of the final model (model 3) used in the analysis. Please note that the mediators representing discrimination, support, stress and trust were allowed to covary. Covariates included age, sex, ethnicity and hallucinatory experiences. The mediating variables (discrimination, support, stress and trust) were regressed onto the IV - the index of multiple deprivation (IMD) variable (path a). The DVs (paranoia and depression) were regressed onto the mediating variables (path b) and the DVs were also regressed onto the IV IMD (path c') simultaneously. The effects from IMD to the mediating variables were linear regression estimates and the effects from the mediators to the symptoms were logistic estimates reported as odds ratios.

Results

Simple bivariate associations between IMD and mental health outcomes are summarized in Table 1. The general trend suggests that as deprivation increases the presence of mental health difficulties also increases. This is reflected in the logistic regression analyses (Table 2), when controlling for age, sex, ethnicity, drug use in the last year and education level achieved, IMD predicts definite and probable psychosis ($\beta = 34$, $p < .01$; $\beta = .26$, $p < .01$ respectively), as well as depression ($\beta = .16$, $p < .001$). However when we investigated specific symptoms experienced within psychosis (paranoia, AVHs and mania/hypomania) direct associations were found for paranoia ($\beta = .15$, $p < .01$) and not for either AVHs or mania/hypomania.

The odds ratios (ORs) from the multivariate binary logistic regression analysis are presented in Table 3. Model 1 estimated the direct effect of IMD on paranoia and depression. For this model the likelihood ratio chi-square was statistically significant ($X^2 = 54.94$, df = 12, $p < .01$). The addition of the covariates (model 2; change in $X^2(\Delta X^2) = 186.61$, change in df (Δdf) = 12, $p < .01$) and the mediator variables (model 3; $\Delta X^2 = 2583.82$, Δdf = 38, $p < .01$) made significant improvements to the overall model (Table 3).

In model 1, the IMD variable significantly predicted each symptom (paranoia and depression). The effect was highest for paranoia, with an OR of 1.44 (95% CI [1.25, 1.66]). The OR for depression was 1.29 (95% CI [1.16, 1.44]). The introduction of the covariate variables in model 2 resulted in a slight decrease in the ORs, however remained statistically significant (paranoia OR = 1.26, 95% CI [1.07, 1.47]; depression OR 1.23, 95% CI [1.09, 1.39]).

In model 3, the IMD variables significantly predicted the mediating variables stress, (standardised $B = 0.03$, $SE = 0.01$, $p = .01$) lack of trust ($B = 0.23$, $SE = 0.01$, $p < .001$), lack of social support ($B = 0.04$, $SE = 0.01$, $p < .001$), and discrimination ($B = 0.03$, $SE = 0.01$, $p = .02$). Each of the potential mediators significantly predicted the symptom measures with the exception of the path from lack of support to paranoia, which was non-significant. The largest effect for paranoia was discrimination (OR = 1.47, 95% CI [1.07, 2.03]) and the smallest effect was stress

Table 1. Simple bivariate associations, showing percentages (%) and actual numbers (n) between the index of multiple deprivation (IMD) and mental health outcomes (psychosis, depression, paranoia, auditory-verbal hallucinations (AVHs) and mania).

Diagnoses/Symptom	Level of deprivation											
	Least deprived						Most deprived					
	0.59>8.35		8.35>13.72		13.72>21.16		21.16>34.21		34.21>86.36		Total	
	%	(n)	%	(n)	%	(n)	%	(n)	%	(n)	%	(n)
Definite Psychosis	4.3	(1)	8.7	(2)	17.4	(4)	17.4	(4)	52.2	(12)	100	(23)
Probable Psychosis	5.0	(2)	10.0	(4)	22.5	(9)	22.5	(9)	40.0	(16)	100	(40)
Depression	12.5	(32)	11.0	(28)	14.9	(38)	27.5	(70)	34.1	(87)	100	(255)
Paranoia	6.4	(8)	9.6	(12)	24.8	(31)	28.0	(35)	31.2	(39)	100	(125)
AVHs	14.7	(10)	10.3	(7)	20.6	(14)	26.5	(18)	27.9	(19)	100	(68)
Hypomania	9.1	(4)	15.9	(7)	22.7	(10)	22.7	(10)	29.5	(13)	100	(44)

(OR = 1.41, 95% CI [1.13, 1.75]). With the DV depression, the largest effect was between stress and depression (OR = 2.30, 95% CI [1.95, 2.70]). The smallest effect was between lack of social support and depression (OR = 1.10, 95% CI [1.04, 1.16]). Model 3 indicates that *partial mediation* occurred between IMD and paranoia through discrimination, stress and lack of trust. This is due to the fact that c′ (the relationship between IMD and paranoia) remained significant, but reduced between models 2 and 3 (from OR = 1.26, $p<.01$, to OR = 1.19, $p<.05$). However, in the case of depression, *full mediation* occurred as model 3 shows that c′ became non-significant when the mediators were included.

Discussion

Consistent with our first hypothesis neighbourhood deprivation significantly predicted psychosis and depression. When focussing on specific symptoms, again as we hypothesised, IMD was associated with both paranoia and depression, but not with AVHs or mania. In our multivariate mediation model, when controlling for comorbidity between the symptoms and other background variables (age, sex, ethnicity, drug use and education level), IMD was associated with all four mediators; lack of trust, social support and stress and discrimination. Examination of the final model (model 3) indicated that the ORs for the direct effects between deprivation and symptoms reduced once the mediators were entered into the model. In the case of depression the OR became statistically insignificant, indicating full mediation between IMD and depression through discrimination, trust, lack of support and stress [75]. In the case of paranoia, the OR reduced in magnitude but remained statistically significant therefore indicating partial mediation through discrimination, trust, and stress. Overall, this study is generally consistent with previous findings of an association between social and economic deprivation and psychosis [11,17,27–29] but our analyses add to previous studies by indicating that this association relates to specific symptoms and can be at least partially explained by several potential underlying mechanisms.

The absence of significant affects for both hallucinations and mania are as worthy of note as the positive findings. As discussed earlier, impairment in the ability to discriminate between self-generated thoughts and external verbal stimuli, a process known as source monitoring, is a crucial mechanism in vulnerability to auditory hallucinations [59,76]. Although it is well known that childhood trauma is associated with hallucinations in adulthood [33], and although we had previously found an association between childhood IMD and hallucination-proneness in early adulthood, there was no reason to believe that source monitoring would be affected by current exposure to urban environments as measured in this study.

Very little is known about environmental risk factors for mania, but there is evidence that manic episodes can be triggered by goal achievement life events [77] which are, if anything, less likely to be experienced in deprived versus affluent areas. Previous research has failed to find any association between bipolar disorder and urban environments [67] and our findings appear to confirm this observation.

Two findings from covariates included in our analyses are also worth considering. Female sex was associated with an increased risk of depression, as shown in many previous studies [78]. This observation therefore testifies to the validity of our approach. Perhaps more intriguingly, belonging to an ethnic minority group was strongly associated with paranoia but not depression. It has been well-demonstrated that ethnic minority status is a risk factor for psychosis [79] but we are not aware of attempts to tease out

Table 2. Summary of logistic regression analysis for variables predicting mental health outcomes, controlling for background variables (age, sex, ethnicity, education and drug use).

	Unstandardised		Standardised		
Index of Multiple Deprivation to:	**ß**	**SE**	**ß**	**SE**	**OR (95% CI)**
Definite Psychosis	.57*	.20	.34*	.11	1.8* (1.2–2.6)
Probable Psychosis	.39*	.14	.26*	.08	1.5** (1.1–1.9)
Depression	.21**	.06	.16**	.04	1.2** (1.1–1.4)
Paranoia	.22*	.08	.15*	.05	1.2** (1.1–1.5)
AVHs	.12	.11	.09	.08	1.1 (0.9–1.4)
Mania	.09	.14	.06	.10	1.1 (0.8–1.4)

Note:
**p<.001,
*p<.01 Definitive Psychosis was weighted using specific weight designed for this variable; all other variables were weighted using phase one data weights.

Table 3. Logistic regression odds ratios of symptoms by IMD and fit indices for the mediation model.

Variable		Model 1 OR (95% CI)	Model 2 OR (95% CI)	Model 3 OR (95% CI)
Paranoia	IMD	1.44** (1.25–1.66)	1.26** (1.07–1.47)	1.19* (1.02–1.40)
	Age	-	0.97** (0.96–0.99)	0.99* (0.97–1.00)
	Sex	-	1.35 (0.88–2.09)	1.36 (0.87–2.11)
	Ethnicity	-	2.47** (1.48–4.13)	2.24** (1.32–3.78)
	Education	-	0.93 (0.83–1.04)	0.97 (1.14–3.63)
	Drug use	-	2.35** (1.34–4.11)	2.03 (1.14–3.63)
	AVHs	-	22.78** (10.21–50.85)	12.08** (5.07–28.81)
	Discrimination	-	-	1.47** (1.07–2.03)
	Stress	-	-	1.41** (1.13–1.75)
	Trust	-	-	1.45** (1.19 - 1.76)
	Support	-	-	1.05 (0.98–1.14)
Depression	IMD	1.29** (1.16–1.44)	1.23** (1.09–1.39)	1.11 (0.98–1.26)
	Age	-	0.99** (0.99–1.00)	1.01 (1.00–1.02)
	Sex	-	0.66** (0.49–0.90)	0.63 (0.45–0.87)
	Ethnicity	-	0.85 (0.53–1.38)	0.62 (0.37–1.05)
	Education	-	0.88** (0.81–0.95)	0.91* (0.84–0.99)
	Drug use	-	2.02 (1.29–3.18)	1.54 (0.92–2.57)
	AVHs	-	7.18** (3.43–15.02)	2.15 (0.92–5.01)
	Discrimination	-	-	1.96** (1.56–2.46)
	Stress	-	-	2.30** (1.95–2.70)
	Trust	-	-	1.34** (1.18–1.53)
	Support	-	-	1.10** (1.04–1.16)
Loglikelihood		-39894	-39801	-38509
# Free Parameters		12	24	62
AIC		79813	79650	77142
BIC		79895	79815	77568
ssaBIC		79857	79739	77371

Note:
**p<.01,
*p<.05.
IMD (Index of multiple deprivation), AVHs (auditory-verbal hallucinations), AIC = Akaike information criterion, BIC = Bayesian information criterion, SSABIC = sample size adjusted BIC.

which positive symptoms of psychosis are most sensitive to this effect. Because this observation emerged in models which also include trust, stress, social support and discrimination, the implication is that this increased risk from ethnicity cannot be explained by these variables. Further research is required with other datasets to determine whether a specific link between ethnic status and paranoia can be replicated, and what mechanisms might be involved.

A number of limitations to the study need to be considered. Firstly, the PSQ used in the APMS2007 dataset concerns experiences in the last year, rather than across the lifetime. It is possible that people classified as not experiencing paranoia or AVHs in our analyses in fact had these experiences in the more distant past. However, it is worth noting that focusing on recent experiences of psychosis as opposed to lifetime experiences will have most likely led us to underestimate the association between deprivation and symptoms. Second, the measure of social deprivation used in the APMS2007 dataset, IMD scores was divided into quintiles, producing an ordinal scale; due to data protection restrictions raw IMD data was unavailable to us. This loss of information may have attenuated some relationships. Moreover, the measure pertained to current living circumstances, rather than those of, say, childhood or the time of onset of psychotic experiences. Hence we hypothesize that the findings reflect the provocation of psychotic symptoms by the current environment (as in the case of the experimental studies of the effects of the urban environment on paranoia, [43,44]), rather than developmental pathways to psychotic symptoms. Third, the reliability of our measure of stress may be compromised as it used a single item relating to work stress. Arguably, the findings related to stress need to be assessed using an established measure of stress to incorporate other forms of stress (e.g. emotional and home stressors).

Fourth, and perhaps most importantly, the present study is cross-sectional and correlational, and direction of causality cannot be tested using the statistical models we have employed. Therefore, we cannot exclude the possibility that symptoms may affect people's judgments about discrimination, trust, stress and social support or, indeed, that, when answering questions about paranoia and depression, feelings of discrimination, mistrust, stress and the experience of poor social support influenced their answers. Indeed, it could be argued that there is conceptual overlap between mistrust and paranoia and that, therefore, a close association between the two was inevitable. (We think this argument is harder to make about the other mediators.)

With respect to our meditational models, there is no certainty that our mediators were temporally consequent to exposure to a deprived urban environment or that they preceded the onset of symptoms. However, it seems unlikely that people suffering specifically from paranoia and depression (as opposed to AVHs and mania/hypomania) would seek out deprived neighbourhoods to live in. Moreover, our findings are not only consistent with our meditational hypotheses, but also with our previous findings on the relationship between perceived social disadvantage and paranoia [42], with current understandings of the psychological mechanisms underlying paranoid beliefs [39,40], and, as already noted, with experimental studies which show that short-term exposure to deprived environments tends to provoke paranoid thoughts [43,44]. A further caveat is that epidemiological findings, particularly involving mediation analysis [80], are vulnerable to unmeasured covariates. This is a problem in most areas of research that can only be addressed by considering other potential covariates in future studies.

It might be argued that our results offer some support to the SD hypothesis and related concepts [54,56], suggesting that living at the bottom end of an unequal society breeds stress and a lack of trust and support a constellation of experiences which might be described as socially defeating. However, one criticism of the SD model is that it is fairly non-specific in terms of what characterises social defeat, which symptoms are most affected and likely mediating mechanisms.

To our knowledge this is the first study to test for specific symptom relationships (paranoia and depression) with deprivation, as opposed to the broadly defined diagnostic categories which have been identified as particularly problematic when researching social determinants of psychopathological phenomena [81]. It will be useful to replicate these findings in other samples to further assess the specific associations identified here. Longitudinal designs would also help clarify the direction of causality. If supported by future research the present findings have important social implications.

Although the effects found in paranoid and depressive symptoms in this study might be described as modest, at the population level the impact of deprivation on mental health is potentially large. If we consider the UK as an example, the inevitable outcome of experiences of deprivation indicates that more people are being pushed towards mental illness [82]. In much of the developed world, income inequalities have increased since the 1970s with current disparities at an all-time high [2]. It may be possible that efforts to reverse this trend, for example through progressive taxation or through enhanced benefits to poor families will, in the long-term, positively impact on public mental health but devising such policies, and gaining popular support for their implementation may prove to be a very considerable challenge for all concerned, particularly as individuals tend to justify the status quo in more unequal societies [83,84]. It may be more viable to tackle the social stressors that inequality produces through psychological treatments (e.g. cognitive-behaviour therapy (CBT) and interpersonal psychotherapy) which already aim to address self-esteem and are thought to be effective in depression [85], and in the case of CBT at least, effective for psychosis (CBTp [86]). It is possible that these might be enhanced by specifically targeting the mediating mechanisms outlined in the current study, namely support, trust and stress. At a societal level, our findings suggest that public mental health might be promoted by either addressing inequalities, ameliorating the social stressors that arising from inequalities, or both.

Author Contributions

Conceived and designed the experiments: SLW PJT MS RPB. Performed the experiments: SLW PJT MS RPB. Analyzed the data: SLW PJT MS RPB. Contributed reagents/materials/analysis tools: SLW PJT MS RPB. Contributed to the writing of the manuscript: SLW PJT MS RPB.

References

1. Toynbee P, Walker D (2008) Unjust rewards: Ending the greed that is bankrupting Britain. London: Granta Books.
2. Marmot MG, Allen J, Goldblatt P, Boyce T, McNeish D, et al. (2010) Fair society, healthy lives: The Marmot review. Strateg Rev Heal Inequalities Engl Post 2010.
3. Marmot MG, Stansfeld S, Patel C, North F, Head J, et al. (1991) Health inequalities among British civil servants: the Whitehall II study. Lancet 337: 1387–1393. Available: http://www.sciencedirect.com/science/article/B6T1B-49K5F0V-506/2/2dc5b634b421e8988be6ae5c15ce2be8.
4. Wilkinson RG, Pickett KE (2009) The spirit level: Why more equal societies almost always do better. London: Penguin Group.

5. Kirkbride J (2010) Impact of contextual environmental mechanisms on the incidence of schizophrenia and other psychoses. In: Gattaz WF, Busatto G, editors. Advances in Schizophrenia Research 2009. Springer New York. pp. 67–96. Available: http://dx.doi.org/10.1007/978-1-4419-0913-8_4.
6. Lee H (2011) Inequality as an explanation for obesity in the United States. Sociol Compass 5: 215–232. Available: http://doi.wiley.com/10.1111/j.1751-9020.2010.00355.x.
7. Kim D, Kawachi I, Hoorn S . Vander, Ezzati M (2008) Is inequality at the heart of it? Cross-country associations of income inequality with cardiovascular diseases and risk factors. Soc Sci Med 66: 1719–1732. Available: http://www.ncbi.nlm.nih.gov/pubmed/18280021. Accessed 2014 March 27.
8. Fryers T, Melzer D, Jenkins R, Brugha T (2005) The distribution of the common mental disorders: social inequalities in Europe. Clin Pract Epidemiol Ment Health 1: 14. Available: http://www.cpementalhealth.com/content/1/1/14. Accessed 2014 Feb 5.
9. Lorant V, Croux C, Weich S, Deliège D, Mackenbach J, et al. (2007) Depression and socio-economic risk factors: 7-year longitudinal population study. Br J Psychiatry 190: 293–298. Available: http://www.ncbi.nlm.nih.gov/pubmed/17401034. Accessed 2014 Feb 25.
10. Gilman SE, Bruce ML, Have T Ten, Alexopoulos GS, Mulsant BH, et al. (2013) Social inequalities in depression and suicidal ideation among older primary care patients. Soc Psychiatry Psychiatr Epidemiol 48: 59–69. doi:10.1007/s00127-012-0575-9
11. Kirkbride J, Jones PB (2011) The prevention of schizophrenia–what can we learn from eco-epidemiology? Schizophr Bull 37: 262–271. Available: http://www.pubmedcentral.nih.gov/articlerender.fcgi?artid = 3044619&tool = pmcentrez&rendertype = abstract. Accessed 2012 Nov 6.
12. Wilkinson RG, Pickett KE (2009) Income inequality and social dysfunction. Annu Rev Sociol 35: 493–511. Available: http://www.annualreviews.org/doi/abs/10.1146/annurev-soc-070308-115926. Accessed 2012 Oct 26.
13. Zimmerman FJ, Bell JF (2006) Income inequality and physical and mental health: Testing associations consistent with proposed causal pathways. J Epidemiol Community Health 60: 513–521. doi:10.1136/jech.2005.040154
14. Dickerson SS, Kemeny ME (2004) Acute stressors and cortisol responses: a theoretical integration and synthesis of laboratory research. Psychol Bull 130: 355–391. Available: http://www.ncbi.nlm.nih.gov/pubmed/15122924. Accessed 2012 Oct 26.
15. Marwaha S, Broome M, Bebbington PE, Kuipers E, Freeman D (2014) Mood instability and psychosis: analyses of British national survey data. Schizophr Bull 40: 269–277.
16. Lorant V, Deliège D, Eaton W, Robert A, Philippot P, et al. (2003) Socioeconomic inequalities in depression: A meta-analysis. Am J Epidemiol 157: 98–112. Available: http://aje.oxfordjournals.org/content/157/2/98.abstract.
17. Kirkbride J, Jones PB, Ullrich S, Coid J (2014) Social deprivation, inequality, and the neighborhood-level incidence of psychotic syndromes in East london. Schizophr Bull 40: 169–180. Available: http://www.pubmedcentral.nih.gov/articlerender.fcgi?artid = 3885290&tool = pmcentrez&rendertype = abstract. Accessed 2014 Jan 21 January.
18. Andersen I, Thielen K, Nygaard E, Diderichsen F (2009) Social inequality in the prevalence of depressive disorders. J Epidemiol Community Health 63: 575–581. Available: http://www.ncbi.nlm.nih.gov/pubmed/19293167. Accessed 2014 Feb 24.
19. Crump C, Sundquist K, Sundquist J, Winkleby MA (2011) Neighborhood deprivation and psychiatric medication prescription: A Swedish national multilevel study. Ann Epidemiol 21: 231–237. Available: http://www.sciencedirect.com/science/article/pii/S1047279711000263.
20. Croudace TJ, Kayne R, Jones PB, Harrison G (2000) Non-linear relationship between an index of social deprivation, psychiatric admission prevalence and the incidence of psychosis. Psychol Med 30: 177–185. Available: http://dx.doi.org/10.1017/S0033291799001464.
21. Fone DL, Dunstan F (2006) Mental health, places and people: a multilevel analysis of economic inactivity and social deprivation. Health Place 12: 332–344. Available: http://www.ncbi.nlm.nih.gov/pubmed/16546698. Accessed 2012 Nov 27.
22. Goldberg EM, Morrison SL (1963) Schizophrenia and social class. Br J Psychiatry 109: 785–802.
23. Wicks S, Hjern A, Gunnell D, Lewis G, Dalman C (2005) Social adversity in childhood and the risk of developing psychosis: A national cohort study. Am J Psychiatry 162: 1652–1657. Available: http://ajp.psychiatryonline.org/cgi/content/abstract/162/9/1652.
24. Harrison G, Gunnell D, Glazebrook C, Page K, Kwiecinski R (2001) Association between schizophrenia and social inequality at birth: Case–control study. Br J Psychiatry 179: 346–350. Available: http://bjp.rcpsych.org/cgi/content/abstract/179/4/346.
25. Pedersen CB, Mortensen PB (2001) Evidence of a dose-response relationship between urbanicity during upbringing and schizophrenia risk. Arch Gen Psychiatry 58: 1039–1046. Available: http://www.ncbi.nlm.nih.gov/pubmed/11695950.
26. Heinz A, Deserno L, Reininghaus U (2013) Urbanicity, social adversity and psychosis. World Psychiatry 12: 187–197. doi:10.1002/wps.20056
27. Wicks S, Hjern A, Dalman C (2010) Social risk or genetic liability for psychosis? A study of children born in sweden and reared by adoptive parents. Am J Psychiatry 167: 1240–1246. Available: http://ajp.psychiatryonline.org/cgi/content/abstract/167/10/1240.
28. Burns JK, Esterhuizen T (2008) Poverty, inequality and the treated incidence of first-episode psychosis: An ecological study from South Africa. Soc Psychiatry Psychiatr Epidemiol 43: 331–335. Available: http://www.ncbi.nlm.nih.gov/pubmed/18253683. Accessed 2012 Nov 20.
29. Burns JK, Tomita A, Kapadia AS (2014) Income inequality and schizophrenia: Increased schizophrenia incidence in countries with high levels of income inequality. Int J Soc Psychiatry 60: 185–196. Available: http://www.ncbi.nlm.nih.gov/pubmed/23594564. Accessed 2014 March 20.
30. Tsai K-Y, Chung T-C, Lee C-C, Chou Y-M, Su C-Y, et al. (2014) Is low individual socioeconomic status (SES) in high-SES areas the same as low individual SES in low-SES areas: a 10-year follow-up schizophrenia study. Soc Psychiatry Psychiatr Epidemiol 49: 89–96. Available: http://www.ncbi.nlm.nih.gov/pubmed/23728232. Accessed 2014 Jan 30.
31. Van Os J, Kapur S (2009) Schizophrenia. Lancet 374: 635–645. Available: http://www.ncbi.nlm.nih.gov/pubmed/19700006. Accessed 2014 March 19.
32. Bentall RP (2003) Madness explained: Psychosis and human nature. London: England: Penguin Group.
33. Bentall RP, Wickham S, Shevlin M, Varese F (2012) Do specific early-life adversities lead to specific symptoms of psychosis? A study from the 2007 adult psychiatric morbidity survey. Schizophr Bull 38: 734–740. Available: http://www.pubmedcentral.nih.gov/articlerender.fcgi?artid = 3406525&tool = pmcentrez&rendertype = abstract. Accessed 2014 Jan 30.
34. Sitko K, Bentall RP, Shevlin M, O'Sullivan N, Sellwood W (2014) Associations between specific psychotic symptoms and specific childhood adversities are mediated by attachment styles: An analysis of the National Comorbidity Survey. Psychiatry Res 217: 202–209. doi:10.1016/j.psychres.2014.03.019
35. Oher F, Demjaha A, Jackson D, Morgan C, Dazzan P, et al. (2014) The effect of the environment on symptom dimensions in the first episode of psychosis: A multilevel study. Psychol Med 44: 2419–2430. doi:10.1017/S0033291713003188
36. Cooper C, Morgan C, Byrne M, Dazzan P, Morgan K, et al. (2008) Perceptions of disadvantage, ethnicity and psychosis. Br J Psychiatry 192: 185–190. Available: http://www.ncbi.nlm.nih.gov/pubmed/18310577. Accessed 2014 March 23.
37. Rippy A, Newman E (2006) Perceived religious discrimination and its relationship to anxiety and paranoia among muslim americans. J Muslim Ment Health 1: 5–20.
38. Combs DR (2006) Perceived racism as a predictor of paranoia among african Americans. J Black Psychol 32: 87–104. Available: http://jbp.sagepub.com/cgi/doi/10.1177/0095798405283175. Accessed 2014 March 19.
39. Bentall RP, Corcoran R, Howard R, Blackwood N, Kinderman P (2001) Persecutory delusions: A review and theoretical integration. Clin Psychol Rev 21: 1143–1192. Available: http://www.ncbi.nlm.nih.gov/pubmed/11702511.
40. Freeman D, Garety P, Kuipers E, Fowler D, Bebbington PE (2002) A cognitive model of persecutory delusions. Br J Clin Psychol 41: 331–347. doi:10.1348/014466502760387461
41. Mirowsky J, Ross CE (1983) Paranoia and the structure of powerlessness. Am Sociol Rev 48: 228–239. Available: http://www.jstor.org/stable/2095107.
42. Wickham S, Lyons M, Dickins T, Shyrane N, Bentall RP (2014) Why does relative deprivation affect mental health? The role of justice, trust and social rank in psychological wellbeing and paranoid ideation. J Public Ment Health 13: 114–126. doi:10.1108/JPMH-06-2013-0049
43. Ellett L, Freeman D, Garety P (2008) The psychological effect of an urban environment on individuals with persecutory delusions: the Camberwell walk study. Schizophr Res 99: 77–84. Available: http://www.ncbi.nlm.nih.gov/pubmed/18061407. Accessed 2014 March 27.
44. Nettle D, Pepper G V, Jobling R, Schroeder KB (2014) Being there: a brief visit to a neighbourhood induces the social attitudes of that neighbourhood. PeerJ 2: e236. doi:10.7717/peerj.236
45. Harrison G, Fouskakis D, Rasmussen F, Tynelius P, Sipos A, et al. (2003) Association between psychotic disorder and urban place of birth is not mediated by obstetric complications or childhood socio-economic position: a cohort study. Psychol Med 33: 723–731. doi:10.1017/S0033291703007591
46. Yolken RH, Torrey EF (2008) Are some cases of psychosis caused by microbial agents? A review of the evidence. Mol Psychiatry 13: 470–479. doi:10.1038/mp.2008.5
47. Mednick SA, Machon RA, Huttunen MO, Bonett D (1988) Adult schizophrenia following prenatal exposure to an influenza epidemic. Arch Gen Psychiatry 45: 189–192. doi:10.1001/archpsyc.1988.01800260109013
48. Varma VK, Wig NN, Phookun HR, Misra AK, Khare CB, et al. (1997) First-onset schizophrenia in the community: relationship of urbanization with onset, early manifestations and typology. Acta Psychiatr Scand 96: 431–438. Available: http://www.ncbi.nlm.nih.gov/pubmed/9421339.
49. Brown AS, Derkits EJ (2010) Prenatal infection and schizophrenia: A review of epidemiologic and translational studies. Am J Psychiatry 167: 261–280. Available: http://www.pubmedcentral.nih.gov/articlerender.fcgi?artid = 3652286&tool = pmcentrez&rendertype = abstract.
50. Walker E, Mittal V, Tessner K (2008) Stress and the hypothalamic pituitary adrenal axis in the developmental course of schizophrenia. Annu Rev Clin Psychol 4: 189–216. Available: http://www.ncbi.nlm.nih.gov/pubmed/18370616. Accessed 2012 Nov 16.

51. Walker E, Diforio D (1997) Schizophrenia: a neural diathesis-stress model. Psychol Rev 104: 667–685. doi:10.1037/0033-295X.104.4.667
52. Singh-Manoux A, Marmot MG, Adler NE (2001) Does subjective social status predict health and change in health status better than objective status? Psychosom Med 67: 855–861. Available: http://www.ncbi.nlm.nih.gov/pubmed/16314589. Accessed 2012 Nov 26.
53. Marmot MG (2006) Status syndrome: A challenge to medicine. JAMA J Am Med Assoc 295: 1304–1307. Available: http://dx.doi.org/10.1001/jama.295.11.1304
54. Selten J-P, Cantor-Graae E (2005) Social defeat: Risk factor for schizophrenia? Br J Psychiatry 187: 101–102. Available: http://bjp.rcpsych.org/content/187/2/101.abstract.
55. Barry B (2002) Social exclusion, social isolation and the distribution of income. In: Hills J, Le Grand J, Piachaud D, editors. Understanding Social Exclusion. Oxford University Press. pp. 13–29.
56. Selten J-P, van der Ven E, Rutten BPF, Cantor-Graae E (2013) The social defeat hypothesis of schizophrenia: an update. Schizophr Bull 39: 1180–1186. Available: http://www.ncbi.nlm.nih.gov/pubmed/24062592. Accessed 2014 Jan 22.
57. McManus S, Meltzer H, Brugha T, Bebbington PE (2009) Adult Psychiatric Morbidity in England, 2007: Results of a Household Survey. London: The NHS Information Centre.
58. Galea S, Ahern J, Nandi A, Tracy M, Beard J, et al. (2007) Urban neighborhood poverty and the incidence of depression in a population-based cohort study. Ann Epidemiol 17: 171–179. Available: http://www.pubmedcentral.nih.gov/articlerender.fcgi?artid=2442459&tool=pmcentrez&rendertype=abstract. Accessed 2014 March 31.
59. Brookwell ML, Bentall RP, Varese F (2013) Externalizing biases and hallucinations in source monitoring, self-monitoring and signal detection studies: A meta-analytic review. Psychol Med 43: 2465–2475. doi:10.1017/S0033291712002760
60. Sherazi R, McKeon P, McDonough M, Kennedy N (2006) What's new: The clinical epidemiology of bipolar disorder. Harv Rev Psychiatry 14: 274–284.
61. Kaymaz N, van Os J, de Graaf R, Ten Have M, Nolen W, et al. (2007) The impact of subclinical psychosis on the transition from subclinicial mania to bipolar disorder. J Affect Disord 98: 55–64. Available: http://www.ncbi.nlm.nih.gov/pubmed/16934874. Accessed 2014 March 31.
62. Freeman D, McManus S, Brugha T, Meltzer H, Jenkins R, et al. (2011) Concomitants of paranoia in the general population. Psychol Med 41: 923–936. doi:10.1017/S0033291710001546
63. Gayer-Anderson C, Morgan C (2013) Social networks, support and early psychosis: a systematic review. Epidemiol Psychiatr Sci 22: 131–146. Available: http://www.ncbi.nlm.nih.gov/pubmed/22831843. Accessed 2014 April 1.
64. Doucet DJ (2003) Poverty, inequality, and discrimination as sources of depression among U.S. women. Psychol Women Q 27: 101–113. doi:10.1111/1471-6402.00090
65. Grav S, Hellzèn O, Romild U, Stordal E (2012) Association between social support and depression in the general population: the HUNT study, a cross-sectional survey. J Clin Nurs 21: 111–120. Available: http://www.ncbi.nlm.nih.gov/pubmed/22017561. Accessed 2014 March 27.
66. Aylaz R, Aktürk Ü, Erci B, Öztürk H, Aslan H (2012) Relationship between depression and loneliness in elderly and examination of influential factors. Arch Gerontol Geriatr 55: 548–554. Available: http://www.ncbi.nlm.nih.gov/pubmed/22487148. Accessed 2014 March 20.
67. Kirkbride J, Errazuriz A, Croudace TJ, Morgan C, Jackson D, et al. (2012) Incidence of schizophrenia and other psychoses in England, 1950–2009: A systematic review and meta-analyses. PLoS One 7: e31660. Available: http://www.pubmedcentral.nih.gov/articlerender.fcgi?artid=3310436&tool=pmcentrez&rendertype=abstract. Accessed 2014 March 20.
68. Bebbington PE, Nayani T (1995) The psychosis screening questionnaire. Int J Methods Psychiatr Res 5: 11–19.
69. Wing JK, Babor T, Brugha T, Burke J, Cooper JE, et al. (1990) SCAN: Schedules for clinical assessment in neuropsychiatry. Arch Gen Psychiatry 47: 589–593. doi:10.1001/archpsyc.1990.01810180089012
70. Lewis G, Pelosi AJ, Araya R, Dunn G (1992) Measuring psychiatric disorder in the community: a standardized assessment for use by lay interviewers. Psychol Med 22: 465–486. doi:10.1017/S0033291700030415
71. Muthén LK, Muthén BO (n.d.) Mplus user's guide. Sixth. Los Angeles: Muthén & Muthén.
72. Akaike H (1987) Factor analysis and AIC. Psychometrika 52: 317–332. doi:10.1007/BF02294359
73. Schwarz G (1978) Estimating the dimension of a model. Ann Stat 6: 461–464. doi:10.1214/aos/1176344136
74. Sclove SL (1987) Application of model-selection criteria to some problems in multivariate analysis. Psychometrika 52: 333–343. doi:10.1007/BF02294360
75. Baron RM, Kenny DA (1986) The moderator-mediator variable distinction in social psychological research: conceptual, strategic, and statistical considerations. J Pers Soc Psychol 51: 1173–1182. doi:10.1037/0022-3514.51.6.1173
76. Bentall RP (1990) The illusion of reality: a review and integration of psychological research on hallucinations. Psychol Bull 107: 82–95. doi:10.1037/0033-2909.107.1.82
77. Johnson SL, Sandrow D, Meyer B, Winters R, Miller I, et al. (2000) Increases in Manic Symptoms After Life Events Involving Goal Attainment. 109: 721–727. doi:10.1037//Q021-843X.1G9.4.721
78. Nolen-Hoeksema S (2001) Gender differences in depression. Curr Dir Psychol Sci 10: 173–176. Available: http://cdp.sagepub.com/lookup/doi/10.1111/1467-8721.00142. Accessed 2014 July 3.
79. Veling W (2013) Ethnic minority position and risk for psychotic disorders. Curr Opin Psychiatry 26: 166–171. Available: http://www.ncbi.nlm.nih.gov/pubmed/23286992. Accessed 2014 July 3.
80. Bullock JG, Green DP, Ha SE (2010) Yes, but what's the mechanism? (don't expect an easy answer). J Pers Soc Psychol 98: 550–558. doi:10.1037/a0018933
81. Harper DJ (2011) Social inequality and the diagnosis of paranoia. Heal Sociol Rev 20: 423–436. Available: http://pubs.e-contentmanagement.com/doi/abs/10.5172/hesr.2011.20.4.423.
82. Dorling D (2011) So you think you know Britain? The surprising truth about modern Britain. UK: Constable.
83. Kay AC, Gaucher D, Peach JM, Laurin K, Friesen J, et al. (2009) Inequality, discrimination, and the power of the status quo: Direct evidence for a motivation to see the way things are as the way they should be. J Pers Soc Psychol 97: 421–434. Available: http://www.ncbi.nlm.nih.gov/pubmed/19685999. Accessed 2012 Oct 27.
84. Dorling D (2010) Injustice: Why social inequality persists. Bristol: The Policy Press.
85. Cuijpers P, van Straten A, Andersson G, van Oppen P (2008) Psychotherapy for depression in adults: A meta-analysis of comparative outcome studies. J Consult Clin Psychol 76: 909–922. doi:10.1037/a0013075
86. Wykes T, Steel C, Everitt B, Tarrier N (2008) Cognitive behavior therapy for schizophrenia: effect sizes, clinical models, and methodological rigor. Schizophr Bull 34: 523–537. Available: http://www.pubmedcentral.nih.gov/articlerender.fcgi?artid=2632426&tool=pmcentrez&rendertype=abstract. Accessed 2014 Feb 4.

19

Age-Associated Epigenetic Upregulation of the FKBP5 Gene Selectively Impairs Stress Resiliency

Jonathan J. Sabbagh[1], John C. O'Leary III[1], Laura J. Blair[1], Torsten Klengel[2,3], Bryce A. Nordhues[1], Sarah N. Fontaine[1], Elisabeth B. Binder[2,3], Chad A. Dickey[1]*

1 Department of Molecular Medicine, Byrd Alzheimer's Research Institute, University of South Florida, Tampa, Florida, United States of America, **2** Department of Psychiatry and Behavioral Sciences, Emory University School of Medicine, Atlanta, Georgia, Unites States of America, **3** Department of Translational Research, Max Planck Institute of Psychiatry, Munich, Germany

Abstract

Single nucleotide polymorphisms (SNPs) in the FK506 binding protein 5 (*FKBP5*) gene combine with traumatic events to increase risk for post-traumatic stress and major depressive disorders (PTSD and MDD). These SNPs increase FKBP51 protein expression through a mechanism involving demethylation of the gene and altered glucocorticoid signaling. Aged animals also display elevated FKBP51 levels, which contribute to impaired resiliency to depressive-like behaviors through impaired glucocorticoid signaling, a phenotype that is abrogated in *FKBP5*$^{-/-}$ mice. But the age of onset and progressive stability of these phenotypes remain unknown. Moreover, it is unclear how *FKBP5* deletion affects other glucocorticoid-dependent processes or if age-associated increases in FKBP51 expression are mediated through a similar epigenetic process caused by SNPs in the *FKBP5* gene. Here, we show that FKBP51-mediated impairment in stress resiliency and glucocorticoid signaling occurs by 10 months of age and this increased over their lifespan. Surprisingly, despite these progressive changes in glucocorticoid responsiveness, *FKBP5*$^{-/-}$ mice displayed normal longevity, glucose tolerance, blood composition and cytokine profiles across lifespan, phenotypes normally associated with glucocorticoid signaling. We also found that methylation of *Fkbp5* decreased with age in mice, a process that likely explains the age-associated increases in FKBP51 levels. Thus, epigenetic upregulation of FKBP51 with age can selectively impair psychological stress-resiliency, but does not affect other glucocorticoid-mediated physiological processes. This makes FKBP51 a unique and attractive therapeutic target to treat PTSD and MDD. In addition, aged wild-type mice may be a useful model for investigating the mechanisms of *FKBP5* SNPs associated with these disorders.

Editor: Takeo Yoshikawa, Rikagaku Kenkyūsho Brain Science Institute, Japan

Funding: This work was supported by the National Institutes of Health/National Institutes of Neurological Disease and Stroke R01 NS073899 and the American Federation for Aging Research. The funders had no role in study design, data collection and analysis, decision to publish, or preparation of the manuscript.

Competing Interests: The authors have declared that no competing interests exist.

* Email: cdickey@health.usf.edu

Introduction

Late-life depression (LLD) is a debilitating disorder that can accelerate aging and mortality [1–3]. LLD is associated with reduced stress resiliency [4], a phenomenon that is influenced by the FK506 binding protein 51 (FKBP51) [5,6]. Importantly, FKBP51 levels increase with age in humans and mice [7,8]. This raises the possibility that senescence-related deficits in stress resiliency or coping ability may be due in part to increasing FKBP51 expression with age. Moreover, single nucleotide polymorphisms (SNPs) in the *FKBP5* gene that increase its expression through a mechanism involving demethylation increase susceptibility to anxiety disorders, post-traumatic stress disorder (PTSD) and major depression [9–12], further implicating a role for increased levels of this protein in psychiatric illnesses.

A role for FKBP51 in stress-related disorders was first suggested by its functional control of glucocorticoid receptor (GR) signaling [13]. FKBP51 has an inhibitory effect on GR, decreasing the affinity of cortisol or corticosterone (CORT) for GR [14] and impairing GR translocation [15]. This inhibition delays negative feedback of the hypothalamic-pituitary-adrenal (HPA) axis, prolongs the stress response and leads to elevated circulating CORT levels and glucocorticoid resistance. Previous work from our laboratory and others has shown that ablation of *FKBP5* in mice leads to an age-dependent anti-depressive phenotype, more robust coping behavior following stress, and reduced stress-induced circulating CORT levels without altering cognitive function [5,6,16]. *FKBP5*$^{-/-}$ mice are more responsive to the dexamethasone suppression test, suggesting HPA axis negative feedback is accelerated in the absence of FKBP51 [6]. Normalizing the HPA axis hyperactivity observed in depressed patients may be of critical importance for treatment outcome; individuals that display persistently elevated cortisol levels following treatment have higher rates of relapse [17–19]. Therefore, attenuating the effect of FKBP51 on HPA axis dysregulation is an attractive therapeutic strategy for depression, especially in aged individuals.

The current study sought to determine the effects of FKBP51 on behavioral and neuroendocrine changes across lifespan. We also examined whether FKBP51 affects stress-related phenotypes such as mortality, glucose tolerance, blood composition, cognitive flexibility, and inflammatory markers. Our data demonstrate that *FKBP5* deletion prevents the progressive age-associated increases in depression-like behavior and circulating CORT levels observed in wild-type mice. Furthermore, *FKBP5*$^{-/-}$ mice exhibited normal longevity, glucose tolerance, blood composition, and cytokine levels across lifespan, while even displaying enhanced cognitive flexibility in a reversal paradigm. We also show for the first time that wild-type mice display decreased DNA methylation of *Fkbp5* with age, modeling human disease. These findings support the viability of FKBP51 as a therapeutic target to treat stress-related disorders and suggest aged wild-type mice may have utility for studying SNP-like epigenetic changes in *FKBP5*.

Results

Fkbp5 deletion reduced depression-like behavior and serum CORT levels across lifespan

FKBP5$^{-/-}$ mice have previously demonstrated protection from depression-like behavior at 17–20 months of age [5], but not at 10–16 weeks [6]. Because FKBP51 levels increase with age, we hypothesized that a critical load of FKBP51 was necessary to produce this phenotype, but this was not known. To determine the age at which FKBP51 levels were sufficient to cause depression-like behavior and whether this phenotype was dependent on FKBP51 across lifespan, separate cohorts of wild-type and *FKBP5*$^{-/-}$ mice were examined at 6, 10, and 21 months of age for depression-like behavior in the forced swim test (FST) and tail suspension test (TST) and stress reactivity via post-restraint CORT sampling. At 6 months, no differences were found in the FST (Figure 1A), TST (Figure 1B), or in serum CORT levels (Figure 1C). However, at 10 months, increased immobility in the FST and TST, as well as elevated serum CORT levels following restraint stress emerged in wild-type mice, but not in *FKBP5*$^{-/-}$ mice (Figure 1A–C). These phenotypes remained in 21 month old wild-type mice, but again *FKBP5*$^{-/-}$ mice were protected. In fact, across whole lifespan, *FKBP5* ablation significantly reduced serum CORT levels ($p<0.001$) and immobility time in the FST ($p<0.0001$) and TST ($p<0.001$) as measured by two way analysis of variance (ANOVA). Collectively, these data suggest that FKBP51 levels reach a critical load somewhere around 10 months of age, culminating in slowed negative feedback of the HPA axis, higher circulating CORT levels, and increased vulnerability to depressive-like phenotypes.

FKBP5 deletion does not impact other GR-dependent physiologies

Based on these results, we speculated that *FKBP5* deletion would impact other phenotypes related to HPA axis regulation. First, since the degree of HPA axis hyperactivity correlates with overall lifespan in rodents [20], such that shorter-lived strains are more reactive to stress and have elevated circulating glucocorticoids compared to longer-lived ones, we suspected that *FKBP5*$^{-/-}$ mice might have a longer lifespan than wild-type littermates. However, when we examined the survival curves of wild-type and *FKBP5*$^{-/-}$ mice, no differences were found in mouse survival up to 28 months of age, suggesting that FKBP51 neither increases or decreases longevity up to this point (Figure 2); but it is possible that differences between genotypes may emerge if animals are permitted to age longer.

Next, since GR signaling and FKBP51 have a prominent role in energy metabolism [21], we examined the effects of *FKBP5* deletion on glucose metabolism. A glucose tolerance test was performed in 10.5 month old wild-type and *FKBP5*$^{-/-}$ mice, wherein blood glucose levels were measured out to 120 minutes after glucose injection. No significant differences in glucose metabolism were observed between genotypes ($p>0.05$; Figure 3). Moreover, *FKBP5* deletion did not produce any deleterious effects on blood composition compared to wild-type mice. As shown in Table 1, there were no differences between genotypes in mass, the composition of red or white blood cells, or platelets.

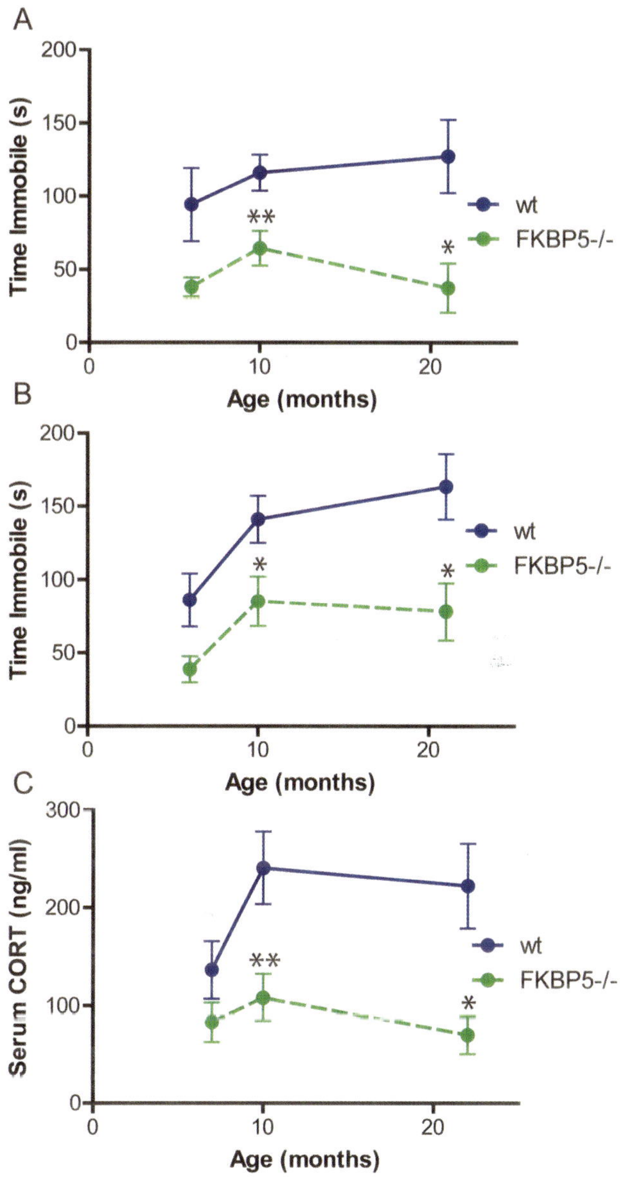

Figure 1. Ablation of *FKBP5* reduces depressive-like behavior and serum corticosterone (CORT) levels across lifespan. (A) *FKBP5*$^{-/-}$ mice display reduced immobility time in the forced swim test at 10 and 21 months. (B) *FKBP5*$^{-/-}$ mice have reduced immobility time in the tail suspension test at 10 and 21 months. (C) *FKBP5*$^{-/-}$ mice display reduced serum CORT levels following acute restraint stress at 10 and 21 months. **$p<0.01$, *$p<0.05$ as measured by two-way ANOVA. wild-type (wt). FST: n at 6 months: wt = 9, *FKBP5*$^{-/-}$ = 10; n at 10 months: wt = 30, *FKBP5*$^{-/-}$ = 33; n at 21 months: wt = 9, *FKBP5*$^{-/-}$ = 9. TST: n at 6 months: wt = 7, *FKBP5*$^{-/-}$ = 9; n at 10 months: wt = 18, *FKBP5*$^{-/-}$ = 19; n at 21 months: wt = 9, *FKBP5*$^{-/-}$ = 9. CORT ELISA: n at 6 months: wt = 8, *FKBP5*$^{-/-}$ = 10; n at 10 months: wt = 12, *FKBP5*$^{-/-}$ = 13; n at 21 months: wt = 5, *FKBP5*$^{-/-}$ = 6.

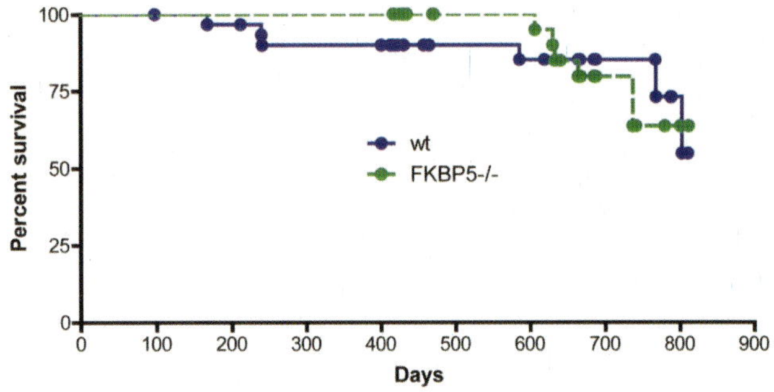

Figure 2. FKBP51 does not affect longevity. No significant differences were found in the percent survival of wild-type (wt) and *FKBP5*$^{-/-}$ mice, p>0.05. wt, n = 34 (18 male and 16 female); *FKBP5*$^{-/-}$, n = 32 (18 male and 14 female).

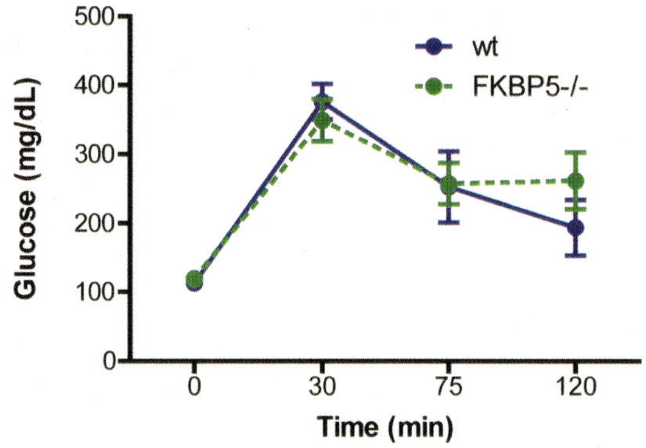

Figure 3. Deletion of *FKBP5* does not alter glucose metabolism. *FKBP5*$^{-/-}$ mice displayed normal glucose tolerance up to 120 minutes following glucose injection compared to wild-type (wt) mice, p>0.05. wt, n = 7; *FKBP5*$^{-/-}$, n = 10.

We then suspected that FKBP51 could impact immune function and inflammation given its role as an immunophilin and the known ability of GR to regulate transcription of inflammatory mediators [22]. Serum cytokines known to be affected by GR were examined from 6, 10, and 21 month old wild-type and *FKBP5*$^{-/-}$ mice (Figure 4). Levels of interleukin (IL)-1β ($p<0.01$; Figure 4A) and IL-5 ($p<0.05$; Figure 4D) were decreased at 6 months as measured by t-test but no other differences were observed. Across lifespan, no changes were found in any of the markers as measured by two-way ANOVA ($p>0.05$), suggesting the absence of FKBP51 does not adversely affect basal immune function. Taken together, these findings suggest that *FKBP5* deletion selectively protects aging mice from depressive-like behavior without impacting other important GR-mediated physiological effects.

FKBP5 deletion enhanced cognitive flexibility

FKBP5$^{-/-}$ mice do not display any cognitive deficits [5]; however, given the role of FKBP51 in resiliency, we suspected that these mice might be able to adapt better to a changing environment or paradigm. To test this, 6 month old mice were trained for three days to find the location of a hidden platform in the radial arm water maze (RAWM). They were then trained for three additional days to locate a hidden platform placed 180° from the original location. Although there were no differences in RAWM acquisition training to find the first location of the platform ($p>0.05$; Figure 5A), *FKBP5*$^{-/-}$ mice were able to find the new location of the platform significantly faster than wild-type littermates as measured by two-way ANOVA ($p<0.05$; Figure 5B). Thus, FKBP51 can interfere with stress-based learning and cognitive flexibility. These findings indicate that increasing levels of FKBP51 exacerbate stress-responsiveness, particularly to psychological stimuli, to the point of pathogenesis. While a degree of FKBP51 expression may be necessary for threat assessment [23], overabundance of FKBP51 can be problematic. Therefore, we next sought to examine how *FKBP5* expression was increasing with age in an effort to identify ways to reduce the expression of this gene.

The *Fkbp5* gene is demethylated with age

Several studies have shown that SNPs linked to the *FKBP5* gene or stress each increase FKBP51 expression through a process involving demethylation of the *FKBP5* gene. We suspected that this same mechanism was responsible for the increased expression of FKBP51 in aging mice. We performed bisulfite pyrosequencing on isolated DNA from wild-type mouse frontal cortex to examine age-dependent *Fkbp5* methylation in intron 5, which contains a functional glucocorticoid response element (GRE) [24,25]. As expected, linear regression analyses revealed that *Fkbp5* methylation decreased with age at multiple CpG sites (CPG_3: $r = -0.3890$, $p<0.05$; CPG_4: $r = -0.4004$, $p<0.05$; CpG_5: $r = -0.5044$, $p<0.01$; Figure 6). Demethylation in intron 5 has been shown to increase *Fkbp5* mRNA expression [25], suggesting this epigenetic phenomenon is also likely responsible for the age-related increase in FKBP51 levels previously observed in mice [8].

Discussion

The *FKBP5* gene is associated with depression [10], PTSD [9], anxiety [11,26] and Alzheimer's disease (AD) [7,8], but little is known about its role in aging. Here we demonstrate that the abundance of FKBP51 by 10 months of age is sufficient to increase depression-like behavior and stress-induced serum CORT levels without adversely affecting other glucocorticoid-dependent processes. Our data also show for the first time a learning enhancement following *FKBP5* deletion in a task dependent upon cognitive flexibility in a stressful environment. Finally, we have shown progressive *Fkbp5* demethylation occurs with age in wild-type mice, elucidating a mechanism by which FKBP51 levels increase throughout life. These findings suggest that aging acts as an epigenetic milieu similar to how SNPs interact with early life events to promote vulnerability to depression and other disorders.

Prolonged exposure to glucocorticoids is considered a potential driving factor for depression [27], suggesting elevations in FKBP51 due to age or SNPs could facilitate onset of the disorder. Our data demonstrated that wild-type mice have an age-dependent increase in depression-like behavior and circulating CORT levels that was absent in *FKBP5*$^{-/-}$ mice, indicating these age-related changes were mediated by increasing FKBP51 expression with age. Glucocorticoid signaling is also vital for a number of physiological processes, raising the possibility that deleting *FKBP5* could affect some of these pathways. For example, longevity can be influenced by stress and depression [2,3,28,29], leading us to hypothesize that reducing FKBP51 levels could be beneficial for survival. Aberrant glucose metabolism is observed in patients with major depression and Cushing's disease and following chronic CORT exposure in rodents [30–32]. Furthermore, overexpression of FKBP51 in the hypothalamus impaired glucose tolerance, while food deprivation increased *Fkbp5* mRNA expression in mice [21], suggesting FKBP51 may play a role in energy metabolism. Finally, because FKBP51 is an immunophilin and it has been implicated in the dysregulation of

Table 1. Blood composition and animal mass of wild-type versus FKBP5$^{-/-}$ mice do not differ.

	Wild-type	*FKBP5*$^{-/-}$	P value
Animal Mass (g)	43.04±3.35	38.82±2.32	0.3043
WBC (10^3/μl)	4.16±0.69	3.30±0.82	0.4394
RBC (10^6/μl)	7.05±0.89	4.76±0.90	0.0852
Lym (10^3/μl)	3.12±0.53	2.43±0.62	0.4155
Mono (10^3/μl)	0.32±0.04	0.24±0.04	0.2013
Gran (10^3/μl)	0.72±0.13	0.63±0.17	0.6726
HGB (g/dl)	11.02±1.37	7.52±1.42	0.0921
PLT (10^3/μl)	569.3±84.57	445.70±105.97	0.3779

WBC: white blood cells, RBC: red blood cells, Lym: lymphocytes, Mono: monocytes, Gran: granulocytes, HGB: hemoglobin, PLT: platelets. Wild-type, n = 11; FKBP5$^{-/-}$, n = 12. Values are listed as the mean ± the standard error of the mean.

nuclear factor kappa-light-chain enhancer of activated B cells (NF-κB) signaling [33], its deletion could alter levels of GR-regulated inflammatory markers. However, our data reveal that *FKBP5*$^{-/-}$ mice display normal longevity, glucose tolerance, blood composition, and cytokine profile. These findings are important for determining the potential adverse effects of therapeutically targeting FKBP51.

Thus far FKBP51 has not been implicated in the regulation of synaptic plasticity or learning. However, its expression has been linked to EphB2/NR1 signaling [26], while others have shown that individuals with the rs1360780 *FKBP5* SNP have altered hippocampal function and morphology [23]. We have previously shown that deletion of *FKBP5* does not affect basic hippocampal function in mice [5], but we predicted that perhaps a behavior influenced by stress could be modulated by FKBP51. Using a reversal paradigm in the RAWM, we were able to discriminate differences in behavior between wild-type and *FKBP5*$^{-/-}$ mice. In fact, *FKBP5*$^{-/-}$ mice made fewer errors than wild-type mice, indicative of enhanced cognitive flexibility. Chronic stress and aging have been demonstrated to independently impair cognitive flexibility in rodents and humans [31–37]. Together with our data, these findings suggest progressively increasing FKBP51 expression with age may attenuate the ability to rapidly shift strategy and retain cognitive flexibility under stressful conditions.

While demethylation of *FKBP5* has been identified as a potential mechanism for FKBP51 upregulation in humans [7,12], it was not known if this was contributing to the progressive increases in FKBP51 that we observed in aged mice [8]. We demonstrated that *Fkbp5* methylation decreases with age in wild-type mice, underscoring the validity of utilizing aged mouse models to study *Fkbp5* gene x environment interactions. Interestingly, chronic CORT treatment decreases *Fkbp5* methylation in mice similar to aging [25], linking the effects of stress and aging through FKBP51. Previous work has shown that functional SNPs in *FKBP5* lead to demethylation of the gene in an interaction with early environmental factors [12]. Our data suggest that aging acts similarly to the SNPs, leading to epigenetic changes in *FKBP5* regulation across lifespan. Because GR stimulation leads to *FKBP5* demethylation [12,38], it is possible that stress throughout life may lead to progressively decreased methylation and difficulty regulating the HPA axis and the stress response with age.

Elderly depressed patients suffer from increased treatment resistance and frequency of depressive episodes [39,40]. Depression is frequently comorbid with AD and may be a risk factor for development of AD [41,42]. Moreover, expression of *FKBP5* increases with age and is even further elevated in AD, providing a putative link between LLD and AD [7,8]. Therefore, inhibition of FKBP51 is a desirable strategy for stress-related disorders such as depression and age-related diseases. Although the development of FKBP51 ligands has been difficult due to the similarity between FKBP51 and its homologues, it is considered a tractable, viable drug target [43]. Our data support the need for continued research into FKBP51 biology and the advancement of its therapeutic development. Furthermore, we provide data supporting the idea that aging activates an epigenetic mechanism that increases FKBP51 expression, leading to impaired HPA axis function and LLD-like phenotypes. Thus, aged wild-type mice may model human conditions caused by SNPs in the *FKBP5* gene.

Materials and Methods

Animals and experimental design

FKBP5$^{-/-}$ and wild-type littermate mice were generated and genotyped as described previously [5]. All animals were naïve to each procedure performed. For *Fkbp5* methylation studies, a separate cohort of wild-type mice aged to 1, 3.5, 4, 5, 6, or 12 months of age was used. Longevity was compared between wild-type and *FKBP5*$^{-/-}$ mice in a subset of animals used for behavioral analyses. Glucose tolerance was measured in 10.5 month old mice that had previously been tested at 6 months of age in the TST, FST, and the RAWM. The complete blood composition analysis was performed in a separate cohort of 14 month old mice that were previously tested in the TST and FST at 10 months of age. A final cohort was tested in the TST and FST at 21 months of age. CORT and cytokine levels were examined from the serum of animals used for behavioral analyses. All animal studies were approved by the University of South Florida Institutional Animal Care and Use Committee and carried out in accordance with the National Institutes of Health (NIH) guidelines for the care and use of laboratory animals. Mice were group housed under a 12 hour light-dark cycle (lights on at 06:00) and permitted *ad libitum* access to food and water.

DNA methylation analyses

DNA was isolated from 15 mg of flash frozen frontal cortex brain tissue from wild-type mice aged 1, 3.5, 4, 5, 6 and 12 months old using a QuickGene DNA tissue kit (Autogen; Holliston, MA). Briefly, tissue was incubated overnight on a shaking incubator at 70°C in tissue lysis buffer supplemented with Proteinase K (Autogen). DNA was isolated following complete tissue lysis as directed by the manufacture, with RNase treatment to remove

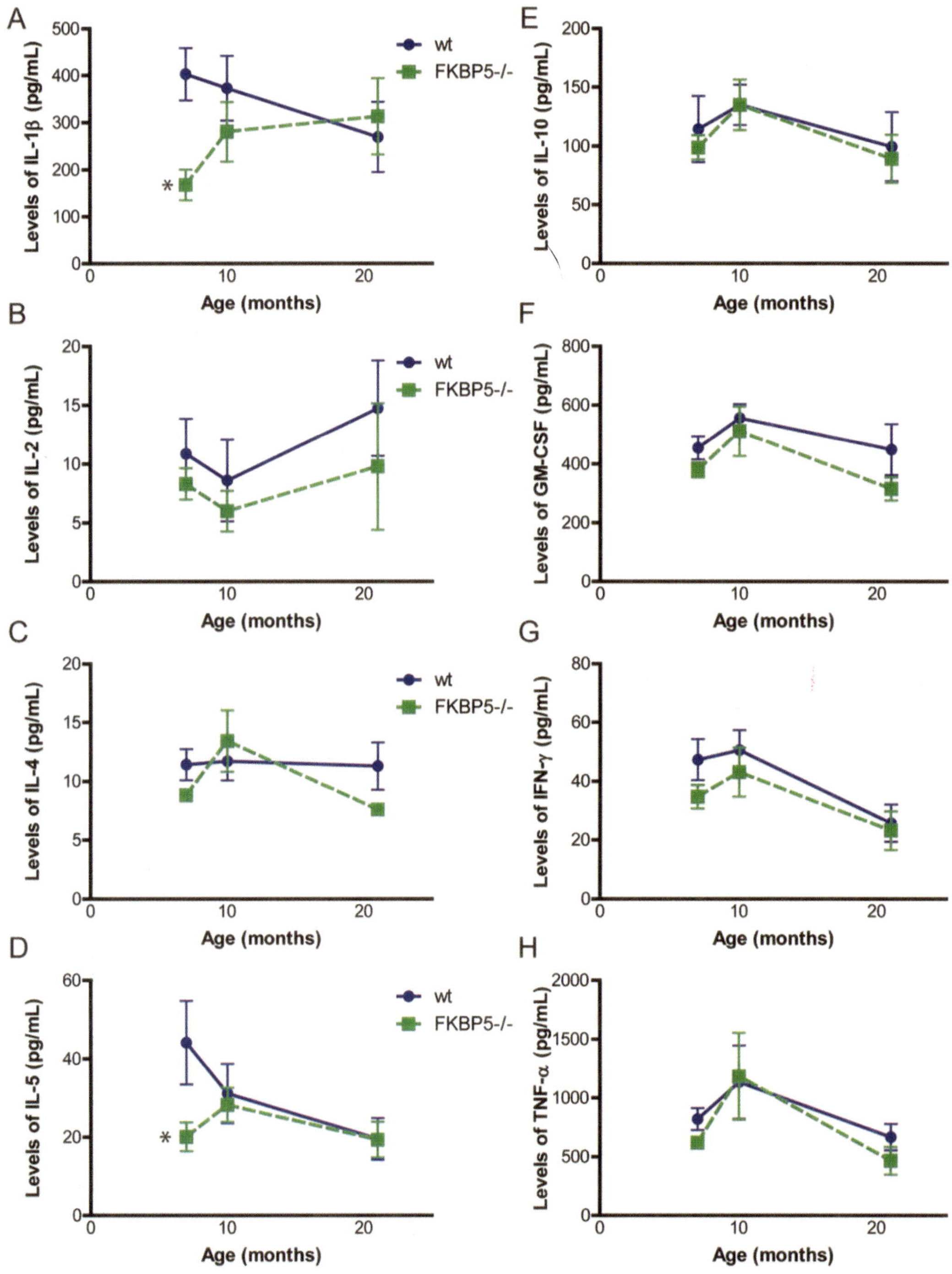

Figure 4. Ablation of *FKBP5* does not alter cytokine levels over time. Serum levels of interleukin-1β (A) and interleukin-5 (D) were decreased at 6 months ($p<0.05$ via t-test) but not across time ($p>0.05$ by two-way ANOVA). Levels of interleukin-2 (B), interleukin-4 (C), interleukin-10 (E), granulocyte-macrophage colony-stimulating factor (F), interferon gamma (G), or tumor necrosis factor alpha (H) did not differ between genotypes across lifespan, $p>0.05$. *$p<0.05$. wild-type (wt), n = 6 for each age; *FKBP5*$^{-/-}$, n = 7 at 7 and 10 months, n = 6 at 21 months.

residual RNA. Isolated DNA was purified through provided columns in a QuickGene Mini80 (Autogen). Following isolation, DNA concentration and purity were determined using a Qubit 1.0 Fluorometer (Invitrogen; Grand Island, NY) and Nanodrop (Thermo Scientific; Wilmington, DE), confirmed by visualization on a 1% agarose DNA gel. Pure DNA was then subjected to bisulfite pyrosequencing as previously described [7,12]. Mouse *Fkbp5* DNA was evaluated at 5 CpG sites across intron 5 [25]. Specifically, DNA methylation was interrogated in the intron 5 region of mouse *Fkbp5* harboring functional GREs and previously shown to be demethylated in response to GR activation [25]. Sequenom EpiTYPER DNA methylation analysis was performed according to the instructions of the manufacturer. Primer sequences for amplification of a 412 bp *Fkbp5* fragment from bisulfite converted DNA were: F_mouse-I5 5′-aggaagagagAA-TATTTTGTTTTGAATGTGGTTGG-3′ and R_mouse-I5 5′-

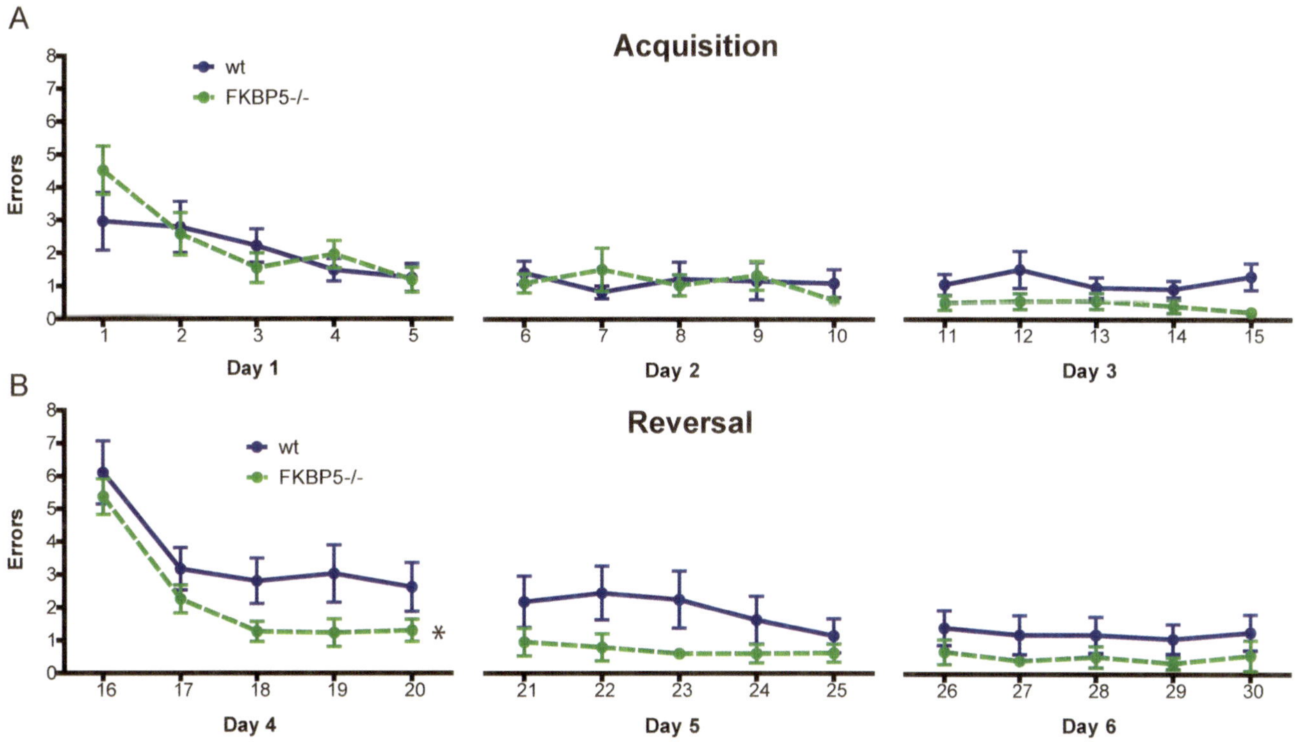

Figure 5. *FKBP5*$^{-/-}$ mice display enhanced cognitive flexibility in the radial arm water maze. (A) No differences were found in acquisition learning between genotypes ($p>0.05$). (B) There was a main effect of genotype ($p<0.05$) during reversal training, indicating *FKBP5*$^{-/-}$ mice made fewer errors across sessions. Data points represent a session of three trials. *$p<0.05$. wild-type (wt), n = 9; *FKBP5*$^{-/-}$, n = 10.

cagtaatacgactcactatagggagaaggctCTCTCCTAAAAACCCTTAC-CCAATA-3′. Uncertainty threshold was set to 0.1.

Survival analysis

To measure longevity, an independent cohort of wild-type and *FKBP5*$^{-/-}$ mice was monitored until death or euthanasia was deemed necessary by veterinarian assessment. The survival curve was plotted using the Kaplan-Meier method and statistically analyzed by GraphPad Prism software. Animals were aged to 28 months of age, at which point all surviving animals were humanely euthanized.

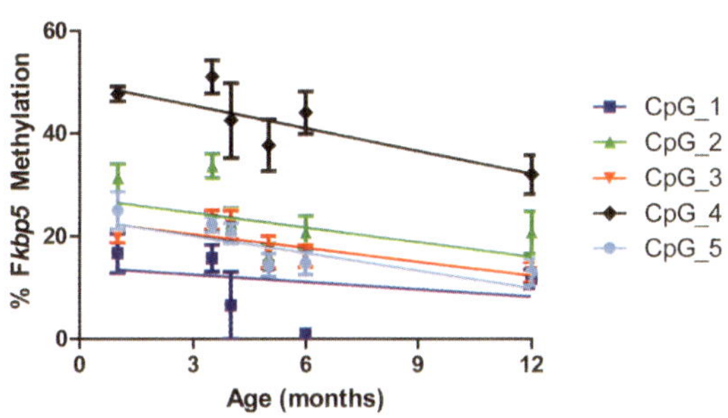

Figure 6. *Fkbp5* DNA methylation decreases with age in mice. Isolated DNA samples from wild-type mice aged 1 (n = 3), 3.5 (n = 3), 4 (n = 6), 5 (n = 7), 6 (n = 6), and 12 (n = 3) months were subjected to bisulfite pyrosequencing. Multiple CpG sites in intron 5 were analyzed for *Fkbp5* methylation. Significant demethylation was found at CPG_3 ($r = -0.3890$, $p<0.05$), CPG_4 ($r = -0.4004$, $p<0.05$) and CpG_5 ($r = -0.5044$, $p<0.01$) as measured by linear regression analyses.

Glucose tolerance test

Mice were fasted overnight by removing food at 18:00. The following day, animals were injected intraperitoneally with glucose (2 g/kg) and blood was extracted from the tail vein prior to and 30, 75, and 120 minutes after injection. Blood glucose levels were measured with a True Track blood glucose meter (NIPRO Diagnostics, Fort Lauderdale, FL).

Radial arm water maze

The RAWM was adapted from previous studies [44]. Briefly, a circular black tank with a six arm metal insert was filled with water. A platform was submerged 1 cm below the surface of the water at the end of a designated goal arm. Animals were permitted 60 seconds to locate the platform during which time an observer blind to genotype manually scored the number of errors. An error was defined as an entry into an incorrect arm. Mice were trained for 15 trials per day, which were divided into 5 sessions of 3 trials each. Following 3 days of acquisition training with a consistent platform location, the platform was moved 180° to test reversal learning, a measure of cognitive flexibility.

Tail suspension test

The TST was conducted as previously described [5]. Mice were suspended from the tail for one 6 minute session which was video recorded (ANY-maze Software, Stoelting Co., Wood Dale, IL). The amount of time spent immobile was recorded by a trained observer blind to genotype.

Forced swim test

The FST was performed as previously reported [5]. Mice were placed in a clear glass cylinder 23 cm high and 15 cm wide, filled with room temperature water to a depth of 13 cm. Each session lasted 6 minutes and was video recorded. The amount of time spent immobile was measured by a trained observer blind to genotype.

Enzyme-linked immunosorbent assays

Blood was collected from mice through the submandibular vein one hour after the start of the light cycle. For measurement of CORT, blood was collected 30 minutes following a 10 minute tube restraint. Serum was separated from blood using BD Microtainer serum separator tubes (BD Biosciences, Sparks, MD) and centrifuged at 1,300× g. CORT levels were measured using a CORT enzyme-linked immunosorbent assay (ELISA) kit (Enzo Life Sciences, Farmingdale, NY) and cytokines were analyzed with a Bio-Plex Pro Mouse Cytokine 8-plex Assay (Bio-Rad, Hercules, CA) according to manufacturer's instructions.

Statistical analyses

Statistical significance for each analysis was determined with linear regression, Student's *t* tests, or two-way ANOVA with Bonferroni post-tests to compare groups where appropriate. All figures and statistics were generated using GraphPad Prism software; each graph represents the mean ± the standard error of the mean (SEM).

Author Contributions

Conceived and designed the experiments: JJS JO CAD. Performed the experiments: JO LJB BAN TK EBB. Analyzed the data: JJS LJB. Contributed to the writing of the manuscript: JJS SNF TK EBB CAD.

References

1. Lenze EJ, Schulz R, Martire LM, Zdaniuk B, Glass T, et al. (2005) The course of functional decline in older people with persistently elevated depressive symptoms: longitudinal findings from the Cardiovascular Health Study. J Am Geriatr Soc 53: 569–575.
2. Gump BB, Matthews KA, Eberly LE, Chang YF, Group MR (2005) Depressive symptoms and mortality in men: results from the Multiple Risk Factor Intervention Trial. Stroke 36: 98–102.
3. Wolkowitz OM, Epel ES, Reus VI, Mellon SH (2010) Depression gets old fast: do stress and depression accelerate cell aging? Depress Anxiety 27: 327–338.
4. Freret T, Gaudreau P, Schumann-Bard P, Billard JM, Popa-Wagner A (2014) Mechanisms underlying the neuroprotective effect of brain reserve against late life depression. J Neural Transm.
5. O'Leary JC 3rd, Dharia S, Blair LJ, Brady S, Johnson AG, et al. (2011) A new anti-depressive strategy for the elderly: ablation of FKBP5/FKBP51. PLoS One 6: e24840.
6. Touma C, Gassen NC, Herrmann L, Cheung-Flynn J, Bull DR, et al. (2011) FK506 binding protein 5 shapes stress responsiveness: modulation of neuroendocrine reactivity and coping behavior. Biol Psychiatry 70: 928–936.
7. Blair LJ, Nordhues BA, Hill SE, Scaglione KM, O'Leary JC 3rd, et al. (2013) Accelerated neurodegeneration through chaperone-mediated oligomerization of tau. J Clin Invest 123: 4158–4169.
8. Jinwal UK, Koren J 3rd, Borysov SI, Schmid AB, Abisambra JF, et al. (2010) The Hsp90 cochaperone, FKBP51, increases Tau stability and polymerizes microtubules. J Neurosci 30: 591–599.
9. Binder EB, Bradley RG, Liu W, Epstein MP, Deveau TC, et al. (2008) Association of FKBP5 polymorphisms and childhood abuse with risk of posttraumatic stress disorder symptoms in adults. JAMA 299: 1291–1305.
10. Binder EB, Salyakina D, Lichtner P, Wochnik GM, Ising M, et al. (2004) Polymorphisms in FKBP5 are associated with increased recurrence of depressive episodes and rapid response to antidepressant treatment. Nat Genet 36: 1319–1325.
11. Minelli A, Maffioletti E, Cloninger CR, Magri C, Sartori R, et al. (2013) Role of allelic variants of FK506-binding protein 51 (FKBP5) gene in the development of anxiety disorders. Depress Anxiety 30: 1170–1176.
12. Klengel T, Mehta D, Anacker C, Rex-Haffner M, Pruessner JC, et al. (2013) Allele-specific FKBP5 DNA demethylation mediates gene-childhood trauma interactions. Nat Neurosci 16: 33–41.
13. Galigniana NM, Ballmer LT, Toneatto J, Erlejman AG, Lagadari M, et al. (2012) Regulation of the glucocorticoid response to stress-related disorders by the Hsp90-binding immunophilin FKBP51. J Neurochem 122: 4–18.
14. Denny WB, Valentine DL, Reynolds PD, Smith DF, Scammell JG (2000) Squirrel monkey immunophilin FKBP51 is a potent inhibitor of glucocorticoid receptor binding. Endocrinology 141: 4107–4113.
15. Wochnik GM, Ruegg J, Abel GA, Schmidt U, Holsboer F, et al. (2005) FK506-binding proteins 51 and 52 differentially regulate dynein interaction and nuclear translocation of the glucocorticoid receptor in mammalian cells. J Biol Chem 280: 4609–4616.
16. Hartmann J, Wagner KV, Liebl C, Scharf SH, Wang XD, et al. (2012) The involvement of FK506-binding protein 51 (FKBP5) in the behavioral and neuroendocrine effects of chronic social defeat stress. Neuropharmacology 62: 332–339.
17. Appelhof BC, Huyser J, Verweij M, Brouwer JP, van Dyck R, et al. (2006) Glucocorticoids and relapse of major depression (dexamethasone/corticotropin-releasing hormone test in relation to relapse of major depression). Biol Psychiatry 59: 696–701.
18. Lok A, Mocking RJ, Ruhe HG, Visser I, Koeter MW, et al. (2012) Longitudinal hypothalamic-pituitary-adrenal axis trait and state effects in recurrent depression. Psychoneuroendocrinology 37: 892–902.
19. Zobel AW, Nickel T, Sonntag A, Uhr M, Holsboer F, et al. (2001) Cortisol response in the combined dexamethasone/CRH test as predictor of relapse in patients with remitted depression. a prospective study. J Psychiatr Res 35: 83–94.
20. Gilad GM, Gilad VH (1995) Strain, stress, neurodegeneration and longevity. Mech Ageing Dev 78: 75–83.
21. Yang L, Isoda F, Yen K, Kleopoulos SP, Janssen W, et al. (2012) Hypothalamic Fkbp51 is induced by fasting, and elevated hypothalamic expression promotes obese phenotypes. Am J Physiol Endocrinol Metab 302: E987–991.
22. Storer CL, Dickey CA, Galigniana MD, Rein T, Cox MB (2011) FKBP51 and FKBP52 in signaling and disease. Trends Endocrinol Metab 22: 481–490.
23. Fani N, Gutman D, Tone EB, Almli L, Mercer KB, et al. (2013) FKBP5 and attention bias for threat: associations with hippocampal function and shape. JAMA Psychiatry 70: 392–400.
24. Magee JA, Chang LW, Stormo GD, Milbrandt J (2006) Direct, androgen receptor-mediated regulation of the FKBP5 gene via a distal enhancer element. Endocrinology 147: 590–598.
25. Lee RS, Tamashiro KL, Yang X, Purcell RH, Harvey A, et al. (2010) Chronic corticosterone exposure increases expression and decreases deoxyribonucleic acid methylation of Fkbp5 in mice. Endocrinology 151: 4332–4343.
26. Attwood BK, Bourgognon JM, Patel S, Mucha M, Schiavon E, et al. (2011) Neuropsin cleaves EphB2 in the amygdala to control anxiety. Nature 473: 372–375.
27. Sterner EY, Kalynchuk LE (2010) Behavioral and neurobiological consequences of prolonged glucocorticoid exposure in rats: relevance to depression. Prog Neuropsychopharmacol Biol Psychiatry 34: 777–790.
28. Epel ES, Blackburn EH, Lin J, Dhabhar FS, Adler NE, et al. (2004) Accelerated telomere shortening in response to life stress. Proc Natl Acad Sci U S A 101: 17312–17315.
29. Simon NM, Smoller JW, McNamara KL, Maser RS, Zalta AK, et al. (2006) Telomere shortening and mood disorders: preliminary support for a chronic stress model of accelerated aging. Biol Psychiatry 60: 432–435.
30. Weber B, Schweiger U, Deuschle M, Heuser I (2000) Major depression and impaired glucose tolerance. Exp Clin Endocrinol Diabetes 108: 187–190.
31. Chanson P, Salenave S (2010) Metabolic syndrome in Cushing's syndrome. Neuroendocrinology 92 Suppl 1: 96–101.
32. Karatsoreos IN, Bhagat SM, Bowles NP, Weil ZM, Pfaff DW, et al. (2010) Endocrine and physiological changes in response to chronic corticosterone: a potential model of the metabolic syndrome in mouse. Endocrinology 151: 2117–2127.
33. Romano S, Mallardo M, Romano MF (2011) FKBP51 and the NF-kappaB regulatory pathway in cancer. Curr Opin Pharmacol 11: 288–293.
34. Naegeli KJ, O'Connor JA, Banerjee P, Morilak DA (2013) Effects of milnacipran on cognitive flexibility following chronic stress in rats. Eur J Pharmacol 703: 62–66.
35. Ohira H, Matsunaga M, Kimura K, Murakami H, Osumi T, et al. (2011) Chronic stress modulates neural and cardiovascular responses during reversal learning. Neuroscience 193: 193–204.
36. Beas BS, Setlow B, Bizon JL (2013) Distinct manifestations of executive dysfunction in aged rats. Neurobiol Aging 34: 2164–2174.
37. West RL (1996) An application of prefrontal cortex function theory to cognitive aging. Psychol Bull 120: 272–292.
38. Yang X, Ewald ER, Huo Y, Tamashiro KL, Salvatori R, et al. (2012) Glucocorticoid-induced loss of DNA methylation in non-neuronal cells and potential involvement of DNMT1 in epigenetic regulation of Fkbp5. Biochem Biophys Res Commun 420: 570–575.
39. Luijendijk HJ, van den Berg JF, Dekker MJ, van Tuijl HR, Otte W, et al. (2008) Incidence and recurrence of late-life depression. Arch Gen Psychiatry 65: 1394–1401.

40. Naismith SL, Norrie LM, Mowszowski L, Hickie IB (2012) The neurobiology of depression in later-life: clinical, neuropsychological, neuroimaging and pathophysiological features. Prog Neurobiol 98: 99–143.
41. Palmer K, Di Iulio F, Varsi AE, Gianni W, Sancesario G, et al. (2010) Neuropsychiatric predictors of progression from amnestic-mild cognitive impairment to Alzheimer's disease: the role of depression and apathy. J Alzheimers Dis 20: 175–183.
42. Starkstein SE, Mizrahi R, Power BD (2008) Depression in Alzheimer's disease: phenomenology, clinical correlates and treatment. International review of psychiatry (Abingdon, England) 20: 382–388.
43. Schmidt MV, Paez-Pereda M, Holsboer F, Hausch F (2012) The prospect of FKBP51 as a drug target. ChemMedChem 7: 1351–1359.
44. Alamed J, Wilcock DM, Diamond DM, Gordon MN, Morgan D (2006) Two-day radial-arm water maze learning and memory task; robust resolution of amyloid-related memory deficits in transgenic mice. Nat Protoc 1: 1671–1679.

20

Emotional Reactions of Mothers Facing Premature Births: Study of 100 Mother-Infant Dyads 32 Gestational Weeks

Julien Eutrope[1]*, Aurore Thierry[2], Franziska Lempp[1], Laurence Aupetit[3], Stéphanie Saad[4], Catherine Dodane[5], Nathalie Bednarek[6], Laurence De Mare[3], Daniel Sibertin-Blanc[4], Sylvie Nezelof[5], Anne-Catherine Rolland[1]

1 CHU Reims, Hôpital Robert Debré, Structure interne de Psychothérapie de l'Enfant et de l'Adolescent, Reims, F-51092, France, **2** CHU Reims, Hôptal Robert Debré, Unité d'aide méthodologique, REIMS, F-51092, France, **3** Centre d'Action Médico-Sociale Précoce, Reims, F-51100, France, **4** CHU Nancy, Centre psychothérapique de Nancy, Service de pédopsychiatrie, Laxou, F-54521, France, **5** CHU de Besançon, Hôpital Saint Jacques, Service de psychiatrie de l'enfant et de l'adolescent, Besancon, F-25030, France, **6** CHU de Reims, Hôpital Maison Blanche, Structure Interne de Pédiatrie B, Reims, F-51092, France

Abstract

Objectives: This current study has been conducted to clarify the relationship between the mother's post-traumatic reaction triggered by premature birth and the mother-infant interactions. In this article, the precocious maternal feelings are described.

Methods: A multicenter prospective study was performed in three French hospitals. 100 dyads with 100 very premature infants and their mothers were recruited. Mothers completed, at two different times self-questionnaires of depression/ anxiety, trauma and social support. The quality of interactions in the dyads was evaluated.

Results: Thirty-nine percent of the mothers obtained a score at HADS suggesting a high risk of depression at the first visit and approximately one-third at visit two. Seventy-five percent of the mothers were at risk of suffering from an anxiety disorder at visit one and half remained so at visit two. A "depressed" score at visits one and two correlated with a hospitalization for a threatened premature labor. We noted a high risk of trauma for 35% of the mothers and high interactional synchrony was observed for approximately two-thirds of the dyads. The mothers' psychological reactions such as depression and anxiety or postnatal depression correlate strongly with the presence of an initial trauma. At visit one and visit two, a high score of satisfaction concerning social support correlates negatively with presence of a trauma. A maternal risk of trauma is more frequent with a C-section delivery.

Conclusions: Mothers' psychological reactions such as depression and anxiety correlate greatly with the presence of an initial trauma. The maternal traumatic reaction linked to premature birth does not correlate with the term at birth, but rather with the weight of the baby. Social support perceived by the mother is correlated with the absence of maternal trauma before returning home, and also seems to inhibit from depressive symptoms from the time of the infant's premature birth.

Editor: Kenji Hashimoto, Chiba University Center for Forensic Mental Health, Japan

Funding: This study was supported by grants from the Hospital Clinical Research Program of the French Ministry of Health (PHRC 2008). The funders had no role in study design, data collection and analysis, decision to publish, or preparation of the manuscript.

Competing Interests: The authors have declared that no competing interests exist.

* Email: jeutrope@chu-reims.fr

Introduction

In January 2008, in an article titled, "Preterm: What Can be Done?"[1], The Lancet announced a series of three articles series by Robert Goldenberg, to focus on a rising public health issue by studying causes as well as interventions to reduce infant morbidity and mortality, which according to the author was being neglected. According to this editorial, premature births account for 12–13% of births in the United States, and 5–9% in a number of other developed countries. Remarkably, the numbers of very premature births has increased over the last decade. An epidemiological birth study from 2005 [2] states that the United States has a premature birth rate (<37 Gestational Weeks) of 12.7% compared to 10.6% in 1990 and only 9.5% in 1981. Another objective study [3] also shows a 20% rise in premature births between 1990 and 2005. In Europe, the rate increased by 22% [4], concerning first-time mothers in particular, a trend also found in Australia [5]. The rise in medically assisted procreation partly explains this increase in which mothers pregnant with multiples are often induced or have ovary stimulation [6]. The risk of a very preterm birth is considerably higher in the case of multiples: in 1995 7% of twins and 25% of triplets were born before 33 weeks. Furthermore, cases of prematurity are higher in single pregnancies done with in vitro fertilization.

In this article we want to discuss very preterm births or births occurring before 32 Gestational Weeks (GW). An infant, who is born very preterm, worries neonatologists as to his/her viability and his/her pathologies for the short-term outlook. Premature births are considered to be responsible for 75% of perinatal mortality, and more than 75% of the long-term perinatal morbidity [7].

Our intervention in the maternity and neonatal wards sensitized us to the immediate parental reaction of the premature birth. Among these reactions, most often the parents are what they call "stressed", which is the origin of trauma. The unexpected confrontation with a baby is far from what the parents had anticipated; the shock experienced during a rapid chain of events taking place, an experience of emptiness when the baby is placed in the intensive care unit, the feeling of powerlessness when facing the real risk of the infant's death, the invasive treatments, etc. The parents worry about the viability and future of their premature infant. Their parental reactions and more specifically those of the mother facing the premature birth could have repercussions on the development of the infant, due to complex and atypical interactions.

These observations have driven us to elaborate on a hypothesis that distinguishes itself separate to the lesion model commonly applied to premature infants, and shifts the psychopathological approach to the post-traumatic reaction of the mother following the premature birth; it repositions the question of behavioral disorders of the child in the mother-infant interactions. In a second phase, we think that a premature birth can bring about post-traumatic symptoms as described in the post-traumatic stress state, and most notably in the mother. Therefore, this reaction could have effects on the mother-infant interactions.

We have conducted this current study to clarify the relationship between the mother's post-traumatic reaction triggered by the premature birth and the mother-infant interactions. In this article, our research aims to describe precocious maternal feelings when the mother has to face the premature birth of her infant.

Methods

1. Design

This present study is part of the larger research program that was a multicenter prospective study performed in 3 French hospitals (Reims, Nancy and Besançon) between January 2008 and January 2011. The follow-up period was 18 months for each participant. The entire research program covers 5 visits: the first visit, in the maternity service following the birth of the child, and the second visit, in the neonatology service, right before the discharge. The three following visits with the same design took place at 6, 12 and 18 months, within the framework of the systematic tracking of premature babies within the early medico-social actions' center (CAMSP). The study described in this article analyses the results of the first two visits of the research program.

2. Sample and procedure

All the preterm infants who were admitted to one of the NICU of the 3 investigation centres (Reims, Besancon and Nancy) from January 2008 to January 2010 and who matched our principal inclusion criteria (<32 gestational weeks) were considered for inclusion in the study. Exclusion criteria were for the mothers with an evident psychiatric illness, drug or alcohol abuse, aged <18 years, and language barriers; for the newborn: unfavourable vital prognosis evaluated with the Perinatal Risk Inventory [8] (a PRI score ≥10 identifies infants at risk of significant developmental disabilities and constitutes as an infant exclusion criteria), malformation and/or genetic anomaly diagnosed before the inclusion.

The 3 maternities and NICU are levels 3B (a NICU that provides mechanical ventilation without restrictions but does not provide major surgery) or 3C (a NICU that provides major neonatal surgery but neither open-heart surgery nor extracorporeal membrane oxygenation). These definitions are based on the American Academy of Paediatrics report on NICU levels of care [9]. Regarding the location of the family's city, 30% of the infants considered for inclusion were excluded. Undoubtedly the area of the family had to be close to the investigation centre to allow the routine follow-up proposed to preterm infants linked to our study. For the mother exclusion criteria concerning a psychiatric illness, we based it on a standard clinical interview performed by a psychiatrist investigator responsible for the inclusions. For the infant exclusion criteria, pediatricians connected to NICU recorded the PRI (Perinatal Risk inventory) and decided whether to allow the inclusion or not. To consider infant and mothers exclusion criteria, it excluded 20% of the dyads divided as: for the mothers: evident psychiatric illness (n = 4), drug or alcoholic abuse (n = 2), age <18 years (n = 2) and language barriers (n = 7); for the newborn: PRI ≥10 (n = 60), malformation and/or genetic anomaly diagnosed before the inclusion (n = 5). Following these restrictions of location and exclusion criteria, this study was explained and proposed to 50% of the population relating to our principal inclusion criteria (birth <32GW). Sixty-five percent of the mothers accepted to participate in this study (130 mothers). There were 26 cases of multiple births (22 twins, and 4 triples); only one child (randomly selected) was kept for the study; 30 children were then removed. Limited by our financial funding, we decided to stop the inclusions when reaching a population of 100 dyads, a number considered high enough by the statisticians. The second visit was completed by 93 dyads, 2 infants died, 2 infants were transferred to another hospital ward because their family moved away and 3 mothers dropped out.

3. Ethics

Given the observational nature of the study, which is not governed by French biomedical law, it could not be approved by the Committee for the Protection of Persons. Given the guidelines of publishers focused on the ethics of the investigations published, CHU de Reims has established an IRB since 2007. This study has been approved globally for all the centers (Reims, Nancy and Besançon) and all the participating patients. It received the approval of the local Institutional Review Board: IRB of Reims University Hospital. The study was conducted in compliance with good clinical practice, as indicated in the Declaration of Helsinki. Written consent was obtained from all the patients after providing specific information on the study. After a premature birth below 32 gestational weeks, NICU pediatricians contacted our research team and one of the practicians/author in charge of the clinical part of the research, met the mother and her baby to introduce the research program. Therefore, some of the authors have been in contact with participants as expected in a clinical research. Patients were free to refuse to take part in the study or to withdraw from it at any stage on simple request, without any alteration to the care provided to them. Data collection was made anonymous.

4. Data collection

4.1 Sociodemographic and clinical data. Sociodemographic variables recorded during the study were age, marital status, level of education and profession.

For the mothers, clinical data were: number of childbirths, number of pregnancies, medical history of the pregnancy (threatened premature labor, hospitalization), obstetric history (miscarriage, medical interruption of pregnancy, termination of pregnancy, in vitro fertilization, threatened premature labor, prematurity, hospitalization), delivery conditions (C-section or vaginal), multiple pregnancy (number of babies), anesthesia type (none, epidural, total), personal histories (medical, surgical, psychiatric, family).

For the infants, clinical data were: date of birth, term of birth, weight, size, cranial perimeter, Apgar score at five and ten minutes, necessity or not of a neonatal resuscitation, method of feeding (breast-, bottle-, mixed-feeding).

For the dyads, clinical data was the presence or absence of specific care (psychologist, psychomotor therapist).

4.2 Measures. The design of this study's two visits is described in table 1.

For the mothers, the evaluation of the mother's trauma was done by using *mPPQ (modified PTSD-Perinatal Posttraumatic Stress Disorder-Questionnaire)* [10,11]. This self-report questionnaire consists of 14 items, specially adapted to the parents of perinatal high-risk children, in order to evaluate the presence of traumatic elements concerning the birth. For this measurement, we decided to use a cut-off score of ≥19 [10,12], which identifies a high risk of trauma in the maternal population needing specific care (referral for therapy) when the PPQ has reached 19 or more.

In order to compensate for the biases identified, we also evaluated the maternal co morbidity using:

The *HADS (Hospital Anxiety and Depression Scale)* [13,14], which is a self-report questionnaire frequently used in international literature, and divided into 2 sub-scales, which are anxiety and depression HADS scales. This scale, which is easy to use, makes it possible to evaluate anxious and depressive symptoms in people who have somatic diseases. It allows episodes of recent anxiety and depression to be evaluated and to attribute to an overall score for each one. The result is given as a score. We have used a cut-off score of 8 or above, which is suggestive of clinically significant anxious (HADS anxiety sub-scale) or depressive (HADS depression sub-scale) symptomatology [15].

The *EPDS (Edinburgh Post-natal Depression Scale)* [16] consists of a self-report questionnaire that tracks postnatal depression and includes 10 items, which we propose to the mother from the fourth week of postpartum. A score of 12 or above is suggestive of clinically significant depressive symptomatology. The EPDS cutoff has been found to identify major depression in women, with a sensitivity of 86%, a specificity of 78%, and a positive predicative value of 73% [17].

The Social Support Questionnaire (SSQ) of Sarason [18] is a self-report questionnaire which includes 2 scales: availability (the number of people of whom the subject can rely on), and satisfaction (the level of fulfillment concerning this support).

For the infants, we identified some who were at risk of significant developmental abnormalities by using the *Perinatal Risk Inventory (PRI)* [8]. This scale uses 18 items to describe the weight of the perinatal problems and the severity of the perinatal risk, based on perinatal factors such as the Apgar score, the gestational age, the weight or the cranial perimeter. The score can be from o to 51. An inventory score ≥10 identifies infants at risk of significant developmental disabilities. The performances of the Perinatal Risk Inventory are: sensitivity 76%, specificity 79%, positive predictive value 47,7%, and negative predictive value 92,9%.

In the dyad, Censullo's DMC (Dyadic Mutuality Code) instrument [19] can be used for the first 6 months of the baby's life. After a 5-minute observation of the dyad interacting, the observer codes 6 items (mutual attention, positive affect, reciprocity, maternal pauses, clearness of the signals of the baby, and receptivity/maternal sensitivity). A score of 1 or 2 is given for each

Table 1. Design of the two first visits of the study.

	Place	Date	PPQ	HADS	EPDS	SSQ	PRI	DMC
Visit 1	Maternity	Day1 to day 15		X		X	X	
Visit 2	Neonatalogy	15 days before output	X	X	X	X	X	X

item and a total score is rated as synchronous or low synchronous. The total score ranges from 6 to 12. A score of 6 to 9 is ranked as low synchronous; and 10 to 12, as synchronous. The summary ratings use combinations of all 6 items as an operational definition of the levels of synchrony, because included in the 6 items are the relevant components of synchronous interaction established in specialized literature, and collectively they represent the concept of synchrony. The validation of the DMC has been constructed by Censullo on relevant findings of interrater reliability, items analysis, concurrent to 38 videotapes of mother-infant face-to-face interaction, compared to cross-spectral analyses of the Monadic Phase Scale [20].

5. Statistical analysis

The quantitative variables are the average, the standard deviation, and the minimal and maximal values. The qualitative variables are the number of observations and the associated frequency. The search for a link between the quantitative and qualitative variables was accomplished by using the Mann-Whitney/Wilcoxon or Kruskal-Wallis test. We did Spearman's correlation analysis between two quantitative variables. For all statistical tests, a p value<0.05 was considered statistically significant. Analyses were performed using the SAS software (version 9.0; SAS Institute Inc., Cary, N.C., USA).

Results

1. Patient characteristics

We included 100 dyads (100 babies and their mothers). The average age of the mothers is just under 30 years old (29.8±6 [17–45], and 92% of them lived with a partner at the time of birth. The majority have a higher education (79.29%) and work (69%). Most of the mothers (88.8%) have been hospitalized for a risk of premature labor. The majority of them (58.2%) have obstetrical antecedents (miscarriage, medical termination of pregnancy, IVF, premature birth). It is generally a first (48%) or a second pregnancy (32%), with a small majority of births by C-section (54%) and a rather homogeneous distribution of the method of feeding (40.82% breast-, 33.67% bottle-, 25.51% mixed-feeding). The average term is from 29 weeks of amenorrhea and 6 days (29.84±6 [17–45], with a very small majority of boys and an average birth weight of 1320g.

2. Mother evaluation

Table 2 represents the scores of evaluation scales at visit 1 and visit 2.

Our first results show that 39% of the mothers obtained a score at HADS suggesting a high risk of depression at the first visit and approximately one-third at the second visit (HADS depression sub-score: 26%, EPDS: 34%). HADS anxiety sub-score reveals that 75% of the mothers were at risk of suffering from an anxiety disorder at visit one and half (50%) were still at risk at visit two [21]. A high score at visits one and two correlated with a hospitalization for a risk of premature labor ($p_{V1}=0.0392$; $p_{V2}=0.0282$) and did not correlate with the babies' birth term ($p=0.64$) or birth weight ($p=0.55$) at visit two.

We noted a high risk of trauma in 35% of the mothers and a high interactional synchrony score was observed for approximately two-thirds (66%) of the dyads.

Access to services to a psychologist or a psychomotor therapist was offered to 30.1% of the mothers and their babies.

In Table 3, the data concerning the mothers' and babies' clinical characteristics correlated significantly with the mother's trauma.

The mothers' psychological reactions at visit one and two such as a high risk of depression and/or anxiety disorder or postnatal depression at visit two correlated strongly with the high probability of initial trauma ($p<0.0001$).

At visit one ($p=0.03$) and visit two ($p=0.04$) a high score of satisfaction concerning social support correlates negatively with a high score on the PPQ scale (which indicates a mother's trauma). A high score obtained on the PPQ is significantly ($p=0.0092$) more frequent with a C-section delivery (vs. vaginal delivery) and the majority of the mothers with a high risk of trauma (PPQ's high score) belong to the dyads having specific psychological care with psychologists or psychomotor therapists ($p=0.0026$).

3. Baby evaluation

The babies' health characteristics correlate with the presence of an initial trauma: state of health of the newborn (PRI score to V2) ($p=0.04$), his or her's evolution of state of health ($p=0.04$) and his or her birth weight ($p=0.03$).

4. Dyad interaction

We looked for correlations between the quality of interactions in the dyads (evaluated with the DMC on Visit 1 and 2) and the characteristics collected on Visit 1 as: pregnancy conditions (medically assisted procreation or not), delivery conditions (C-section or vaginal), babies' clinical characteristics (birth weight, intrauterine growth restriction, term at birth), and the infant's measures (PRI score), and also the mothers' measures (HADS, EPDS and PPQ scores) for evaluating states of mind of the mothers; but we did not find any significant correlation.

Discussion

Prerequisite

As clinicians, it's essential to underline the complexity of the subject. Prematurity, depending on the term at birth, takes many different forms. Many innate and acquired factors, outside of the gestation period itself, intervene in clinical prematurity. It would be simplistic and inexact to consider clinical prematurity as a well-defined entity. Also, for facilitating the reading, in this discussion, we will use the terminology of depressed or anxious for mothers with high scores on specific self questionnaires (HADS and EPDS), allowing them enough substantial to assess anxious and depressive symptomatology, especially by using the cutoff mentioned in the method paragraph.

The general characteristics (sociodemographic and clinical data, main psychological reactions) of our population were comparable with other studies also addressing the maternal reactions after a premature birth [22–24].

We didn't find any significant correlations between maternal distress and dysfunctional interactions, whereas our hypothesis was that a maternal traumatic reaction would be correlated with difficulties in parent-child interactions, especially as the general sense of this hypothesis has been partially confirmed by some studies [25–27]. By the second visit we observed the mother-infant interactions, but no significant correlation was found between low-quality interactions nor with certain maternal emotional reactions such as traumatism, or with any of the factors related to the child (term, weight, health). It seems that the assessment tool (DMC) is not sensitive enough. We could also question the timing of the observation at visit two, which is just before the infant returns home so the mother is very enthusiastic and in a hurry to return home. It probably would have been more efficient to observe interactions at home.

Table 2. Mean scores of evaluation scales at visit 1 and visit 2.

	N[a]	m (sd)[b]
Visit 1	*100*	
PRI[1]	95	4.7 (2.5)
HADS[2] Depression	98	6.8 (4.3)
HADS[2] Anxiety	98	10.2 (4.4)
HADS[2] Global	98	17.0 (7.9)
SSQ[3] Disponibility	98	21.6 (12.3)
SSQ[3] Satisfaction	98	31.5 (4.8)
Visit 2	*93*	
PRI[1]	72	6.8 (7.1)
HADS[2] Depression	89	5.4(3.2)
HADS[2] Anxiety	89	8.5 (3.7)
HADS[2] Global	89	13.9 (6.2)
SSQ[3] Disponibility	87	22.0 (12.6)
SSQ[3] Satisfaction	88	31.9 (4.3)
mPPQ[4]	88	16.4 (9.9)
EPDS[5]	89	9.2 (5.1)
DMC[6]	90	10.2 (1.2)

[a]N: Number of dyads.
[b]m(sd): mean (standard deviation).
[1]PRI: Perinatal Risk Inventory.
[2]HADS: Hospital Anxiety and Depression Scale.
[3]SSQ: Social Support Questionnaire of Sarason.
[4]mPPQ: modified Perinatal PTSD (Post Traumatic Stress Disorder) Questionnaire.
[5]EPDS: Edimburgh Postnatal Depression Scale.
[6]DMC: Dyadic Mutuality Code.

Nonetheless, the findings of this study about precocious, maternal and emotional reactions are interesting and consistent with previous studies which suggest that the premature birth of an infant has repercussions on maternal emotional responses [28]. In many studies, elevated scores affirming postnatal depression were found to be significantly more often associated with the mothers of infants born prematurely [22,29]. In this study, during the 15 days after birth, 39% of the mothers attained scores on the HADS that suggested a high risk of depressive symptoms and about one third of the mothers remained at risk of depression during the few days before the discharge from the NICU. This evolution of depression scores approves with an American longitudinal study [30] in which

Table 3. Mothers' and babies' clinical characteristics and the high risk of maternal trauma.

	High risk of initial trauma[3] r (p)
State of health of the child (PRI to V2)	0.25 (0.04)
Evolution of the state of health of the child (PRI V2 - PRI V1)	0.25 (0.04)
Birth Weight	−0.23 (0.03)
HADS[1] depression score V1	0.54 (<.0001)
HADS[1] depression score V2	0.48 (<.0001)
HADS[1] anxiety score V1	0.54 (<.0001)
HADS[1] anxiety score V2	0.52 (<.0001)
HADS[1] global score V1	0.60 (<.0001)
HADS[1] global score V2	0.56 (<.0001)
Satisfaction of perceived social support (SSQ Satisfaction V1)	−0.23 (0.03)
Satisfaction of perceived social support (SSQ Satisfaction V2)	−0.22 (0.04)
EPDS[2] (postnatal depression V2)	0.50 (<.0001)

[1]HADS = Hospital Anxiety and Depression Scale.
[2]EPDS = Edimburgh Postnatal Depression Scale.
[3]Score at modified Perinatal PTSD (Post Traumati Stress Disorder) Questionnaire (mPPQ) ≥19 suggesting a maternal trauma.

more than half of the population of mothers with premature babies were considered depressed (60%) according to the study criteria, with a progressive improvement of the symptomatology reaching stability at the infant's sixth month. The correlation between positive scores of depression's risk and threatened premature labor confirm the results of previous studies [31,32] which find psychological origins in more than 50% of those at risk of premature labor.

A large majority of mothers (75%) present a post-natal symptomatology of anxiousness in the early post-natal period following the premature birth of their child and before their child goes home. The results are in concordance with a New Zealand study [33] that finds that anxiety dominated in the group where parents were confronted with the hospitalization of their infant versus the second group where the infants were never placed in the NICU. However, in the first group, a significant difference was found depending on the reason for the infant's hospitalization: premature births lead to more depressive symptomatology in NICU admissions than infants that were born at term. The premature birth itself plays its own role, independent of only stress linked to the infant's state of health.

Traumatism, measured by the PPQ scale after the birth and before the return home, is objective among 35% of the mothers. Our results confirm those of previous studies [23,24]. For all of the parents, the premature birth of their infants is an intense experience, shattering their psychological reserves. A one year French prospective study [34] shows that the feeling about this experience changed little during the infant's first year of life: memories remain vivid and raise strong emotions. Certain parents retell the birth story using exactly the same words with the same effects one year later. A birth like this could therefore be considered as a traumatic event. In an article co-written by Léon Kreisler and Michel Soulé [35], the mothers' emotional response and the initial circumstances surrounding the premature infant is studied by evaluating the pregnancy, delivery, separation, and subsequent evolution. This is a psychological storm that bears on the mother. Once objectified, the presence and extent of this maternal trauma reaction following the premature birth of her child makes it important to attempt to correlate certain factors. According to our results, the method of delivery, and more specifically when a cesarean occurs, correlates significantly with signs of a traumatic reaction, objectified and quantified during the second visit of our research protocol. The same was also found regardless of the term at birth [36,37].A Norwegian study [38] shows that the mothers having undergone a caesarean section are 12% less likely to have a second baby than other mothers. We can reasonably assume that the psychological trauma of a cesarean section therefore remains an obstacle into having another pregnancy. A premature birth and delivery requiring a cesarean section would be two factors predisposing parturient women to the development of a traumatic reaction.

According to our results and the results of another recent study [23], the maternal traumatic reaction linked to the premature birth does not correlate to the term at birth, but rather to the weight of the baby. This point is also witnessed in medical consultations, even a long time after the premature birth, because the parents, or sometimes even the child, report the weight to indicate the severity of the birth and their worries, and not the term. Parents remain sensitive to the news of "low weight" at birth (500, 600 grams), and also by the image of this weight, which seems to actively participate in the emergence of an anxious and traumatic symptomatology in the mother. We have also looked for a correlation with the presence of an intrauterine growth restriction (IUGR) by using applicable scales. We know that in terms of developmental evolution of a premature infant, the existence of intrauterine growth restriction increases the risk of mortality, morbidity, and sequelae, because of chronic anoxia, cerebral malnutrition, and even the causes that led to the IUGR. But we did not find any correlation between the negative maternal emotional responses and the existence or lack of IUGR. Only the infant's weight at birth, a factor perceived visually by the mother, is a factor of the emergence of the mother's negative emotions.

Our results show a correlation between the somatic state of health of the baby quantified by the Perinatal Risk Inventory (PRI), and the maternal trauma (measured by the PPQ). During the premature infant's hospitalization in the NICU, the parents are worried and are constantly listening to the information being relayed to them several times a day by the professionals in regards to the state of their infant's health. Daniel Sibertin-Blanc [39] describes certain premature infant's parents as vigilant guardians of their infant's bodies. Catherine Druon [40] alludes to the possible risk of passing from a "maternal preoccupation" to a "primarily medical preoccupation". Submerged in an atypical medical universe, mothers learn how to become good technicians, leaving aside normal maternal preoccupations.

Social support perceived by the mother, both in the number of people recognized to support the mother and the quality of this support is essential and is significantly correlated with the absence of maternal trauma before returning home, and also seems to protect from depressive symptoms from the time of the infant's premature birth.

One of the most interesting results on the clinical level of our research involves the support given to mothers in neonatal units. The identified mothers as having psychological distress in the aftermath of the premature birth through the study's questionnaires (PPQ, HADS) are those who have benefited from support. They benefit from care by a psychologist or psychomotor therapist during the hospitalization of their infant in the NICU, without the results of their self-questionnaires being known by professionals.

Limitations

By not using structural interviews for the mothers' assessments at the time of the inclusion to respond categorically to the mother exclusion criteria, and also to diagnostic depression symptoms in the two visits, is a main limitation of our study. However, structured assessments might have been too intense, even too emotionally difficult for the mothers having just experienced the premature birth of their infant, and have to continue to live with this supposed traumatic event. About the representation of our population, the location restrictions (explained in the "Sample and Procedure" paragraph), could appear as a limitation to our study, because our population most probably live in big cities or nearby. Concerning our data collection, we didn't have any data concerning mother anxiety and or depressive symptoms before the infant's birth, so this remains a limitation for us to discuss our results. Also it would have been pertinent to investigate the mother's smoking habits, so as to correlate to the infant's characteristics. At least, as for any study, a control group would have permitted the results to be more consistent.

Conclusion and Clinical Implications

The mother is the central figure of anxiety related to premature birth. She experiences and expresses her feelings about it (not necessarily), and it is up to the clinical staff to hear what she is feeling. In our study, we observed that professionals have been sensitive to the expression of maternal suffering, and have proposed specific support. This kind of intervention is now well described in literature (38), so we believe that being able to express suffering is a good prognosis in the evolution of trauma for the mother.

Author Contributions

Conceived and designed the experiments: ACR. Performed the experiments: JE ACR FL LA SS CD NB LDM DSB SN. Analyzed the data: JE ACR AT. Contributed reagents/materials/analysis tools: AT. Wrote the paper: JE ACR.

References

1. The Lancet (2008) Preterm birth: what can be done? The Lancet 371(9606): 2.
2. Brady E, Hamilton D, Joyce A (2006) Births: preliminary data for 2005. Natl Vital Stat Rep 55(11): 1–19.
3. Martin J, Hamilton B, Ventura S, Menacker F, Kirmeyer S (2006) Births: final data for 2004. Natl Vital Stat Rep 55(1): 1–101.
4. Langhoff-Ross J, Kesmodel U, Jacobson B, Rasmussen S, Vogel I (2006) Spontaneous preterm delivery in primarous women at low risk in Denmark; population based study. BMJ 332: 937–939.
5. Tracy S, Tracy M, Dean J, Laws P, Sullivan E (2007) Spontaneous preterm birth of liveborn infants in women at low risk in Australia over 10 years: a population-based study. BJOG 114: 731–735.
6. Jakobsson M, Paavonen J, Tapper A (2008) The incidence of preterm deliveries decreases in Finland. BJOG 115: 38–43.
7. Goldenberg R, Culhan J, Iams J, Romero R (2008) Epidemiology and causes of preterm birth. The Lancet 371: 75–84.
8. Scheiner A, Sexton M (1991) Prediction of developmental outcome using a perinatal risk inventory. Pediatrics 88(6): 1135–1143.
9. Stark AR (2005) Levels of neonatal care. Pediatrics 115: 1118.
10. Callahan J, Borja S, Hynan M (2006) Modification of the Perinatal PTSD Questionnaire to enhance clinical utility. J Perinatol 26(9): 533–539.
11. Pierrehumbert B, Borghini A, Forcada-Guex M, Jaunin L, Muller-Nix C, et al. (2004) French validation of the "Perinatal PTSD Questionnaire" assessing parent's posttraumatic stress reactions following the birth of a high risk infant. Ann Médico-psychol 162(9): 711–721.
12. Hynan MT, Mounts KO, Vanderbilt DL (2013) Screening parents of high-risk infants for emotional distress: rationale and recommendations. J Perinatol 33:748–753.
13. Zigmond A, Snaith R (1983) The hospital anxiety and depression scale. Acta psychiatr scand 67(6): 361–370.
14. Lepine JP, Godchau M, Brun P, Lemperière T (1985) Evaluation de l'anxiété et de la dépression chez des patients hospitalisés dans un service de médecine interne. Ann Médico-Psychol 2: 175–189.
15. Hinz A, Brähler E (2011) Normative values for the Hospital Anxiety and Depression Scale (HADS) in the general German population. J Psychosom Res 71(2): 74–78.
16. Cox JL, Holden JM, Sagovsky R (1987) Detection of postnatal depression: development of the 10-item Edimburgh Postnatal Depression Scale. Br J Psychiatry 150: 782–786.
17. Holden JM (1991) Posnatal depression: It's nature, effects and identity using the Edinburg Postnatal Depression Scale. Birth 18: 211–221.
18. Sarason IG, Levine HM, Basham RB, Sarason BR (1983) Assessing social support: the social support questionnaire. J Personnal Soc Psychol 44(1): 127–139.
19. Censullo M, Bowler R, Lester B, Brazelton TB (1987) An instrument of the measurement of infant-adult synchrony. Nurs Res 36(4): 244–248.
20. Tronick E, Als H, Brazelton TB (1980) Monadic phases: A structural descriptive analysis of infant-mother face-to-face interaction. Merrill-Palmer Quaterly 26: 3–24.
21. Bjelland I, Dahl AA, Haug TT, Neckelmann D (2011) The validity of the Hospital Anxiety and Depression Scale: An updated literature review. J Psychosom Res 52(2): 69–77.
22. Davis L, Edwards H, Moyah H, Wollin J (2003) The impact of very premature birth on the psychological health of mothers. Early Hum Dev 73(1–2): 61–70.
23. Gamba Szijarto S, Forcada-Guex M, Borghini A, Pierrehumbert B, Ansermet F, et al. (2009) Prematurity and parental post-traumatic stress disorder: Similarities and differences. Neuropsychiatr Enfance Adolesc 57(5): 385–391.
24. Feeley N, Zelkowitz P, Cormier C, Charbonneau L, Lacroix A, et al. (2011) Posttraumatic stress among mothers of very low birthweight infants at 6 months after discharge from the neonatal intensive care unit. Appl Nurs Res 24(2): 114–117.
25. Pierrehumbert B, Nicole C, Muller-Nix C, Forcada-Guex M, Ansermet F (2003) Parental post-traumatic reactions after premature birth: implications for sleeping and eating problems in the infant. Arch Dis Child Fetal Neonatal Ed 88(5): F400–404.
26. Muller-Nix C, Forcada-Guex M, Pierrehumbert B, Jaunin L, Borghini A, et al. (2004) Prematurity, maternal stress and mother-child interacions. Early Hum Dev 79(2): 145–158.
27. Cohen SE, Parmelee AH (1983) Prediction of five-year Standford-Binet scores in preterm infants. Child dev 54(5): 1242–1253.
28. Singer L, Salvator A, Guo S, Collin M, Lilien L, et al. (1999) Maternal Psychological Distress and Parenting Stress after Birth of very low-birth-weight Infant. JAMA 281(9): 799–805.
29. Drewett R, Blair P, Emmet P, Edmond A (2004) Failure to thrive in the term and preterm infants of mothers depressed in the postnatal period: population-based birth cohort study. J Child Psychol Psychiatry 45(2): 359–366.
30. Miles M, Holditch-Davis D, Schwartz T, Scher M (2007) Depressive symptoms in mother of prematurely born infants. J Dev Behav Pediatr 28(1):36–44.
31. Précelle F (2004) Problematic of depression, first pregnancy and risk of premature birth. Neuropsychiatr Enfance Adolesc 52(5): 279–283.
32. De Muylder X (1989) Psychological factors and preterm labour. J. Reprod. Inf. Psychol 7: 55–57.
33. Carter J, Mulder R, Bartarm A, Darlow B (2005) Infants in neonatal intensive care unit: parental response. Arch Dis Child Fetal Neonatal Ed 90: F109–113.
34. Pavoine S, Azémar E, Rajon A, Raynaud JP (2004) Parents of premature children: what future for the first year of life? Neuropsychiatr Enfance Adolesc 52(6): 398–404.
35. Kreisler L, Soulé M (1976) L'enfant prématuré et sa mère in P. Satgé et M. Soulé, L'accueil et la prise en charge des parents dans un centre de néonatologie. L'expansion scientifique ed. pp. 8–25.
36. Creedy D (2000) Childbirth and the development of acute trauma symptom symptoms following: incidence and contributing factors. Birth 27: 104–111.
37. Soet J, Brack G, Dilorio C (2003) Prevalence and predictors of women's experience of psychological trauma during childbirth. Birth 30: 36–46.
38. Daltveit A, Tollanes M, Philstorm H, Irgens L (2008) Cesarean delivery and subsequent pregnancies. Obstet Gynecol 11(6): 1327–1334.
39. Sibertin-Blanc D, Tchenio D, Vert P (2002) To be born "very-low-birth-weight children", and after? La psychiatrie de l'enfant 2(45): 437–482.
40. Druon C (1996) A l'écoute du bébé prématuré, une vie aux portes de la vie. Paris: Flammarion.198 p.

The Influence of Work-Related Chronic Stress on the Regulation of Emotion and on Functional Connectivity in the Brain

Armita Golkar[1], Emilia Johansson[1], Maki Kasahara[1], Walter Osika[1,2], Aleksander Perski[3], Ivanka Savic[4]*

1 Department of Clinical Neuroscience, Karolinska Institute, Stockholm, Sweden, 2 Center for Social Sustainability, Department of Neurobiology, Care Sciences and Society, Karolinska institute, Stockholm, Sweden, 3 Stress Research Institute, Stockholm University, Stockholm, Sweden, 4 Department of Women's and children's health, and Neurology Clinic, Karolinska Institute and Hospital, Stockholm, Sweden

Abstract

Despite mounting reports about the negative effects of chronic occupational stress on cognitive and emotional functions, the underlying mechanisms are unknown. Recent findings from structural MRI raise the question whether this condition could be associated with a functional uncoupling of the limbic networks and an impaired modulation of emotional stress. To address this, 40 subjects suffering from burnout symptoms attributed to chronic occupational stress and 70 controls were investigated using resting state functional MRI. The participants' ability to up- regulate, down-regulate, and maintain emotion was evaluated by recording their acoustic startle response while viewing neutral and negatively loaded images. Functional connectivity was calculated from amygdala seed regions, using explorative linear correlation analysis. Stressed subjects were less capable of down-regulating negative emotion, but had normal acoustic startle responses when asked to up-regulate or maintain emotion and when no regulation was required. The functional connectivity between the amygdala and the anterior cingulate cortex correlated with the ability to down-regulate negative emotion. This connectivity was significantly weaker in the burnout group, as was the amygdala connectivity with the dorsolateral prefrontal cortex and the motor cortex, whereas connectivity from the amygdala to the cerebellum and the insular cortex were stronger. In subjects suffering from chronic occupational stress, the functional couplings within the emotion- and stress-processing limbic networks seem to be altered, and associated with a reduced ability to down-regulate the response to emotional stress, providing a biological substrate for a further facilitation of the stress condition.

Editor: Daniel Margulies, Max Planck Institute for Human Cognitive and Brain Sciences, Germany

Funding: The Swedish Council for Working Life and Social Research (FAS), the Swedish Research Council, and VINNOVA are acknowledged for their financial support. The funders had no role in study design, data collection and analysis, decision to publish, or preparation of the manuscript.

Competing Interests: The authors have declared that no competing interests exist.

* Email: ivanka.savic-berglund@ki.se

Introduction

Stress is common and hard to avoid. When stress becomes chronic, it may have negative effects on cognitive functioning and even lead to psychiatric conditions such as anxiety and depression [1–2]. In recent years, the mounting reports about occupational stress and the substantial costs for society that are associated with it, mainly due to impaired mental health, have been gaining more attention [3]. These worldwide reports signal the pressing need for scientific investigations of the underlying pathophysiological mechanisms.

Cognitive and emotional dysfunctions attributed to occupational stress – 'the burnout syndrome'

Occupational 'burnout' is characterized by stress-related symptoms among otherwise healthy and high-performing persons who report that they have not experienced any major negative life events [4–8]. The described symptoms are attributed to occupational stress. They are stereotyped, and include memory and concentration problems, sleeplessness, diffuse aches, profound fatigue, irritability, anxiety, and a feeling of being emotionally drained. The underlying mechanisms are largely unknown. Measurements of cortisol levels after awakening in these subjects have hitherto yielded inconclusive results [9], with reports of normal [10–11], reduced [12–15], and elevated levels [16–18]. Recent data from brain imaging studies, although still limited, suggest, however, that burnout from occupational stress is associated with an affection of the limbic structures, the amygdala, and the mesial prefrontal cortex (mPFC), in particular [19–23]. These initial findings call for further research, considering the amygdala's key role in evoking stress responses [24–25] and considering that the regulation of stress responses during emotional conflict is processed via functional connectivity between the amygdala and the mPFC and anterior cingulate cortex (ACC) [26–30]. During the cognitive reappraisal of emotion, it has, for example, been demonstrated that the activity of the amygdala is down-regulated (measured as change in BOLD signal), whereas the activity in portions of the lateral and medial prefrontal cortex is upregulated [31–36]. Moreover, it was recently shown that the ability to cognitively down- regulate negative emotion was severely jeopardized after stress exposure [37]. It is, thus, possible that subjects reporting cognitive and emotional dysfunction due to chronic occupational stress could have an impaired ability to modulate emotional stress and emotionally stressful stimuli, rendering them less apt to cope with psychosocial stress. Furthermore, in these individuals, the amygdala connectivity with the mPFC and ACC, and perhaps also to the hippocampus and the insular cortex, could have undergone alterations. Such changes could constitute a stress vulnerability factor, or be a consequence of prolonged occupational stress. Both scenarios would be in line with our previous observations of structural and neuroreceptor changes along the limbic circuits in affected subjects [20–23]. These limbic changes, and their apparent overlap with the networks that are reported to be involved in emotional regulation led us to design a combined behavioral and MR study to test two specific hypothesis: (1) That subjects suffering from occupational stress have an impaired ability to modulate stressful emotions; and (2) That these subjects show altered amygdala functional connectivity. To test these, forty subjects with occupational burnout along with seventy unstressed healthy controls were investigated using a cognitive emotion regulation task as well as resting state fMRI.

Emotion regulation and the acoustic startle reflex

In order to assess emotion regulation, we measured the magnitude of the fear-potentiated startle reflex, which is a highly conserved, fast defensive reflex that consists of a series of muscular contractions and is mediated by a well-characterized neural circuitry [38–39]. In humans, this reflex can be elicited by a sudden and intense auditory stimulus (acoustic startle probe). The amplitude of this reflex is measured through facial electromyography (EMG), [40], and is potentiated when the individual is in an aversive or fearful state [41]. The startle reflex is a reliable and well-validated measure of emotion modulation [40] and has previously been successfully used as an index of cognitive emotion regulation in a healthy population [42–43].

In the present study the acoustic startle reflex was measured to investigate possible group differences in emotional reactions to negative visual stimuli and in the ability to regulate negative emotion. We also measured functional resting state connectivity from the amygdala, paying special attention to the connectivity to other nodes of the limbic system and to the mPFC and ACC in particular. In addition, a possible association between the ability to modulate emotion and the resting state functional connectivity was tested with linear regression analysis.

Methods

Participants

Forty right-handed [44] subjects (27 females; age 38±6 years, range 19–46 years; education 17±3 years), who had been diagnosed as having a 'reaction to severe stress and an adjustment disorder' according to the International Classification of Diseases (ICD-10, F43), were recruited from the Stress Research Institute at Stockholm University. The selection was limited to subjects who attributed their illness to prolonged work-related stress, after working 60 to 70 hours per week continuously over several years prior to the onset of symptoms. Inclusion criteria consisted of a characteristic symptom course of sleeplessness, diffuse aches, palpitations and fatigue, a subsequent onset of irritability, anxiety, memory and concentration problems, feeling of depersonalization, and reduced work capacity (confirmed by the employers) [8],[19]. All of the subjects attributed their symptoms to chronic stress and had no other known etiology for their distress.

Subjects were also required to have had a symptom duration of at least one year (their histories of stress-related burnout symptoms ranged from 1.5 to 3.5 years), to have been on sick leave (≥50%) for stress-related symptoms for a minimum of 6 months before entering the study, and to have an average stress-burnout score of ≥*3.0* on the Maslach Stress-Burnout Inventory – General Survey (MBI-GS) [45]. This 7-point rating scale, ranging from 0 (never) to 6 (daily), consists of three subscales: exhaustion (five items), cynicism (five items) and lack of professional efficacy (six items). When rating perceived stress, subjects were asked to take into consideration the last six months, and not only the actual time-point. The average scores for Scandinavian populations are around 2 for MBI-GS [4],[46].

Subjects were excluded if they had a previous history of psychosis, personality disorder, major or bipolar depression, alcohol or substance abuse, chronic fatigue, chronic pain, fibromyalgia, or neurological or endocrine disease. Those who had experienced prominent stress factors in their private life or a major traumatic event at any time in their life, including sexual abuse, were also excluded. No daily medication was allowed during the two months prior to the study, except contraceptives. According to a review of their pharmacological treatment histories, none of them had taken drugs that are known to affect brain structure (e.g., psychopharmaca). Subjects who were sleep deprived the night before the scan/testing procedures were rescheduled, in order to exclude the acute effects of sleep deprivation.

Seventy healthy, right-handed, non-smoking volunteers (45 females; age 33±6 years, range 24–45 years; education 17±3 years) with no history of chronic stress or heredity for neuropsychiatric disorders comprised the control group. The patient and control groups had similar gender distributions, and both were predominately female to accord with the female-dominated epidemiology of the condition studied [4].

The two groups were matched for socioeconomic status assessed on the basis of years of education, type of occupation, and organizational position (employee, middle management, supervisor). The study was approved by the Ethics Committee at the Karolinska Institute and written informed consent was received from each participant.

Before the interview, participants completed questionnaires in order to evaluate their stress symptoms and assess their previous life events [47]. In addition, the occurrence of major life events among the subjects was assessed through a clinical psychiatric interview based on the non-work-related items of the Holmes and Rahe Scale [48]. The participants were asked to answer yes or no to whether they had experienced any non-work- related stressful life events (e.g., death of a relative or spouse, recent divorce, forced family relocation). Subjects were excluded if they answered positively to having experienced such an event in their lives. Patients also received a medical screening (physical examination, test of thyroid and liver function). A structured interview, the Swedish version of the Mini-International Neuropsychiatric Interview, MINI [49] was performed, along with a test for depression using the Montgomery-Asberg Depression Rating Scale [50]. Although some subjects had high scores in the MADRS they did not fulfill the MINI criteria for depression, and were therefore not excluded.

Out of the participants who matched the inclusion criteria, 8 subjects with occupational burnout and 9 controls failed to display a startle response to the probe. The results from the emotion regulation experiment and the correlation analyses with fMRI are therefore based on data from the remaining 32 subjects with occupational burnout (20 females; mean age = 37.6 years,

SD = 6.5) and 61 controls (33 females; mean age = 30.9 years, SD = 6.7), whereas the analysis of resting state amygdala connectivity is based on the entire study group.

Salivary cortisol

Salivary cortisol was sampled according to a previously established protocol [51]. Saliva sampling was chosen because the method is simple, non-invasive, and non- stressful; the samples are shown to readily reflect the levels of the free fraction of cortisol in plasma [52]. Participants were instructed carefully on how to collect their own salivary samples. Samples were collected seven times on an ordinary weekday using Salivette cotton rolls (Sarstedt, Rommelsdorf, Germany), which participants were instructed to place in the mouth for 2 minutes. The first sample was collected immediately upon awakening in the morning, irrespective of time. The second sample was collected 15 minutes later, before eating or brushing teeth, and the third sample was collected 15 minutes after that. The fourth sample was collected around noontime, before lunch. The fifth sample was collected at about 3 p.m., the sixth at 8 p.m., and the seventh at bedtime, after having rested in bed for 15 minutes, before falling asleep. The samples were frozen (−18°C) until analyzed. The levels of salivary cortisol were measured with radioimmunoassay using the Spectria (^{125}I) coated tubes radioimmunoassay kit (Orion Diagnostica, FIN-02101 Espoo, Finland). The within-assay coefficients of variation ranged from 0.8 to 0.9, and those between assays never exceeded 10 percent. All samples from each group were analyzed simultaneously in duplicate.

Emotion regulation task

Before the experiment, the participants were given written as well as verbal explanations of the task and instructions. Participants were informed that they would receive three different instructions during the experiment and that these instructions would be symbolically represented by three different arrows: (1) an upward arrow indicated that the participant should make an effort to reinforce the feelings that are elicited by the picture, so that he/she experiences the image as more emotionally charged ("up-regulate"); (2) a horizontal arrow indicated that the participant should focus on the feeling the picture elicits, without trying to manipulate the emotion ("maintain"); and (3) a downward arrow indicated that the participant should make an effort to down-regulate the feelings that the picture elicits, so that he/she experiences the image as less emotionally charged, or as neutral as possible ("down-regulate"). Participants were thoroughly informed of the importance of following the instructions during the experiment and not distracting themselves from their feelings by thinking of something else or by looking away from the image or closing their eyes. The subjects were however free to choose the strategy to regulate their emotion.

The experiment began with a practice session during which the participants were first subjected to the auditory startle probe six times to allow for habituation to the sound. This was followed by twelve practice trials that mirrored the experimental procedure. After the practice session, the participants were asked to describe the strategy they had used to regulate emotion. None of the participants reported that they were confused about how to adopt a reappraisal strategy for the neutral and negative trials before or after completing the experimental task.

An example of an experimental trial is shown in Figure 1. During each trial, the participant was presented with a picture for 5 s, which was then replaced by an instruction cue for 1 s. For negative pictures, participants were instructed to suppress (down-regulate), enhance (up-regulate) or maintain their emotional response. Based on previous work [42] and to avoid confusion due to ambiguous instructions (e.g., to suppress emotional reactions to neutral pictures), neutral pictures were only coupled with the instruction to maintain the emotional response. Immediately following the instruction cue, the same picture was presented again for 5 s, during which time the participants carried out the regulation instruction. During each trial, startle probes were presented 3 s after picture onset during the first (pre-instruction) and the second (post-instruction) picture-viewing phases. Lastly, the participants were given 4 s to rate on a scale of 1–7 how well they had managed to carry out the instructions. Between each trial, a fixation cross was presented for 4–6 s (mean 5 s). Each trial lasted for 20 s. There were 60 trials, and the entire testing session lasted approximately twenty minutes, with a 15-second pause after the first 30 trials. The presentation of pictures was synchronized with the monitor's refresh rate and presented with the software Presentation (Neurobehavioural systems, www.neurobs.com).

Material

We selected three sets of 15 negative pictures and one set of 15 neutral pictures from the International Affective Picture Set (IAPS) [53]. Each of the three sets of negative pictures was assigned to one of the three task instructions (maintain, down-regulate, up-regulate), and this assignment was counterbalanced between participants (male and female controls, and patients). Pictures were selected to match valence and arousal scores of pictures used in a similar report [54].

Electromyographic recordings: response definition and data reduction

The eye-blink component of the startle response was measured through electromyographic (EMG) recordings of the left orbicularis oculi muscle using two miniature Ag/AgCl electrodes prepared with electrolyte gel. A third ground electrode was placed behind the left ear over the mastoid. Startle probes were 50-ms bursts of approximately 95-db[A] white noise with a near instantaneous rise time (<1 ms), delivered through sound-proof headphones (Bose AE21, Bose Co. Framingham, Massachusetts). The raw EMG signal was amplified and filtered through a 28–50 Hz bandpass filter, rectified and integrated with a time constant of 20 ms. Startle eye-blink magnitude (microvolts) was measured as the amplitude from onset to peak, and trials with excessive baseline activity or recording artifacts were rejected. To assess initial, unaltered startle responses, pre-instruction (Startle 1) startle scores for negative and neutral images were normalized using z-standardization to ensure that all participants contributed equally to the group means, as has been described previously [55–56]. The z-score calculation is a within-individual normalization, resulting in a distribution with an overall mean of 0 and a standard deviation of 1 for each participant. To assess the regulation of the startle response according to instruction, for each participant, we calculated the change in startle response by subtracting the raw startle 1 response from the raw startle 2 response separately for each instruction (maintain neutral, maintain negative, down-regulate negative, up-regulate negative) of the task. This way, we defined emotion regulation ability as the magnitude during emotion regulation controlling for baseline levels before the regulation cues.

Statistical analyses

Initial startle reactions were assessed in a 2×2 repeated measures analysis of variance (ANOVA) with Valence (Negative,

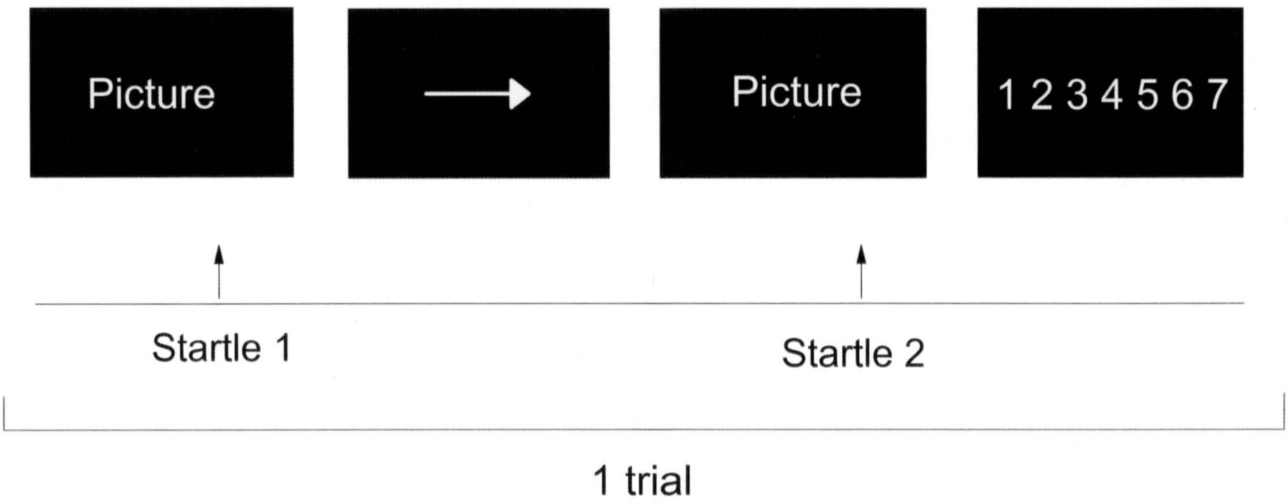

Figure 1. Overview of one experimental trial with the maintain instruction. Participants were presented with a picture, which was replaced by an instruction cue. For negative picture trials, this cue indicated whether the participants' task was to maintain (horizontal arrow), down- regulate (downward arrow) or enhance (upward arrow) their emotional response. Immediately following the instruction cue, participants implemented the regulation instruction while being exposed to the same picture again. Lastly, participants rated how well they managed to implement the regulation instruction on a scale of 1–7.
doi:10.1371/journal.pone.0104550.g001

Neutral) as a within-subjects variable and Group (Burnout, Control) as a between subjects variable. To test the hypothesis that burnout patients would differ from controls in their startle responses during down-regulation of negative emotion, we ran a 2×2 repeated measures ANOVA with Instruction (Down-regulate, Maintain) as the within-subject variable and Group (Burnout, Control) as the between-subject variable. As a control, we similarly assessed whether there were any group differences in startle responses during up-regulation of negative emotions in a 2 (Up-regulate, Maintain)×2 (Burnout, Control) repeated-measures ANOVA. Possible group difference in salivary cortisol levels was tested with a repeated measure ANOVA ($p < .05$).

fMRI data acquisition

MR experiments were carried out on a separate day to avoid contamination by possible effects of the emotional regulation tasks. Functional MRI time series data were collected from all of the participants at rest over 8 minutes in a 3 Tesla MR scanner Discovery 750 (GE Healthcare), using a 32-channel head coil. Resting fMRI blood oxygenation-level dependent (BOLD) data were acquired in a standard gradient echo-planar-imaging (EPI) acquisition, TR = 2.5 s, TE = 30 ms, flip angle = 90°, resolution = 3×3×3 mm, whole-head coverage. The participants were asked to lie with their eyes closed, to think of nothing in particular, and not to fall asleep. Structural brain images were acquired using a T1-weighted 3D brain imaging volume imaging sequence with whole-head coverage, TR = 7.91 s, TE = 3.06 s, flip angle = 12°, and resolution 1×1×1 mm. These structural images were used to aid the registration of the functional data into a common standard brain coordinate system (MNI152).

Seed region analysis

Seed region analysis is based on calculating cross-correlation coefficients of the time series in a particular seed region-of-interest (ROI) with all other voxels in the brain, which reveals the strength of functional connectivity with respect to this seed region [57]. The seed regions consisted of the right and left amygdala, and were delineated with the guidance of the WFU-pick atlas, and after adaptation to the gray matter template of our own population. The MNI coordinates for the amygdala seeds where (sphere of 5 mm radius, co-ordinate −22, −7 −19, and 22 −7 −19); the seed regions covered the amygdala, with the exception of the most medial 2 mm of the basomedial amygdala, which was excluded to avoid the susceptibility artifact that was detected in some subjects.

Given the amygdala's pivotal role in stress perception, we first evaluated whether and how the functional connectivity from the amygdala seeds differed between patients and controls. We then used multiple regression analysis to investigate whether the degree of perceived stress interacted with the pattern of connectivity from the amygdala seed. Spatial preprocessing and statistical analysis of functional images were performed using SPM8 (Welcome Department of Cognitive Neurology). Functional images were slice-timed and realigned, and then registered to structural T1 SPGR (spoiled gradient) images for each subject. Next, the individual T1 SPGR images were segmented into gray matter, white matter, and cerebrospinal fluid, and the gray matter image was used to determine the parameters of normalization for the standard Montreal Neurological Institute gray matter template. The spatial parameters were then applied to the slice-timed and realigned functional volumes that were finally resampled to 2×2×2 mm voxels and smoothed with a 6-mm full-width at half-maximum kernel. Each voxel's time series was corrected for noise using standard resting-state low-pass filtering with a cut-off frequency of 0.1 Hz. In addition, voxel-wise multidimensional regression analysis was employed in a standardized manner to remove artifacts due to motion and changes in ventricle and white matter signals. This was done by adding six movement regressors obtained from rigid-body head motion correction (SPM 8 statistical package). Segmented WM (white matte) and CSF (cerebro spinal fluid) were used as ROI for correction of signals from non-gray matter tissue. To ensure that signals from WM and CSF ROIs did not contain signals from gray matter, these ROIs were superimposed on the individual EPIs and, when needed, adapted to the respective subject, based on intensity differences between white matter, gray matter, and ventricular regions. Global signal correction was not employed, as it has been reported that regression against the global signal may artificially introduce anticorrelations into fMRI data sets [58]. For each subject, the average fMRI time course within the seed region was used as the regressor of interest. Individual time series in each seed region were extracted with MarsBar toolbox (http://marsbar.sourceforge.net/). Each subject's seed region time course was then regressed voxel-wise against the subject's fMRI time course using the entire brain as search space. The t-values of the corresponding regression coefficients at each voxel were used as each subject's connectivity map.

Statistical analysis

Group comparisons between stressed subjects and healthy controls were carried out in SPM8 using one-way ANOVA, with $p<.001$ voxel threshold, FWE corrected at cluster level, $p<.05$, and controlling for age and gender, which were used as nuisance covariates.

Results

Demographics

No group differences were found with regard to education or gender distribution. The controls were younger than the stressed subjects (Table 1). The subjects with occupational burnout scored significantly higher on the MBI-GS scale (3.8±0.8 vs. 2.5±0.7 $p=.001$; $F=64.3$) as well as on the MADRS (16.8±5.5 vs. 3.8±3.8; $p=.001$, $F=206.8$) (Table 1). However, no group difference was detected in cortisol levels ($p=.56$, $F=.08$).

Emotion regulation task

To verify that the data could be collapsed across female and male controls, we first confirmed that there was no significant difference between female and male controls in their initial startle response to negative and neutral pictures (Valence×Group interaction: $F(1,30)=.13$, $p=.72$). Furthermore, no sex differences were found regarding the startle response to negative and neutral pictures across instructions (Instruction×Group interaction: $F(2,60)=2.23$, $p=.12$). Because no significant differences were detected between male and female controls, all of the comparisons with the subjects with burnout were based on data from the entire gender-mixed control group.

The burnout group and control group did not differ in their initial startle response to negative and neutral pictures (Main effect of Valence: $F(1,91)=39.97$, $p<.001$; Valence×Group interaction: $F<1$); both groups showed significantly higher startle responses to negative images than to neutral images (burnout: $t(31)=3.87$, $p=.001$; control: $t(60)=5.65$, $p<.001$). However, group differences emerged in the emotional regulation task (see Figure 2). A 2×2 repeated measures ANOVA with Instruction (Down-regulate, Maintain) as the within-subject variable and Group (burnout, control) as the between-subject variable revealed that the burnout population showed overall higher startle responses across instructions (Main effect of Instruction: $F(1,91)=16.32$, $p<.001$ and Group, $F(1,91)=5.55$, $p=.02$). As predicted, follow-up analysis revealed that compared to the controls, the startle response among the burnout patients was significantly higher during negative down-regulation, [$t(91)=2.38$, $p=.02$], but did not reach significance during the negative maintain instruction, [$t(91)=1.55$, $p=.13$]. No significant group difference in startle response was detected during the up-regulate negative condition, [$F(1,91)=6.04$, $p=.02$], or during the maintain neutral condition [$t(91)=.06$; $p=.96$]. Lastly, we compared the emotion regulation success ratings of the burnout patients and the controls (see Figure 3). The burnout patients differed from the controls (Instruction×Group: $F(2,160)=4.63$, $p=.01$): the burnout patients had overall lower success ratings after viewing negative images, an effect that was particularly pronounced with regard to being instructed to down-regulate [$t(80)=4.70$, $p<.001$] and maintain negative emotion [$t(80)=3.12$, $p=.003$] but that did not reach significance for up-regulation of negative emotion [$t(80)=1.77$; $p=.08$]. These results parallel those observed with the startle response. Critically, there were no differences between groups with respect to rating after viewing neutral images [$t(80)=.94$, $p=.35$].

To test for possible effects of stress (MBI-GS) and depression (MADRS) scores on the ability to down-regulate negative emotion, two separate correlational analyses were run (Pearsson's linear correlation analysis). Bonferroni correction was not employed

Table 1. Demographics.

	Stressed subjects (n = 40)	Controls (n = 70)	P and F values
Age (years)	38.2±6.8	33.2±5.8	p = 0.00 F = 17.4
Education (years)	16.9±3.4	16.8±2.9	p = 0.88 F = 0.22
MBI- GS (score)	3.8±0.8	2.5±0.7	p = 0.00 F = 64.3
• exhaustion	4.4±1.1	1.2±0.8	p = 0.00 F = 269.0
• cynicism	3.3±1.3	1.3±1.0	p = 0.00 F = 75.6
MADRS (score)	16.8±5.5	3.8±3.8	p = 0.00 F = 206.8
Cortisol sample 1	15.8±12.6	5.7±3.9	p = 0.86 F = 0.33
Cortisol sample 2	24.2±15.7	15.2±8.5	p = 0.78 F = 0.08
Cortisol sample 3	22.9±14.9	20.3±12.2	p = 0.17 F = 1.92
Cortisol sample 4	8.8±10.0	23.1±16.2	p = 0.96 F = 0.00
Cortisol sample 5	5.8±3.5	9.7±13.9	p = 0.73 F = 0.12
Cortisol sample 6	3.6±4.3	3.7±4.9	p = 0.92 F = 0.01
Cortisol sample 7	4.2±10.8	2.6±3.9	p = 0.33 F = 0.86

Age and education are expressed in years; MBI-GS is a questionnaire to score perceived work-related stress. Raw 3 indicates the mean total score, raw 4–5 the sub-scores for the exhaustion and cynicism. MADRS = Montgomery Asberg Depression Scale. There was no overall group difference in cortisol levels (p = 0.56; F = 0.08, repeated measure ANOVA). Time of the day for cortisol samples: *Sample 1*: 06.30–07.30; *Sample 2*: 15 minutes after sample 1; *Sample 3*: 30 minutes after sample 1; *Sample 4*: 12.00–13.00; *Sample 5*: 15.00–16.00; *Sample 6*: 20.00–21.00. *Sample 7*: 22.30–23.30.

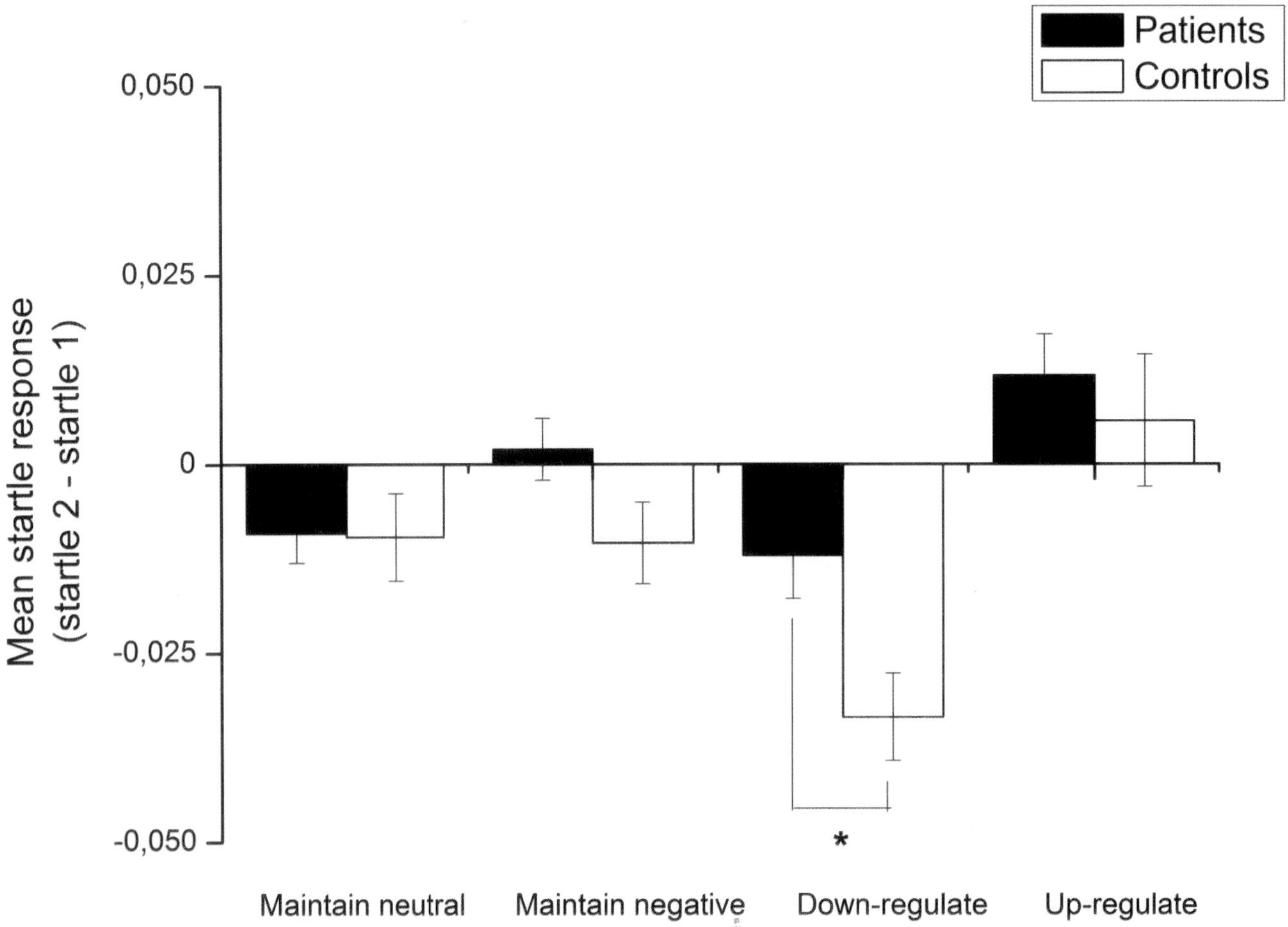

Figure 2. Comparison between burnout patients and controls regarding startle reactions across task instructions. The burnout group displayed overall higher responses when implementing instructions during negative pictures and this pattern was particularly pronounced during down- regulation of negative emotion. Note that the y-axis represents post-instruction response – pre- instruction response; * = $p<.05$.

because significant correlations were hypothesized for both score types. Correlation analyses were carried out using both groups, and also within each separate group. Both higher stress scores (MGI-GS: $r = 22$, $p = .02$) and higher depression scores (MADRS: $r = .37$, $p = .02$) were related to a decreased ability to down-regulate negative emotion, as indexed by higher differential startle responses during the negative down-regulation condition. However, neither of these scores correlated with the differential startle responses during down-regulation of negative emotion within the burnout or control groups (both p's>.1).

Seed region fMRI connectivity

There was a significant difference between stressed subjects and controls with respect to functional connectivity of the right and left amygdala. Stressed subjects showed significantly weaker correlations with clusters in the mPFC, the dorsolateral prefrontal cortex (dlPFC), and the motor cortex, whereas their functional connectivity during resting state with clusters in the cerebellum (vermis cerebelli and the anterior cerebellum in particular) and the insular cortex were stronger than in controls (Table 2, Figure 4a and 4b, clusters calculated at $p = .001$, cluster level FWE correction at $p< .05$). These differences were constitutes by differences in positive connectivity and not anticorrelations (please see Figure 4c, which shows within group connectivity patterns).

Post hoc analyses

Because the co-variation pattern from the amygdala differed between the two groups of participants, we explored if this could be related to degree of perceived stress or, perhaps, to the MADRS scores. Each subject's MGI-GS and MADRS scores were, therefore, regressed on the individual connectivity maps from the right and left amygdala seed (voxel threshold corresponded to $p = .001$, FWE cluster correction at $p<.05$). In addition, given the pivotal role of the mPFC and the ACC in emotional regulation, we tested in the same manner whether the ability to down-regulate negative emotion could be linked to the connectivity between the amygdala and these two regions. Because this analysis was hypothesis based, we employed small volume correction (FWE corrected peak level at $p<.05$), using a search area defined by a box covering both the ACC and the mPFC, according to Montreal Neurological Institutes (MNI) atlas, the MNI co-ordinates $x = -10$ to 10; $y = 16$ to 66; $z = 4$ to 24.

Only correlational data from the entire study group (thus, without subdivision into burnout subjects and controls) are presented. The subject groups were too limited to allow explorative calculations of possible group differences in the interaction between functional connectivity and emotional regulation or to investigate the respective correlations in each group separately.

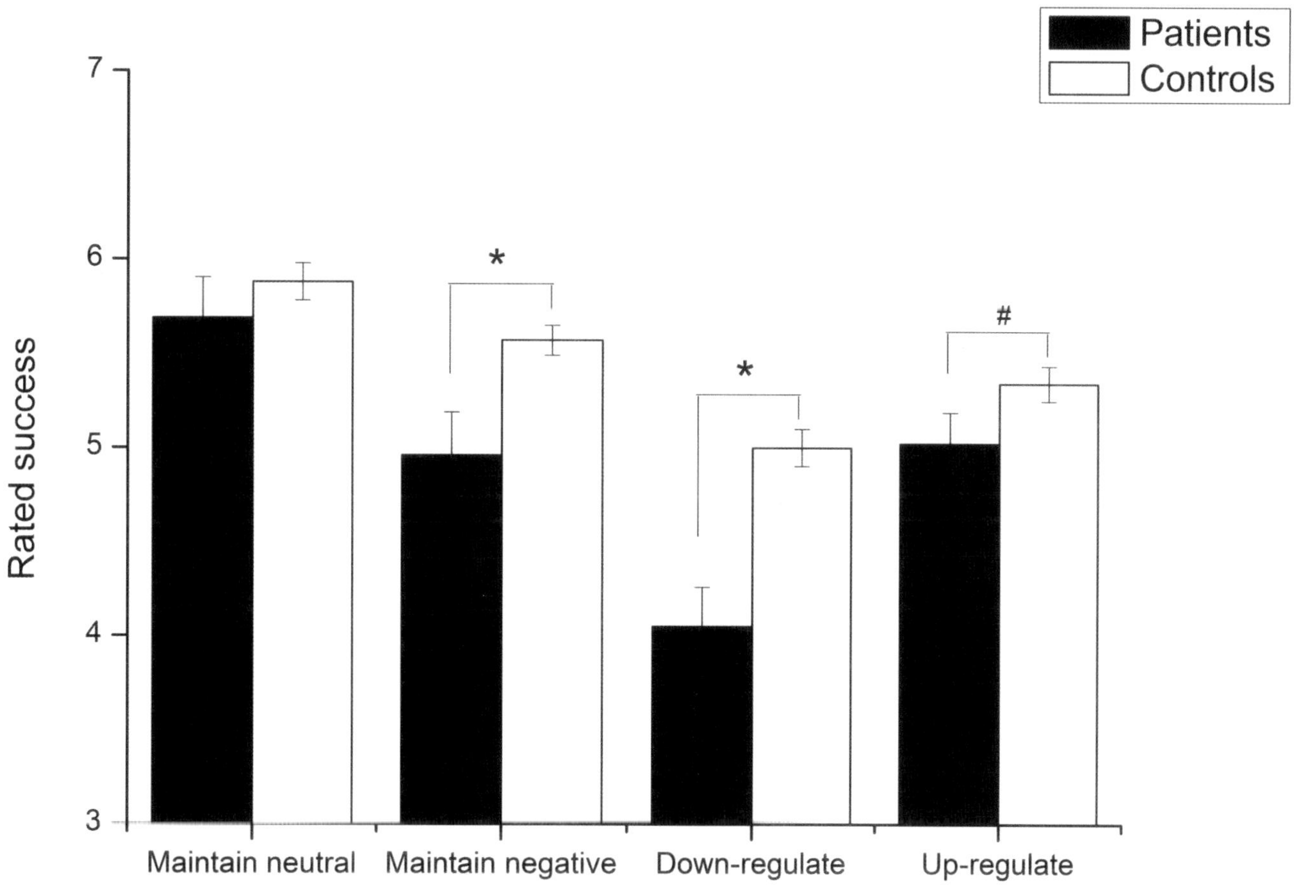

Figure 3. Comparison between burnout patients and controls regarding rated regulation success across task instructions. The burnout group rated themselves as generally less successful at implementing the task instruction after viewing negative pictures. * = $p<.05$, # = $p<.1$.

The MBI-GS scores (total mean scores) were found to be positively correlated to the functional connectivity between the left amygdala and the insular cortex, and the thalamus (covering a portion of the hypothalamus); the more pronounced the stress perception, the stronger the functional connection was (Table 3, Figure 5). The corresponding analysis involving the right amyg-

Table 2. Group differences in functional resting state connections from the amygdala.

Region	Z level	Size, cm^3	Coordinates
Controls>stressed subjects, R amygdala			
R PFC+motor cortex	3.8	3.2	44 6 34
Controls>stressed subjects, L amygdala			
L mPFC+L dlPFC	4.3	4.8	−48 20 10
			−18 50 22
Stressed subjects>controls, R amygdala			
R insular cortex	4.2	4.0	44 14 2
L insular cortex	3.9	3.2	−28 20 6
Cerebellum	4.1	8.0	−22 −22 −28
			26 −32 −26
Stressed subjects>controls, L amygdala			
Cerebellum	4.3	3.3	−22 −44 −28

Clusters calculated using voxel threshold at $p = 0.001$, cluster level FWE correction at $p<0.05$.
R = right; L = left. The cerebellar clusters covered the anterior cerebellum and the vermis.

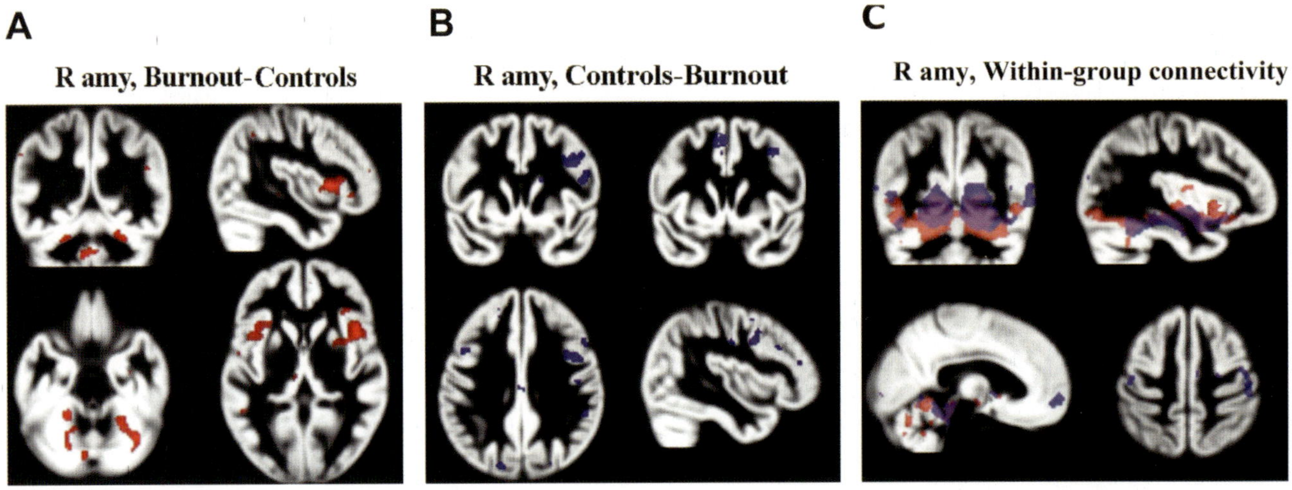

Figure 4. Group difference in resting state functional connectivity from the right amygdala (R amy). Red clusters were calculated from the burnout group - control-group contrast (A), and blue clusters from the reverse contrast (B), ($p<0.05$ FWE corrected). Clusters are superimposed on the grey matter template (in the MNI space) from the entire study group. (C) Within group connectivity (positive) from the right amygdala. Blue clusters show connectivity clusters in controls, red clusters in the burnout group.

dala did not show any significant clusters. There were no negative correlations with the stress scores, nor any interactions with MADRS scores. The ability to down-regulate negative emotion was associated with an increased functional connection between the right amygdala seed and the ACC (the MNI co-ordinate was 6 26 14, $z = 3.6$, $p = .027$, FWE corrected, small volume correction).

Discussion

The present study represents part of a larger effort to characterize the potential neurobiological underpinnings of occupational burnout, an increasingly reported condition in Western societies. The finding that subjects suffering from chronic occupational stress had an impaired ability to modulate emotion, and weaker functional connectivity between the amygdala and the mPFC (two key structures for orchestrating defensive reactions to environmental threats including stress) supports our previous notion that we are dealing with a condition affecting the limbic system.

Notably, stressed subjects showed higher startle responses specifically during down-regulation of negative emotion, whereas no group difference was detected in the initial response to negative images or in the startle response during up-regulation of negative emotion. Cortisol response during the image presentation was not specifically measured, and it was not possible to objectively verify that the images eliciting negative emotions were perceived as stressful. Such an association has, however, been documented in several previous studies which showed increased cortisol levels as well as increased skin conductance responses during the presentation of negatively valenced IAPS images [59–60]. It is, therefore, reasonable to assume that the higher startle response among the burnout group during negative down-regulation reflected an impaired ability to modulate a stressful emotion, although we cannot exclude that this effect was accompanied by differences in attentional resources required to perform the tasks Emotion regulation, as well as stress relies on an intact functional connection between the amygdala, the mPFC, and the ACC [24],[35]. The presently detected functional disconnection between the amygdala and the mPFC in the burnout group as well as the detected interaction between the ability to down-modulate negative emotion and the amygdala–ACC connection confirm this notion. These findings are in line with our previous observation based on PET measurements of resting state connectivity [22], although the methodology and participant sample were different. They are also in accordance with the reduction of gray matter volume in the dlPFC and ACC and the cortical thinning of the mPFC observed in subjects suffering from occupational stress [21],[23]. Taken together, these data support the postulation that

Table 3. Functional resting state connections from the amygdala in relation to stress perception.

Region	Z level	Size, cm^3	Coordinates
L amygdala connectivity and MBI-GS			
L hypothalamus+thalamus	3.9	1.5	−8 −20 6
			−6 −6 6
L insular cortex	4.0	1.0	−32 24 4
R amygdala connectivity vs MBI-GS			
R insular cortex	3.7	3.0	36 22 0

The interaction with MBI-GS is calculated at voxel threshold corresponding to $p = 0.001$, cluster level FWE correction at $p<0.05$. R = right; L = left. There were no negative covariations from the amygdala seed regions.

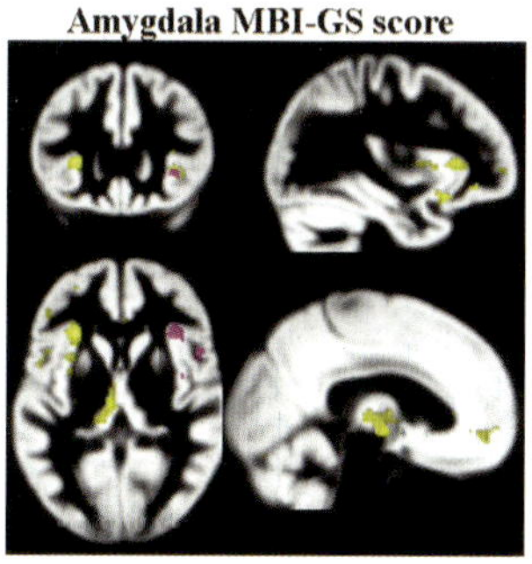

Figure 5. Yellow clusters denote significant interaction between the left amygdala connectivity map and the MBI-GS score merging both groups. Pink clusters denote corresponding clusters from the right amygdala. Clusters calculated at $p<0.05$ FWE corrected, and superimposed on the grey matter template (in the MNI space) from the entire study group.

stress-processing limbic networks are affected in subjects suffering from occupational burnout.

The cluster showing impaired functional connectivity from the amygdala in the burnout population comprised portions of the motor cortex, which may be due to the fact that our groups were gender mixed. In men there are strong connectivity between the amygdala and motor cortex, while women have strong connectivity between the amygdala and both the mPFC and ACC [61]. Thus, assuming that the amygdala–frontal lobe connectivity were impaired in both sexes among the burnout population, it is not surprising that a cluster encompassing both the mPFC and the motor cortex was observed when comparing the entire control group with the entire burnout group.

The MGI-GS scores interacted with functional connectivity between the amygdala, the thalamus, and a minor portion of the hypothalamus (Figure 5); thus, the more stressed the subject, the stronger the connectivity was. This finding is congruent with the well-established finding that stress leads to the activation of the HPA via amygdala connectivity with the paraventricular hypothalamic nuclei. It also fits well with the notion that the insular cortex relays stress signals from the amygdala to the autonomous nervous system. The observance of a stress-related enhancement of the amygdala–insular cortex connection is in accordance with previous findings for other stress conditions [62].

The enhanced connectivity observed between the amygdala and the cerebellum in the stressed group was, on the other hand, not directly expected. Nevertheless, there are several previous reports suggesting that cerebellum may have a modulatory role in the processing of psychosocial stress. The amygdala relays the emotional salience of incoming signals to the rest of the brain, and via cholinergic connections to the pontine nuclei and the cerebellum, the neuronal traffic from the amygdala leads to increased arousal [24–25]. The cerebellum is part of the amygdala's resting state connectivity network [63], and via inhibitory (GABAergic) output from Purkinje, the excitation of the amygdala is modulated by the cerebellum. Via this ability to modulate the excitation of the amygdala the cerebellum is involved in the processing of emotion, and potentially also the psychosocial stress. Interestingly, the cerebellum has dense glucocorticoid binding sites as well as reciprocal monosynaptic connections to the hypothalamus, that provide a biological substrate for the regulation of HPA, and the stress response. Animal experiments show an enlargement of Purkinje cell spines in response to corticotropin-releasing factor [64]. The involvement of the cerebellum in stress is also indicated by reports about a reduction in the cerebellar volume in patients with PTSD [65–67]. Thus, although there have not been any comparable previous studies showing stress- related increases in the functional connectivity between the amygdala and cerebellum, one may speculate that, in our burnout population, a compensatory enhancement of the modulatory pathway from the cerebellum could have occurred due to weakened amygdala–mPFC connectivity.

Methodological limitations and future directions

The amygdala seed covered the entire amygdala except for its most medial portion, which was excluded because of the signal loss in the fMRI images; thus, no differentiation could be made between the basomedial and dorsolateral nuclei. In previous studies of stress with resting state fMRI, primarily carried out in patients with PTSD, it has been reported that amygdala–mPFC (and also the amygdala-ACC) connectivity is decreased when seeding from the entire amygdala [68–69]. However, when separating the medial and lateral portions of the amygdala, Brown et al. found elevated connectivity between the basomedial-amygdala and the insular and dorsomedial PFC in PTDS patients, whereas the connection between the lateral amygdala and the inferior frontal cortex was stronger in controls [70]. It is, thus, possible that the results with respect to amygdala connectivity would be slightly different if the two major portions of the amygdala were separated. In this initial study, our priority was, however, to minimize the noise in the seed ROI. Also, there was no primary hypothesis that the mesial and lateral portions of the amygdala would be affected differently in the burnout population.

The relatively small size of the subject sample did not allow us to test for possible gender-related differences in our results among the burnout group. This important issue will be investigated in a separate study. The groups were, however, matched with respect to gender distribution.

One important question worth discussing is whether and to what extent the present findings could reflect depression. For several reasons we find this to be unlikely. First of all, none of the stressed subjects reported dysthymia, and none were judged to be depressed according to the psychiatrist in charge and the SCID-MINI ratings. Although the depression scores were significantly higher among the stressed group, for those subjects who had high MADRS scores, the only items that contributed to these scores were anxiety and poor sleep, which does not necessarily imply depression. Higher MADRS scores were related to a decreased ability to down-regulate negative emotion, but these scores covaried highly with the stress scores, and did not moderate the ability to down-regulate negative emotion within the burnout group. While the MGI-GS scores interacted with the amygdala connectivity with the insular cortex and the thalamus, no such interaction was detected with the MADRS scores, not even when employing small volume correction. Finally, the cortisol levels were normal in our stressed subjects, whereas they have been found to be high in a large portion of patients with genuine depression [71]. We recently also found that women suffering from chronic occupational stress had an elevated reaction to allopregnanolone [20] which differed from the diminished allopregnanolone response that has been observed among depressed women [72]. Emotional reactions to chronic stress and major depression may, thus, represent separate constructs. They share, however, certain symptoms perhaps due to the affection of similar limbic networks. Indeed, the higher MADRS scores among the stressed subjects who were not diagnosed as depressed could be an effect of this comorbidity. Stress may lead to depression, and the impaired ability to specifically down-regulate negative emotions that was demonstrated in the present study may by itself render stressed individuals more prone to depressive thoughts and explain the comorbidity between the two conditions. Because the study was cross-sectional, it is difficult to know whether the detected changes represent effects of stress or of a pre-existing condition that could have rendered the brain more vulnerable to the development of pathological stress responses and reduced the ability to modulate emotion.

Conclusion

In subjects suffering from chronic emotional stress, there seems to be a dysregulation of the emotion- and stress-processing networks, which prevents the restoration of internal homeostasis in response to negative emotional stress. An impairment of the ability to down-regulate negative emotions in subjects suffering from occupational stress may render them more vulnerable to depressive symptoms. This finding needs to be further explored, as it may potentially explain the link between stress and psychological ill health.

Acknowledgments

Tom Perski, Edin Fazlic, and Alexander Berglund are acknowledged for excellent data collection.

Author Contributions

Conceived and designed the experiments: AG MK WO AP IS. Performed the experiments: MK EJ. Analyzed the data: MK AG EJ. Wrote the paper: IS AG.

References

1. Eisler RM, Polak PR (1971) Social stress and psychiatric disorder. J Nerv Ment Dis 153: 227–233.
2. Weber K, Miller GA, Schupp HT, Borgelt J, Awiszus B, et al. (2009) Early life stress and psychiatric disorder modulate cortical responses to affective stimuli. Psychophysiology 46: 1234–1243.
3. Kalia M (2002) Assessing the economic impact of stress–the modern day hidden epidemic. Metabolism: clinical and experimental 51: 49–53.
4. Ahola K, Honkonen T, Isometsa E, Kalimo R, Nykyri E, et al. (2006) Burnout in the general population. Results from the Finnish Health 2000 Study. Soc Psychiatry Psychiatr Epidemiol 41: 11–17.
5. Copertaro A, Barbaresi M, Tarsitani L, Battisti F, Baldassari M, et al. (2007) [Fast stress evaluation in nurses]. Giornale italiano di medicina del lavoro ed ergonomia 29: 350–352.
6. Copertaro A, Bracci M, Amati M, Mocchegiani E, Barbaresi M, et al. (2010) [Biological risk and health care workers: analysis of the effects of work chronobiology on the immune system]. Med Lav 101: 427–436.
7. Fernandez Torres, B, Roldan Perez LM, Guerra Velez A, Roldan Rodriguez T, Gutierrez Guillen A, et al. (2006) [Prevalence of burnout among anesthesiologists at Hospital Universitario Virgen Macarena de Sevilla]. Rev Esp Anestesiol Reanim 53: 359–362.
8. Rydmark I, Wahlberg K, Ghatan PH, Modell S, Nygren A, et al. (2006) Neuroendocrine, cognitive and structural imaging characteristics of women on longterm sickleave with job stress-induced depression. Biological psychiatry 60: 867–873.
9. Fries E, Dettenborn L, Kirschbaum C (2009) The cortisol awakening response (CAR): facts and future directions. Int J Psychophysiol 72: 67–73.
10. Langelaan S, Bakker AB, Schaufeli WB, van Rhenen W, van Doornen LJ (2007) Is burnout related to allostatic load? Int J Behav Med 14: 213–221.
11. Mommersteeg PM, Heijne CJ, Verbraak MJ, van Doornen, LJ(2006a) Clinical burnout is not reflected in the cortisol awakening response, the day-curve or the response to a low-dose dexamethasone suppression test. Psychoneuroendocrinology 31: 216–225.
12. Chida Y, Steptoe A (2009) Cortisol awakening response and psychosocial factors: a systematic review and meta-analysis. Biol Psychol 80: 265–278.
13. Moch SL, Panz VR, Joffe BI, Havlik I, Moch JD (2003) Longitudinal changes in pituitary- adrenal hormones in South African women with burnout. Endocrine 21: 267–272.
14. Mommersteeg PM, Keijsers GP, Heijnen CJ, Verbraak MJ, van Doornen LJ (2006b) Cortisol deviations in people with burnout before and after psychotherapy: a pilot study. Health Psychol 25: 243–248.
15. Pruessner JC, Hellhammer DH, Kirschbaum C (1999) Burnout, perceived stress, and cortisol responses to awakening. Psychosom Med 61: 197–204.
16. Grossi G, Perski A, Ekstedt M, Johansson T, Lindstrom M, et al. (2005) The morning salivary cortisol response in burnout. J Psychosom Res 59: 103–111.
17. Grossi G, Perski A, Evengard B, Blomkvist V, Orth-Gomer K (2003). Physiological correlates of burnout among women. J Psychosom Res 55: 309–316.
18. Melamed S, Ugarten U, Shirom A, Kahana L, Lerman Y, Froom P (1999) Chronic burnout, somatic arousal and elevated salivary cortisol levels. J Psychosom Res 46: 591–598.
19. Sandstrom A, Rhodin IN, Lundberg M, Olsson T, Nyberg L (2005) Impaired cognitive performance in patients with chronic burnout syndrome. Biological psychology 69: 271–279.
20. Backstrom T, Bixo M, Nyberg S, Savic I (2013) Increased neurosteroid sensitivity–an explanation to symptoms associated with chronic work related stress in women? Psychoneuroendocrinology 38: 1078–1089.
21. Blix E, Perski A, Berglund H, Savic I (2013) Long-term occupational stress is associated with regional reductions in brain tissue volumes. PLoS ONE 8: e64065.
22. Jovanovic H, Perski A, Berglund H, Savic I (2011) Chronic stress is linked to 5-HT(1A) receptor changes and functional disintegration of the limbic networks. Neuroimage 55: 1178–1188.
23. Savic I. Structural changes of the brain in relation to occupational stress. Cereb Cortex 2013 Dec 18. [Epub ahead of print]
24. LeDoux JE (2000) Emotion circuits in the brain. Annual review of neuroscience 23: 155–184.
25. Phillips ML, Drevets WC, Rauch SL, Lane R (2003) Neurobiology of emotion perception I: The neural basis of normal emotion perception. Biological Psychiatry 54: 504–514.
26. Egner T, Etkin A, Gale S, Hirsch J (2008) Dissociable neural systems resolve conflict from emotional versus nonemotional distracters. Cereb Cortex 18: 1475–1484.
27. Etkin A, Egner T, Peraza DM, Kandel ER, Hirsch J (2006) Resolving emotional conflict: A role for the rostral anterior cingulate cortex in modulating activity in the amygdala. Neuron 51: 871–882.
28. Gianaros PJ, Sheu LK, Matthews KA, Jennings JR, Manuck SB, et al. (2008) Individual differences in stressor-evoked blood pressure reactivity vary with activation, volume, and functional connectivity of the amygdala. J Neurosc 28: 990–999.
29. Pezawas L, Meyer-Lindenberg A, Drabant EM, Verchinski BA, Munoz KE, et al. (2005) 5-HTTLPR polymorphism impacts human cingulate-amygdala interactions: a genetic susceptibility mechanism for depression. Nature neuroscience 8: 828–834.
30. Wager TD, Davidson ML, Hughes BL, Lindquist MA, Ochsner KN (2008) Prefrontal-subcortical pathways mediating successful emotion regulation. Neuron 59: 1037–1050.
31. Goldin PR, McRae K, Ramel W, Gross JJ (2008) The neural bases of emotion regulation: Reappraisal and suppression of negative emotion. Biological Psychiatry 63: 577–586.
32. Golkar A, Lonsdorf TB, Olsson A, Lindstrom KM, Berrebi J, et al. (2012) Distinct contributions of the dorsolateral prefrontal and orbitofrontal cortex during emotion regulation. PLoS ONE 7: e48107.
33. Koenigsberg HW, Fan J, Ochsner KN, Liu X, Guise K, et al. (2010) Neural correlates of using distancing to regulate emotional responses to social situations. Neuropsychologia 48: 1813–1822
34. Levesque J, Eugene F, Joanette Y, Paquette V, Mensour B, et al. (2003) Neural circuitry underlying voluntary suppression of sadness. Biological Psychiatry 53: 502–510.
35. Ochsner KN, Bunge SA, Gross JJ, Gabrieli JDE (2002) Rethinking feelings: An fMRI study of the cognitive regulation of emotion. Journal of Cognitive Neuroscience 14: 1215–1229.
36. Ochsner KN, Ray RD, Cooper JC, Robertson ER, Chopra S, et al. (2004) For better or for worse: neural systems supporting the cognitive down- and up-regulation of negative emotion. Neuroimage 23: 483–499.
37. Raio CM, Orederu TA, Palazzolo L, Shurick AA, Phelps EA (2013) Cognitive emotion regulation fails the stress test. Proc Natl Acad Sci U S A 110: 15139–15144.
38. Davis M, Parisi T, Gendelman DS, Tischler M, Kehne JH (1982) Habituation and sensitization of startle reflexes elicited electrically from the brain-stem. Science 218: 688–690.
39. Yeomans JS, Frankland PW (1995) The acoustic startle reflex: Neurons and connections. Brain research reviews 21: 301–314.
40. Lang PJ, Bradley MM, Cuthbert BN (1990) Emotion, attention, and the startle reflex. Psychological Review 97: 377–395.
41. Bradley MM, Cuthbert BN, Lang PJ (1990) Startle reflex modification - emotion or attention. Psychophysiology 27: 513–522.
42. Dillon DG, LaBar KS (2005). Startle modulation during conscious emotion regulation is arousal- dependent. Behav Neurosci 119: 1118–1124.

43. Jackson DC, Malmstadt JR, Larson CL, Davidson RJ (2000) Suppression and enhancement of emotional responses to unpleasant pictures. Psychophysiology 37: 515–522.
44. Oldfield RC (1971) The assessment and analysis of handedness: the Edinburgh inventory. Neuropsychologia 9: 97–113.
45. Schaufeli WB, Van Dierendonck D (1995) A cautionary note about the cross-national and clinical validity of cut-off points for the Maslach Burnout Inventory. Psychological reports 76: 1083–1090.
46. Stenlund T, Ahlgren C, Lindahl B, Burell G, Knutsson A (2007) Patients with burnout in relation to gender and a general population. Scandinavian journal of public health 35: 516–523.
47. Deykin EY, Keane TM, Kaloupek D, Fincke G, Rothendler J, et al. (2001) Posttraumatic stress disorder and the use of health services. Psychosom Med 63: 835–841.
48. Holmes TH, Rahe RH (1967) The Social Readjustment Rating Scale. J Psychosom Res 11: 213–218.
49. Sheehan DV, Lecrubier Y, Sheehan KH, Amorim P, Janavs J (1998) The Mini-International Neuropsychiatric Interview (M.I.N.I.): the development and validation of a structured diagnostic psychiatric interview for DSM-IV and ICD-10. J Clin Psychiatry 59 Suppl 20: 22–33;quiz 34–57.
50. Montgomery S, Asberg M, Traskman L, Montgomery D (1978) Cross cultural studies on the use of CPRS in English and Swedish depressed patients. Acta Psychiatrica Scandinavica Suppl 271: 33–37.
51. Karlamangla AS, Friedman EM, Seeman TE, Stawksi RS, Almeida DM (2013) Daytime trajectories of cortisol: Demographic and socioeconomic differences-Findings from the National Study of Daily Experiences. Psychoneuroendocrinology 38: 2585–2597.
52. Galbois A, Rudler M, Massard J, Fulla Y, Bennani A, et al. (2010) Assessment of adrenal function in cirrhotic patients: salivary cortisol should be preferred. J Hepatol 52: 839–845.
53. Lang PJ, Bradley MM, Cuthbert BN (1997) International Affective Picture System (IAPS): Technical manual and affective ratings. Gainesville, FL: NIMH Center for the Study of Emotion and Attention, University of Florida.
54. Jackson DC, Mueller CJ, Dolski I, Dalton KM, Nitschke JB, et al. (2003) Now you feel it, now you don't: Frontal brain electrical asymmetry and individual differences in emotion regulation. Psychological science 14: 612–617.
55. Golkar A, Bellander M, Ohman A (2013) Temporal properties of fear extinction–does time matter? Behav Neurosci 127: 59–69.
56. Weike AI, Schupp HT, Hamm AO (2007) Fear acquisition requires awareness in trace but not delay conditioning. Psychophysiology 44: 170–180.
57. Biswal B, Yetkin FZ, Haughton VM, Hyde JS (1995) Functional connectivity in the motor cortex of resting human brain using echo-planar MRI. Magn Reson Med 34: 537–541.
58. Weissenbacher A, Kasess C, Gerstl F, Lanzenberger R, Moser E, et al. (2009) Correlations and anticorrelations in resting-state functional connectivity MRI: a quantitative comparison of preprocessing strategies. Neuroimage 47: 1408–1416.
59. Bradley MM, Codispoti M, Cuthbert BN, Lang PJ (2001) Emotion and Motivation I: Defensive and Appetitive Reactions in Picture Processing. Emotion, 1: 276–298.
60. Gerra G, Somaini L, Manfredini M, Raggi MA, Saracino MA, et al. (2014) Dysregulated responses to emotions among abstinent heroin users: Correlation with childhood neglect and addiction severity, Progress in Neuro-Psychopharmacology and Biological Psychiatry, 48: 220–228.
61. Savic I, Lindstrom P (2008) PET and MRI show differences in cerebral asymmetry and functional connectivity between homo- and heterosexual subjects. Proc Natl Acad Sci U S A 105: 9403–9408.
62. Hong JY, Kilpatrick LA, Labus J, Gupta A, Jiang Z, et al. (2013) Patients with chronic visceral pain show sex-related alterations in intrinsic oscillations of the resting brain. J Neurosci 33: 11994–12002.
63. Sang L, Qin W, Liu Y, Han W, Zhang Y, et al. (2012) Resting-state functional connectivity of the vermal and hemispheric subregions of the cerebellum with both the cerebral cortical networks and sub.cortical structures. Neuroimage 61: 1213–1225.
64. Gounko NV, Swinny JD, Kalicharan D, Jafari S, Corteen N, et al. (2013) Corticotropin-releasing factor and urocortin regulate spine and synapse formation: structural basis for stress-induced neuronal remodeling and pathology. Molecular psychiatry 18: 86–92.
65. Anderson CM, Teicher MH, Polcari A, Renshaw PF (2002) Abnormal T2 relaxation time in the cerebellar vermis of adults sexually abused in childhood: potential role of the vermis in stress-enhanced risk for drug abuse. Psychoneuroendocrinology 27: 231–244.
66. De Bellis MD, Kuchibhatla M (2006) Cerebellar volumes in pediatric maltreatment-related posttraumatic stress disorder. Biol Psychiatry 60: 697–703.
67. Baldacara L, Jackowski AP, Schoedl A, Pupo M, Andreoli SB, et al. (2011) Reduced cerebellar left hemisphere and vermal volume in adults with PTSD from a community sample. J Psychiatr Res 45: 1627–1633.
68. Rabinak CA, Angstadt M, Welsh RC, Kenndy AE, Lyubkin M, et al. (2011) Altered amygdala resting-state functional connectivity in post-traumatic stress disorder. Frontiers in psychiatry 2: 62.
69. Sripada RK, King AP, Garfinkel SN, Wang X, Sripada C.S, et al. (2012). Altered resting-state amygdala functional connectivity in men with posttraumatic stress disorder. J Psychiatry Neurosci 37: 241–249.
70. Brown VM, Labar KS, Haswell CC, Gold AL, Mid-Atlantic MIRECC Workgroup, et al. (2014) Altered resting-state functional connectivity of basolateral and centromedial amygdala complexes in posttraumatic stress disorder. Neuropsychopharmacology 39: 351–359.
71. Kasckow JW, Baker D, Geracioti TD Jr (2001) Corticotropin-releasing hormone in depression and post-traumatic stress disorder. Peptides 22: 845–851.
72. Girdler SS, Klatzkin R (2007) Neurosteroids in the context of stress: implications for depressive disorders. Pharmacology & therapeutics 116: 125–139.

Permissions

All chapters in this book were first published in PLOS ONE, by The Public Library of Science; hereby published with permission under the Creative Commons Attribution License or equivalent. Every chapter published in this book has been scrutinized by our experts. Their significance has been extensively debated. The topics covered herein carry significant findings which will fuel the growth of the discipline. They may even be implemented as practical applications or may be referred to as a beginning point for another development.

The contributors of this book come from diverse backgrounds, making this book a truly international effort. This book will bring forth new frontiers with its revolutionizing research information and detailed analysis of the nascent developments around the world.

We would like to thank all the contributing authors for lending their expertise to make the book truly unique. They have played a crucial role in the development of this book. Without their invaluable contributions this book wouldn't have been possible. They have made vital efforts to compile up to date information on the varied aspects of this subject to make this book a valuable addition to the collection of many professionals and students.

This book was conceptualized with the vision of imparting up-to-date information and advanced data in this field. To ensure the same, a matchless editorial board was set up. Every individual on the board went through rigorous rounds of assessment to prove their worth. After which they invested a large part of their time researching and compiling the most relevant data for our readers.

The editorial board has been involved in producing this book since its inception. They have spent rigorous hours researching and exploring the diverse topics which have resulted in the successful publishing of this book. They have passed on their knowledge of decades through this book. To expedite this challenging task, the publisher supported the team at every step. A small team of assistant editors was also appointed to further simplify the editing procedure and attain best results for the readers.

Apart from the editorial board, the designing team has also invested a significant amount of their time in understanding the subject and creating the most relevant covers. They scrutinized every image to scout for the most suitable representation of the subject and create an appropriate cover for the book.

The publishing team has been an ardent support to the editorial, designing and production team. Their endless efforts to recruit the best for this project, has resulted in the accomplishment of this book. They are a veteran in the field of academics and their pool of knowledge is as vast as their experience in printing. Their expertise and guidance has proved useful at every step. Their uncompromising quality standards have made this book an exceptional effort. Their encouragement from time to time has been an inspiration for everyone.

The publisher and the editorial board hope that this book will prove to be a valuable piece of knowledge for researchers, students, practitioners and scholars across the globe.

List of Contributors

Jin-Ha Yoon, Jong-Uk Won, Wanhyung Lee, Pil Kyun Jung and Jaehoon Roh
The Institute for Occupational Health, Yonsei University College of Medicine, Seoul, Korea
Department of Preventive Medicine and Public Health, Yonsei University
College of Medicine, Seoul, Korea, 3 Graduate School of Public Health, Yonsei University College of Medicine, Seoul, Korea

Zhan-Zhan Li and Lizhang Chen
Department of Epidemiology and Health Statistics, School of Public Health, Central South University, Changsha, China

Ya-Ming Li
Department of Nursing, Central South University, Changsha, Hunan Province, China
The Second Affiliated Hospital, Xiangya Medical School, Central South University, Changsha, Hunan Province, China

Xian-Yang Lei
The Second Affiliated Hospital, Xiangya Medical School, Central South University, Changsha, Hunan Province, China

Dan Zhang, Li Liu and Si-Yuan Tang
Department of Nursing, Central South University, Changsha, Hunan Province, China

Ruth Chan and Jean Woo
Department of Medicine and Therapeutics, The Chinese University of Hong Kong, Shatin, Hong Kong

Dicken Chan
The Jockey Club School of Public Health and Primary Care, The Chinese University of Hong Kong, Shatin, Hong Kong

Michael A. Sugarman, Amy M. Loree, Boris B. Baltes and Emily R. Grekin
Wayne State University, Department of Psychology, Detroit, Michigan, United States of America

Irving Kirsch
Harvard Medical School, Boston, Massachusetts, United States of America

Christina L. Nemeth and Constance S. Harrell
Department of Psychiatry and Behavioral Sciences, Emory University, Atlanta, Georgia, United States of America
Department of Physiology, Emory University, Atlanta, Georgia, United States of America

Erica R. Glasper
Department of Psychology, University of Maryland, College Park, Maryland, United States of America

Sanjana A. Malviya
Department of Physiology, Emory University, Atlanta, Georgia, United States of America

Jeffrey S. Otis
Division of Pulmonary, Allergy and Critical Care Medicine, Emory University, Atlanta, Georgia, United States of America

Gretchen N. Neigh
Department of Psychiatry and Behavioral Sciences, Emory University, Atlanta, Georgia, United States of America
Department of Physiology, Emory University, Atlanta, Georgia, United States of America
Center for Behavioral Neuroscience, Emory University, Atlanta, Georgia, United States of America

Ricardo Cáceda and Zachary N. Stowe
Psychiatric Research Institute, University of Arkansas for Medical Sciences, Little Rock, Arkansas, United States of America

Tori Moskovciak, Stefania Prendes-Alvarez, Justyna Wojas, Anzhelika Engel and Samantha H. Wilker
Department of Psychiatry and Behavioral Sciences, University of Miami Miller School of Medicine, Miami, Florida, United States of America

Jorge L. Gamboa
Department of Medicine, Vanderbilt University, Nashville, Tennessee, United States of America

Miyeon Choi
Department of Biochemistry and Molecular Biology, College of Medicine, Hanyang University, Seoul, Korea

Sung Eun Wang, Seung Yeon Ko, Seung Yeun Chae and Seung Hoon Lee
Graduate School of Biomedical Science and Engineering, Hanyang University, Seoul, Korea

Hyo Jung Kang
Department of Life Science, Chung-Ang University, Seoul, Korea

Yong-Seok Kim and Hyeon Son
Department of Biochemistry and Molecular Biology, College of Medicine, Hanyang University, Seoul, Korea
Graduate School of Biomedical Science and Engineering, Hanyang University, Seoul, Korea

Ronald S. Duman
Laboratory of Molecular Psychiatry, Center for Genes and Behavior, Departments of Psychiatry, Neurobiology, and Laboratory Medicine, Yale University School of Medicine, New Haven, Connecticut, United States of America

Janna N. Vrijsen, Iris van Oostrom and Anne Speckens
Department of Psychiatry, Radboud University Medical Centre, Nijmegen, the Netherlands

Alejandro Arias-Vásquez
Department of Psychiatry, Radboud University Medical Centre, Nijmegen, the Netherlands
Donders Institute for Brain, Cognition and Behaviour, Radboud University Medical Centre, Nijmegen, the Netherlands
Department of Cognitive Neuroscience, Radboud University Medical Centre, Nijmegen, The Netherlands
Department of Human Genetics, Radboud University Medical Centre, Nijmegen, The Netherlands

Barbara Franke
Department of Psychiatry, Radboud University Medical Centre, Nijmegen, the Netherlands
Donders Institute for Brain, Cognition and Behaviour, Radboud University Medical Centre, Nijmegen, the Netherlands
Department of Human Genetics, Radboud University Medical Centre, Nijmegen, The Netherlands

Eni S. Becker
Behavioural Science Institute, Radboud University Nijmegen, Nijmegen, The Netherlands

Daniel Wiswede
Department of Neurology, University of Lübeck, Lübeck, Germany
Hanse Institute for Advanced Study, Delmenhorst, Germany

Svenja Taubner
Department of Psychology, Alpen-Adria-University of Klagenfurt, Klagenfurt, Austria
Hanse Institute for Advanced Study, Delmenhorst, Germany

Anna Buchheim
Institute of Psychology, University of Innsbruck, Innsbruck, Austria
Hanse Institute for Advanced Study, Delmenhorst, Germany

Thomas F. Münte
Department of Neurology, University of Lübeck, Lübeck, Germany

Michael Stasch and Manfred Cierpka
Institute of Psychosomatic Cooperation Research and Family Therapy, University of Heidelberg, Heidelberg, Germany

Horst Kächele
Department of Psychosomatic Medicine and Psychotherapy, University of Ulm, Ulm, Germany
Hanse Institute for Advanced Study, Delmenhorst, Germany

Gerhard Roth
Brain Research Institute, University of Bremen, Bremen, Germany
Hanse Institute for Advanced Study, Delmenhorst, Germany

Peter Erhard
Brain Research Institute, University of Bremen, Bremen, Germany

Henrik Kessler
Department of Psychosomatic Medicine and Psychotherapy, LWL University Hospital, Ruhr-University Bochum, Bochum, Germany
Hanse Institute for Advanced Study, Delmenhorst, Germany

Kamaldeep Bhui
Wolfson Institute of Preventive Medicine, Barts and The London School of Medicine and Dentistry, Queen Mary University of London, London, United Kingdom

Brian Everitt
Institute of Psychiatry King's College London, London, United Kingdom

Edgar Jones
King's Centre for Military Health Research, Institute of Psychiatry, King's College London, London, United Kingdom

Kelly Rowe Bijanki, Brendan Hodis, Michael C. Brumm, Emily L. Harlynn and Laurie M. McCormick
Department of Psychiatry, University of Iowa Roy J. and Lucille A. Carver College of Medicine, Iowa City, Iowa, United States of America

Chih-Chao Hsu and Ti Lu
Department of Psychiatry, Kaohsiung Veterans General Hospital, Kaohsiung, Taiwan

San-Chi Chen
Division of Hematology and Oncology, Department of Medicine, Taipei Veterans General Hospital, Taipei, Taiwan

Chia-Jen Liu
Division of Hematology and Oncology, Department of Medicine, Taipei Veterans General Hospital, Taipei, Taiwan
Institute of Public Health and School of Medicine, National Yang-Ming University, Taipei, Taiwan

Cheng-Che Shen
Department of Psychiatry, Chiayi Branch, Taichung Veterans General Hospital, Chiayi, Taiwan

Yu-Wen Hu
Institute of Public Health and School of Medicine, National Yang-Ming University, Taipei, Taiwan
Cancer Center, Taipei Veterans General Hospital, Taipei, Taiwan

Chiu-Mei Yeh
Department of Family Medicine, Taipei Veterans General Hospital, Taipei, Taiwan

Pan-Ming Chen
Department of Psychiatry, Yuanshan Branch, Taipei Veterans General Hospital, Yilan, Taiwan

Tzeng-Ji Chen
Department of Family Medicine, Taipei Veterans General Hospital, Taipei, Taiwan
School of Medicine, National Yang-Ming University, Taipei, Taiwan

Li-Yu Hu
Department of Psychiatry, Kaohsiung Veterans General Hospital, Kaohsiung, Taiwan
Institute of Public Health and School of Medicine, National Yang-Ming University, Taipei, Taiwan

Nicolas Carvalho and Gilles Chopard
Department of Clinical Psychiatry, University Hospital, Besançon, France
E.A. 481, Laboratory of Neurosciences, University of Franche-Comté, Besançon, France

Nicolas Noiret
Department of Clinical Psychiatry, University Hospital, Besançon, France
E.A. 3188, Laboratory of Psychology, University of Franche-Comté, Besançon, France

Pierre Vandel and Julie Monnin
Department of Clinical Psychiatry, University Hospital, Besançon, France
E.A. 481, Laboratory of Neurosciences, University of Franche-Comté, Besançon, France
CICIT 808 Inserm, Besançon University Hospital, Besançon, France

Eric Laurent
E.A. 3188, Laboratory of Psychology, University of Franche-Comté, Besançon, France
UMSR 3124/FED 4209 MSHE Ledoux, CNRS and University of Franche-Comté, Besançon, France

Stéphane Jamain, Nora Zidane, Lucie Chevallier, Aude Nicolas, Annabelle Henrion and Flavie Mathieu
Institut National de la Santé et de la Recherche Médicale U955, Psychiatrie Génétique, Créteil, France
Université Paris-Est, Faculté de Médecine, Créteil, France
Fondation Fonda Mental, Créteil, France

Sven Cichon
Institute of Neuroscience and Medicine (INM-1), Research Center Juelich, Juelich, Germany
Institute of Human Genetics, University of Bonn, Bonn, Germany
Department of Genomics, Life and Brain Center, University of Bonn, Bonn, Germany
Division of Medical Genetics, University Hospital and Department of Biomedicine, University of Basel, Basel, Switzerland

Bruno Etain, Chantal Henry and Marion Leboyer
Institut National de la Santé et de la Recherche Médicale U955, Psychiatrie Génétique, Créteil, France
Université Paris-Est, Faculté de Médecine, Créteil, France
Fondation Fonda Mental, Créteil, France
Assistance Publique - Hôpitaux de Paris, Hôpital Henri Mondor-Albert Chenevier, Pôle de Psychiatry, Créteil, France

Alexander Georgi and Marcella Rietschel
Department of Genetic Epidemiology in Psychiatry, Central Institute of Mental Health, Mannheim, Germany
Department of Psychiatry, University of Bonn, Bonn, Germany

Jasmine Deshommes
Institut National de la Santé et de la Recherche Médicale U955, Psychiatrie Génétique, Créteil, France
Université Paris-Est, Faculté de Médecine, Créteil, France
Fondation Fonda Mental, Créteil, France
Assistance Publique - Hôpitaux de Paris, Hôpital Henri Mondor-Albert Chenevier, Plate-forme de Resources Biologiques, Créteil, France

Institut National de la Santé et de la Recherche Médicale Centre d'Investigation Clinique 006, Hôpital Henri Mondor-Albert Chenevier, Pôle Recherche Clinique Santé Publique, Créteil, France

Franziska Degenhardt, Lutz Priebe, Markus M. Nöthen and Thomas W. Mühleisen
Institute of Human Genetics, University of Bonn, Bonn, Germany
Department of Genomics, Life and Brain Center, University of Bonn, Bonn, Germany

Manuel Mattheisen
Institute of Human Genetics, University of Bonn, Bonn, Germany
Department of Genomics, Life and Brain Center, University of Bonn, Bonn, Germany
Department of Biomedicine and the Centre for Integrative Sequencing, Aarhus University, Aarhus, Denmark

Jean-Pierre Kahn
Fondation Fonda Mental, Créteil, France
Département de Psychiatrie et de Psychologie Clinique, Centre Hospitalier Universitaire de Nancy, Hôpital Jeanne-d'Arc, Toul, France

Anne Boland, Diana Zelenika, Ivo Gut, Simon Heath and Mark Lathrop
Commissariatà l'Energie Atomique, Institut Génomique, Centre National de Génotypage, Evry, France

Wolfgang Maier
Department of Psychiatry, University of Bonn, Bonn, Germany

Thomas G. Schulze
Department of Genetic Epidemiology in Psychiatry, Central Institute of Mental Health, Mannheim, Germany
Department of Psychiatry and Psychotherapy, University Medical Center, Georg-August-Universitä, Göttingen, Germany

Francis J. McMahon
Unit on the Genetic Basis of Mood and Anxiety Disorders, National Institute of Mental Health, National Institutes of Health, US Department of Health and Human Services, Bethesda, MD, United States of America

John R. Kelsoe
Department of Psychiatry, University of California San Diego, La Jolla, CA, United States of America

Margot Albus
Department of Genetic Epidemiology in Psychiatry, Central Institute of Mental Health, Mannheim, Germany

Marian Hamshere and Nicholas Craddock
MRC Centre for Neuropsychiatric Genetics and Genomics, School of Medicine, Cardiff University, Heath Park, Cardiff, United Kingdom

Frank Bellivier
Institut National de la Santé et de la Recherche Médicale U955, Psychiatrie Génétique, Créteil, France
Fondation Fonda Mental, Créteil, France
Assistance Publique - Hôpitaux de Paris, Groupe Hospitalier Lariboisière-F. Widal, Pôle de Psychiatrie, Paris, France
Université Paris Diderot, Paris, France

Ulrich S. Tran, Tobias M. Glück and Theresa von Moy
University of Vienna, Vienna, Austria

Ausiàs Cebolla
University Jaume I, Castelló de la Plana, Spain
Ciber Fisiopatologia de la obesidad y la nutrición (CIBEROBN), Santiago de Compostela, Spain

Joaquim Soler
Department of Psychiatry, Hospital de la Santa Creu i Sant Pau, Barcelona, Spain
Universitat Autònoma de Barcelona (UAB), Centro de Investigación Biomédica en Red de Salud Mental (CIBERSAM), Institut d'Investigació Biomèdica-Sant Pau (IIB-SANT PAU), Barcelona, Spain

Javier Garcia-Campayo
University of Zaragoza, Instituto Aragones de Ciencias de la Salud, Red Investigación Atención Primaria (RD 12/005/006), Zaragoza, Spain

Shinn-Won Lim and Hong-Hee Won
Center for Clinical Research, Samsung Biomedical Research Institute, Seoul, Korea

Hyeran Kim, Woojae Myung and Doh Kwan Kim
Department of Psychiatry, Samsung Medical Center, Sungkyunkwan University School of Medicine, Seoul, Korea

Seonwoo Kim
Biostatistics Unit, Samsung Biomedical Research Institute, Seoul, Korea

Ka-Kyung Kim and Jong-Won Kim
Department of Laboratory Medicine and Genetics, Samsung Medical Center, Sungkyunkwan University School of Medicine, Seoul, Korea

Bernard J. Carroll
Pacific Behavioral Research Foundation, Carmel, California, United States of America

Peter A. Coventry and Linda Gask
Collaboration for Leadership in Applied Health Research and Care, Centre for Primary Care and Manchester Academic Health Science Centre, University of Manchester, Manchester, United Kingdom

Joanna L. Hudson
Health Psychology Section, Psychology Department, Institute of Psychiatry, King's College London, London, United Kingdom

Evangelos Kontopantelis and Peter Bower
NIHR School for Primary Care Research, Centre for Primary Care and Manchester Academic Health Science Centre, University of Manchester, Manchester, United Kingdom

Janine Archer and Karina Lovell
School of Nursing, Midwifery and Social Work, University of Manchester, Manchester, United Kingdom

David A. Richards and Chris Dickens
Institute of Health Service Research, University of Exeter Medical School, University of Exeter, Exeter, United Kingdom

Simon Gilbody
Mental Health Research Group, Department of Health Sciences and Hull York Medical School, University of York, York, United Kingdom

Waquas Waheed
Lancashire Care NHS Foundation Trust, Preston, United Kingdom

Sophie Wickham, Peter Taylor and Richard P. Bentall
Institute of Psychology, Health and Society, University of Liverpool, Liverpool, Merseyside, United Kingdom

Mark Shevlin
School of Psychology, University of Ulster, Magee Campus, Londonderry, Northern Ireland, United Kingdom

Jonathan J. Sabbagh, John C. O'Leary III, Laura J. Blair, Bryce A. Nordhues, Sarah N. Fontaine and Chad A. Dickey
Department of Molecular Medicine, Byrd Alzheimer's Research Institute, University of South Florida, Tampa, Florida, United States of America

Torsten Klengel and Elisabeth B. Binder
Department of Psychiatry and Behavioral Sciences, Emory University School of Medicine, Atlanta, Georgia, Unites States of America
Department of Translational Research, Max Planck Institute of Psychiatry, Munich, Germany

Julien Eutrope, Franziska Lempp and Anne-Catherine Rolland
CHU Reims, Hôpital Robert Debré, Structure interne de Psychothérapie de l'Enfant et de l'Adolescent, Reims, F-51092, France

Aurore Thierry
CHU Reims, Hôptal Robert Debré, Unitéd'aide méthodologique, REIMS, F-51092, France

Laurence Aupetit and Laurence De Mare
Centre d'Action Médico-Sociale Précoce, Reims, F-51100, France

Stéphanie Saad and Daniel Sibertin-Blanc
CHU Nancy, Centre psychothérapique de Nancy, Service de pédopsychiatrie, Laxou, F-54521, France

Catherine Dodane and Sylvie Nezelof
CHU de Besançon, Hôpital Saint Jacques, Service de psychiatrie de l'enfant et de l'adolescent, Besancon, F-25030, France

Nathalie Bednarek
CHU de Reims, Hôpital Maison Blanche, Structure Interne de Pédiatrie B, Reims, F-51092, France

Armita Golkar, Emilia Johansson and Maki Kasahara
Department of Clinical Neuroscience, Karolinska Institute, Stockholm, Sweden

Walter Osika
Department of Clinical Neuroscience, Karolinska Institute, Stockholm, Sweden
Center for Social Sustainability, Department of Neurobiology, Care Sciences and Society, Karolinska institute, Stockholm, Sweden

Aleksander Perski
Stress Research Institute, Stockholm University, Stockholm, Sweden

Ivanka Savic
Department of Women's and children's health, and Neurology Clinic, Karolinska Institute and Hospital, Stockholm, Sweden

Index